Study Guide

for

Medical-Surgical Nursing: Assessment and Management of Clinical Problems, 6th edition

Sharon Mantik Lewis, RN, PhD, FAAN
Professor, Schools of Nursing and Medicine
Castella Distinguished Professor of Nursing
University of Texas Health Science Center
Clinical Nurse Scientist
Geriatric Research, Education, and Clinical Center
South Texas Veterans Health Care System
San Antonio, Texas

Margaret M. Heitkemper, RN, PhD, FAAN
Professor, Biobehavioral Nursing and Health Systems
School of Nursing
Adjunct Professor, Division of Gastroenterology
School of Medicine
University of Washington
Seattle, Washington

Shannon Ruff Dirksen, RN, PhD
Associate Professor, College of Nursing
Arizona State University
Tempe, Arizona

Prepared by

Patricia Graber O'Brien, RNCS, MSN, MA
Instructor, College of Nursing
University of New Mexico
Clinical Resource Coordinator
Lovelace Scientific Resources
Albuquerque, New Mexico

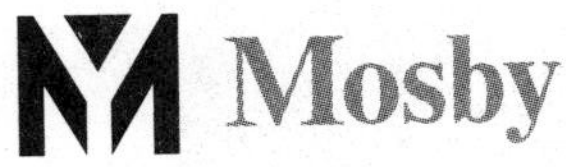

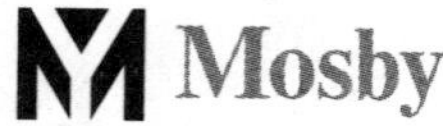

An Affiliate of Elsevier

11830 Westline Industrial Drive
St. Louis, Missouri 63146

Study Guide for Medical-Surgical Nursing:
Assessment and Management of Clinical Problems,
6th Edition

NOTICE

Nursing is an ever-changing field. Standard safety precautions must be followed, but as new research and clinical experience broaden our knowledge, changes in treatment and drug therapy may become necessary or appropriate. Readers are advised to check the most current product information provided by the manufacturer of each drug to be administered to verify the recommended dose, the method and duration of administration, and contraindications. It is the responsibility of the licensed prescriber, relying on experience and knowledge of the patient, to determine dosages and the best treatment for each individual patient. Neither the publisher nor the author assumes any liability for any injury and/or damage to persons or property arising from this publication.

The Publisher

ISBN-13: 978-0-323-01855-5

ISBN-10: 0-323-01855-6

Executive Publisher: Robin Carter
Developmental Editor: Kristin Geen
Publishing Services Manager: Gayle May
Cover Art: Studio Montage

Printed in the United States of America

Last digit is the print number: 9 8 7 6 5 4 3

Contents

Worksheets

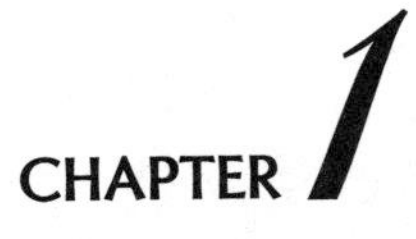

CHAPTER 1 CRITICAL THINKING IN THE NURSING PROCESS

1. Using the American Nurses Association's definition of nursing, identify which of the following activities are the domain of nursing.

_____ a. Writing an order for intake and output for a patient who is vomiting

_____ b. Explaining the risks associated with the planned surgical procedure when a preoperative patient asks

_____ c. Teaching a postoperative patient relaxation and meditation techniques to manage pain

_____ d. Preventing pneumonia in an immobile patient by ordering frequent turning, coughing, and deep breathing

_____ e. Determining and administering fluid replacement therapy needed for a patient with serious burns

_____ f. Assessing the abdomen of an immobile patient for bowel motility

2. In the following situation, identify 5 human responses to actual or potential health problems that are identified nursing diagnoses (see list of nursing diagnoses on inside back cover).

A 36-year-old woman is admitted to the hospital for a breast biopsy and possible mastectomy. The patient tells the nurse she has known about the mass in her breast for about 8 months but had not seen her doctor because she was afraid it might be cancer. She paces the room, telling the nurse she has a 4-year-old son she wants to be able to care for and that she does not know what to expect if surgery is done. The following morning she undergoes a right modified radical mastectomy after a frozen section reveals cancer. Postoperatively, she experiences much incisional pain and swelling and limited movement of her right arm. She glances at the surgical site once when the dressings are changed and comments how awful she looks. When the doctor informs her that four of the lymph nodes were positive for cancer and she will have to undergo chemotherapy and radiation, she begins to cry. She says she had been worried that she would not be attractive to her husband, but now she just needs to focus on being able to live.

a.

b.

c.

d.

e.

3. Identify which of the following are the advantages of a national certification standard for advanced practice nursing.

_____ a. All advanced practice nurses would receive Medicaid reimbursement for their practice.

_____ b. Qualifications for advanced practice nurse would be ensured through graduate education and national examination.

_____ c. The legal status of advanced practice nurses would be the same throughout the country.

_____ d. The public would have a better understanding of the scope of advanced practice nursing.

_____ e. Prescriptive authority for advanced practice nurses would be universal.

4. The nurse knows that the use of evidence-based nursing practice

   a. is the same thing as research utilization.
   b. does not consider the individual patient's preferences.
   c. improves the quality of patient care and patient outcomes.
   d. provides clinical practice guidelines that eliminate the need to make decisions about patient care.

5. Classification of nursing interventions and outcomes is a process designed to

   a. standardize nursing care for patients with specific nursing diagnoses.
   b. identify patient problems that are the specific domain of nursing practice.
   c. develop a standardized language for nursing planning, implementation, and evaluation.
   d. eliminate the need for nurses to identify individualized outcomes and interventions for patients.

6. Identify the three nursing languages that specifically relate to the steps of the nursing process.

   a.

   b.

   c.

7. Match the phases of the nursing process with the descriptions (answers may be used more than once).

_____	a. Analysis of data	1. Assessment
_____	b. Priority setting	2. Diagnosis
_____	c. Nursing interventions	3. Planning
_____	d. Data collection	4. Implementation
_____	e. Identifying patient strengths	5. Evaluation
_____	f. Measuring patient achievement of goals	
_____	g. Setting goals	
_____	h. Identifying health problems	
_____	i. Nursing interventions	
_____	j. Modifying the plan of care	
_____	k. Documenting care provided	

8. A 62-year-old patient hospitalized with heart failure has been receiving large doses of diuretics. The nurse notes that the patient has increasing weakness, flabby muscles, increased irritability, and a weak, rapid pulse. The nurse notifies the physician regarding these findings, and asks the doctor if the patient's potassium level should be checked. The physician orders a laboratory test for serum electrolytes. The results indicate a hypokalemia, and the nurse calls the physician to report the results. The physician orders potassium supplements, daily serum electrolyte levels, and a high-potassium diet. The nurse administers the medication and discusses the dietary order and the patient's status with the dietician. The dietician sees the patient and does initial teaching regarding dietary intake of potassium. The nurse helps the patient choose high potassium foods from the daily menu and evaluates the patient's ability to make correct choices. The nurse also monitors the patient's response to the potassium supplements with the daily lab results and physical assessment findings.

What are the independent, collaborative, and dependent functions that the nurse performed in this situation?

a. Independent

b. Collaborative

c. Dependent

9. The following is a list of two-part nursing diagnoses. Identify if each statement is correctly (C) or incorrectly (I) written. If it is incorrectly written, explain what is incorrect.

_____ a. Need for activity related to social isolation

_____ b. Inability to turn related to traction

_____ c. Dyspnea related to activity intolerance

_____ d. Body image disturbance related to loss of breast

_____ e. Pain related to surgery

_____ f. Ineffective individual coping related to inadequate support system

_____ g. Constipation related to bowel obstruction

_____ h. Cardiac monitoring related to cardiac arrhythmias

10. For the following problems, write "ND" in front of those that are nursing diagnoses and "CP" in front of those that are collaborative problems.

_____ a. Infection related to immunosuppression

_____ b. Ineffective airway clearance related to excessive mucus

_____ c. Constipation related to irregular defecation habits

_____ d. Deficient fluid volume related to NPO status

_____ e. Fatigue related to sleep deprivation

_____ f. Excess fluid volume related to high sodium intake

_____ g. Imbalanced nutrition: less than body requirements related to anorexia

_____ h. Risk for cardiac arrhythmias related to potassium deficiency

_____ i. Stress urinary incontinence related to weak pelvic floor muscles

_____ j. Hypoxia related to chronic obstructive pulmonary disease

11. Read all of the data for the case history below and write a three-part nursing diagnosis statement that clearly describes the problem.

A 52-year-old patient has been on prolonged bed rest following a fractured pelvis. When he begins ambulation, he develops the following signs and symptoms: shortness of breath on exertion; reports inability to carry out usual activities of daily living because of weakness and fatigue; pulse remains elevated after activity for more than 5 minutes.

12. Identify four guidelines that may be used in setting priorities of intervention for nursing diagnoses.

    a.

    b.

    c.

    d.

13. Describe how planned nursing interventions would differ between these two nursing diagnoses: (a) imbalanced nutrition: less than body requirements related to anorexia and (b) imbalanced nutrition: less than body requirements related to difficulty in swallowing.

14. Identify the expected patient outcomes that are correctly (C) written, and identify what criteria are not met in those outcomes that are incorrectly (I) written.

    _____ a. The patient will recognize the importance of taking the medications as prescribed.

    _____ b. The patient lists the supplies needed to change the dressing by discharge.

    _____ c. The patient maintains a low-sodium diet.

    _____ d. The patient's activity tolerance will be increased by discharge.

    _____ e. The patient will ambulate with a walker from the room to the nurse's station 3 times a day without assistance.

15. For the nursing diagnoses and patient outcomes listed below, write a specific nursing order indicated to help the patient reach the outcome.

    a. Nursing Diagnosis: Risk for impaired skin integrity related to immobility
    Patient Outcome: Patient will demonstrate skin integrity free of pressure ulcers

    b. Nursing Diagnosis: Constipation related to inadequate fluid and fiber intake
    Patient Outcome: Patient will have daily soft bowel movements in 1 week

16. A patient with a seizure disorder is admitted to the hospital following a sustained seizure. When the patient tells the nurse that she has not taken her medication regularly, the nurse makes a nursing diagnosis of ineffective therapeutic regimen management related to lack of knowledge regarding medication regimen, and identifies an expected patient outcome of "Takes prescribed medication as directed."

    When the nurse tries to teach the patient about the medication regimen, the patient tells the nurse that she knows about the medications but she does not always have the money to refill the prescriptions. Where was the mistake made in the nursing process with this patient?

    How would the nurse revise the care plan based on this evaluation?

17. Identify four advantages of computerized documentation, especially when nursing languages are integrated in the computer programming.

    a.

    b.

    c.

    d.

CHAPTER 2 CULTURALLY COMPETENT CARE

1. Match the following terms with their descriptions.

_____	a. Culture	1. Identification with a group whose members share a common social and cultural heritage passed through generations
_____	b. Values	2. Modification of one's culture as a result of contact with another culture
_____	c. Subculture	3. Forcing one's own cultural beliefs and practices on others without regard for their culture
_____	d. Acculturation	4. Principles and standards that serve as bases for beliefs, attitudes, and behaviors
_____	e. Assimilation	5. The knowledge, values, beliefs, laws, and customs of members of a society
_____	f. Ethnicity	6. Divisions of humankind sharing common ancestry and physical characteristics
_____	g. Race	7. Large groups of people who have shared characteristics that are not common to all members of the culture
_____	h. Ethnocentricity	8. The assumption that all members of a culture or ethnic group share the same values and beliefs
_____	i. Cultural imposition	9. Loss of one's cultural identity in the process of adaptation to the dominant culture
_____	j. Stereotyping	10. The belief that one's own values, beliefs, and behaviors are the only right and natural way

2. List the four basic characteristics of culture.

a.

b.

c.

d.

3. Identify the specific process of acquiring cultural competence reflected in the following examples.

   a. Asking the patient what caused the illness and what treatment would be appropriate.

   ____

   b. Identifying one's own biases toward people of another culture.

   ____

   c. Working directly with persons from different cultures over a period of time.

   ____

   d. Creating a safe environment in which collection of relevant cultural data can be obtained during the health history and physical examination.

   ____

4. During the physical examination of a patient from Southeast Asia, the nurse notes a number of round red bruises on the patient's chest, back, and abdomen. The best response to this finding by the nurse is to ask the patient

   a. "What has caused all these bruises you have on your body?"
   b. "Has someone been hitting you or abusing you in some way?"
   c. "Have you used any traditional treatments for your condition?"
   d. "Did these bruises appear when you became ill with this condition?"

5. Identify one example of how each of the following cultural factors may affect the nursing care of a patient of a different culture.

   a. Time orientation ______________________________

   b. Economic factors ______________________________

   c. Nutrition ______________________________

   d. Personal space ______________________________

   e. Beliefs and values ______________________________

6. A hospitalized Native American patient tells the nurse that later in the day a medicine man from his tribe is coming to perform a healing ceremony to return his world to balance. The nurse recognizes that

   a. the patient does not adhere to an organized, formal religion.
   b. the patient's spiritual needs may be met by traditional rituals.
   c. the patient may be putting his health in jeopardy by relying on rituals.
   d. Native American medicine cannot alter the progression of the patient's physical illness.

7. When the nurse takes a surgical consent form to an Asian woman for a signature after the surgeon has provided the information about the recommended surgery, the patient refuses to sign the consent form. The best response by the nurse is

   a. "Didn't you underst[illegible]d what the doctor told you about the surgery?"
   b. "Are there other [illegible] ou want to talk with before making this decision?"
   c. "You are the [illegible] o can sign this consent. It is your decision to make."
   d. "I'll have [illegible] on and have your surgery canceled until you can make a decision."

8. A male nurse would be providing culturally competent care by requesting that a female nurse provide nursing care for a(n)

   a. Arabic male.
   b. Arabic female.
   c. Hispanic female.
   d. African-American male.

9. The disease that often occurs more frequently and has higher mortality rates in ethnic populations other than white populations is ____________________.

10. Identify at least six classes of drugs that are known to respond differently in other ethnic groups when compared with whites.

   a.

   b.

   c.

   d.

   e.

   f.

11. In a Latin American patient who claims to have *susto*, the nurse would expect assessment findings to include

   a. abdominal pain and cramping.
   b. anxiety, insomnia, anorexia, and social isolation.
   c. nightmares, weakness, and a sense of suffocation.
   d. headaches, stomach problems, and loss of consciousness.

12. During the care of culturally diverse patients, the nurse must be aware that knowledge of cultural beliefs and behaviors may inadvertently lead to

   a. stereotyping patients of one culture.
   b. the tendency to develop ethnocentricity.
   c. unconsciously imposing one's own culture on others.
   d. confusing the values and beliefs of one culture with another.

13. Using the information presented in the textbook, identify the cultural characteristics that the nurse might find in the following areas during assessment of a Native American patient and a traditional Hispanic patient.

	Native American Patient	**Traditional Hispanic Patient**
Communication		
Illness factors		
Culture-bound syndromes		

CHAPTER 3 HEALTH HISTORY AND PHYSICAL EXAMINATION

1. A newly admitted patient has a medical history in his record file. Is it necessary for the nurse to complete a nursing history of the patient? Why or why not?

2. While being admitted to the nursing unit from the emergency department, a patient tells the nurse she is short of breath and has pain in her chest when she breathes. Her respiratory rate is 28 per minute, and she is coughing up yellow sputum. Her skin is hot and moist, and her temperature is 102.2° F (39° C). She says that coughing makes her head hurt and she aches all over. Identify the subjective and objective assessment findings in this patient.

Subjective	**Objective**

3. Give an example of a sensitive way to ask a patient the following questions.

   a. Is a patient on antihypertensive medication having a side effect of impotence?

   b. Has a patient with a history of alcoholism had recent alcohol intake?

   c. Who are the sexual contacts of a patient with gonorrhea?

   d. What complementary and alternative therapies are used by the patient?

4. The nurse prepares to interview a patient for a nursing history but finds the patient in obvious pain. The best action by the nurse at this time is to

   a. delay the interview until the patient is pain free.
   b. administer pain medication before initiating the interview.
   c. gather as much information as quickly as possible by using closed questions that require brief answers.
   d. ask only those questions pertinent to the specific problem and complete the interview when the patient is more comfortable.

5. During an interview the patient tells the nurse, "I am so tired and wrung-out I don't know what to do." The nurse's best action at this time is to

   a. arrange another time with the patient to complete the interview.
   b. stop the interview and leave the patient alone to be able to sleep.
   c. question the patient further about the characteristics of the symptoms.
   d. reassure the patient that the symptoms will improve when treatment has time to be effective.

6. Rewrite each question asked by the nurse so that it is an open-ended question designed to gather information about the patient's functional health patterns.

   a. Are you having any pain?

   b. Do you have a good relationship with your wife?

   c. How long have you been ill?

   d. Do you exercise regularly?

7. The following data are obtained from a patient during a nursing history. Organize this data according to Gordon's functional health patterns. Patterns may be used more than once, and some data may apply to more than one pattern.

_____ a. 78-year-old woman

_____ b. Married, 3 grown children live out of town

_____ c. Cares for invalid husband in home with help of daily homemaker

_____ d. Vision corrected with glasses; hearing normal

_____ e. Ht. 5 ft 10 in; wt. 172 lb

_____ f. VS: T 99.2, HR 82, RR 32, BP 142/88

_____ g. 5-year history of adult-onset asthma; smokes 2-3 cigarettes a day

_____ h. Coughing, wheezing, with stated SOB

_____ i. Moderate, light-yellow sputum

_____ j. Says she now has no energy to care for husband

_____ k. Awakens 3-4 times a night and has to use bronchodilator inhaler

_____ l. Uses a laxative twice a week for bowel function; no urinary problems

_____ m. Feels her health is good for her age

_____ n. Allergic to codeine and aspirin

_____ o. Has esophageal reflux and eats bland foods

_____ p. Can usually handle stress of caring for husband, but if she becomes overwhelmed, asthma becomes worse

_____ q. Has been menopausal for 26 years; no sexual activity

_____ r. Takes medications for asthma, hypertension, hypothyroidism, and uses diazepam (Valium) prn for anxiety

_____ s. Goes out to lunch with friends weekly

_____ t. Says she misses going to church with husband but watches religious services with him on TV

1. Demographic data
2. Important health information
3. Health-perception–health-management pattern
4. Nutrition-metabolic pattern
5. Elimination pattern
6. Activity-exercise pattern
7. Sleep-rest pattern
8. Cognitive-perceptual pattern
9. Self-perception–self concept pattern
10. Role-relationship pattern
11. Sexuality-reproductive pattern
12. Coping–stress tolerance pattern
13. Value-belief pattern

8. An example of a negative finding during a physical examination is

   a. chest pain that does not radiate to the arm.
   b. elevated blood pressure in a patient with hypertension.
   c. pupils that are equal and react to light and accommodation.
   d. clear and full lung sounds in a patient with chronic bronchitis.

9. A screening physical examination is used by the nurse when examining a patient who

   a. is being evaluated during routine health maintenance.
   b. is being seen 2 weeks following treatment of a peptic ulcer.
   c. has generalized weakness and fatigue without specific pain.
   d. wants to know the effectiveness of a prescribed hypertension medication.

10. Match the following data with the assessment technique used to obtain the information.

_____	a. Blood flow through arteries	1. Inspection
_____	b. Enlargement of the liver	2. Palpation
_____	c. Tympany of the abdomen	3. Percussion
_____	d. Pain at a joint	4. Auscultation
_____	e. Cyanosis of the lips	
_____	f. Hyperactive peristalsis	

11. The sequence of examination techniques that should be used when assessing the patient's abdomen is

   a. inspection, palpation, auscultation, percussion.
   b. auscultation, inspection, percussion, palpation.
   c. palpation, percussion, auscultation, inspection.
   d. inspection, auscultation, percussion, palpation.

12. When performing a physical examination, it is most important that the nurse

   a. uses a head-to-toe approach to avoid missing an important area.
   b. uses the same systematic, efficient sequence for all examinations.
   c. follows a sequence that is least revealing and embarrassing for the patient.
   d. allows time to collect the nursing history data while performing the examination.

13. Crossword Puzzle

1	2		3		4	■	■	5	■	6
■		■		■	7					
8						■	■		■	
■		■		■	9	10				
■		■	11	12			■		■	
13		14			■	15	16		17	
	■		■	18	19			■		■
20						■		■		■
	■		■	■	21					
22						■		■		■
	■		■	■	23					

Across

1. SW American Indian requiring cultural considerations
7. What patients do when they come for a physical examination
8. Reddened eardrum may indicate this
9. Upper chamber of the heart
11. Abnormal finding on examination of the skin
13. May be found on nasal examination
15. Rises in midline on "ahhh"
18. Laterally means to the ______
20. Referring to the eyes
21. Normal thyroid finding
22. Direction to a patient to take a deep breath
23. Abnormal findings on abdominal palpation

Down

2. Prefix related to skeletal system
3. Where a pulse is palpated
4. Mouths or openings (var.)
5. Cancer that is localized is termed ______
6. Indicated by decreased hemoglobin and hematocrit
10. Dull sound heard on percussion
12. A mixed-up STAT
13. A drooping eyelid
14. Patient's responses to a joke
16. Blue legs may indicate a ______ obstruction
17. Small or scant
19. Inspected reddened skin; edema massive (abbreviation)

CHAPTER 4 PATIENT AND FAMILY TEACHING

1. In each of the nursing situations described below, identify the specific goal of patient education:

   a. Teaching a new mother how to breast-feed

   b. Discussing recommended lifestyle changes with a patient with newly diagnosed heart disease

   c. Counseling a patient with a breast biopsy that is positive for cancer

   d. Demonstrating condom application to sexually active teenagers

2. In the following examples, indicate what principle(s) of adult education is (are) being used by the nurse in teaching patients.

   a. The nurse explains why it is important for a patient with Parkinson's disease to walk with wide placement of the feet.

      ____

   b. The nurse asks a patient what is most important to her to learn about managing a new colostomy.

      ____

   c. The nurse teaches a patient how to reduce the risks for stroke after the patient has had a transient ischemic attack, warning of carotid artery disease.

      ____

   d. The nurse provides a variety of printed materials and Internet resources for a patient with impaired kidney function to use to learn about the disorder.

      ____

   e. When caring for a patient with newly diagnosed asthma, the nurse explains that asthma is a disorder the patient can control and allows the patient to decide when teaching should be done and who else should be included.

      ____

   f. The nurse arranges for a patient diagnosed with diabetes mellitus to perform self-monitoring of blood glucose and insulin administration in the nurse's presence.

      ____

   g. During preoperative teaching of a patient scheduled for a total hip replacement, the nurse compares the postoperative care with that of the patient's prior back surgery.

      ____

3. When using the Transtheoretical Model of Health Behavior Change during patient teaching, the nurse identifies that the patient who states, "I walked regularly for about a year to help prevent osteoporosis, but recently I haven't been motivated to continue," is in the stage of

   a. action
   b. preparation
   c. termination
   d. maintenance

4. Translate the following medical terms or diagnoses into phrases that a patient with little or no medical knowledge would be able to understand.

   a. Acute myocardial infarction

   b. Intravenous pyelogram

   c. Diabetic retinopathy

5. An empathetic approach to patient teaching is demonstrated when the nurse

   a. assesses the patient's needs before developing the teaching plan.
   b. provides positive nonverbal messages that promote communication.
   c. reads and reviews educational materials before distributing them to patients and families.
   d. can overcome the personal frustration felt when patients are discharged before teaching is complete.

6. The nurse includes the needs of the family and significant others in planning patient teaching because

   a. family support of the patient greatly affects the patient's sense of well-being.
   b. family members will be responsible for continued care of the patient after discharge.
   c. the patient and family often have conflicting views of the illness and treatment options.
   d. family members need to learn about the patient's problems and need to know what to expect.

7. To promote the patient's self-efficacy during the teaching-learning process, the nurse should

   a. emphasize the relevancy of the teaching to the patient's life.
   b. begin with concepts and tasks that are easily learned to promote success.
   c. provide stimulating learning activities that encourage motivation to learn.
   d. encourage the patient to learn independently without instruction from others.

8. Identify what teaching interventions are indicated when the following characteristics are found during assessment of a patient for the purposes of developing a teaching plan.

   a. Impaired hearing

   b. Patient refuses to see a need for a change in health behaviors

   c. Drowsiness caused by use of tranquilizers

   d. Presence of pain

   e. Severe anxiety about self-administering injections

   f. Lack of self-efficacy

   g. Decreased concentration because of cerebral injury

   h. Fatigue and weakness at early discharge from hospital

   i. Reading ability at national average

   j. Visual learning style

9. Upon assessment of a patient's learning needs, the nurse determines that a patient taking potassium-wasting diuretics does not know what foods are high in potassium. An appropriate nursing diagnosis for this patient is

   a. risk for cardiac arrhythmias related to low potassium intake.
   b. deficient knowledge related to lack of recall of high-potassium foods.
   c. imbalanced nutrition: less than body requirements related to lack of intake of potassium-rich foods.
   d. deficient knowledge related to lack of interest regarding dietary requirements when taking diuretics.

10. Write a complete learning objective for the patient taking potassium-wasting diuretics who does not know what foods are high in potassium.

11. Teaching strategies to meet learning objectives should be determined by the

   a. nurse.
   b. patient.
   c. physician.
   d. nurse, patient, and patient's family.

12. Match the following descriptions or characteristics with the appropriate teaching strategy (answers may be used more than once).

_____ a. May require patient to practice between teaching sessions

_____ b. Used to rehearse behaviors or feelings

_____ c. Participants are passive learners

_____ d. Most efficient in terms of time

_____ e. Useful when patients have previous experience with subject

_____ f. Allows for questions and exchange of ideas following content presentation

_____ g. Should be supplementary to the nurse's planned teaching sessions

_____ h. Useful when it is difficult to reach desired objectives of the session

_____ i. Requires patients to learn to identify reliable information

_____ j. Best strategy for teaching motor skills or procedures

_____ k. Nurse must have competency in the technology

_____ l. Requires maturity and confidence of participants

_____ m. May be used in combination with almost any other teaching strategy

_____ k. Offers extensive sources of information

1. Lecture
2. Lecture/discussion
3. Discussion
4. Peer teaching in support groups
5. Demonstration/return demonstration
6. Role play
7. Internet
8. Printed materials

13. When selecting audiovisual and written materials as teaching strategies, it is important for the nurse to

a. provide the patient with these materials before the planned learning experience.
b. ensure that the materials include all the information the patient will need to learn.
c. review the materials before use for accuracy and appropriateness to learning objectives.
d. assess the patient's auditory and visual ability because these functions are necessary for these strategies to be effective.

14. A drug handbook provides the following information about the drug atorvastatin (Lipitor):

- Action: Inhibits HMG-CoA reductase enzyme, which reduces cholesterol synthesis
- Uses: As an adjunct in primary hypercholesterolemia (types Ia, Ib)
- Side effects: Liver dysfunction, dyspepsia, flatus, pancreatitis, rash, pruritus, alopecia, lens opacities, myalgia, and headache
- Precautions: Past liver disease, alcoholism, hypotension, severe acute infections, uncontrolled seizure disorders, severe metabolic disorders, trauma, and electrolyte imbalances
- Interactions: Increased effects of warfarin, digoxin, oral contraceptives; increased myalgia with cyclosporine, gemfibrozil, niacin, erythromycin; decreased effects of atorvastatin with colestipol, antacids, bile acid sequestrants, propranolol; increased effects of atorvastatin with erythromycin, itraconazole

Rewrite the above information as teaching material for a patient with an average adult reading level.

15. Identify what short-term evaluation technique is appropriate to evaluate whether the patient has met the following learning objectives.

a. The patient will demonstrate to the nurse the preparation and administration of a subcutaneous insulin injection to himself with correct technique.

b. The patient will identify five symptoms of digitalis toxicity.

c. The patient will select the foods highest in potassium for each meal from the hospital menu with 80% accuracy.

d. The patient will ambulate unassisted with the walker 100 feet three times a day.

16. The best example of documentation of patient teaching regarding wound care is

a. "The patient was instructed about care of wound and dressing changes."
b. "The patient demonstrated correct technique of wound care following instruction."
c. "The patient and family verbalize that they understand the purposes of wound care."
d. "Written instructions regarding wound care and dressing changes were given to the patient."

CHAPTER 5 OLDER ADULTS

1. Identify two common social conceptions or myths about aging or the aged that illustrate the concept of ageism.

   a.

   b.

2. A 73-year-old man scheduled for surgery tells the nurse that if things do not go well during surgery, he has lived a full life and has no regrets. The nurse recognizes that this statement is consistent with

   a. achievement of the developmental task of ego-integrity described by Erikson.
   b. unsuccessful achievement of earlier developmental tasks described by Havighurst.
   c. the wisdom and judgment that maintains self-esteem in Peck's theory of development.
   d. the changes and redirected growth toward personal goals characteristic of Levinson's late adulthood transition.

3. Match the developmental theorists with their concepts (theorists may be used more than once).

_____	a. Addresses only middle-adult and older adult tasks	1. Erikson
_____	b. Family-oriented tasks	2. Peck
_____	c. Individual life structure	3. Levison
_____	d. Experiences dictate self-adjustment	4. Havighurst
_____	e. Body transcendence vs. body preoccupation	
_____	f. Transitions vs. stability	
_____	g. Ego-integrity vs. despair	

4. A characteristic common to all adult developmental models is that

   a. acceptance of dying is the most important task of adulthood.
   b. development is a continuous process throughout the life span.
   c. the ultimate goal of adult development is to leave a genetic legacy.
   d. chronological age is the most important factor in understanding adult behavior.

5. Match the following characteristics with their related biologic theory of aging.

_____ a. Inherent cellular biologic clock that limits cellular division

_____ b. Increased cellular rigidity related to abnormal joining of metabolites

_____ c. Spontaneous mutation of body cells, eventually causing organ failure

_____ d. Active self-destruction of normal cells by immune system

_____ e. Altered DNA and protein synthesis from oxidative process

_____ f. Loss of DNA enzymes resulting in limited cell division

_____ g. Loss of response of nervous and glandular tissue

_____ h. Gradual loss of genetic regulatory mechanisms resulting in mutational cells

1. Somatic mutation theory
2. Intrinsic mutagenesis theory
3. Free radical theory
4. Cross-link theory
5. Neuroendocrine theory
6. Programmed theory of cell death
7. Immunologic theory
8. Telomere-telomerase theory

6. For each of the nursing diagnoses listed, identify at least two normal expected physiologic changes related to aging that could be etiologic factors of the diagnosis.

   a. Imbalanced nutrition: less than body requirements

      Change:

      Change:

   b. Activity intolerance

      Change:

      Change:

   c. Risk for injury

      Change:

      Change:

   d. Urge urinary incontinence

      Change:

      Change:

   e. Ineffective airway clearance

      Change:

      Change:

   f. Risk for impaired skin integrity

      Change:

      Change:

   g. Ineffective tissue perfusion: peripheral

      Change:

      Change:

   h. Constipation

      Change:

      Change:

7. The nurse identifies the presence of age-associated memory impairment in the older adult who says,

   a. "I just can't seem to remember the name of my new granddaughter."
   b. "I make out lists to help me remember what I need to do, but I can't seem to use them."
   c. "I forget movie stars' names more often now, but I can remember them later after the conversation is over."
   d. "I forgot that I went to the grocery store this morning and didn't realize it until I went again this afternoon."

8. Indicate what the acronym SCALES stands for in assessment of nutrition indicators in frail older adults.

   a. S

   b. C

   c. A

   d. L

   e. E

   f. S

9. When assessing the older adult's health status, the nurse finds a decline in the patient's functional health status. This change often occurs as a result of the patient

   a. manifesting symptoms of delirium.
   b. suffering from asymptomatic pathology.
   c. adjusting for disease symptoms by restricting activities.
   d. treating one symptom with a medication that causes detrimental side effects.

10. Identify one task required for daily living with chronic illness that would specifically apply to the following common chronic conditions present in the older adult.

    a. Diabetes mellitus
    b. Visual impairment
    c. Heart disease
    d. Hearing impairment
    e. Alzheimer's disease
    f. Arthritis
    g. Orthopedic impairment

11. When working with older patients who identify with a specific ethnic group, the nurse recognizes that health care problems may occur because these patients often

    a. live with extended families who isolate the patient.
    b. live in rural areas where services are not readily available.
    c. eat ethnic foods that do not provide all the essential nutrients.
    d. have less income to spend for medications and health care services.

12. An 88-year-old woman is brought to the health clinic for the first time by her 64-year-old daughter. During the initial comprehensive nursing assessment of the patient, the nurse should

    a. ask the daughter whether the patient has any urgent needs or problems.
    b. obtain a health history using a functional health pattern and assess ADLs and mental status.
    c. interview the patient and daughter together so that pertinent information can be confirmed.
    d. refer the patient for an interdisciplinary comprehensive geriatric assessment because she will have multiple needs at her age.

13. A mental status assessment of the older adult is especially important in determining

    a. potential for independent living.
    b. eligibility for federal health programs.
    c. if the person should be classified as frail.
    d. service and placement needs of the individual.

14. The nurse promotes learning activity when teaching older adult patients by providing

    a. written instructions instead of verbal explanations.
    b. information that relates to the patient's actual experience.
    c. a review of basic concepts, because long-term memory is impaired.
    d. numerous repetitive presentations to promote memory retention.

15. One of the most frequent consequences of unscheduled surgery in the older adult is

    a. postoperative infection.
    b. acute confusional state.
    c. fluid and electrolyte imbalances.
    d. anesthesia-induced arrhythmias.

16. An important nursing measure in the rehabilitation of the geriatric patient to prevent loss of function from inactivity and immobility is

    a. performance of active and passive ROM exercises.
    b. using assistive devices such as walkers and canes.
    c. teaching good nutrition to prevent loss of muscle mass.
    d. performance of risk appraisals and assessments related to immobility.

17. A 78-year-old man is admitted to the orthopedic unit from the emergency department with a hip fracture. During the admission process the patient does not complain of pain in the hip. The nurse should

    a. offer the patient pain medication.
    b. ask the patient to keep a pain diary.
    c. recognize that older adults' perception of pain is impaired.
    d. assume that the patient is handling his pain in his own way.

18. An older adult patient has hypertension and congestive heart failure and is treated with enalapril (Vasotec) and digoxin (Lanoxin). The pharmacodynamic and pharmacokinetic properties of these drugs include the following:

	enalapril	**digoxin**
Dynamics:	blocks conversion of angiotensin I to active angiotensin II, causing systemic vasodilation	increases intramedullary calcium, increasing cardiac muscle contraction; parasympathetic stimulation causing decreased heart rate
Kinetics:		
Absorption:	oral absorption 60%	oral absorption 60%-80%
Distribution:	20%-30% plasma protein bound	20%-30% plasma protein-bound
Metabolism:	60% converted by liver to active enalapril	small % metabolized by liver and GI at flora
Excretion:	60% excreted by kidneys, rest by feces	most excreted unchanged by kidneys
Half-life	11 hours	36 hours

a. What physiologic changes in the older adult affect the absorption, metabolism, and excretion of enalapril?

b. Describe the additional effect digoxin may have on the older adult also taking enalapril.

c. What nursing interventions should the nurse plan to monitor for the potential side effects related to administration of these drugs?

19. In view of the fact that most older adults take at least six prescription drugs, what are four nursing interventions that can specifically help prevent problems caused by multiple drug use in older patients?

a.

b.

c.

d.

20. An 80-year-old woman is brought to the emergency department by her daughter, who says her mother has refused to eat for 6 days. The mother says she stays in her room all of the time because the family is mean to her when she eats or watches TV with them. She says her daughter only brings her one meal a day and that meal is cold leftovers from the family's meals days before.

    a. What types of elder abuse may be present in this situation?

    The daughter says her mother is too demanding and she just can not cope with caring for her 24 hours a day.

    b. What might be an appropriate nursing diagnosis for the daughter?

    c. What resources can the nurse suggest to the daughter?

21. An 82-year-old patient with multiple health problems is hospitalized with a fractured hip.

    a. What Medicare coverage will apply to treatment of the fractured hip?

    b. What criteria must be met for the patient to receive Medicare benefits for hospitalization?

    c. The patient is transferred to a skilled nursing facility for rehabilitation. Will Medicare continue to cover the expense of the skilled facility?

    d. The patient is too frail to complete rehabilitation and it is discontinued. Custodial care is indicated. If the patient is placed in a nursing home or taken home to be cared for, what Medicare coverage is available for expenses?

    e. The patient is taken to a daughter's home for custodial care. The daughter and son-in-law are both employed. What community-based service might be appropriate to allow the family members to continue employment?

22. What are three common factors known to precipitate nursing home placement?

    a.

    b.

    c.

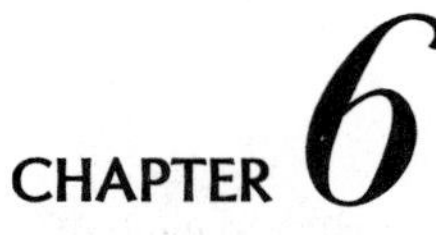

CHAPTER 6 COMMUNITY-BASED NURSING AND HOME CARE

1. The difference between community-based nursing and community-oriented nursing is that in community-based nursing, the nurse

    a. focuses on the health of the community as a whole.
    b. is concerned about the health of individuals, families, and groups in a community.
    c. does not provide direct patient care, but instead coordinates the care provided by other health care professionals.
    d. helps individuals and families manage acute or chronic health problems in the community and home setting.

2. Current changes in health care delivery have been influenced primarily by

    a. institution of systems to provide cost-effective health care.
    b. governmental regulation of the cost of health care services.
    c. the need to meet the health care needs of an aging population.
    d. development of medical technology that has reduced the incidence of illness.

3. Prospective payment systems for health care services

    a. require that health care is provided by preapproved health professionals.
    b. provide payment for health care based on flat predetermined rates regardless of actual cost.
    c. reimburse the expenses of health care only when costs are approved by the system before treatment.
    d. arrange to pay only those health care providers who contract with the system to provide the lowest-priced services.

4. A diagnosis related group (DRG) is

    a. a standard used by health care facilities to determine charges for health care services.
    b. a medical condition classification that determines what Medicare will pay for health care services.
    c. the method that health care institutions use to determine what health care services are needed for patients.
    d. a system used by all third-party health care payers to determine what health care expenses will be covered.

5. Identify five factors that have influenced the shift of acute and long-term chronic care to community-based settings and the home.

    a.

    b.

    c.

    d.

    e.

6. A case manager is responsible for

    a. determining when hospitalization is needed by a patient.
    b. setting limits on the financial expenditures of a patient's illness episode.
    c. coordinating patient care during an entire episode of illness in all care settings.
    d. providing home health care to patients following hospitalization for acute illnesses.

7. Using the following list of health care settings, identify the setting that would be most appropriate in each of the described patient situations.

Settings

acute rehabilitation	long-term acute care
ambulatory care center	residential care facility
home health care	skilled nursing facility
hospice care	subacute care unit
intermediate care facility	

a. An ambulatory patient with Alzheimer's disease needs a segregated, low stimulus environment and activity programming. ______________________

b. A patient requires pain relief and support during the final stages of terminal illness.

____

c. A diabetic patient with a wound infection at an above-the-knee amputation site has exhausted the DRG days and still requires IV antibiotics and frequent complex dressing changes for a short time.

____

d. A stable, comatose patient following a head injury requires tube feedings, IV medications, and continuous nursing support. ______________________

e. A patient with an acute eye infection requires a one-time encounter with health professionals for treatment.

____

f. A patient requires assistance in activities of daily living and medication supervision but is ambulatory and cares for self with direction. ______________________

g. A patient is stable following a stroke but has left-sided paralysis with a potential for return of function.

____

h. A patient requires IV antibiotics and wound care daily and has family members to provide care.

____

i. An alert, middle-aged patient with multiple sclerosis has no immediate family and needs a permanent home in addition to around-the-clock personal care assistance. ______________________

j. A patient has been on a ventilator for 35 days following a diving accident resulting in a cervical fracture and requires extensive medical and nursing intervention. ______________________

8. The patient care setting in which nurses most often perform telephone follow-up with patients is

______________________________.

9. The patient care setting in which nurses are most likely to be required to adapt to a variety of circumstances and make independent decisions is ______________________________.

10. Patient care settings in which professional nurses are most likely to directly supervise personal care of the patient provided by nursing assistants and have limited direct patient contact include

______________________________ and ______________________________.

11. Patient care settings in which nurses are most likely to coordinate patient care with physical therapists, occupational therapists, and speech therapists include ____________________,

______________________________, and ____________________.

12. The primary role of the professional nurse in home health care is to

   a. perform all health and personal care delivered in the home.
   b. coordinate and case-manage all aspects of care in the home.
   c. teach family members to eventually assume all care for the patient.
   d. visit the home at least once a week to evaluate the status of the patient.

13. Continuous quality improvement in home health nursing involves

   a. using clinical or critical pathways to guide patient care.
   b. documenting to ensure legal and professional accountability.
   c. avoiding hospital readmission of patients with chronic conditions.
   d. monitoring patient outcomes with respect to patient progress toward goals.

14. A 72-year old man who has had two strokes is cared for by his wife and daughter in his home. The patient is becoming weaker and is almost bedridden. The wife and daughter are becoming exhausted from the care he requires, but the patient insists that his family care for him at home. What are two nursing diagnoses that might relate to this family situation?

   a.

   b.

CHAPTER 7 COMPLEMENTARY AND ALTERNATIVE THERAPIES

1. Match each description in the left column with its NCCAM classification (in the right column) and with its specific type of therapy (also in the right column).

Descriptions

____ ____ a. Use of hands to direct energy fields

____ ____ b. Nutrition integrated with lifestyle and environment to promote health

____ ____ c. Movement reeducation to promote balanced, graceful movement

____ ____ d. Manipulation of energy channels with fine needles

____ ____ e. Involves assessment of patient's sense of purpose and meaning of life and transcendence beyond context reality

____ ____ f. Emphasizes inherent healing ability of body combined with natural therapies

____ ____ g. Exercise system to manipulate internal energetic movement

____ ____ h. Considers disease as an imbalance of life force and basic metabolic condition

____ ____ i. Involves altering the length and tone of myofascial tissue to realign the body

____ ____ j. Spinal and soft tissue manipulation

____ ____ k. Use of plants or plant parts for specific effects

____ ____ l. System of exercise involving movement integrated with breathing and visualization

____ ____ m. Self-directed practice of focusing, centering, and relaxing

____ ____ n. Uses the principle of "like cures like" with small doses of prepared extracts

NCCAM Classification

1. Alternative medical systems
2. Mind-body interventions
3. Biologic-based therapies
4. Manipulative and body-based methods
5. Energy therapies

Specific Therapies

6. Acupuncture
7. Ayruveda
8. Alexander technique
9. Tai chi
10. Chiropractic therapy
11. Naturopathy
12. Therapeutic touch
13. Phytotherapy
14. Homeopathy
15. Meditation
16. Qigong
17. Spirituality
18. Macrobiotic diet
19. Rolfing

2. Indicate whether the following statements are true or false.

_____ a. The increase in the use of CAM therapies is due primarily to a growing distrust of allopathic medicine by the public.

_____ b. A limitation of the use of CAM therapies is the refusal of insurance companies to reimburse the cost of such therapy.

_____ c. Research and education in CAM therapies are supported by the National Center for Complementary and Alternative Medicine of the National Institutes of Health.

_____ d. Practices that are considered complementary and alternative in one culture or time might be considered conventional in another place or time.

3. Complementary and alternative therapies are advocated by many nurses because these therapies

a. promote self-care and self-determination by patients.
b. are congruent with a view of humans as holistic beings.
c. are less expensive for patients than conventional therapies.
d. cause few adverse effects while achieving positive outcomes.

4. Traditional Chinese medicine holds that disease occurs when

a. yin and yang become imbalanced altering the flow of Qi.
b. acupoints in Qi channels become obstructed preventing the release of Qi.
c. the body's natural healing abilities are impaired by obstruction of fluid channels.
d. the elements of earth, metal, water, wood, and fire are restricted from interacting with each other.

5. Acupuncture is used to

a. relieve pain by causing counterirritation in another area of the body.
b. reestablish the flow of Qi through meridians to simulate the body's self-healing mechanism.
c. create an inflammatory response at an acupoint, increasing blood circulation and healing energy.
d. stimulate the electrical activity of the central nervous system, promoting movement of vital energy through the body.

6. The most common complications of acupuncture are those related to

a. cardiac arrhythmias.
b. infection transmission.
c. post-treatment drowsiness.
d. bleeding from needle sites.

7. Identify three interventions that are frequently used by nurses to help the patient use the mind to affect bodily function.

a.

b.

c.

8. The primary goal of biofeedback is to

   a. measure the physiologic responses to stress.
   b. demonstrate the effect of stress reduction therapies on physiologic function.
   c. teach the patient to voluntarily control physiologic processes that are usually involuntary.
   d. increase the patient's awareness of autonomic nervous system responses to thoughts and feelings.

9. A complementary and alternative therapy shown to be effective in treatment of a patient with chemotherapy-related nausea and vomiting is

   a. rolfing.
   b. acupuncture.
   c. aromatherapy.
   d. electromagnetic therapy.

10. Therapeutic touch is contraindicated in patients

    a. who are pregnant.
    b. who are immunosuppressed.
    c. who are receiving cancer chemotherapy.
    d. with critical or unstable conditions.

11. A patient tells the nurse that she uses regular chiropractic therapy for treatment of dysmenorrhea. The nurse recognizes that chiropractic therapy

    a. is contraindicated for pain of visceral origin.
    b. is effective only for musculoskeletal abnormalities.
    c. involves the prescription of mild antiinflammatory drugs for the menstrual pain.
    d. uses manipulation to correct spinal alterations that cause organ dysfunction and pain.

12. When discussing herbal therapy with a patient, the nurse should advise the patient that

    a. preparations should be purchased only from reputable manufacturers.
    b. herbs rarely cause harm or side effects because they are natural plants.
    c. there are no known contraindications or conditions for which herbal therapy cannot be used.
    d. most herbal preparations have been clinically tested for safety and efficacy before marketing.

13. While the nurse is obtaining a health history for a patient, the patient tells the nurse that he uses a number of herbs to maintain his health. The most important thing the nurse can do to address the patient's use of these products is to

    a. ask the patient what effects the various products have.
    b. have a working knowledge of commonly used herbs and dietary supplements.
    c. reassure the patient that the products can continue to be used with conventional therapies.
    d. warn the patient that there is limited research concerning the therapeutic and harmful effects of herbal products.

14. Crossword Puzzle: Have You Met Herb?

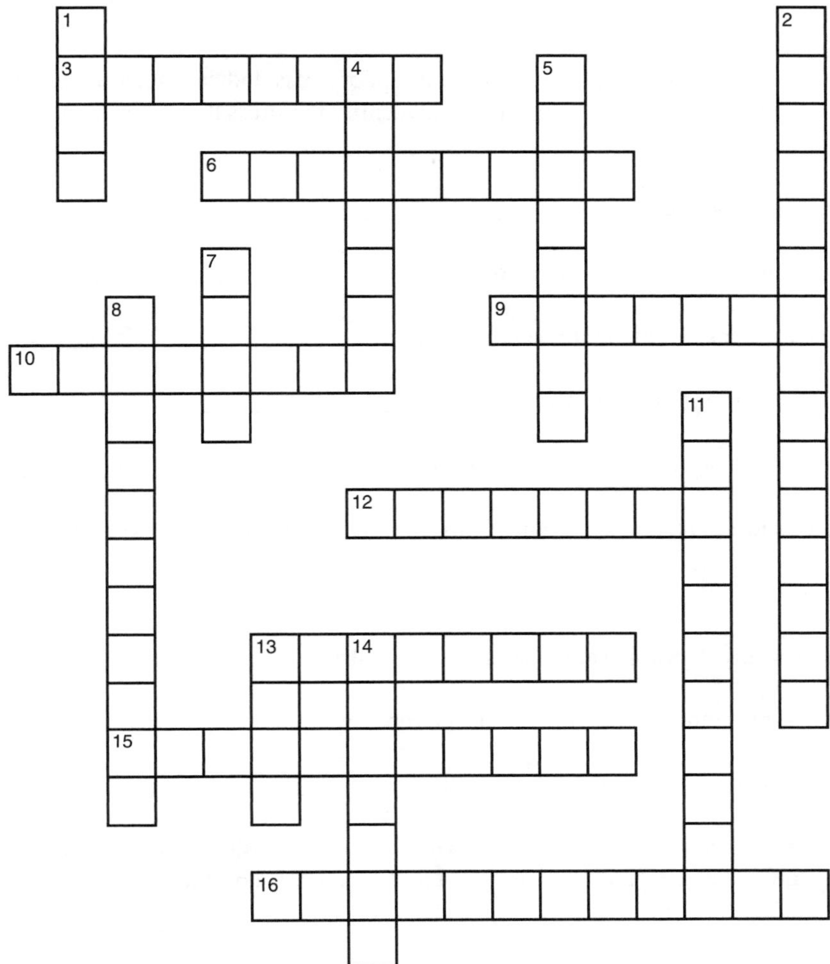

Down

1. As a skeletal muscle relaxant useful for fibromyalgia
2. Affects metabolism of fatty acids and useful in wound healing
4. Safe when used externally for wound healing
5. Sedative and antianxiety effects may interact with CNS depressants
7. Converted to androgens and should not be used in those with reproductive cancers
8. Often used for its estrogen effects by perimenopausal women
11. Slows prostate cell multiplication and used for benign prostatic hyperplasia
13. Common agent used for burns and wound healing
14. Used for its ability to increase endurance and stamina

Across

3. Used for menstrual disorders because of its antispasmodic effects
6. Antibacterial and anti-inflammatory effects that are contraindicated in those with immunosuppression
9. You saw this one before, but it also increases serum cortisol and ability to respond to stress
10. Increases microcirculation in the eyes and used for eye problems
12. Another anti-inflammatory herb that inhibits prostaglandins and histamine
13. You saw this one before, but it also increases the risk for cancer while balancing the effects of estrogen
15. A commonly used herb for depression and anxiety
16. Promotes brain blood flow and memory

CHAPTER 8 STRESS

1. Below are common statements associated with the concept of stress. Indicate whether the term *stress* is used as a stimulus (S), response (R), or transaction (T), and identify the stress theorist(s) associated with the use of the term.

_____ a. "I am so stressed out." ______________________________

_____ b. "She is under a lot of stress right now." ______________________________

_____ c. "What methods do you use to cope with stress?" ______________________________

_____ d. "This job causes too much stress." ______________________________

_____ e. "I always get sick at Christmas—it must be stress." ______________________________

2. The stage of the general adaptation syndrome (GAS) in which the nurse would expect to observe the fewest signs and symptoms is the __________________.

3. A patient who is critically ill briefly shows an increase in pulse, respirations, and blood pressure and becomes more alert, followed by a return of previous vital signs and level of consciousness. The nurse identifies the patient as being in which stage of GAS? ______________________________.

4. Complete a personal inventory of your life events with the Social Readjustment Rating Scale in the textbook. What does your score indicate regarding your risk of developing a major illness?

5. Continuing research in the Stress as a Stimulus theory has shown that the factor that has a closer relationship with somatic illness than the life-event scale is

   a. threat demands.
   b. daily-hassle score.
   c. sense of coherence.
   d. challenge demands.

6. The nurse assesses that a patient with a newly diagnosed chronic illness has a strong sense of coherence. The nurse anticipates that the patient will probably

   a. be able to handle stress without help from health care professionals.
   b. require much emotional and psychologic support to cope with the stress.
   c. ask for much information regarding the illness, its treatment, course, and expected outcome.
   d. go through a formal process of deciding what coping mechanisms and resources are available to manage the stress.

7. A 46-year-old patient is told by his doctor that he has adult-onset diabetes and will require treatment and life-long changes in his lifestyle. The patient is very distressed, but asks for information about the illness, visits the local office of the American Diabetes Association, and elicits help and suggestions from his family in planning lifestyle changes.

   Using the Stress as a Transaction theory, identify the following elements in the above situation.

   a. Stimulus

   b. Primary appraisal outcome

   c. Type of demand

   d. Secondary appraisal

8. Using the word and phrase list on the next page, fill in the boxes below with the numbers of the words or phrases that illustrate the physiologic response to stress.

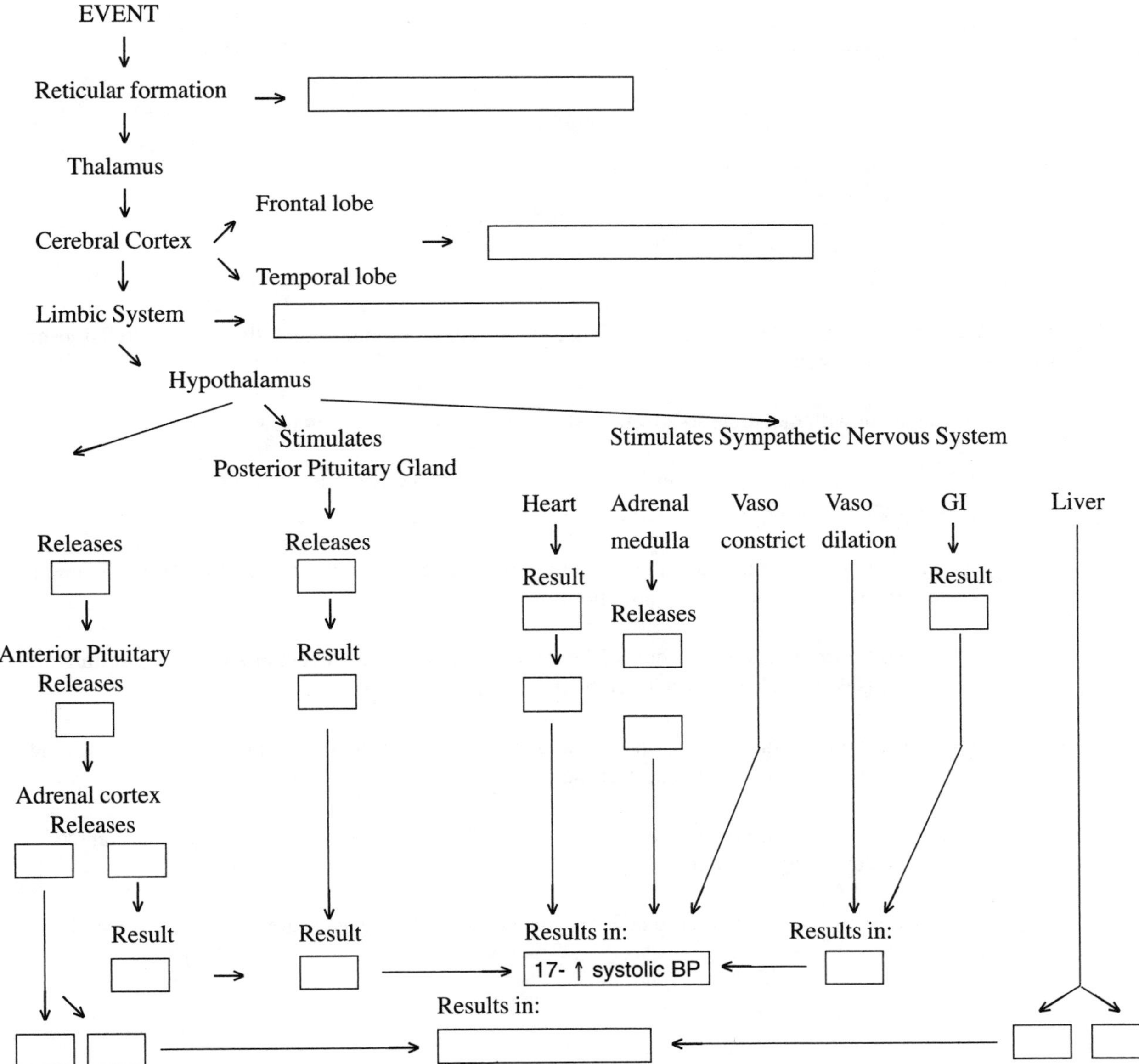

Word and Phrase List

1. Interpretation of event, fear
2. ↑ ADH
3. Cortisol
4. ↑ blood volume
5. ↑ HR and stroke volume
6. ↑ water retention
7. Wakefulness and alertness
8. ↑ sympathetic response
9. Behavior change, ↑ pain perception
10. ↑ cardiac output
11. Corticotropin releasing hormone
12. Aldosterone
13. ACTH
14. ↑ gluconeogenesis
15. ↑ epinephrine and norepinephrine
16. ↓ digestion
17. ↑ systolic blood pressure
18. ↓ inflammatory response
19. Glycogenolysis
20. ↑ blood to vital organs and large muscles
21. ↑ blood glucose
22. ↑ Na nd H_20 reabsorption

9. From the diagram above and the physiologic responses that are noted, identify 8 objective clinical manifestations that the nurse might expect, and 3 or 4 subjective findings.

a. ______________________________

b. ______________________________

c. ______________________________

d. ______________________________

e. ______________________________

f. ______________________________

g. ______________________________

h. ______________________________

i. ______________________________

j. ______________________________

k. ______________________________

l. ______________________________

10. Place a check mark in front of each of the following findings or observations that illustrates the relationship between the immune system and stress.

_____ a. A patient with moderate-to-severe postoperative pain experiences slow wound healing.

_____ b. A diabetic patient experiences wide variations in blood glucose levels when he has an upper respiratory infection.

_____ c. After surgery to remove a malignant tumor, reducing the patient's pain and stress may maintain tumor cell surveillance and destruction.

_____ d. The corticosteroids released during the stress response could prevent exacerbations of immune-based diseases such as multiple sclerosis and rheumatoid arthritis.

_____ e. A patient with numerous daily hassles and with high scores on the Social Readjustment Rating Scale develops a urinary tract infection.

_____ f. Patients with metastatic breast cancer who attend a support group have a longer survival rate than patients who do not receive psychologic support.

_____ g. A patient who uses laughter to relieve pain and stress slows the progression of a rheumatoid condition.

11. While caring for a patient with Alzheimer's disease and her husband, the nurse finds that the patient's husband has a progressively increased blood pressure and morning edema of the hands and feet. One explanation for this allostatic load is that

   a. allostasis is impaired during a time of stress.
   b. the husband does not perceive the care of his wife as stressful.
   c. allostatic responses to stress do not terminate when stress is chronic.
   d. chronic diseases always become more pronounced in stressful situations.

12. A patient has recently had a myocardial infarction. Identify two specific problem-focused coping efforts and two specific emotion-focused coping efforts the nurse could encourage him to use to adapt to the physical and emotional stress of his illness.

Problem-Focused	**Emotion-Focused**
a. ______________________________	c. ______________________________
b. ______________________________	d. ______________________________

13. Identify the three major areas to be assessed in a patient with stress, and describe techniques that would be appropriately used by the nurse to evaluate these areas.

	Areas	**Techniques**
a.		
b.		
c.		

14. A 42-year-old patient with rheumatoid arthritis is withdrawn, pulls the covers over her head, and does not initiate conversation with her husband or other visitors. Upon questioning, the patient tells the nurse that she must either withdraw or cry all the time, that she just cannot cope with the chronic nature of the disease. An appropriate nursing diagnosis for the patient is

   a. ineffective denial related to inability to cope.
   b. ineffective coping related to disruption of emotional bonds.
   c. ineffective coping related to inadequate psychologic resources.
   d. impaired adjustment related to unwillingness to modify lifestyle to accommodate chronic illness.

15. List the nine factors that can increase resistance to stress in all individuals.

    a.

    b.

    c.

    d.

    e.

    f.

    g.

    h.

    i.

CASE STUDY

STRESS

Patient Profile

Ms. J., a 26-year-old unmarried secretary, is admitted to the hospital with right lower quadrant pain; 10 to 12 watery, blood-streaked stools in the past 24 hours; and a low grade fever. She has a 7-year history of inflammatory bowel disease.

Subjective Data

Patient relates the following:
- Has been hospitalized 4 times in the past year
- Not currently working because of the illness and has no income
- Has no insurance
- Has a boyfriend who has lived with her for 2 years
- Does not want her boyfriend to visit because she thinks he has enough of his own problems
- Has been in bed the past week because of weakness, nausea, and malaise and has been crying and depressed

Objective Data

Height: 5 ft 6 in (168 cm)
Weight: 104 lb (47.3 kg)
Hemoglobin: 10.5 gm/dl (105 g/L)
Hematocrit: 30%
Temperature: 100° F (37.8° C)

Critical Thinking Questions

1. What physiologic and psychologic stressors can be identified or anticipated in Ms. J.'s situation? Describe the possible effects of these stressors on the course of her illness.

2. What factors identified in Ms. J.'s nursing assessment may affect her current adaptation to stress?

3. What physiologic changes would be expected in Ms. J. as she begins to respond to prescribed treatment?

4. Describe an approach that the nurse could use to assess Ms. J.'s perception of her situation. Include several specific questions to be asked by the nurse.

5. What specific nursing interventions can be implemented with Ms. J. to enhance her adaptation to stress?

6. Based on the assessment data provided, write one or more nursing diagnoses. Are there any collaborative problems?

CHAPTER 9 PAIN

1. The practice by nurses of routinely administering the smallest prescribed opioid analgesic dose when a range of doses is prescribed

   a. protects the patient from addiction and toxic effects of the drug.
   b. prevents hastening or causing a patient's death from respiratory dysfunction.
   c. contributes to unnecessary suffering and physical and psychosocial dysfunction.
   d. indicates that the nurse understands the adage of "start low and go slow" in administering analgesics.

2. *Pain* has been defined as "whatever the person experiencing the pain says it is, existing whenever the patient says it does." The definition is problematic when caring for a patient who has

   a. been placed on a ventilator.
   b. a history of opioid addiction.
   c. decreased cognitive function.
   d. pain resulting from severe trauma.

3. List and briefly describe the five components of pain.

   a.

   b.

   c.

   d.

   e.

4. Match the following afferent nerve fibers with their characteristics (answers may be used more than once).

_____	a. Transmit nociceptive signals at the fastest rate	1. A-alpha fibers
_____	b. Rapid transmission of soft touch to the skin	2. A-beta fibers
_____	c. The smallest peripheral nerve fibers	3. A-delta fibers
_____	d. Slowly transmit nociceptive signals	4. C fibers
_____	e. Myelinated fiber with rapid transmission of vibration and pressure from muscles	
_____	f. Myelinated fiber transmitting sharp, pointed stimulation	
_____	g. Nonmyelinated fiber with slow transmission of dull, burning sensations	
_____	h. The smallest peripheral nerve fibers	

5. Why is the size, myelinization, and conduction velocity of peripheral nerve fibers of significance in pain management?

6. During transmission of an action potential along a primary afferent nociceptor (PAN) to the dorsal root of the spinal cord

a. nothing can stop the action potential along an intact nerve until it reaches the spinal cord.
b. the transmission may be interrupted by drugs such as local anesthetics and anticonvulsants.
c. the fiber produces neurotransmitters that may activate nearby nerve fibers to transmit pain impulses.
d. the action potential must cross several synapses, points at which the impulse may be blocked by drugs.

7. The development of referred pain during dorsal horn processing of nociceptive impulses is believed to occur when these impulses

a. stimulate excitatory projection cells that send the impulse to the brain on the opposite side of the body.
b. cause neural remodeling, increasing the number and excitability of areas activated by peripheral input.
c. stimulate inhibitory interneurons in the dorsal horn that block the perception of pain from the area of stimulus.
d. mix with impulses from A-beta fibers, causing perception of pain in the body part innervated by the A-beta fiber.

8. While caring for an unconscious patient, the nurse knows that

a. perception of pain will not occur.
b. any noxious stimulus should be treated as potentially painful.
c. if pain is perceived, the patient will have a behavioral response.
d. all nociceptive stimuli that are transmitted to the brain result in the perception of pain.

9. During pain modulation

a. opioid receptors in the brain are blocked to prevent the perception of nociceptive input.
b. transmission of nociceptive stimuli is inhibited by inhibitory neurotransmitters released by afferent nerve fibers.
c. descending fibers may release serotonin, epinephrine, and enkephalins that prevent pain transmission to the brain.
d. endorphins released from the cell during tissue damage occupy receptors on the PANs preventing transduction of pain.

10. When teaching a patient with rheumatoid arthritis to avoid repetitive motions such as knitting, the nurse is addressing the

a. sensory component of pain.
b. affective component of pain.
c. cognitive component of pain.
d. behavioral component of pain.

11. A patient with trigeminal neuralgia has neuropathic pain. In helping the patient manage the pain, the nurse recognizes that this type of pain

a. is not as severe as nociceptive pain.
b. is often described as aching and throbbing in nature.
c. is chronic in nature and will require long-term treatment.
d. involves treatment that includes the use of adjuvant analgesics.

12. List the sensory components of pain that should always be assessed in the patient with pain and give an example of a tool that is helpful in measuring these factors.

	Component	Tool
a.		
b.		
c.		
d.		

13. List the eight basic principles that should guide the treatment of all pain.

a.

b.

c.

d.

e.

f.

g.

h.

14. A patient with bowel cancer has continuous, poorly localized abdominal pain. The nurse teaches the patient to use pain medications

a. on an around-the-clock schedule.
b. as often as necessary to keep the pain controlled.
c. by alternating two different types of drugs to prevent tolerance.
d. when the pain cannot be controlled with distraction or relaxation.

15. A patient who has been taking ketoprofen (Orudis) and imipramine (Tofranil) for control of cancer pain is having increased pain. Based on the WHO Analgesic Ladder guidelines, an appropriate change in the medication plan would be to

a. substitute po levorphanol (Levo-Dromoran) for the other medications.
b. add po hydrocodone (Vicodan, Lortab) to the use of the other medications.
c. substitute po oxycodone with acetaminophen (Percocet) for the other medications.
d. add po sustained-release morphine (MS Contin) to the use of the other medications.

16. A patient with chronic cancer-related pain has started using MS Contin for pain control and has developed common side effects of the drug. The nurse reassures the patient that tolerance will develop to most of these effects but that continued treatment will most likely be required for the

    a. pruritis.
    b. dizziness.
    c. constipation.
    d. nausea and vomiting.

17. The use of a continuous infusion of an analgesic with patient-controlled-analgesia (PCA) prevents what disadvantage of PCA?

18. Match each step of the pain process (in the right column) with the measures or drugs (in the left column) that may be effective in controlling pain during that step.

_____	a. NMDA antagonist drugs	1. Transduction
_____	b. Massage	2. Transmission along PAN
_____	c. NSAIDs	3. Dorsal horn processing
_____	d. Local anesthetics	4. Modulation
_____	e. TENS	
_____	f. Tricyclic antidepressants	
_____	g. Corticosteroids	
_____	h. Epidural opiates	
_____	i. Antiseizure medications	
_____	j. baclofen (Lioresal)	

19. Mrs. S. has developed a physical dependence on morphine following a protracted course after abdominal surgery complicated by multiple peritoneal abscesses. She is currently using morphine 30 mg po q2h, and she is to be tapered from the morphine. Plan a tapering schedule to implement with Mrs. S., including specific dosages and frequency over a specific time frame.

20. What is the position of the American Nurses' Association regarding the responsibility of the nurse in providing large doses of pain medications to terminally ill patients?

21. A patient with multiple injuries resulting from an automobile accident tells the nurse that he has "bad" pain but that he can "tough it out" and doesn't require pain medications. To gain the patient's participation in pain management, the nurse explains that

   a. patients have a responsibility to keep the nurse informed about their pain.
   b. unrelieved pain has many harmful effects on the body that can impair recovery.
   c. using pain medications rarely leads to addiction when they are used for actual pain.
   d. nonpharmacologic therapies can be used to relieve his pain since he is afraid to use pain medications.

CASE STUDY

PAIN

Patient Profile

Mr. D., a 62-year-old postal worker, is being evaluated for a change in his pain therapy for chronic malignant pain from metastatic cancer.

Subjective Data

- Desires 0 pain but will accept 3-4 on a 0-10 scale
- Has been taking 2 Percocet tablets q4h while awake but his pain is now usually at 4-5 with the medication
- Reports his pain varies over 24 hours from 5-10
- Always awakens in the morning with pain at 10 with nervousness and nausea and a runny nose
- When pain becomes severe he stays in bed and concentrates on blocking the pain by emptying his mind
- States he is worried that his increased pain means his disease is becoming worse
- States he is afraid to take additional doses or other narcotics because of fear of addiction

Objective Data

- Height: 6 ft 0 in (183 cm); Weight: 150 lb (68 kg)
- Rigid posturing, slow gait

Critical Thinking Questions

1. What additional assessment data should the nurse obtain from Mr. D. before making any decisions about his problem?

2. What data from the nursing assessment is characteristic of the affective, behavioral, and cognitive dimensions of the pain experience?

3. Based on Mr. D.'s lack of pain control with his current dosage of narcotic and his symptoms upon arising in the morning, what changes are indicated in his medication regimen?

4. What information would the nurse include in a teaching plan for Mr. D. to titrate his analgesic dose effectively?

5. How could the nurse best help Mr. D. overcome his fear of addiction to opioid drugs?

6. What additional pain therapies could the nurse plan to help Mr. D. manage his pain?

7. Based on the assessment data provided, write one or more nursing diagnoses. Are there any collaborative problems?

CHAPTER 10 END-OF-LIFE CARE

1. The primary goal of end-of-life care is

   a. comfort and care that promotes a dignified death.
   b. protecting the terminally ill patient from needless grieving.
   c. implementation of measures to sustain physiologic functioning.
   d. enhancing the patient's progression through all stages of grieving.

2. For each of the following systems, identify three physical manifestations that the nurse would expect to see in a patient approaching death.

   Respiratory

   a.

   b.

   c.

   Skin

   a.

   b.

   c.

   Gastrointestinal

   a.

   b.

   c.

   Musculoskeletal

   a.

   b.

   c.

3. A terminally ill patient is unresponsive and has Cheyne-Stokes respiration. The patient's husband and two grown children are arguing at the bedside about where the patient's funeral should be held. The nurse should

   a. ask the family members to leave the room if they are going to argue.
   b. take the family members aside and explain that the patient may be able to hear them.
   c. tell the family members that this decision is premature since the patient has not yet died.
   d. remind the family that this should be the patient's decision and to ask her if she regains consciousness.

4. A 20-year-old patient with a massive head injury is on life support including a ventilator to maintain respirations. What three criteria for brain death are necessary to discontinue life support?

   a.

   b.

   c.

5. A 62-year-old woman has been diagnosed with metastatic lung cancer and is told that with therapy she may live for 12 to 18 months. Within the first month after her diagnosis, she prepares photo albums for her adult children, organizing and labeling all the photos of her family she has accumulated over the years. The nurse recognizes that this activity illustrates the psychosocial response of

   a. life review.
   b. peacefulness.
   c. saying goodbye.
   d. anxiety about unfinished business.

6. A patient with end-stage liver failure tells the nurse, "If I can just live to see my first grandchild that is expected in 5 months, then I can die happy." The nurse recognizes that the patient is demonstrating

   a. Rando's phase of avoidance.
   b. Kübler-Ross's stage of bargaining.
   c. Martocchio's stage of shock and disbelief.
   d. Martocchio's stage of reorganization and restoration.

7. Match the following types of grief with their characteristics.

_____ a. Anticipatory grief

_____ b. Pathologic grief

_____ c. Conflicted grief

_____ d. Adaptive grief

_____ e. Absent grief

_____ f. Dysfunctional grief

1. Appearance of coping and carrying on as if nothing has happened
2. Exaggerated feelings and behaviors that are disruptive to the person's lifestyle
3. Grieving based on perception of potential loss
4. Unresolved ambivalent feelings toward the deceased
5. Helps in acceptance of the reality of death
6. Chronic grief that does not decrease after the first year

8. A terminally ill man tells the nurse, "I have never believed there is a God or an afterlife, but now it is too terrible to imagine that I will not exist. Why was I here in the first place?" The nurse recognizes that the patient

   a. is experiencing spiritual distress.
   b. most likely will not have a peaceful death.
   c. needs to be reassured that his feelings are normal.
   d. should be referred to a clergyman for a discussion of his beliefs.

9. Identify the legal document or other term described by each of the following.

   a. A lay term for statements that give instructions about future treatment if the person is unable to do so for self: ______________________________

   b. A term used to describe a document designating the person or persons who should make health care decisions if a patient cannot make informed decisions for self: ______________________________

   c. A written document to a physician stating the patient's wish to be allowed to die without heroic or extraordinary measures: ______________________________

   d. Specific state laws that include a variety of directives related to an individual's wishes regarding medical treatment and prolongation of life: ______________________________

   e. The federal law specifying that institutions participating in Medicare must provide written information to patients concerning their rights to accept or refuse treatment: ______________________________

   f. A general term used to describe all documents that give instructions about future medical care and treatments: ______________________________

10. A patient is receiving care to manage symptoms of a terminal illness when the disease no longer responds to treatment. This type of care is known as

    a. terminal care.
    b. palliative care.
    c. supportive care.
    d. maintenance care.

11. A patient with advanced cancer is referred for hospice care. The nurse explains to the patient and the family that the goal of hospice care differs from the goal of traditional care in that hospice care

    a. provides for more complete pain control.
    b. focuses on helping the patient and family prepare for death.
    c. more readily recognizes advance directives related to "right to die."
    d. is delivered in the home and does not rely on the technology of hospitals.

12. End-of-life nursing care involves

    a. constant assessment for changes in physiologic functioning.
    b. administering large doses of analgesics to keep the patient sedated.
    c. providing as little physical care as possible to prevent disturbing the patient.
    d. encouraging the patient and family members to verbalize their feelings of sadness, loss, and forgiveness.

CASE STUDY

END-OF-LIFE CARE

Patient Profile

Mrs. J., a 42-year-old housewife, had unsuccessful treatment for cancer of the breast 1 year ago and now has metastasis to the lung and vertebrae. She lives at home with her husband, a 15-year-old daughter, and a 12-year-old son. She has been referred to hospice because of her deteriorating condition and increasing pain. Her husband is an accountant and tries to do as much of his work at home as possible so that he can help care for his wife. Their children have become withdrawn, choosing to spend as much time as possible at their friends' homes and in outside activities.

Subjective Data

- Mrs. J. reports that she stays in bed most of the time because it is too painful to stand and sit
- She reports her pain as an 8 while taking oral MS Contin q12h.
- She reports shortness of breath with almost any activity, such as getting up to go to the bathroom.
- Mrs. J. says she knows she is dying, but her greatest suffering results from her children not caring about her.
- She and her husband have not talked about her dying with the children.
- Her husband reports that he just doesn't know how to help his wife anymore and that he feels guilty sometimes when he just wishes it were all over.

Objective Data

- Height: 5 ft 2 in (157 cm); Weight: 97 lb (44 kg)
- Skin intact
- Vital signs: T 99° F (37.2° C); HR 92; RR 30; BP 102/60

Critical Thinking Questions

1. What additional assessment data should the nurse obtain from Mr. and Mrs. J. before making any decisions about the care of the family?

2. What types of grieving appear to be occurring in the family?

3. What physical care should the nurse include in a plan for Mrs. J. at this time?

4. What is the best way to facilitate healthy grieving in this family?

5. What resources of a hospice team are available to assist this patient and her family?

6. Based on the assessment data provided, write one or more nursing diagnoses.

CHAPTER 11 ADDICTIVE BEHAVIORS

1. Match the following terms with their definitions.

_____	a. Addiction	1. Absence of a substance will cause withdrawal symptoms
_____	b. Abuse	2. Responses occurring after abrupt cessation of a substance
_____	c. Craving	3. Return to drug use after a period of abstinence
_____	d. Physical dependence	4. Drug use for purposes other than that intended
_____	e. Tolerance	5. Compulsive need to experience pleasure
_____	f. Withdrawal	6. Overuse and dependence on substance that negatively affects functioning
_____	g. Abstinence	7. Refraining from substance use
_____	h. Detoxification	8. Decreased effect of substance following repeated exposure
_____	i. Relapse	9. Overwhelming desire for substance after decreased use
_____	j. Misuse	10. Removal of the drug and its effects from the body
_____	k. Psychologic dependence	11. Compulsive use of substances for physical and psychologic effects

2. The neurotransmitter that appears to have a dominant effect on the process of addiction is

   a. serotonin.
   b. dopamine.
   c. norepinephrine.
   d. gamma-aminobutyric acid (GABA).

3. A patient is admitted to the emergency department with chest pain and cardiac arrhythmias related to cocaine use. The patient's wife tells the nurse she didn't suspect a problem because her husband generally functioned normally, even though she now realizes he was using cocaine. The nurse explains to the wife that when addiction occurs, tolerance causes the individual to

   a. use the drug to feel and function normally.
   b. maintain normal behavior to prevent detection of addiction.
   c. experience different behavior only when the substance is not available.
   d. need less drug for the desired effects, decreasing the signs of drug use.

4. In working with culturally diverse populations, the nurse recognizes that health problems related to addiction include high rates of

   a. AIDS in Hispanic women.
   b. hepatitis C in Asian populations.
   c. alcoholism in Native Americans.
   d. marijuana use in women of all cultures.

5. List two major health problems commonly seen in the acute care setting related to the abuse of the following substances.

Nicotine/tobacco

a.

b.

Cocaine and amphetamines

a.

b.

Alcohol

a.

b.

Cannabis

a.

b.

6. Match the following commonly abused substances with the physiologic effects associated with their use (answers may be used more than once).

_____	a. Increase in appetite	1. Cocaine/amphetamines
_____	b. Sexual arousal	2. Opioids
_____	c. Depersonalization	3. Cannabis
_____	d. Tachycardia with hypertension	4. Hallucinogens
_____	e. Reddened eyes	
_____	f. Constricted pupils	
_____	g. Nasal damage	
_____	h. Decreased respirations	
_____	i. Altered perception	
_____	j. Euphoria and sedation	

7. Use the words below to fill in the blanks in the following statements.

sedative-hypnotic(s)	narcotic(s)
stimulant(s)	hallucinogen(s)

a. Seizures may be a symptom of toxicity in ______________ addiction and a symptom of withdrawal in ______________ addiction.

b. Assessment findings of tremors, chills and sweating, and nausea and cramps are most likely to be found in the patient with ______________ withdrawal.

c. The patient who abuses ______________ is least likely to have withdrawal symptoms.

d. Suicidal thoughts and proneness to violence should be assessed in patients during withdrawal from ______________.

e. The safest and most effective method to withdraw the patient from large doses of ______________ is with hospitalization and gradual reduction of the drug.

f. A patient with severe central nervous system depression with slow and shallow breathing and coma will respond to treatment with naloxone (Narcan) in acute ______________ toxicity, but not in acute ______________ toxicity.

8. When the nurse is encouraging a woman who smokes 1½ packs of cigarettes a day to quit with the use of nicotine replacement therapy, the woman asks how the nicotine in a patch or gum is different from the nicotine she gets from cigarettes. The nurse explains that that nicotine replacements

a. include a substance that eventually creates an aversion to nicotine.
b. provide a noncarcinogenic nicotine, unlike the nicotine in cigarettes.
c. prevent the weight gain that is of concern to women who stop smoking.
d. eliminate the thousands of toxic chemicals that are inhaled with smoking.

9. Match the following drugs used for treatment of cocaine toxicity with their uses (answers may be used more than once).

_____	a. Haloperidol (Haldol)	1. Tachycardia
_____	b. IV lidocaine	2. Hallucinations
_____	c. IV diazepam (Valium)	3. Arrythmias
_____	d. Propranolol (Inderal)	4. Seizures
_____	e. Bretylium (Bretylol)	
_____	f. IV lorazepam (Ativan)	
_____	g. Procainamide (Pronestyl)	

10. A patient who is a heavy caffeine user has been NPO all day in preparation for a late afternoon surgery. The nurse recognizes that the patient may be experiencing caffeine withdrawal when the patient complains of

    a. a headache.
    b. nervousness.
    c. mild tremors.
    d. shortness of breath.

11. A patient admits to the nurse that she used to take diazepam (Valium) 5 mg twice a day when she became nervous, but recently has been taking 10 mg of the drug several times a day to keep herself calm. The nurse identifies that the pattern of abuse in this patient is most likely that of

    a. illegal, intermittent social use that leads to daily use and rapid tolerance.
    b. early prescription use of the drug with increasing dose and frequency without medical indication.
    c. a psychologic dependence that results in anxiety but not physical symptoms if the drug is stopped.
    d. learned behavior from parents who demonstrated substance abuse for solutions to problems.

12. The third day after an alcohol-dependent patient was admitted to the hospital for pancreatitis, the nurse determines that the patient is experiencing alcohol withdrawal. Identify the four characteristic signs of withdrawal on which the nurse bases this judgment.

    a.

    b.

    c.

    d.

13. The best approach by the nurse to assess a newly admitted patient's use of addictive drugs is to ask the patient

    a. "How do you relieve your stress?"
    b. "You don't use any illegal drugs, do you?"
    c. "What alcohol or recreational drugs do you use?"
    d. "Do you have any addictions we should know about to prevent complications."

14. A patient who abuses a variety of depressants and narcotics minimizes the amount and frequency of substances used, as well as the specific agents taken, and tells the nurse that a recent overdose episode was a result of experimentation. An appropriate nursing diagnosis for the patient is

    a. defensive coping.
    b. ineffective denial.
    c. ineffective coping.
    d. ineffective health maintenance.

15. To stop the behavior that leads to the most preventable cause of death in the United States, the nurse should support programs that

    a. prohibit alcohol use in public places.
    b. prevent tobacco use in children and adolescents.
    c. motivate individuals to enter addiction treatment.
    d. recognize addictions as illnesses rather than crimes.

16. A young woman is brought to the emergency department by police who found her lying on a downtown sidewalk. Initial assessment finds that she is unresponsive and has a weak pulse of 112, shallow respirations of 8 per minute, and cold, clammy skin. Identify the two drugs that would most likely be given immediately to this patient, and explain why.

    a.

    b.

17. A patient with a history of alcohol abuse is admitted to the hospital following an automobile accident. To plan care for the patient, it is most important for the nurse to assess

    a. when the patient last had alcohol intake.
    b. how much alcohol has recently been used.
    c. what type of alcohol has recently been ingested.
    d. the patient's current blood alcohol concentration.

18. A patient in alcohol withdrawal has a nursing diagnosis of risk for injury related to sensorimotor deficits, seizure activity, and confusion. An appropriate nursing intervention for the patient is to

    a. provide a darkened, quiet environment free from external stimuli.
    b. force fluids to assist in diluting the alcohol concentration in the blood.
    c. use restraints as necessary to prevent the patient from reacting violently to hallucinations.
    d. monitor vital signs frequently as an indicator of an extreme autonomic nervous system response.

19. What are four precautions indicated for the alcoholic patient who is alcohol intoxicated and is undergoing emergency surgery?

    a.

    b.

    c.

    d.

20. During admission to the emergency department, a patient with chronic alcoholism is intoxicated and very disoriented and confused. The nurse anticipates that the patient's management will initially include administration of

    a. intravenous thiamine.
    b. D_5 in ½ NS at 100 ml/hr.
    c. intravenous benzodiazepines.
    d. intravenous haloperidol (Haldol).

21. The nurse uses motivational interviewing with a patient dependent on alcohol who is hospitalized for gastritis. When the patient says she doesn't really think her use of alcohol is a problem because she can control her drinking when she wants, it would be most appropriate for the nurse to

    a. help the patient consider the positive and negative factors of drinking.
    b. refrain from talking about her alcohol use while the patient is in denial.
    c. explain that the gastritis is evidence that alcohol is affecting her health.
    d. reassure the patient that she can quit drinking when she finally decides she wants to.

22. When assessing an older patient for substance abuse, the nurse recognizes that abuse problems in older persons are most often related to the use of alcohol with

    a. opiates.
    b. sedative-hypnotics.
    c. central nervous system stimulants.
    d. prescription and over-the-counter medications.

CASE STUDY

COCAINE TOXICITY

Family Profile

Mr. C. is a 34-year-old man who was admitted to the emergency department with chest pain, tachycardia, dizziness, nausea, and severe migraine-like headache.

Subjective Data

- Is extremely nervous and irritable
- Thinks he is having a heart attack
- Admits that he was at a party earlier in the evening drinking alcohol, smoking pot, and snorting cocaine
- Noted a change in personality, including irritability and restlessness
- Experienced an increased need for cocaine in the past few months

Objective Data

Physical examination
- Appears pale and diaphoretic
- Has tremors
- BP 210/110, HR 100, RR 30

Critical Thinking Questions

1. What other information is needed to assess Mr. C.'s condition?

2. How should questions regarding these areas be addressed?

3. What other clues should the nurse be alert for in assessing Mr. C.'s drug use?

4. What emergency conditions must be carefully monitored?

5. What nursing interventions are appropriate?

6. What is the best way to approach Mr. C. to engage him in a treatment program?

7. Based on the assessment data presented, write one or more nursing diagnoses. Are there any collaborative problems?

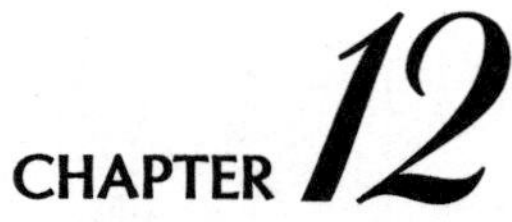

CHAPTER 12 INFLAMMATION, INFECTION, AND HEALING

1. Match the definitions of cell adaptation and maladaptation to sublethal injury to their types.

_____	a. Decrease in size or number of cells	1. Hypertrophy
_____	b. Increase in size of cells	2. Hyperplasia
_____	c. Transformation of one cell type to another	3. Atrophy
_____	d. Change in size, shape, and appearance of cells	4. Metaplasia
_____	e. Increase in number of cells	5. Dysplasia
_____	f. Cells in a more embryonic form	6. Anaplasia

2. A patient has suffered a penetrating injury to the abdomen causing a bowel perforation. The injury was caused by a hot coil flying off a machine. In this situation, four causes of lethal cell injury are

_____________________, ___________________, ________________, and ____________________.

3. For each of the following types of tissues or organs, identify the specific phagocytic cells of the mononuclear phagocyte system that are present, and whether the cells are fixed or free.

   a. Liver

   b. Lung

   c. Central nervous system

   d. Blood

   e. Connective tissue

   f. Bone

   g. Lymph nodes

4. A patient with an inflammatory disease has the following symptoms. Identify the primary chemical mediators involved in producing the symptom and the physiologic change that causes the symptoms.

	Chemical mediators	Physiologic change
a. Fever		
b. Redness		
c. Edema		
d. Leukocytosis		

5. In a patient with leukocytosis with a shift to the left, the nurse recognizes that

   a. monocytes are released into the blood in larger than normal amounts.
   b. the complement system has been activated to enhance phagocytosis.
   c. the response to cellular injury is not adequate to remove damaged tissue and promote healing.
   d. the demand for increased neutrophils causes the release of immature neutrophils from the bone marrow into the circulation.

6. Chemotaxis is a mechanism that

   a. causes the transformation of monocytes into macrophages.
   b. involves a pathway of chemical processes resulting in cellular lysis.
   c. attracts the accumulation of neutrophils and monocytes to an area of injury.
   d. slows the blood flow in a damaged area allowing migration of leukocytes into tissue.

7. A patient with an inflammation has a high eosinophil count. The nurse recognizes that this indicates that

   a. humoral and cell-mediated immunity is being stimulated.
   b. the inflammatory response has been stimulated by infection.
   c. tissue damage has been caused by an allergen-antibody reaction.
   d. the inflammation has become chronic with persistent tissue damage.

8. The action of the complement system in inflammation has the effect of

   a. modifying the inflammatory response to prevent stimulation of pain.
   b. increasing body temperature resulting in destruction of microorganisms.
   c. producing prostaglandins and leukotrienes that increase blood flow, edema, and pain.
   d. increasing inflammatory responses of vascular permeability, chemotaxis, and phagocytosis.

9. Identify whether the following statements are true or false. If a statement is false, correct the bold word(s) to make the statement true.

_____ a. Nonsteroidal antiinflammatory drugs used for inflammation inhibit the **release of leukotrienes from cells**.

_____ b. The primary effect of most **leukotrienes** is formation of the slow-reacting substance of anaphylaxis (SRS-A) that causes bronchial constriction.

_____ c. **Prostaglandins** are responsible for the constitutional symptoms of inflammation such as malaise, fatigue, and anorexia.

_____ d. Complement factors C3a, C5a, and C4a bind to receptors on **basophils**, causing histamine release and anaphylactoid reactions.

_____ e. Interleukin-1 (IL-1) and tumor necrosis factor (TNF) are cytokines that are released from **bacterial cells** during phagocytosis.

10. During the healing phase of inflammation, regeneration of cells would be most likely to occur in

a. neurons.
b. lymph glands.
c. cardiac muscle.
d. skeletal muscle.

11. Place the following events that occur during healing by primary intention in sequential order from 1 to 10:

_____ a. Contraction of healing area by movement of myofibroblasts

_____ b. Fibrin clot serves as meshwork for capillary growth and epithelial cell migration

_____ c. Accumulation of inflammatory debris

_____ d. Epithelial cells migrate across wound surface

_____ e. Fibroblasts migrate to site and secrete collagen

_____ f. Blood clots form

_____ g. Enzymes from neutrophils digest fibrin

_____ h. Avascular, pale, mature scar present

_____ i. Budding capillaries result in pink, vascular friable wound

_____ j. Macrophages ingest and digest cellular debris and red blood cells

12. The primary difference between healing by primary intention and healing by secondary intention is that

a. secondary healing requires surgical debridement for healing to occur.
b. primary healing involves suturing two layers of granulation tissue together.
c. the presence of more granulation tissue in secondary healing results in more scarring.
d. healing by secondary intention takes longer because more steps in the healing process are necessary.

13. Complications of healing that are related to scar formation include ___________, ______________, ________________, ________________, and ______________.

14. The three antibiotic-resistant bacteria that are of most current concern are ________________, ______________, and ______________. The one most important method for nurses to prevent the spread of antibiotic-resistant organisms is ______________________________.

15. The most important instruction the nurse should provide to a patient to prevent the development of antibiotic-resistant bacterial infections is to

    a. wash the hands after toileting and before eating.
    b. avoid crowds and contact with others with infections.
    c. take prescribed antibiotics at the frequency and for the duration directed.
    d. request antibiotic therapy when a cold or the flu does not resolve in 2 to 3 days.

16. A patient's normal calorie requirement is 1800 calories per day. During an infection, the patient's temperature averages 101.2° F (38.5° C). The increase in calories the nurse plans to provide the patient is

    a. 100.
    b. 150.
    c. 300.
    d. 900.

17. Match the characteristics and management techniques of wounds with their types (answers may be used more than once).

_____	a. Serosanguineous drainage	1. Closed wound
_____	b. Adherent gray necrotic tissue	2. Red wound
_____	c. Spray films	3. Yellow wound
_____	d. Creamy ivory to yellow-green exudate	4. Black wound
_____	e. Autolytic debridement	
_____	f. Dry sterile dressing	
_____	g. Soft necrotic slough	
_____	h. Clean, moist granulating tissue	
_____	i. Negative pressure wound therapy	

18. A basic principle of wound management for all open wounds is to

    a. protect new granulation and epithelial tissue.
    b. apply topic antimicrobials to prevent wound infection.
    c. remove wound exudate with frequent dressing changes.
    d. use occlusive dressings to prevent wound contamination.

19. During care of patients, the most important precaution for preventing transmission of infections is

    a. wearing face and eye protection during routine care of the patient.
    b. wearing a gown to protect skin and clothing during patient care activities likely to soil clothing.
    c. wearing nonsterile gloves when in contact with body fluids, excretions, and contaminated items.
    d. hand washing following touching fluids and secretions, removal of gloves, and between patient contacts.

20. The patient who is at greatest risk for developing pressure ulcers is

    a. a 42-year-old obese woman with type 2 diabetes.
    b. a 78-year-old man who is confused and malnourished.
    c. a 65-year-old woman who has urge and stress incontinence.
    d. a 30-year-old man who is comatose following a head injury.

21. The most important nursing intervention for the prevention and treatment of pressure ulcers is

    a. using pressure-reduction devices.
    b. massaging pressure areas with lotion.
    c. repositioning the patient a minimum of every 2 hours.
    d. using lift sheets and trapeze bars to facilitate patient movement.

22. Match the stages of pressure ulcers with their characteristics.

_____	a. Necrosis of subcutaneous tissue to fascia	1. Stage I
_____	b. Skin loss with damage to muscle or bone	2. Stage II
_____	c. Loss of epidermis or dermis	3. Stage III
_____	d. Closed, nonblanchable erythema	4. Stage IV

CASE STUDY

INFLAMMATION

Patient Profile

Kate G., a 23-year-old diabetic, is admitted to the hospital with a cellulitis of her left lower leg. She had been applying heating pads to the leg for the last 48 hours, but the leg has become more painful and she has developed chilling.

Subjective Data

- Complains of pain and heaviness in her leg
- States she cannot bear weight on her leg and has been in bed for 3 days
- Lives alone and has not had anyone to help her with meals

Objective Data

Physical examination:

- Round, yellow-red, 2-cm diameter, 1-cm deep, open wound above the medial malleolus with moderate amount of thick yellow drainage
- Left leg red from knee to ankle
- Calf measurement on left 3 in larger than right
- Temperature: 102° F (38.9° C)
- Height: 5 ft 4 in (160 cm); weight: 184 lb (83.7 kg)

Laboratory:

- WBC: 18,300/μl; 80% neutrophils, 12% bands
- Wound culture: *Staphylococcus aureus*

Critical Thinking Questions

1. What clinical manifestations of inflammation are present in Kate?

2. What type of exudate is draining from the open wound?

3. What is the significance of Kate's WBC count and differential?

4. What factors are present in this situation that could delay wound healing?

5. Kate's physician orders aspirin to be given prn for a temperature above 102° F (38.9° C). How does the aspirin act to interfere with the fever mechanism? Why is the aspirin to be given only if the temperature is above 102° F? To prevent cycling of chills and diaphoresis, how should the nurse administer the aspirin?

6. What type of wound dressing would promote healing of the open wound?

7. What precautions to prevent infection transmission are required in the care of Kate's wound?

8. Based on the assessment data provided, write one or more nursing diagnoses. Are there any collaborative problems?

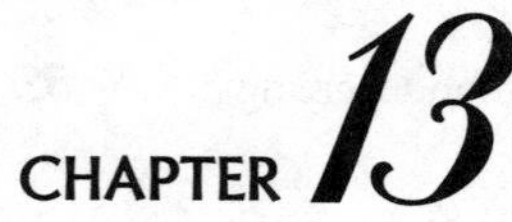

GENETICS AND ALTERED IMMUNE RESPONSES

1. Match the following genetic terms with their descriptions.

_____ a. Phenotype
_____ b. Locus
_____ c. Allele
_____ d. Chromosome
_____ e. Dominant allele
_____ f. Genotype
_____ g. Recessive allele
_____ h. Autosomes
_____ i. DNA
_____ j. RNA
_____ k. Gene

1. The 22 homologous pairs of chromosomes
2. Double-stranded molecule-forming gene; stores genetic information
3. Position of a gene on a chromosome
4. Gene that has no noticeable effect on the phenotype in a heterozygous individual
5. Structure in cell nucleus that carries genes
6. Basic unit of heredity; arranged on chromosome
7. One of two or more alternative forms of a gene on a particular locus
8. Gene that is expressed in the phenotype of a heterozygous individual
9. Genetic physical traits expressed by an individual
10. Actual genetic make-up of an individual
11. Single-stranded nucleic acid that transfers genetic information for protein synthesis

2. When a pair of chromosomes fails to completely separate during meiosis, it may result in

a. the formation of oncogenes.
b. the creation of new autosomal recessive disorders.
c. chromosomal abnormalities such as Down syndrome.
d. a greater diversity in the genetic make-up of oocytes and sperm.

3. When the father has Huntington's chorea, the nurse uses Punnett squares to illustrate the inheritance patterns and the probability of transmission of the autosomal-dominant disease. Complete the Punnett squares below to illustrate this inheritance pattern, using "H" as the normal gene, and "h" as the gene for Huntington's chorea.

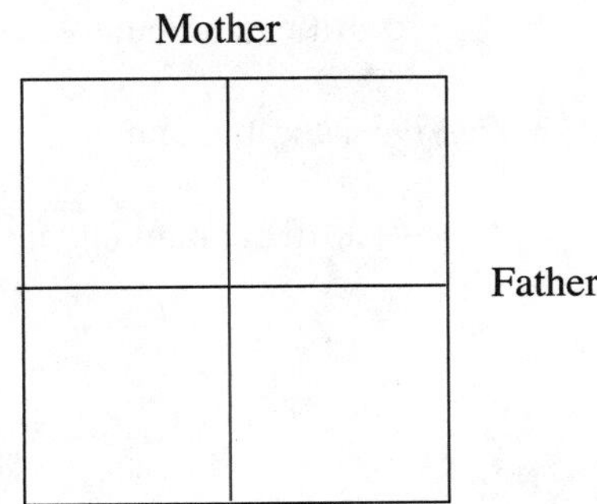

There is a ______ % chance that offspring will be unaffected.

There is a ______ % chance that offspring will be carriers.

There is a ______ % chance that offspring will be affected.

4. The nurse uses Punnett squares to illustrate the inheritance patterns and the probability of transmission of phenylketonuria, an autosomal-recessive gene carried by the mother. Complete the Punnett squares below to illustrate this inheritance pattern, using "P" as the normal gene and "p" as the gene for phenylketonuria.

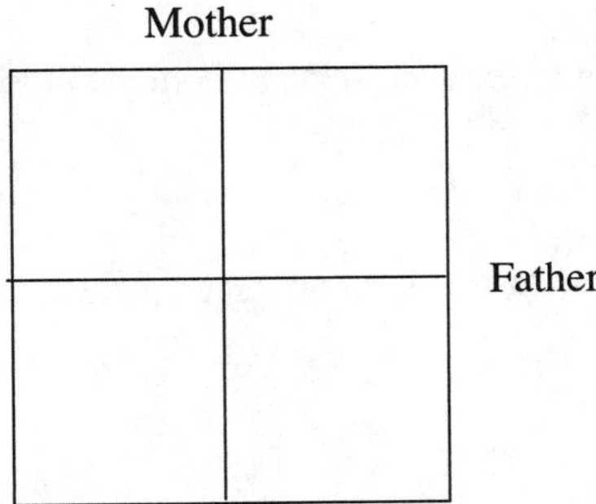

There is a ______% chance that offspring will be unaffected.

There is a ______% chance that offspring will be carriers.

There is a ______% chance that offspring will be affected.

5. The use of a vector to carry genetic material into cells of the body is performed with

a. in vivo methods of gene therapy.
b. ex vivo methods of gene therapy.
c. both in vivo and ex vivo gene therapy.
d. physical transfection of the genetic material.

6. Match the descriptions of acquired specific immunity with their types of immunity (answers may be used more than once).

_____	a. Maternal immunoglobulins in neonate	1. Active natural immunity
_____	b. Contact with antigen through infection	2. Active artificial immunity
_____	c. Immediate, lasting several weeks	3. Passive natural immunity
_____	d. Longest lasting immunity	4. Passive artificial immunity
_____	e. Immunization with antigen	
_____	f. Temporary for several months	
_____	g. Boosters may be needed for extended protection	
_____	h. Pooled gamma globulin	

7. Complete the following statements:

   a. The central organs of the lymphoid system are the ______________ and the ____________________.

   b. The primary cells involved in the immune response are ______________, ______________, and ____________________.

   c. The lymphoid organ primarily responsible for filtering foreign substances from the blood is the ____________________.

   d. Lymphocytes that differentiate into B lymphocytes are processed in the ________________; T lymphocytes are differentiated in the ____________.

8. To stimulate an immune response, an antigen must be

   a. captured, processed, and presented to a lymphocyte by a macrophage.
   b. a foreign protein that has antigenic determinants different from the body.
   c. circulated in the blood where it comes in contact with circulating lymphocytes.
   d. combined with larger molecules that are capable of stimulating production of antibodies.

9. T lymphocytes that are involved in direct attack and destruction of foreign pathogens are

   a. T cytotoxic cells.
   b. natural killer cells.
   c. T helper (CD4) cells.
   d. T suppressor (CD8) cells.

10. Interferon is a cytokine that

    a. directly attacks and destroys virus-infected cells.
    b. augments the immune response by activating phagocytes.
    c. induces production of antiviral proteins in cells that prevent viral replication.
    d. is produced by viral infected cells and prevents the transmission of the virus to adjacent cells.

11. The humoral immune response involves

a. surveillance for malignant cell changes.
b. production of antigen-specific immunoglobulins.
c. direct attack of antigens by activated B lymphocytes.
d. releasing cytokines responsible for destruction of antigens.

12. Activated B lymphocytes differentiate primarily into

a. plasma cells that secrete antibodies.
b. natural killer cells that destroy infected cells.
c. memory B cells that retain a memory of the antigen.
d. helper cells that in turn activate additional B lymphocytes.

13. Match the characteristics of the immunoglobulins with their types (answers may be used more than once).

_____	a. Crosses placenta for fetal protection	1. IgA
_____	b. Predominant in primary immune response	2. IgD
_____	c. Predominant in secondary immune response	3. IgE
_____	d. Responsible for allergic reactions	4. IgG
_____	e. Assists in B lymphocyte differentiation	5. IgM
_____	f. Protects body surfaces and mucous membranes	
_____	g. Antibodies against ABO blood antigens	
_____	h. Passed to neonate in colostrum	
_____	i. Assists in parasitic infections	

14. Identify five important functions of cell-mediated immunity.

a.

b.

c.

d.

e.

15. With advancing age, the immunologic response that is increased is

a. antibody responses.
b. tumor surveillance.
c. autoimmune responses.
d. hypersensitivity responses.

16. Identify the types of hypersensitivity reactions from the following characteristics.

1. Type I: anaphylactoid
2. Type II: cytotoxic
3. Type III: immune-complex mediated
4. Type IV: delayed hypersensitivity

_____ a. Cellular lysis or phagocytosis through complement activation following antigen-antibody binding on cell surfaces

_____ b. Antigen links with specific IgE antibodies bound to mast cells or basophils releasing chemical mediators

_____ c. T lymphocyte attack of antigens or release of lymphokines attract macrophages that cause tissue damage

_____ d. Antigens combined with IgG and IgM too small to be removed by mononuclear phagocytic system deposit in tissue and cause fixation of complement

17. Match the following examples of hypersensitivity to their types (answers may be used more than once).

_____	a. Transfusion reactions	1. Type I
_____	b. Asthma	2. Type II
_____	c. Angioedema	3. Type III
_____	d. Transplant rejection	4. Type IV
_____	e. Rheumatoid arthritis	
_____	f. Allergic rhinitis	
_____	g. Tubercular caseous necrosis	
_____	h. Goodpasture's syndrome	
_____	i. Atopic dermatitis	
_____	j. Acute glomerular nephritis	
_____	k. Anaphylactic shock	
_____	l. Urticaria	
_____	m. Contact dermatitis	

18. A patient was given an IM injection of penicillin in the gluteus maximus and developed dyspnea and weakness within minutes following the injection.

a. What are four additional assessment findings that would indicate that the patient is having an anaphylactoid reaction?

1)

2)

3)

4)

b. Identify five nursing interventions to be taken to treat the patient's problem.

1)

2)

3)

4)

5)

19. The rationale for treatment of atopic allergies with immunotherapy is that this therapy

a. decreases the levels of allergen-specific T-helper cells.
b. decreases the level of IgE so that it does not react as readily with an allergen.
c. stimulates increased IgG to bind with allergen-reactive sites, preventing mast cell–bound IgE reactions.
d. gradually increases the amount of allergen in the body until it is no longer recognized as foreign and does not elicit an antibody reaction.

20. When administering immunotherapy to a patient, the nurse must

a. give the injections at the same site each time.
b. give the injection in the upper arm near the shoulder.
c. observe the patient for 1 hour following the injection.
d. have emergency equipment and drugs available for immediate use.

21. A nurse who develops a contact dermatitis from wearing latex gloves

a. is demonstrating an allergy to natural latex proteins.
b. can use powder-free latex gloves to prevent the development of symptoms.
c. should use an oil-based hand cream when wearing gloves to prevent latex allergy.
d. has a type IV allergic reaction to chemicals used in the manufacture of latex gloves.

22. Although the cause of autoimmune disorders is unknown, the two factors believed to be present in most conditions are ____________________ and ____________________.

23. Plasmapheresis is indicated in autoimmune disorders to

a. obtain plasma for analysis and evaluation of specific autoantibodies.
b. decrease high lymphocyte levels in the blood to prevent immune responses.
c. remove autoantibodies, antigen-antibody complexes, and inflammatory mediators of immune reactions.
d. add monocytes to the blood to promote removal of immune complexes by the mononuclear phagocyte system.

24. The human leukocyte antigen type appears to be closely related to

a. sex-linked genetic immunodeficiency disorders.
b. hereditary tendencies for immune or autoimmune disorders.
c. development of idiopathic environmental intolerances (IEI).
d. susceptibility to viral infection of the lymphoid organs and cells.

25. Explain what the term *histocompatibility complex* means, and identify which genes (of what chromosome) are involved in histocompatibility.

26. Currently, HLA typing can be used to

a. determine paternity and predict risk for certain diseases.
b. match tissue types for transplantation and determine paternity.
c. establish racial background and predict risk for certain diseases.
d. predict risk for certain diseases and match tissue types for transplantation.

27. The most common cause of secondary immunodeficiency disorders is ______________________________.

28. The disorder in which viable T lymphocytes infused into an immunodeficient patient destroy vulnerable host cells is ______________________________.

29. A common combination of immunosuppressive agents used to prevent rejection of transplanted kidneys is

a. cyclosporine, sirolimus, and muromonab-CD3.
b. everolimus, mycophenolate mofetil, and sirolimus.
c. tacrolimus, prednisone, and mycophenolate mofetil.
d. prednisone, polyclonal antibodies, and cyclosporine.

CASE STUDY

ALLERGY

Patient Profile

Mr. W., age 54, has been diagnosed as having perennial allergic rhinitis. He is to undergo skin testing to identify specific allergens. His physician has prescribed oral antihistamines for control of his symptoms.

Subjective Data

- Itching of eyes, nose, and throat
- Stuffy nose, head congestion

Objective Data

- Physical examination: clear nasal drainage; reddened eyes and lacrimation

Critical Thinking Questions

1. What immunoglobulins and chemical mediators are involved in Mr. W.'s allergic reaction?

2. Describe the procedure the nurse uses to perform the skin testing. What results indicate a positive response?

3. What precautions should be taken by the nurse during skin testing?

4. How do antihistamines act to relieve allergic symptoms? What information should the nurse include in teaching Mr. W. about using his antihistamines?

5. Skin testing indicates Mr. W. has an allergy to household dust. What information should the nurse include in teaching Mr. W. to control his exposure to this allergen?

6. Mr. W. is to begin immunotherapy. What precautions does the nurse use during the administration of the allergen extract?

7. Based on the assessment data provided, write one or more nursing diagnoses. Are there any collaborative problems?

CHAPTER 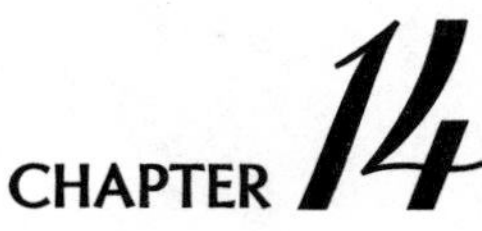

HUMAN IMMUNODEFICIENCY VIRUS INFECTION

1. The most common method of transmission of HIV infection is

   a. sexual contact with a HIV-infected partner.
   b. sharing HIV-contaminated injection equipment.
   c. fetal exposure to infection from HIV-infected mother.
   d. transfusion of HIV-contaminated blood or blood products.

2. Underline the factors in the following situations in which the risk for HIV transmission is highest.

   a. Women compared with men during sexual intercourse

   b. Hollow-bore needle used for vascular access or used for IM injection

   c. Vaginal intercourse or anal intercourse

   d. Transfusion of whole blood or clotting factors

   e. First 2 to 6 months of infection or 1 year after infection

   f. Perinatal transmission from HIV-infected mothers taking antiretroviral therapy or HIV-infected mothers using no therapy

   g. A splash exposure of HIV-infected blood on skin with an open lesion or a needle-stick exposure to HIV-infected blood

3. Place the following events of HIV infection of a cell in sequence from 1 to 7.

   ____ a. Viral RNA is converted to single-strand viral DNA with assistance of reverse transcriptase

   ____ b. Viral DNA is spliced into cell genome using the enzyme integrase

   ____ c. gp 120 proteins on viral envelope combine with CD4 receptors of body cells

   ____ d. Cell replicates infected daughter cells and makes more HIV

   ____ e. Viral RNA and reverse transcriptase enzyme enter host cell

   ____ f. Long strands of viral RNA are cut in the presence of protease

   ____ g. Single-strand viral DNA replicates into double-stranded DNA

4. In the previous question, indicate what two events of HIV infection of a cell can be controlled with current drugs.

   a.

   b.

5. A primary reason that the normal immune response fails to contain HIV infection is that

   a. CD8+ T cells are stimulated, causing suppression of B lymphocyte activity.
   b. the virus inactivates B lymphocytes, preventing the production of HIV antibodies.
   c. activated CD4+ T cells drawn to HIV become infected and support viral replication.
   d. monocytes ingest infected cells, differentiate into macrophages, and shed viruses in body tissues.

6. List three methods by which HIV destroys CD4+ T cells.

   a.

   b.

   c.

7. Match the following characteristics with the corresponding stage of progression of HIV infection.

3	a. CD4+ T cells <600/μl	1. Acute retroviral syndrome
1	b. Flulike symptoms	2. Early chronic infection
2	c. May last up to 10 years	3. Intermediate chronic infection
1	d. HIV seroconversion	4. AIDS or late chronic infection
3	e. Median length is 2 years	
2	f. CD4+ T cell count usually normal	
1	g. Lasts 1 to 2 weeks	
3	h. Persistent fevers and night sweats	
4	i. Reversal of CD4+ T cell to CD8+ T cell ratio	
3	j. Oral hairy leukoplakia	

8. A diagnosis of AIDS can be made in a patient with HIV when there is

   a. a CD4+ T cell count of <500/μl.
   b. a WBC count <3000/μl (3 x 10^9/L).
   c. development of oral candidiasis (thrush).
   d. onset of *Pneumocystis carinii* pneumonia.

9. Match the following characteristics with opportunistic diseases associated with AIDS.

3 a. Hyperpigmented lesions of skin, lungs, and gastrointestinal tract
6 b. Maculopapular, pruritic rash treated with acyclovir
8 c. Common yeast infection involving mouth, esophagus, GI tract
2 d. Viral infection affecting skin, eyes, and oral and esophageal mucosa
5 e. May cause meningitis
7 f. Diagnosed with lymph node biopsy
1 g. Pneumonia with dry, nonproductive cough
4 h. Viral retinitis, stomatitis, esophagitis, gastritis, colitis

1. *Pneumocystis carinii* infection
2. Herpes simplex 1 infection
3. Kaposi's sarcoma
4. Cytomegalovirus infection
5. *Cryptococcus* infection
6. Varicella-zoster virus infection
7. Non-Hodgkin's lymphoma
8. *Candida albicans*

10. Opportunistic diseases develop in AIDS because these disorders are

a. side effects of drug treatment of AIDS.
b. sexually transmitted to individuals during exposure to HIV.
c. characteristic in individuals with stimulated B and T lymphocytes.
d. infections or tumors that occur when there is impaired immune function.

11. Identify whether the following statements are true or false. If a statement is false, correct the bold word(s) to make the statement true.

T a. An individual with a positive result with the EIA is not considered HIV-antibody positive until confirmed with a repeat positive EIA and positive **Western blot or immunofluorescence assay (IFA) testing**.

F b. **Polymerase chain reaction (PCR) tests** or **viral cultures** are done to confirm repeatedly positive ELISA testing for HIV antibodies.

F c. The progression of HIV infection is monitored with the use of **Western blot** or **immunofluorescence assay (IFA)**.

T d. An individual with HIV infection may have a **negative ELISA** for 6 months following infection.

T e. **PCR and viral cultures** may be done to diagnose HIV infection in infants.

12. A newborn infant of a mother with HIV infection has a positive HIV antibody test. This indicates that the newborn

a. has HIV infection.
b. will require treatment for AIDS.
c. will most likely develop AIDS within 15 months.
d. has maternal HIV antibodies but may not have HIV infection.

13. Treatment with two nucleoside reverse transcriptase inhibitors (NRTIs) and a protease inhibitor (PI) is prescribed for a patient with HIV infection who has a $CD4^+$ T cell count of <400/μl. The patient asks why three drugs are necessary for treatment. The nurse explains that the primary rationale for combination therapy is that

   a. cross resistance between specific antiretroviral drugs is reduced when drugs are given in combination.
   b. combinations of antiretroviral drugs decrease the potential for development of antiretroviral-resistant HIV variants.
   c. side effects of the drugs are reduced when smaller doses of three different drugs are used rather than large doses of one drug.
   d. when $CD4^+$ T cell counts are below 500/μl, a combination of drugs that have different actions is more effective in slowing HIV growth.

14. One of the most significant factors in determining when to start antiretroviral therapy in a patient with HIV infection is

   a. whether the patient has high levels of HIV antibodies.
   b. the confirmation that the patient has contracted HIV infection.
   c. the patient's readiness to commit to a complex, life-long, uncomfortable drug regimen.
   d. whether the patient has a support system to help manage the costs and side effects of the drugs.

15. After teaching a patient with HIV infection about using antiretroviral drugs, the nurse recognizes that further teaching is needed when the patient says

   a. "I should never skip doses of my medication, even if I develop side effects."
   b. "If my viral load becomes undetectable, I will no longer be able to transmit HIV to others."
   c. "I should not use any over-the-counter drugs without checking with my health care provider."
   d. "If I develop a constant headache that is not relieved with aspirin or acetominophen, I should report it within 24 hours."

16. Prophylactic measures that are routinely used as early as possible in HIV infection to prevent opportunistic and debilitating secondary problems include administration of

   a. isoniazid (INH) to prevent tuberculosis.
   b. trimethoprim-sulfamethoxazole (TMP-SMX) for toxoplasmosis.
   c. vaccines for pneumococcal pneumonia, influenza and hepatitis A and B.
   d. varicella zoster immune globulin (VZIG) to prevent chickenpox or shingles.

17. A patient identified as HIV-antibody–positive 1 year ago manifests early HIV infection but does not want to start antiretroviral therapy at this time. An appropriate nursing intervention for the patient at this stage of illness is to

   a. assist with end-of-life issues.
   b. provide care during acute exacerbations.
   c. provide physical care for chronic diseases.
   d. educate the patient regarding immune enhancement.

18. Identify three methods to eliminate or reduce the risk for HIV transmission related to sexual intercourse and drug use.

Sexual intercourse

a.

b.

c.

Drug use

a.

b.

c.

19. A patient with advanced AIDS has diarrhea and wasting syndrome. An appropriate nursing diagnosis for the patient is

a. diarrhea related to opportunistic infection.
b. risk for fluid volume deficit related to diarrhea.
c. risk for infection related to immunosuppression.
d. risk for impaired skin integrity related to altered nutritional status and frequent stools.

20. A patient with advanced AIDS has a nursing diagnosis of altered thought processes related to neurologic changes. In planning care for the patient, the nurse sets the highest priority on

a. providing a quiet, nonstressful environment to avoid overstimulation.
b. using memory cues such as calendars and clocks to promote orientation.
c. providing written instructions of directions to promote understanding and orientation.
d. maintaining a safe patient environment.

CASE STUDY

HIV INFECTION

Patient Profile

Doug K., a 28-year-old single man, had HIV antibody screening performed 2 weeks ago when he was seen at a health clinic for flulike symptoms. At that time, he revealed that he had a history of multiple sexual partners. He has returned to the clinic for the results of his screening.

Subjective Data

- Vague symptoms of fatigue and headache
- Reports occasional night sweats

Objective Data

- Positive Western blot test
- Temperature: 100° F (37.8° C)
- Enlarged cervical and femoral lymph nodes

Critical Thinking Questions

1. What specific post-test counseling activities should be performed by the nurse during Doug's visit?

2. Doug's $CD4^+$ T cell count is 650/μl. What stage of HIV infection is he most likely experiencing?

3. What additional diagnostic tests might be performed at this visit?

4. What prophylactic treatments should be used at this time to prevent the development of opportunistic diseases?

5. The physician encourages Doug to consider starting combination antiretroviral therapy. What can the nurse tell Doug about the expected effect of this therapy?

6. If Doug does not respond to treatment with an increased $CD4^+$ T cell count and a decreased viral load, what tests could be used to identify resistance to the antiretroviral agents?

7. Based on the assessment data presented, write one or more appropriate nursing diagnoses. Are there any collaborative problems?

CHAPTER 15 CANCER

1. When presenting a community education program related to cancer prevention, the nurse stresses that the leading cause of cancer death in both men and women is

   a. lung cancer.
   b. colorectal cancer.
   c. leukemias and lymphomas.
   d. cancer of the reproductive organs.

2. The defect in cellular proliferation that occurs in the development of cancer involves

   a. a rate of cell proliferation that is more rapid than that of normal body cells.
   b. shortened phases of cell life cycles with occasional skipping of G_1 or S phases.
   c. rearrangement of stem cell RNA that causes abnormal cellular protein synthesis.
   d. indiscriminate and continuous proliferation of cells with loss of contact inhibition.

3. The presence of carcinoembryonic antigens (CEAs) and alpha fetoprotein (AFP) on cell membranes is an indication that cells have

   a. shifted to more immature metabolic pathways and functions.
   b. spread from areas of original development to different body tissues.
   c. become more differentiated as a result of repression of embryonic functions.
   d. produced abnormal toxins or chemical that indicate abnormal cellular function.

4. The major difference between benign tumors and malignant tumors is that malignant tumors

   a. grow at a faster rate.
   b. are often encapsulated.
   c. invade and metastasize.
   d. cause death while benign tumors do not.

5. Match the following malignancies with the carcinogenic factors associated with their initiation.

_____	a. Skin cancer	1. Alkylating agents
_____	b. Acute myelogenous leukemia	2. Genetic susceptibility
_____	c. Breast cancer	3. Epstein-Barr virus
_____	d. Cervical cancer	4. Ultraviolet light
_____	e. Burkitt's lymphoma	5. Ionizing radiation
_____	f. Thyroid cancer	6. Human papillomavirus

6. Identify whether the following statements are true or false. If a statement is false, correct the bold word(s) to make the statement true.

_____ a. **Initiation** is the stage of cancer development in which there is an irreversible alteration in the cell's DNA.

_____ b. Tobacco smoke is a complete carcinogen that is capable of both **initiation** and **promotion**.

_____ c. The promotion stage of cancer is characterized by the **irreversible** proliferation of altered, initiated cells.

_____ d. Obesity is an example of a **promoting factor**.

_____ e. The latent period of cancer is the same as **promotion**.

_____ f. Withdrawal of promoting factors will **reduce** the risk of cancer development.

_____ g. Metastasis of malignant cells to distant sites is promoted by the cell's production of **growth factor**.

_____ h. During cancer progression, metastatic cells become more **heterogenous**, making treatment more difficult.

7. List three capabilities of tumor cells that facilitate spread of the tumor from the original site.

a.

b.

c.

8. Match the following terms with their descriptions.

_____ a. Mutations of protooncogens that normally limit cell regulation

_____ b. Substance that promotes blood vessel development within tumors

_____ c. Tumor cell antigens that stimulate an immune response

_____ d. Capable of causing cellular alterations associated with cancer

_____ e. Antigens on tumor cells that reflect a return to embryonic cell differentiation

_____ f. Programmed cellular death

_____ g. Lesion with histologic features of cancer except invasion

_____ h. Evasion of the immune system by cancer cells

1. Tumor-associated antigens
2. Immunologic escape
3. Apoptosis
4. Oncofetal antigens
5. Oncogenes
6. Carcinoma in situ
7. Oncogenic
8. Tumor angiogenesis factor

9. Indicate the source and function of the following cytokines in immunologic surveillance.

	Source	Function
a. Interleukin 1 (IL-1)		
b. Interleukin 2 (IL-2)		
c. Alpha-interferon		
d. Gamma-interferon		
e. Tumor necrosis factor		
f. Colony-stimulating factors		

10. Compare a meningioma and a meningeal sarcoma according to the anatomic site classification system for tumors.

    a. Tissue of origin:

    b. Anatomic site:

    c. Behavior:

11. A patient's tumor has been classified as grade II, $T_1N_1M_0$ carcinoma of the breast. What does this tell the nurse about the tissue of origin and the extent of the disease process?

    a. Carcinoma:

    b. Grade II:

    c. $T_1N_1M_0$:

12. The nurse is counseling a group of individuals over the age of 50 about screening tests for cancer. What are six specific tests that should be performed by health professionals for the people in this group and at what frequency?

    a.

    b.

    c.

    d.

    e.

    f.

13. The definitive method of diagnosing cancer is

   a. x-rays.
   b. biopsy.
   c. CT scan.
   d. presence of oncofetal antigens.

14. Match the surgical procedures with their primary purposes in cancer treatment (answers may be used more than once).

_____	a. Colostomy to bypass bowel obstruction	1. Cure, control, or both
_____	b. Bowel resection	2. Supportive care
_____	c. Mammoplasty	3. Palliation
_____	d. Debulking procedure	4. Rehabilitation
_____	e. Insertion of suprapubic catheter	
_____	f. Cordotomy for pain control	
_____	g. Mastectomy	
_____	h. Insertion of feeding tube into stomach	

15. Normal tissues that may manifest early, acute responses to radiation therapy include

   a. spleen and liver.
   b. kidney and nervous tissue.
   c. bone marrow and gastrointestinal mucosa.
   d. hollow organs such as the stomach and bladder.

16. The rationale for treatment of cancer with radiation includes the knowledge that

   a. radiation damages cellular DNA only in abnormal cells.
   b. malignant cells respond to the effects of radiation because they more frequently go through mitosis.
   c. damage to cells will occur only during M and G_2 phases of the cell cycle, necessitating a series of treatment.
   d. normal cells are able to repair radiation-induced damage to DNA and do not have permanent radiation damage.

17. When a patient is undergoing brachytherapy, it is important for the nurse to recognize that

   a. the patient will undergo simulation to identify and mark the field of treatment.
   b. the patient is a source of radiation and personnel must wear film badges during care.
   c. the goal of this treatment is only palliative and the patient should be aware of the expected outcome.
   d. computerized dosimetry is used to determine the maximum dose of radiation to the tumor within an acceptable dose to normal tissue.

18. A common side effect of radiation therapy that is not associated with the effect of radiation in the treatment field is

   a. fatigue.
   b. alopecia.
   c. skin reactions.
   d. bone marrow suppression.

19. Chemotherapy for the treatment of cancer would be most effective in

a. a small tumor of the bone.
b. a young tumor of the brain.
c. a large tumor in a highly vascular area.
d. malignant changes in hemopoietic cells.

20. Match the following descriptions of chemotherapeutic drugs with their classifications.

_____	a. Cell cycle–specific drugs that mimic essential cellular metabolites	1. Alkylating agents
_____	b. Cell cycle–nonspecific drugs that break DNA strands	2. Antimetabolites
_____	c. Cell cycle–specific drugs that cause mitotic arrest in metaphase	3. Antitumor antibiotics
_____	d. Bind with DNA to block RNA production	4. Plant alkaloids
_____	e. Cell cycle–nonspecific drugs that block purine synthesis	5. Nitrosureas

21. The nurse uses many precautions during intravenous administration of vesicant chemotherapeutic agents primarily to prevent

a. septicemia.
b. extravasion.
c. catheter occlusion.
d. anaphylactic shock.

22. Match the following malignancies with their associated routes of regional chemotherapeutic administration.

_____	a. Bladder	1. Intraoperitoneal
_____	b. Osteogenic sarcoma	2. Intra-arterial
_____	c. Metastasis to the brain	3. Intravenous
_____	d. Metastasis from a primary colorectal cancer	4. Intravesical
_____	e. Leukemia	5. Intrathecal

23. A patient is scheduled to have placement of a silastic right atrial catheter for administration of chemotherapy for breast cancer. When preparing the patient for the catheter insertion, the nurse explains that this method of administration

a. decreases the risk for extravasion at the infusion site.
b. reduces the incidence of systemic side effects of the drug.
c. does not become occluded as peripherally inserted catheters can.
d. allows continuous infusion of the drug directly to the area of the tumor.

24. When teaching the patient with cancer about chemotherapy, the nurse should

  a. avoid telling the patient about possible side effects of the drugs to prevent anticipatory anxiety.
  b. explain that antiemetics, antidiarrheals, and analgesics will be provided as needed to control side effects.
  c. assure the patient that the side effects from chemotherapy are merely uncomfortable, not life-threatening.
  d. inform the patient that chemotherapy-related alopecia is usually permanent but can be managed with life-long use of wigs.

25. The late effects of chemotherapy and high-dose radiation may include

  a. third space syndrome.
  c. persistent myelosuppression.
  b. chronic nausea and vomiting.
  d. resistant secondary malignancies.

26. The primary use of biologic therapy in cancer treatment is to

  a. prevent the fatigue associated with chemotherapy and high-dose radiation.
  b. enhance or supplement the effects of the host's immune responses to tumor cells.
  c. depress the immune system and circulating lymphocytes, as well as increasing a sense of well-being.
  d. protect normal rapidly reproducing cells of the gastrointestinal system from damage during chemotherapy.

27. A side effect common to all of the biologic therapies is

  a. flulike syndrome.
  b. bone marrow suppression.
  c. central nervous system deficits.
  d. nausea, vomiting, anorexia, and diarrhea.

28. To prevent the most frequent cause of death in patients undergoing radiation therapy and chemotherapy for treatment of cancer, the nurse implements measures to

  a. prevent infection.
  b. maintain nutrition.
  c. monitor kidney function.
  d. control vomiting and diarrhea.

29. An allogenic bone marrow transplant is considered as treatment for a patient with acute myelogenous leukemia. The nurse explains that during this procedure

  a. there is no risk for graft-versus-host disease because the donated marrow is treated to remove cancer cells.
  b. bone marrow is obtained from a donor who has a human leukocyte antigen (HLA) match with the patient.
  c. the patient's bone marrow will be removed, treated, stored, and then reinfused after intensive chemotherapy.
  d. there is no need for post-transplant protective isolation because the stem cells are infused directly into the blood.

30. During initial chemotherapy a patient with leukemia develops hyperkalemia and hyperuricemia. The nurse recognizes these symptoms as the oncologic emergency of

  a. hypercalcemia.
  b. third space syndrome.
  c. tumor lysis syndrome.
  d. syndrome of inappropriate antidiuretic hormone (SIADH).

31. Identify five factors that will assist a patient to cope positively with having cancer.

a.

b.

c.

d.

e.

CASE STUDY

CANCER

Patient Profile

Mr. M. is a 45-year-old patient who has recently been diagnosed with acute myelogenous leukemia. He began treatment with chemotherapy through a peripherally inserted central venous catheter 5 days ago.

Subjective Data

- States he has almost continuous nausea, which becomes severe and causes vomiting following his dose of chemotherapy
- States he has no appetite
- Expresses no hope that the chemotherapy will have a positive effect

Objective Data

- Temperature: 99.4° F (37.4° C)
- WBC: 3200/μl (3.2×10^9/L)
- Neutrophils: 500/μl (0.5×10^9/L)
- Skin warm with decreased turgor

Critical Thinking Questions

1. What factors may be responsible for Mr. M.'s decreased WBC and neutrophil count?

2. What assessment data indicate that Mr. M. may be experiencing an infection?

3. What additional assessment data should be collected from Mr. M. to determine the presence of an infection?

4. What factors may contribute to Mr. M.'s negative attitude toward the chemotherapy?

5. Identify nursing measures that could be instituted to help control his anorexia, nausea, and vomiting.

6. What should be included in the teaching plan for Mr. M. and his family to prevent infection?

7. Based on the assessment data presented, write one or more appropriate nursing diagnoses. Are there any collaborative problems?

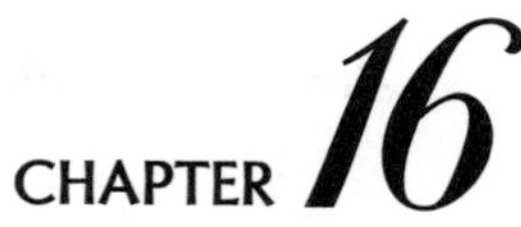

FLUID, ELECTROLYTE, AND ACID-BASE IMBALANCES

1. Identify whether the following statements are true or false. If a statement is false, correct the bold word(s) to make the statement true.

_____ a. A patient with consistent dietary intake who loses 1 kg of weight in 1 day has lost **500** ml of fluid.

_____ b. A man who weighs 90 kg has a total body water content of approximately **60 L**.

_____ c. Major tissue damage that causes release of intracellular electrolytes into extracellular fluid will cause **hypernatremia**.

_____ d. The primary difference in the electrolyte composition of intravascular fluid and interstitial fluid is the higher content of **protein** in plasma.

_____ e. The different concentrations of sodium and potassium between interstitial fluid and intracellular fluid is maintained by the **sodium-potassium pump**.

_____ f. A cell that is surrounded by a hypoosmolar fluid will **shrink and die** as water moves **out of** the cell.

_____ g. Third spacing refers to the abnormal movement of fluid into **interstitial spaces**.

_____ h. The primary hypothalamic mechanism of water intake is **thirst**.

2. Match the following descriptions with the mechanisms of fluid and electrolyte movement.

_____ a. Pressure exerted by proteins

_____ b. ATP required

_____ c. Flow of water from low solute concentration to high solute concentration

_____ d. Force exerted by a fluid

_____ e. Passive movement of molecules from a high concentration to lower concentration

_____ f. Uses a carrier molecule

_____ g. Force determined by osmolality of a fluid

1. Facilitated diffusion
2. Diffusion
3. Osmotic pressure
4. Oncotic pressure
5. Active transport
6. Osmosis
7. Hydrostatic pressure

3. A patient has a serum Na^+ of 147 mEq/L (147 mmol/L) and a blood glucose level of 126 mg/dl (7.0 mmol/L).

The patient's effective serum osmolality is ____________ mOsm/kg. Is the patient's serum osmolality increased, decreased, or normal? __________.

4. As fluid circulates through the capillaries, there is movement of fluid between the capillaries and the interstitium. In the following descriptions, match the direction of fluid movement and the location of the movement in the capillary.

_____ a. Plasma hydrostatic pressure is less than plasma oncotic pressure

_____ b. Interstitial hydrostatic pressure is lower than plasma hydrostatic pressure

_____ c. Plasma hydrostatic pressure is less than interstitial hydrostatic pressure

_____ d. Plasma hydrostatic pressure is higher than plasma oncotic pressure

1. Movement into capillary
2. Movement into interstitium
3. Occurs at arterial end
4. Occurs at venous end

5. Fill in the blanks *preceding* a–g below with 1, 2, 3, or 4 to indicate whether fluid shifts

1) from vessels to interstitium
2) from extracellular compartment to the cell
3) from cell to extracellular compartment
4) from interstitium to vessels

In each of the blanks *following* a–g, identify which mechanism of fluid movement is involved.

_____ a. Low serum albumin _____________________________

_____ b. Hyponatremia _________________________

_____ c. Administration of 10% glucose _______________________

_____ d. Dehydration ______________________________

_____ e. Burns _____________________________

_____ f. Fluid overload ______________________

_____ g. Application of elastic bandages _________________________

6. A woman has ham with gravy and green beans cooked with salt pork for dinner.

a. What could happen to the woman's serum osmolality as a result of this meal?

b. What fluid regulation mechanisms are stimulated by the intake of these foods?

7. Aldosterone is secreted by the adrenal cortex in response to

   a. excessive water intake.
   b. loss of serum potassium.
   c. loss of sodium and water.
   d. increased serum osmolality.

8. A major effect of aldosterone is increased

   a. water loss from kidney.
   b. reabsorption of sodium from the kidney.
   c. reabsorption of potassium from the kidney.
   d. permeability to water in the distal convoluted tubule and collecting duct.

9. A patient at risk for hypernatremia is one who

   a. has a deficiency of aldosterone.
   b. has prolonged vomiting and diarrhea.
   c. receives excessive 5% dextrose solution intravenously.
   d. has impaired consciousness and decreased thirst sensitivity.

10. Manifestations of sodium imbalances are primarily manifested through altered

   a. kidney function.
   b. cardiovascular function.
   c. neuromuscular function.
   d. central nervous system function.

11. Match the electrolyte imbalances with their associated causes (answers may be used more than once).

_____	a. Alcohol withdrawal	1. Hypernatremia
_____	b. Metabolic alkalosis	2. Hyponatremia
_____	c. Parathyroidectomy	3. Hyperkalemia
_____	d. Diabetes insipidus	4. Hypokalemia
_____	e. Fleet's enemas	5. Hypercalcemia
_____	f. Primary polydipsia	6. Hypocalcemia
_____	g. Milk of Magnesia use in renal failure	7. Hyperphosphatemia
_____	h. Early burn stage	8. Hypophosphatemia
_____	i. Chronic alcoholism	9. Hypermagnesemia
_____	j. Vitamin D deficiency	10. Hypomagnesemia
_____	k. Osmotic diuresis	
_____	l. Prolonged immobilization	

12. Several conditions will cause multiple imbalances of electrolytes. Identify three electrolyte imbalances that are caused by the following:

    a. Hyperaldosteronism

        1)

        2)

        3)

    b. Chronic renal failure

        1)

        2)

        3)

    c. Loop and thiazide diuretics

        1)

        2)

        3)

13. A patient is taking diuretic drugs that cause sodium loss from the kidney. The fluid or electrolyte imbalance most likely to occur in this patient is

    a. hyperkalemia.
    b. hyponatremia.
    c. hypocalcemia.
    d. isotonic fluid loss.

14. A common collaborative problem that is indicated for both hyperkalemia and hypokalemia is

    a. potential complication: seizures.
    b. potential complication: paralysis.
    c. potential complication: arrhythmias.
    d. potential complication: acute renal failure.

15. Hyperkalemia is frequently associated with

    a. hypoglycemia.
    b. metabolic acidosis.
    c. respiratory alkalosis.
    d. decreased urine potassium levels.

16. In a patient with a positive Chvostek's sign, the nurse would anticipate the intravenous administration of

    a. calcitonin.
    b. vitamin D.
    c. loop diuretics.
    d. calcium gluconate.

17. A patient with chronic renal failure has hyperphosphatemia. A commonly associated electrolyte imbalance is

a. hypokalemia.
b. hyponatremia.
c. hypocalcemia.
d. hypomagnesemia.

18. The normal pH range of the blood is __________ to ____________. This reflects a ratio of base to acid of

__________ to __________.

19. pH is a negative logarithm that is a measure of ____________________ in a solution.

20. Match the components of the buffer system with their characteristics (answers may be used more than once).

	Characteristic		Buffer
_____	a. Neutralizes a strong base to a weak base and water		1. Carbonic acid–bicarbonate
_____	b. Free acid radicals dissociate into H^+ and CO_2, buffering excess base		2. Phosphate buffer
_____	c. Shifts chloride in and out of red blood cells in exchange for sodium bicarbonate, buffering both acids and bases		3. Hemoglobin buffer
_____	d. Resultant sodium biphosphate is eliminated by kidneys		4. Protein buffer
_____	e. Neutralizes HCl to yield carbonic acid and salt		5. Cellular buffer
_____	f. Free basic radicals dissociate into ammonia and OH^- that combines with H^+ to form water		
_____	g. Resultant CO_2 is eliminated by the lungs		
_____	h. Neutralizes a strong acid to yield sodium biphosphate, a weak acid, and salt		
_____	i. Shifts H^+ in and out of cell in exchange for other cations such as potassium and sodium		
_____	j. H_2CO_3 formed by neutralization dissociates into H_2O and CO_2		

21. A patient who has a large amount of carbon dioxide in the blood has a

a. large amount of carbonic acid and low hydrogen ion concentration.
b. small amount of carbonic acid and low hydrogen ion concentration.
c. large amount of carbonic acid and high hydrogen ion concentration.
d. small amount of carbonic acid and high hydrogen ion concentration.

22. List the three ways that kidneys eliminate acids to maintain acid-base balance.

a.

b.

c.

23. Match the acid-base imbalances with their mechanisms.

_____	a. Increased base bicarbonate	1. Respiratory acidosis
_____	b. Decreased carbonic acid (CO_2)	2. Respiratory alkalosis
_____	c. Increased carbonic acid (CO_2)	3. Metabolic acidosis
_____	d. Decreased base bicarbonate	4. Metabolic alkalosis

24. Identify the compensatory mechanism that occurs in each of the following.

a. Respiratory acidosis

b. Metabolic acidosis

c. Metabolic alkalosis

25. Match the acid-base imbalances with their common causes (answers may be used more than once).

_____	a. Prolonged vomiting	1. Respiratory acidosis
_____	b. Renal failure	2. Respiratory alkalosis
_____	c. Response to anxiety, fear, and pain	3. Metabolic acidosis
_____	d. Respiratory failure	4. Metabolic alkalosis
_____	e. Baking soda use as antacid	
_____	f. Severe shock	
_____	g. Diabetic ketosis	
_____	h. Mechanical overventilation	
_____	i. Sedative or narcotic overdose	

26. A patient with a pH of 7.29 has metabolic acidosis. A value that is useful in determining whether the cause of the acidosis is due to an acid gain or due to a bicarbonate loss is the

a. $PaCO_2$.
b. anion gap.
c. serum Na^+ level.
d. bicarbonate level.

27. Identify the acid-base imbalances represented by the following laboratory values.

a. pH 7.50
$PaCO_2$ 30 mm Hg
HCO_3^- 24 mEq/L

Interpretation:

____

b. pH 7.2
$PaCO_2$ 25 mm Hg
HCO_3^- 15 mEq/L

Interpretation:

____

c. pH 7.26
$PaCO_2$ 56 mm Hg
HCO_3^- 24 mEq/L

Interpretation:

____

d. pH 7.62
$PaCO_2$ 48 mm Hg
HCO_3^- 45 mEq/L

Interpretation:

____

e. pH 7.44
$PaCO_2$ 54 mm Hg
HCO_3^- 36 mEq/L

Interpretation:

____

f. pH 7.35
$PaCO_2$ 60 mm Hg
HCO_3^- 40 mEq/L

Interpretation:

____

28. An example of an intravenous solution that is used to provide free water and intracellular fluid hydration is

a. lactated Ringer's.
b. dextrose 5% in water.
c. dextrose 10% in water.
d. dextrose 5% in normal saline (0.9%).

29. An example of an intravenous solution that would be appropriate to treat an extracellular fluid volume deficit is

a. D_5W.
b. 3% saline.
c. D_5W in 1/2 NS (0.45%).
d. lactated Ringer's solution.

CASE STUDY

FLUID AND ELECTROLYTE IMBALANCE

Patient Profile

Kathleen B., a 74-year-old woman who lives alone, is admitted to the hospital because of weakness and confusion. She has a history of chronic heart failure and chronic diuretic use.

Objective Data

- Neurologic: confusion, slow to respond to questioning, generalized weakness
- Cardiovascular: BP 90/62, HR 112 and irregular, peripheral pulses weak; ECG indicates sinus tachycardia
- Pulmonary: respirations 12 per minute and shallow
- Additional findings: decreased skin turgor; dry mucous membranes

Significant Laboratory Results

- Serum electrolytes:
  - Na^+ 141 mEq/L (141 mmol/L)
  - K^+ 2.5 mEq/L (2.5 mmol/L)
  - Cl^- 85 mEq/L (85 mmol/L)
  - HCO_3^- 43 mEq/L (43 mmol/L)
- BUN 42 mg/dl (15 mmol/L)
- Hct 49%
- Arterial blood gases:
  - pH 7.52
  - $PaCO_2$ 55 mm Hg
  - PaO_2 88 mm Hg
  - HCO_3^- 42 mEq/L (42 mmol/L)

Critical Thinking Questions

1. Evaluate Kathleen's fluid volume and electrolyte status. Which physical assessment findings support your analysis? Which laboratory results support your analysis? What is the most likely etiology of these imbalances?

2. Explain the reasons for Kathleen's ECG changes.

3. Analyze the arterial blood gas results. What is the etiology of the primary imbalance? Is the body compensating for this imbalance?

4. Why has Kathleen's advanced age placed her at risk for her fluid imbalance?

5. Discuss the role of aldosterone in the regulation of fluid and electrolyte balance. How will changes in aldosterone affect Kathleen's fluid and electrolyte imbalances?

6. Develop a plan of care for Kathleen while she is in the hospital. What daily assessments should be included in this plan of care?

7. Based on the assessment data presented, write one or more appropriate nursing diagnoses. Are there any collaborative problems?

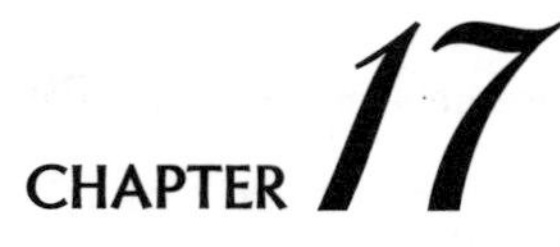

CHAPTER 17 NURSING MANAGEMENT: PREOPERATIVE CARE

1. Indicate the common purpose of surgery in the following procedures.

   a. Gastroscopy

   b. Rhinoplasty

   c. Tracheotomy

   d. Herniorrhaphy

   e. Cholecystectomy

2. A patient is scheduled for a hemorrhoidectomy at an ambulatory day surgery center. An advantage of performing surgery at an ambulatory center is a decreased need for

   a. laboratory tests and perioperative medications.
   b. preoperative and postoperative teaching by the nurse.
   c. psychologic support to alleviate fears of pain and discomfort.
   d. preoperative nursing assessment related to possible risks and complications.

3. A patient who is being admitted for a hysterectomy to the surgical unit paces the floor, repeatedly saying, "I just want this over." To promote a positive surgical outcome for the patient, the nurse should

   a. ask the patient what her specific concerns are about the surgery.
   b. redirect the patient's attention to the necessary preoperative preparations.
   c. reassure the patient that the surgery will be over soon and she will be fine.
   d. tell the patient she has no reason to be so anxious because she is having a common, safe surgery.

4. List six herbal products that the nurse should recognize as possibly increasing the risk for bleeding in a surgical patient.

   a.

   b.

   c.

   d.

   e.

   f.

5. When the nurse asks a preoperative patient about allergies, the patient reports a history of seasonal environmental allergies and allergies to a variety of fruits. The nurse should

   a. note this information in the patient's record as hayfever and food allergies.
   b. place an allergy alert wristband on the patient identifying the specific allergies.
   c. ask the patient to describe the nature and severity of any allergic responses experienced to these agents.
   d. notify the anesthetic care provider (ACP) because the patient may have an increased risk for allergies to anesthetics.

6. During preoperative assessment of a patient, the nurse obtains subjective data related to the patient's functional health patterns. Identify one finding and a related surgical risk factor or need for nursing intervention for the following patterns:

	Finding	Risk/Nursing Need
a. Health perception–health management		
b. Nutrition-metabolic		
c. Elimination		
d. Activity-exercise		
e. Sleep-rest		
f. Cognitive-perceptive		
g. Self-perception–self-concept		
h. Coping–stress tolerance		

7. During a preoperative systems review, the patient reveals a history of renal disease. This finding suggests the need for preoperative diagnostic tests of

   a. FBS and CBC.
   b. ECG and chest x-ray.
   c. ABGs and coagulation tests.
   d. BUN, creatinine, and electrolytes.

8. During a preoperative physical examination, the nurse is alerted to the possibility of compromised respiratory function during or after surgery in the patient with

   a. obesity.
   b. dehydration.
   c. an enlarged liver.
   d. decreased peripheral pulse volume.

9. Preoperative instruction that is appropriate for all patients includes

   a. techniques of deep breathing and coughing.
   b. descriptions of the planned surgical procedure.
   c. physical procedures or preparation required before surgery.
   d. the withholding of all oral fluids or food after midnight on the day of surgery.

10. The nurse asks a preoperative patient to sign a surgical consent form as specified by the surgeon and signs the form after the patient. By this action the nurse is

    a. witnessing the patient's signature.
    b. obtaining informed consent from the patient.
    c. verifying that the consent for surgery is truly voluntary and informed.
    d. ensuring that the patient is mentally competent to sign the consent form.

11. When the nurse prepares to administer a preoperative medication to a patient, the patient tells the nurse that she really does not understand what the surgeon plans to do.

    a. What action should be taken by the nurse?

    b. What criterion of informed consent has not been met in this situation?

12. Preoperative checklists are used on the day of surgery to ensure that

    a. the patient is correctly identified.
    b. patients' families have been informed where they may accompany and wait for patients.
    c. all preoperative orders and procedures have been carried out and records are complete.
    d. preoperative medications are the last procedure carried out before the patient is transported to the operating room.

13. A patient has the following preoperative medication order: morphine 10 mg with atropine 0.4 mg IM. The nurse informs the patient that this injection will

    a. decrease nausea and vomiting during and after surgery.
    b. decrease oral and respiratory secretions, drying the mouth.
    c. decrease anxiety and produce amnesia of the preoperative period.
    d. induce sleep so the patient will not be aware during transport to the operating room.

14. The nurse recognizes that extra time may be necessary when preparing an older adult for surgery because of

    a. ineffective coping.
    b. limited adaptation to stress.
    c. diminished vision and hearing.
    d. the need to include family members in preoperative activities.

CASE STUDY

PREOPERATIVE PATIENT

Patient Profile

Mr. Nathan J., a 49-year-old construction worker, is scheduled for a bronchoscopy. He initially sought medical care for hemoptysis and increasing fatigue. When the nurse asked him to sign the operative permit, he stated he was not certain if he should go ahead with the test because he feared a diagnosis of cancer.

Subjective Data

- Has never been hospitalized
- Has had no medical problems except mild obesity
- Has a cigarette smoking history of 40 pack-years
- Is married with two children, ages 6 and 8; both children have cystic fibrosis
- Is fearful that his wife will not be able to manage without him

Objective Data

- Diagnostic studies: Chest x-ray revealed mass in upper lobe of right lung
- Hematocrit: 31%

Critical Thinking Questions

1. What factors in Nathan's background or personal situation may influence his emotional response and physical reactions to this surgery?

2. What should he know if his consent for surgery is to be truly informed?

3. As Nathan will be an outpatient for this surgery, what preoperative teaching must be done to prepare him for surgery?

4. What risk factors for surgical and anesthetic complications might you anticipate for Nathan? What are the potential interventions that might minimize the risks?

5. Based on the assessment data provided, write one or more appropriate nursing diagnoses. Are there any collaborative problems?

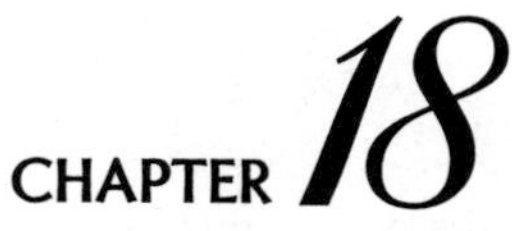

CHAPTER 18 NURSING MANAGEMENT: INTRAOPERATIVE CARE

1. The physical environment of a surgery suite is designed primarily to promote

   a. electrical safety.
   b. medical and surgical asepsis.
   c. comfort and privacy of the patient.
   d. communication among the surgical team.

2. When transporting an inpatient to the surgical department, the nurse from another area of the hospital has access to

   a. the clean core.
   b. the holding area.
   c. corridors of the surgical suite.
   d. an unprepared operating room.

3. Match the surgical team members with their appropriate roles (answers may be used more than once).

_____ a. Gowns and gloves self and other members of the surgical team

_____ b. Admits patient to the operating room

_____ c. Responsible for maintenance of physiologic homeostasis during surgery (MD)

_____ d. Checks mechanical and electrical equipment

_____ e. Passes instruments to surgeon and assistants

_____ f. Supervises postanesthesia recovery of patient in PACU (nurse)

_____ g. Coordinates all activities in room with team members

_____ h. Works with surgeon, assisting with hemostasis and suturing

_____ i. Chooses surgical procedure and management of patient

_____ j. Prepares instrument table

_____ k. Administers anesthesia under supervision of a physician

1. Circulating nurse
2. Scrub nurse
3. Surgeon
4. Anesthesiologist
5. Nurse anesthetist
6. Registered nurse first assistant

4. Identify five examples of data collected during the perioperative nurse's assessment of the patient that indicate special consideration of the patient's needs during surgery.

   a.

   b.

   c.

   d.

   e.

5. During the admission of the patient to the holding area or operating room before surgery, the perioperative nurse must

   a. identify the patient with a formal identification process.
   b. verify the patient's understanding of the risks of surgery.
   c. prepare the skin by scrubbing the surgical site with an antimicrobial agent.
   d. perform a preoperative assessment with a patient history and physical examination.

6. The primary goal of the circulating nursing during preparation of the operating room, transferring and positioning the patient, and assisting the anesthesia team is

   a. avoiding any type of injury to the patient.
   b. maintaining a clean environment for the patient.
   c. providing for patient comfort and sense of well-being.
   d. preventing breaks in aseptic technique by the sterile members of the team.

7. A break in sterile technique during surgery would occur when the scrub nurse touches

   a. the mask with gloved hands.
   b. gloved hands to the gown at chest level.
   c. the drape at the incision site with gloved hands.
   d. the lower arms to the instruments on the instrument tray.

8. During surgery, a patient has a nursing diagnosis of risk for perioperative positioning injury. A common risk factor for this nursing diagnosis is

   a. skin lesions.
   b. break in sterile technique.
   c. musculoskeletal deformities.
   d. electrical or mechanical equipment failure.

9. At the end of the surgical procedure the perioperative nurse evaluates the patient's response to the nursing care delivered during the perioperative period. Which of the following indicates that an outcome related to perioperative safety has been met?

   a. The patient's right to privacy is maintained.
   b. The patient's care is consistent with the perioperative plan of care.
   c. The patient receives appropriate medication(s), safely administered during the perioperative period.
   d. The patient's respiratory function is consistent with or improved from baseline levels established preoperatively.

10. The two short-acting barbiturates most commonly used for induction of general anesthesia are

_____________________ and ________________________.

11. Because of the rapid elimination of halogenated hydrocarbons used for general anesthesia, the nurse should anticipate that early in the anesthesia recovery period, the patient needs

a. warm blankets.
b. analgesic medication.
c. observation for respiratory depression.
d. airway protection in anticipation of vomiting.

12. The primary advantage of the use of midazolam (Versed) as an adjunct to general anesthesia is its

a. amnestic effect.
b. analgesic effect.
c. antiemetic effect.
d. prolonged action.

13. Identify the rationale for the use of each of the following drugs during surgery and one nursing implication indicated in the care of the patient immediately postoperatively related to the drug.

	Use	**Nursing Implication**
a. desflurane (Suprane)		
b. ketamine (Ketalar)		
c. fentanyl (Sublimaze)		
d. succinylcholine (Anectine)		

14. Match the methods of local anesthetic administration with their descriptions.

_____	a. Injection of anesthetic agent directly into tissues	1. Nerve block
_____	b. Injection of anesthetic agent into space between two vertebrae	2. IV nerve block
		3. Spinal block
_____	c. Injection of a specific nerve with an anesthetic agent	4. Epidural block
_____	d. Injection of agent into subarachnoid space	5. Local infiltration
_____	e. Injection of agent into veins of extremity after limb exsanguinated	

15. During epidural and spinal anesthesia, the nurse should monitor the patient for

    a. spinal headache.
    b. hypotension and bradycardia.
    c. loss of consciousness and seizures.
    d. downward extension of nervous block.

16. A preoperative patient reveals that an uncle died during surgery because of a fever and cardiac arrest. The perioperative nurse alerts the surgical team, knowing that if the patient is at risk for malignant hyperthermia

    a. the surgery will have to be cancelled.
    b. specific precautions can be taken to safely anesthetize the patient.
    c. dantrolene (Dantrium) must be given to prevent hyperthermia during surgery.
    d. the patient should be placed on a cooling blanket during the surgical procedure.

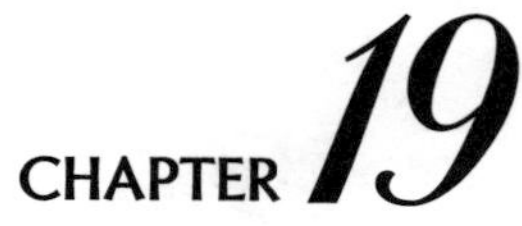

CHAPTER 19 NURSING MANAGEMENT: POSTOPERATIVE CARE

1. In a PACU where fast tracking is used, the postanesthesia nurse

   a. initially admits all patients to phase I recovery areas.
   b. is responsible for determining outcome criteria for discharge from the unit.
   c. transfers patients to appropriate progressive care areas depending on the type of anesthesia used.
   d. collaborates with a postoperative care team to establish standards for admission and progression of patients in recovery areas.

2. Upon admission of a patient to the PACU, the nurse's priority assessment is the patient's

   a. vital signs.
   b. surgical site.
   c. respiratory adequacy.
   d. level of consciousness.

3. To provide care for a surgical patient in the PACU, the nurse needs

   a. a copy of the written operative report.
   b. a verbal report from the circulating nurse.
   c. a verbal report from the anesthesia care provider.
   d. an explanation of the surgical procedure from the surgeon.

4. To prevent confusion during the patient's recovery from anesthesia, the nurse should begin orientation explanations when the patient

   a. is awake.
   b. first arrives in the PACU.
   c. becomes agitated or frightened.
   d. is arousable and recognizes where he or she is.

5. Routine assessment of the patient's cardiovascular function on admission to the PACU includes

   a. ECG monitoring.
   b. monitoring arterial blood gases.
   c. determining fluid and electrolyte status.
   d. direct arterial blood pressure monitoring.

6. Match the postoperative respiratory complications with their associated causes and mechanisms (answers may be used more than once).

_____	a. Pain	1. Airway obstruction
_____	b. Tongue falling back	2. Hypoxemia
_____	c. Medullary depression	3. Hypoventilation
_____	d. Retained secretions	
_____	e. Inhalation of gastric contents	
_____	f. Atelectasis	
_____	g. Laryngospasm	
_____	h. Obesity	

7. To prevent airway obstruction in the postoperative patient who is unconscious or semiconscious, the nurse

   a. encourages deep breathing.
   b. elevates the head of the bed.
   c. administers oxygen per mask.
   d. positions the patient in a side-lying position.

8. While assessing a patient in the PACU, the nurse finds that the patient's blood pressure is below the preoperative base line. An additional assessment finding that indicates the patient has residual vasodilating effects of anesthesia is

   a. an oxygen saturation of 88%.
   b. a urinary output greater than 30 ml/hr.
   c. a normal pulse with warm, dry, pink skin.
   d. a narrowing pulse pressure with normal pulse.

9. A patient in the PACU has an elevated blood pressure and emergence delirium manifested by agitation and thrashing. The nurse should assess the patient for

   a. hypoxemia.
   b. neurologic injury.
   c. a distended bladder.
   d. cardiac arrhythmias.

10. The nurse applies warm blankets to a patient who is shivering and has a body temperature of 96.0° F (35.6° C). The nurse would also anticipate the administration of

    a. oxygen.
    b. vasodilating drugs.
    c. antiarrhythmic drugs.
    d. analgesics or sedatives.

11. List five criteria used to determine when patients are ready for discharge from the PACU.

    a.

    b.

    c.

    d.

    e.

12. Identify six nursing diagnoses or collaborative problems common in postoperative patients for which ambulation of the patient is an appropriate intervention for the problem.

    a.

    b.

    c.

    d.

    e.

    f.

13. To promote effective coughing, deep breathing, and ambulation in the postoperative patient, it is most important for the nurse to

    a. teach the patient controlled breathing.
    b. explain the rationale for these activities.
    c. provide adequate and regular pain medication.
    d. use an incentive spirometer to motivate the patient.

14. In the absence of postoperative vomiting, GI suctioning, and wound drainage, the physiologic responses to the stress of surgery are most likely to cause

    a. diuresis.
    b. hyperkalemia.
    c. fluid overload.
    d. impaired blood coagulation.

15. Describe two independent nursing interventions in addition to ambulation that could be implemented to prevent or treat the following postoperative complications.

    a. Deep venous thrombosis

        1)

        2)

    b. Syncope

        1)

        2)

    c. Urinary retention

        1)

        2)

    d. Abdominal distention

        1)

        2)

    e. Wound infection

        1)

        2)

16. Match the following tubes and drains with their expected drainage (answers may be used more than once).

_____	a. Indwelling catheter	1. Wound drainage
_____	b. Gastrostomy tube	2. Urine
_____	c. Hemovac	3. Bile
_____	d. Penrose drain	4. Gastric contents
_____	e. T-tube	
_____	f. Nasogastric tube	

17. The nurse notes drainage on the surgical dressing when the patient is transferred from the PACU to the clinical unit. The nurse should

    a. change the dressing and assess the wound.
    b. notify the surgeon of the drainage type and amount.
    c. note and record the type, amount, and color of the drainage.
    d. observe the dressing every 15 minutes for an increase in drainage.

18. Thirty-six hours postoperatively a patient has a temperature of 100° F (37.8° C). The nurse recognizes that this finding is most likely a result of

    a. dehydration.
    b. wound infection.
    c. lung congestion and atelectasis.
    d. the normal surgical stress response.

19. The physician has ordered morphine IV q2-4h prn for a patient following major abdominal surgery. The nurse would plan to administer the morphine

    a. before all planned painful activities.
    b. every 2 to 4 hours during the first 48 hours.
    c. every 4 hours as the patient requests the medication.
    d. after assessing the nature and intensity of the patient's pain.

20. Instructions given to the postoperative patient before discharge should include

    a. the need for follow-up care with home care nurses.
    b. directions for maintaining the routine postoperative diet.
    c. written information regarding self-care during recuperation.
    d. the necessity to restrict all activity until surgical healing is complete.

CASE STUDY

POSTOPERATIVE PATIENT

Patient Profile

Mrs. Beverly B., a 28-year-old schoolteacher, is admitted to the PACU following a cystoscopy for recurrent bladder infections and hematuria. The procedure was scheduled as outpatient surgery and was performed under intravenous sedation.

Physician Postoperative Orders

- Vital signs per routine
- D/C IV before discharge
- Patient to void before discharge
- Cipro 500 mg PO q6h × 10 days
- Tylenol #3 1-2 tabs q3-4h prn pain
- Patient to call office to schedule follow-up appointment

Critical Thinking Questions

1. What nursing actions will be required to progress Mrs. B. toward discharge?

2. What precautions will be required in ambulating Mrs. B. after surgery?

3. What problems may interfere with discharging Mrs. B. to home in a timely manner?

4. How will the nurse determine that Mrs. B. is ready to be discharged to home?

5. What are the unique needs of discharging a patient home as opposed to a clinical unit?

6. Based on the data presented, write one or more appropriate nursing diagnoses. Are there any collaborative problems?

CHAPTER 20 NURSING ASSESSMENT: VISUAL AND AUDITORY SYSTEMS

1. Use the following terms to fill in the labels in the illustration below.

List of Terms

Anterior chamber	Optic nerve
Anterior compartment	Posterior chamber
Choroids	Pupil
Ciliary body	Retina
Cornea	Sclera
Iris	Suspensory ligaments
Lens	

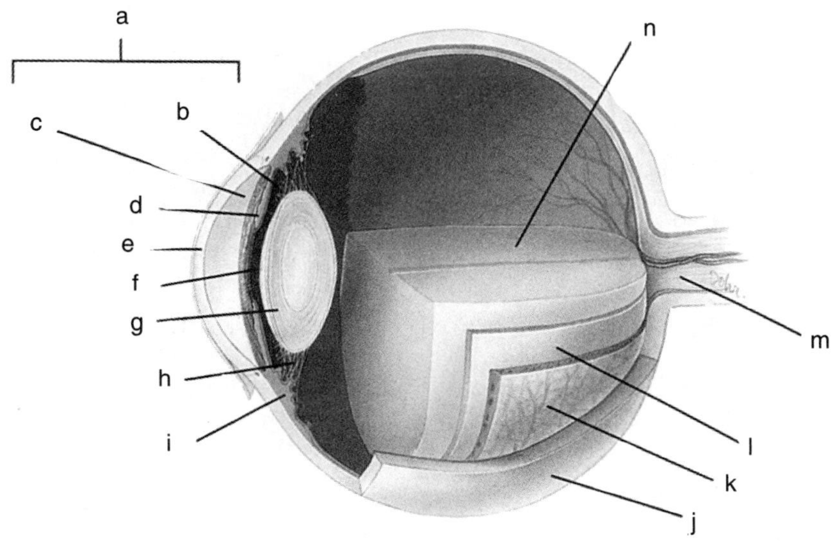

a. ______________________ h. ______________________

b. ______________________ i. ______________________

c. ______________________ j. ______________________

d. ______________________ k. ______________________

e. ______________________ l. ______________________

f. ______________________ m. ______________________

g. ______________________ n. ______________________

2. Word Search. Find the words that are described by the clues given below. The words may be located horizontally, vertically, or diagonally, and may be reversed.

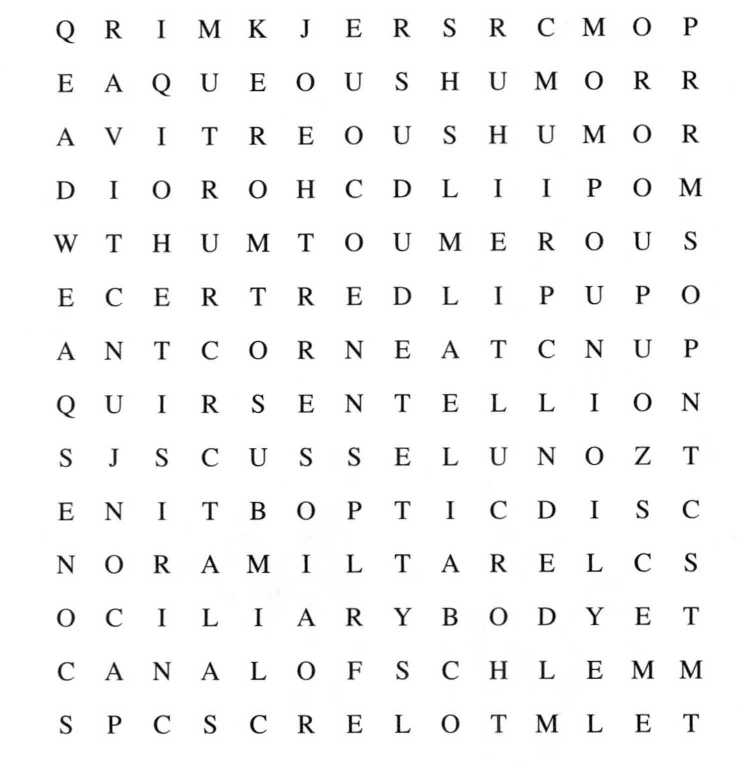

Clues

a. Fibers holding the lens in place
b. Fills anterior cavity of the eye
c. Fills posterior cavity of the eye
d. Clear outer layer of anterior eyeball
e. Secretes aqueous humor
f. Photoreceptor cells stimulated in dim environments
g. Focuses light rays on retina
h. Needed for color vision
i. Protective white outer layer of eyeball
j. Junction of the cornea and sclera
k. Transparent mucous membrane lining the eyelids
l. Drains tears from the surface of the eye into lacrimal canals
m. Point where optic nerve exits eyeball
n. Nourishes ciliary body, iris, and part of retina
o. Drainage path for aqueous humor
p. Colored portion of eye
q. Opening in center of iris

3. Identify whether the following statements are true or false. If a statement is false, correct the bold word(s) to make the statement true.

_____ a. In an individual with **hyperopia** the image is focused in front of the retina and is corrected with a concave lens.

_____ b. Presbyopia is a form of hyperopia that occurs as a result of loss of **lens elasticity**.

_____ c. When the eyeball is too long or there is too much refracting power, the refractive error of **farsightedness** occurs.

_____ d. Based on the visual pathway, a loss of perception in the left visual field results from a lesion in the **right** occipital lobe.

_____ e. The cornea obtains oxygen from **tiny blood vessels in the bulbar conjunctiva**.

4. Match the following eye functions with the appropriate cranial nerve (answers may be used more than once).

_____ a. Medial rectus muscle movement
_____ b. Lateral rectus muscle movement
_____ c. Superior rectus muscle movement
_____ d. Inferior rectus muscle movement
_____ e. Inferior oblique muscle movement
_____ f. Superior oblique muscle movement
_____ g. Eyelid movement
_____ h. Corneal reflex
_____ i. Pupil constriction
_____ j. Pupil dilation
_____ k. Visual acuity

1. CN II (optic)
2. CN III (oculomotor)
3. CN IV (trochlear)
4. CN V (trigeminal)
5. CN VI (abducens)
6. CN VII (facial)

5. Identify the causes of the following assessment findings of the eye that are associated with aging.

a. Ectropium

b. Pinguecula

c. Arcus senilis

d. "Floaters"

e. Changes in color perception

f. Decreased pupil size

g. Yellowish sclera

h. Dry, irritated eyes

6. When obtaining health information from a patient with cataracts, it is important for the nurse to ask about the use of

   a. corticosteroids.
   b. oral hypoglycemic agents.
   c. antihistamine/decongestants.
   d. beta-adrenergic blocking agents.

7. Identify one specific finding identified by the nurse during assessment of each of the patient's functional health patterns that indicates a risk factor for visual problems or the response of the patient to an eye problem.

   a. Health perception–health management

   b. Nutritional-metabolic

   c. Elimination

   d. Activity-exercise

   e. Sleep-rest

   f. Cognitive-perceptual

   g. Self-perception–self-concept

   h. Role-relationship

   i. Sexuality-reproductive

   j. Coping–stress tolerance

   k. Value-belief

8. Describe what is meant by the finding that the patient has a visual acuity of OD: 20/40; OS: 20/50.

9. The nurse documents PERRLA following assessment of a patient's eyes. One finding that supports these data is

   a. slightly oval shape of the pupils.
   b. the presence of nystagmus on far lateral gaze.
   c. dilation of the pupil when a light is shined in the opposite eye.
   d. constriction of the pupils when an object is brought closer to the eyes.

10. Identify the assessment techniques used to obtain the following data.

   a. Peripheral vision field

   b. Extraocular muscle functions

   c. Near visual acuity

   d. Visual acuity

   e. Intraocular pressure

11. A yellow cast to the sclera is a normal assessment finding in

a. infants.
b. dark-skinned persons.
c. persons with brown irises.
d. inflammatory conditions of the eyes.

12. The presence of corneal abrasions or defects may be determined with the use of

a. a tonometer.
b. fluorescein dye.
c. corneal reflex testing.
d. corneal light reflex testing.

13. Match the following assessment abnormalities of the eye with their descriptions.

_____	a. Scotoma	1. Upper lid droop
_____	b. Diplopia	2. Irregularly shaped pupils
_____	c. Exophthalmos	3. Blind spot
_____	d. Chalazion	4. Yellow conjunctival lesion
_____	e. Ptosis	5. Inflamed eyelid
_____	f. Blepharospasm	6. Protrusion of eyeball
_____	g. Pinguecula	7. Double vision
_____	h. Dyscoria	8. Increased blink rate

14. The nurse explains to the patient scheduled for a fluorescein angiography that the test involves

a. anesthetizing the cornea to attach a mirrored lens to examine the anterior chamber angle.
b. application of eyedrops containing a dye that will localize arterial abnormalities in the retina.
c. intravenous injection of a dye to evaluate blood flow through epithelial and retinal blood vessels.
d. measurement of the electrical response of the retina to a flash of light using a contact lens electrode.

15. Match the structures of the ear with their functions.

_____ a. Semicircular canals
_____ b. Tympanic membrane
_____ c. Organ of Corti
_____ d. Cochlea
_____ e. Vestibular portion of CN VIII
_____ f. Acoustic portion of CN VIII
_____ g. External ear
_____ h. Ossicular chain
_____ i. Eustachian tube

1. Sets bones of middle ear in motion
2. Allows for equalization of pressure in middle ear
3. Receives sound waves and transmits to tympanic membrane
4. Converts mechanical sound waves into electrochemical impulse
5. Organ of balance and equilibrium
6. Transmits sound stimuli to brain
7. Receptor organ of sound
8. Amplifies sound waves and transmits vibrations to inner ear
9. Transmits stimuli from semicircular canals to brain

16. Identify one change in the external, middle, and inner ear that can impair hearing in the older adult.

a. External ear

b. Middle ear

c. Inner ear

17. The nurse suspects a patient has presbycusis when she complains of

a. ringing in the ears.
b. a sensation of fullness in the ears.
c. difficulty understanding the meaning of words.
d. a decrease in the ability to hear high-pitched sounds.

18. Describe the significance of the following questions asked of the patient while obtaining subjective data during assessment of the auditory system.

a. Do you have a history of childhood ear infections or ruptured eardrums?

b. Do you use any over-the-counter or prescription medications on a regular basis?

c. Have you ever been treated for a head injury?

d. Is there a history of hearing loss in your parents?

e. Have you been exposed to excessive noise levels in your work or recreational activities?

f. Has there been a change in the amount of social activities you are involved in?

19. Identify whether the following statements are true or false. If a statement is false, correct the bold word(s) to make the statement true.

_____ a. Examination of the external ear involves the techniques of **inspection and palpation**.

_____ b. To straighten the ear canal in an adult before insertion of the otoscope, the nurse grasps the auricle and pulls **downward and backward**.

_____ c. Major landmarks of the tympanic membrane are the **short process of the malleus, the handle of malleus, and the cone of light**.

_____ d. A normal finding upon physical assessment of the ear is the ability to hear a low whisper at **30 cm**.

_____ e. A patient has a negative Rinne test of the left ear. The nurse would expect that with Weber testing the patient would hear the tuning fork sound best in the **right** ear.

_____ f. The presence of a retracted eardrum on otoscopic examination is indicative of **negative pressure in the middle ear**.

_____ g. In **chronic otitis media**, the nurse would expect to find a lack of landmarks and a bulging eardrum on otoscopic examination.

20. Indicate whether conductive hearing loss (CHL) or sensorineural hearing loss (SHL) is associated with the following.

_____ a. Positive Rinne test

_____ b. Negative Rinne test

_____ c. Weber lateralization to impaired ear

_____ d. Weber lateralization to good ear

_____ e. External or middle ear pathology

_____ f. Inner ear or nerve pathway pathology

21. Results of an audiometry indicate that a patient has a 10 dB hearing loss at 8000 Hz. The nurse recognizes that the patient

a. has only a mild hearing loss at high frequencies.
b. will have problems in everyday communication situations.
c. will have difficulty distinguishing high-pitched consonants.
d. will need to use a hearing aid to amplify low-frequency sound.

22. Disease of the vestibular system of the ear is indicated with caloric testing when

a. hearing is improved with irrigation of the external ear canal.
b. no nystagmus is elicited with application of water in the external ear.
c. the patient experiences intolerable pain with irrigation of the external ear.
d. irrigation of the external ear with water produces nystagmus opposite the side of instillation.

CHAPTER 21 NURSING MANAGEMENT: VISUAL AND AUDITORY PROBLEMS

1. Match the refractive conditions with their characteristics (answers may be used more than once).

_____	a. Corrected with cylinder lens	1. Myopia
_____	b. Absence of crystalline lens	2. Hyperopia
_____	c. Corrected with convex lens	3. Emmetropia
_____	d. Image focused behind retina	4. Astigmatism
_____	e. Abnormally long eyeball	5. Aphakia
_____	f. Excessive light refraction	
_____	g. Corrected with concave lens	
_____	h. Unequal corneal curvature	
_____	i. No accommodation for distance vision with accommodation for near vision	
_____	j. Insufficient light refraction	
_____	k. Abnormally short eyeball	
_____	l. Image focused in front of retina	

2. To remove soft contact lenses from the eyes of an unconscious patient, the nurse

   a. uses a small suction cup placed on the lenses.
   b. pinches the lens off the eye after sliding it off the cornea.
   c. lifts the lenses with a dry cotton ball that adheres to the lenses.
   d. tenses the lateral canthus while stimulating a blink reflex by the patient.

3. The most common correction for aphakia is

   a. aphakic spectacles.
   b. aphakic contact lenses.
   c. photorefractive keratectomy.
   d. surgical implantation of intraocular lens.

4. A patient tells the nurse on admission to the health care facility that he recently has been classified as legally blind. The nurse recognizes that the patient

   a. has lost usable vision but has some light perception.
   b. will need time for grieving and adjusting to living with total blindness.
   c. will be dependent on others to ensure a safe environment for functioning.
   d. may be able to perform many tasks and activities with vision enhancement techniques.

5. Identify five nursing measures that should be implemented to increase a visually impaired patient's safety and comfort.

   a.

   b.

   c.

   d.

   e.

6. A patient is admitted to the emergency department with a wood splinter imbedded in the right eye. An appropriate intervention by the nurse is to

   a. irrigate the eye with a large amount of sterile saline.
   b. carefully remove the splinter with a pair of sterile forceps.
   c. cover the eye with a dry sterile patch and a protective shield.
   d. apply light pressure on the closed eye to prevent bleeding or loss of aqueous humor.

7. Match the following extraocular disorders with their descriptions.

_____	a. Acute bacterial conjunctivitis	1. Inflammation of the lid margin
_____	b. Keratoconus	2. Sty
_____	c. Keratitis	3. Blindness-causing keratoconjunctivitis
_____	d. Epidemic keratoconjunctivitis	4. Pinkeye
_____	e. Blepharitis	5. Corneal degeneration
_____	f. Trachoma	6. Spread by direct and sexual contact
_____	g. Hordeolum	7. Inflammation of the cornea

8. The nurse teaches all patients with conjunctival infections to use

   a. artificial tears to moisten and soothe the eyes.
   b. dark glasses to prevent discomfort of photophobia.
   c. warm moist compresses to the eyes to promote drainage and healing.
   d. frequent and thorough hand washing to avoid spreading the infection.

9. A patient with early cataracts tells the nurse that he is afraid that cataract surgery may cause permanent visual damage. The nurse informs the patient that

   a. progression of the cataracts can be prevented by avoidance of UV light and good dietary management.
   b. the cataracts will only become worse with time and they should be removed as early as possible to prevent blindness.
   c. cataract surgery is very safe and with the implantation of intraocular lens the need for corrective lenses will be eliminated.
   d. vision enhancement techniques may improve vision until surgery becomes an acceptable option to maintain desired activities.

10. A 60-year-old patient is being prepared for outpatient cataract surgery. When obtaining admission data from the patient, the nurse would expect to find that the patient has a history of

    a. a painless, sudden, severe loss of vision.
    b. blurred vision, colored halos around lights, and eye pain.
    c. a gradual loss of vision with abnormal color perception and glare.
    d. light flashes, floaters, and a "cobweb" in the field of vision with loss of central or peripheral vision.

11. A patient with bilateral cataracts is scheduled for an extracapsular cataract extraction with an intraocular lens implantation of one eye. Preoperatively, the nurse should

    a. assess the visual acuity in the inoperative eye to plan the need for postoperative assistance.
    b. inform the patient that the operative eye will need to be patched for 3 to 4 days postoperatively.
    c. assure the patient that vision in the operative eye will be improved to near-normal on the first postoperative day.
    d. teach the patient routine coughing and deep-breathing techniques to use postoperatively to prevent respiratory complications.

12. Complete the following sentences:

    a. Retinal tears leading to retinal detachment are most often caused by

    ________________________, ________________________________.

    b. The leakage of vitreous humor into the subretinal space, separating the sensory retina from the pigment epithelium, is termed a ________________ retinal detachment.

    c. Treatments for retinal detachment that are used to create an inflammation and scarring between the retina and the choroid include ____________________ and ________________.

    d. The surgical procedure that involves physical indentation of the globe to bring the pigmented epithelium, the choroid, and sclera in contact with a detached retina is known as ____________________.

13. Following a scleral buckling with a pneumatic retinopexy, the nurse plans postoperative care of the patient based on the knowledge that

    a. specific positioning and activity restrictions are likely to be required for several days.
    b. the patient is frequently hospitalized for 7 to 10 days on bed rest until healing is complete.
    c. patients experience little or no pain and development of pain indicates hemorrhage or infection.
    d. reattachment of the retina commonly fails and patients can be expected to grieve for loss of vision.

14. In caring for the patient with age-related macular degeneration (ARMD), it is important for the nurse to

    a. teach the patient how to correctly use topical eyedrops for treatment of ARMD.
    b. emphasize the use of vision enhancement techniques to improve what vision is present.
    c. encourage the patient to undergo laser treatment to slow the deposit of extracellular debris.
    d. explain that nothing can be done to save the patient's vision since there is no treatment for ARMD.

15. A patient with wet ARMD is treated with photodynamic therapy. After the procedure the nurse instructs the patient to

    a. maintain the head in an upright position for 24 hours.
    b. avoid blowing the nose or causing jerking movements of the head.
    c. completely cover all the skin to avoid a thermal burn from sunlight.
    d. expect to experience blind spots where the laser has caused retinal damage.

16. Visual impairment occurring with glaucoma results from

    a. ischemic pressure on the retina and optic nerve.
    b. clouding of aqueous humor in the anterior chamber.
    c. deposition of drusen and degeneration of the macula.
    d. loss of accommodation from paralysis of the ciliary body.

17. An important health promotion nursing intervention that is relevant to glaucoma is

    a. teaching individuals at risk for glaucoma about early signs and symptoms of the disease.
    b. preparing patients with glaucoma for lifestyle changes necessary to adapt to eventual blindness.
    c. promoting regular measurements of intraocular pressure for early detection and treatment of glaucoma.
    d. informing patients that glaucoma is curable if eye medications are administered before visual impairment has occurred.

18. Indicate whether the following characteristics of glaucoma are associated with primary open-angle glaucoma (POAG) or primary angle-closure glaucoma (PACG).

    _____ a. Resistance to aqueous outflow through trabecular meshwork

    _____ b. Treated with iridotomy/iridectomy

    _____ c. Administration of hypertonic oral and IV fluids

    _____ d. Caused by lens blocking pupillary opening

    _____ e. May be caused by increased production of aqueous humor

    _____ f. Causes sudden, severe eye pain associated with nausea and vomiting

    _____ g. Treated with beta-adrenergic blocking agents

    _____ h. Gradual loss of peripheral vision

    _____ i. Treated with trabeculoplasty/trabeculectomy

    _____ j. Causes loss of central vision with corneal edema

19. The physician has prescribed optic drops of betaxolol (Betoptic), dipinefrin (Propine), and carbachol (Isopto Carbachol) in addition to oral acetazolamide (Diamox) for treatment of a patient with chronic open-angle glaucoma. What is the rationale for the use of each of these drugs in the treatment of glaucoma?

   a. betaxolol

   b. dipinefrin

   c. carbachol

   d. acetazolamide

20. Describe the method of removing and inserting an ocular prosthesis.

21. One of the nurse's roles in preservation of hearing includes

   a. advising patients to keep the ears clean of wax with cotton-tipped applicators.
   b. monitoring patients at risk for drug-induced ototoxicity for tinnitus and vertigo.
   c. promoting the use of ear protection in work and recreational activity with noise levels above 120 dB.
   d. advocating MMR (measles, mumps, rubella) immunization in susceptible women as soon as pregnancy is confirmed.

22. Number the following high noise environments from the highest risk for ear injury to the lowest.

   _____ a. Noisy restaurant for 12 hours

   _____ b. Sitting in front of amplifiers at a rock band concert

   _____ c. Listening to music with stereo headphones for 3 hours

   _____ d. Guiding jet planes to and from airport gates

   _____ e. Heavy factory noise for 8 hours

   _____ f. Using a chain saw continuously for 2 hours

23. A 74-year-old man has moderate presbycusis and heart disease. He takes one aspirin a day as an antiplatelet agent and uses quinidine, furosemide (Lasix), and enalapril (Vasotec) for his heart condition. What risk factors are present for ototoxicity in this situation?

24. Nursing management of the patient with external otitis includes

    a. irrigating the ear canal with body temperature saline several hours after instilling lubricating ear drops.
    b. inserting an ear wick into the external canal before each application of eardrops to disperse the medication.
    c. teaching the patient to prevent further infections by instilling antibiotic drops into the ear canal before swimming.
    d. administering ear drops without touching the dropper to the auricle and positioning the ear upward for 2 minutes afterwards.

25. Identify whether the following statements are true or false. If a statement is false, correct the bold word(s) to make the statement true.

    _____ a. Acute otitis media is most commonly treated with a **myringotomy** to resolve the increased pressure and inflammation in the middle ear.

    _____ b. In chronic otitis media, formation of an **acoustic neuroma** may destroy the structures of the middle ear or invade the dura of the brain.

    _____ c. A **tympanoplasty** may be used to insert an ossicular prostheses and a tympanic membrane graft in patients with chronic otitis media.

    _____ d. The patient who has had a myringotomy with placement of a ventilating tube should be instructed to **avoid getting water in the ear**.

    _____ e. **Acute** otitis media is an infection of the middle ear that frequently leads to mastoiditis and meningitis.

    _____ f. Impairment of the **eustachian tube** is most commonly associated with chronic otitis media with effusion.

    _____ g. Following middle ear surgery, the patient should be positioned **flat in bed**.

26. The nurse teaches a patient with chronic otitis media with effusion to equalize atmospheric pressure within the middle ear by

    a. using the Valsalva maneuver to force air into the middle ear.
    b. coughing or sneezing with the mouth open to prevent middle ear pressure.
    c. blowing the nose with both nostrils open to prevent eustachian tube collapse.
    d. keeping the head elevated and in straight alignment to decrease middle ear pressure.

27. While caring for a patient with otosclerosis, the nurse would expect that the patient has

    a. a strong family history of the disease.
    b. symptoms of sensorineural hearing loss.
    c. a positive Rinne test and lateralization to the good or better ear on Weber testing.
    d. an immediate and consistent improvement in hearing at the time of surgical treatment.

28. The nurse identifies a nursing diagnosis of risk for injury for a patient following a stapedectomy based on the knowledge that

    a. nystagmus may result from perilymph disturbances caused by surgery.
    d. stimulation of the labyrinth during surgery may cause vertigo and loss of balance.
    c. blowing the nose or coughing may precipitate dislodgement of the tympanic graft.
    d. postoperative tinnitus may decrease the patient's awareness of environmental hazards.

29. List the triad of symptoms that occur with Ménière's disease.

a.

b.

c.

30. An appropriate nursing intervention for the patient during an acute attack of Ménière's disease includes providing

a. frequent positioning.
b. a quiet, darkened room.
c. a television for diversion.
d. padded side rails on the bed.

31. The nurse counsels the patient with an acoustic neuroma based on the knowledge that

a. widespread metastasis usually occurs before symptoms of the tumor are noticed.
b. facial nerve function will be sacrificed during surgical treatment to preserve hearing.
c. treatment is usually delayed until hearing loss is significant since it is a benign tumor.
d. early diagnosis and treatment of the tumor can preserve hearing and vestibular function.

32. Indicate whether the following characteristics of hearing loss are associated with conductive loss (C) or sensorineural loss (S).

_____ a. Hears best in noisy environment

_____ b. May be caused by impacted cerumen

_____ c. Hearing aid is helpful

_____ d. Speaks softly

_____ e. Caused by noise trauma

_____ f. Associated with otosclerosis

_____ g. Presbycusis

_____ h. Associated with Ménière's disease

_____ i. Result of ototoxic drugs

_____ j. Related to otitis media

33. When teaching a patient to use a hearing aid, the nurse encourages the patient to use the aid initially

a. outdoors where sounds are distinct.
b. at social functions where there are simultaneous conversations.
c. in a quiet, controlled environment to experiment with tone and volume.
d. in public areas such as malls or stores where others will not notice its use.

CASE STUDY

CHRONIC OPEN-ANGLE GLAUCOMA

Patient Profile

Mrs. G. is a 58-year-old African-American woman seen in her ophthalmologist's office for a routine eye examination. Her last examination was 5 years ago.

Subjective Data

- Has no current ocular complaints
- Has not kept annually scheduled examinations because her eyes have not bothered her
- Takes metoprolol tartrate (Lopressor) for hypertension
- Has a family history of glaucoma
- Uses over-the-counter diphenhydramine (Benadryl) for her seasonal allergies

Objective Data

- Blood pressure: 130/78
- Heart rate: 72

Ophthalmic Examination

- Visual acuity: OD 20/20, OS 20/20
- Intraocular pressure: OD 25, OS 28; by Tono-pen tonometry
- Direct and indirect ophthalmoscopy: small, scattered retinal hemorrhages, optic discs appear normal with no cupping
- Visual field perimetry: early glaucomatous changes, OU

Collaborative Care

The physician prescribed betaxolol (Betoptic) gtts 1 OU. The nurse instructed Mrs. G. on the reasons for the drug and how to do punctal occlusion.

Critical Thinking Questions

1. Why should Mrs. G. have been seeing an ophthalmologist on a yearly basis even though she had no ocular complaints?

2. Explain why the nurse instructed Mrs. G. to use punctal occlusion when she uses the drops.

3. Why is it permissible for Mrs. G. to use her antihistamine? What would the nurse have told her if gonioscopy had revealed narrow angles?

4. Will this patient be able to discontinue her eyedrops once her intraocular pressures are within the normal range? Explain your answer.

5. If topical therapy does not control Mrs. G.'s intraocular pressures, what should she be told about alternative therapies?

6. Describe the probable appearance of Mrs. G.'s optic discs in the future if her glaucoma is left untreated. What would her visual complaints be?

7. Based on the assessment data presented, write one or more appropriate nursing diagnoses. Are there any collaborative problems?

CHAPTER 22 NURSING ASSESSMENT: INTEGUMENTARY SYSTEM

1. Use the following terms to fill in the labels in the illustration below.

List of Terms

Adipose tissue	Connective tissue	Hair follicle	Sebaceous gland
Apocrine sweat gland	Dermis	Hair shaft	Stratum corneum
Arrector pili muscle	Eccrine sweat gland	Melanocyte	Stratum germinativum
Blood vessels	Epidermis	Nerves	Subcutaneous tissue

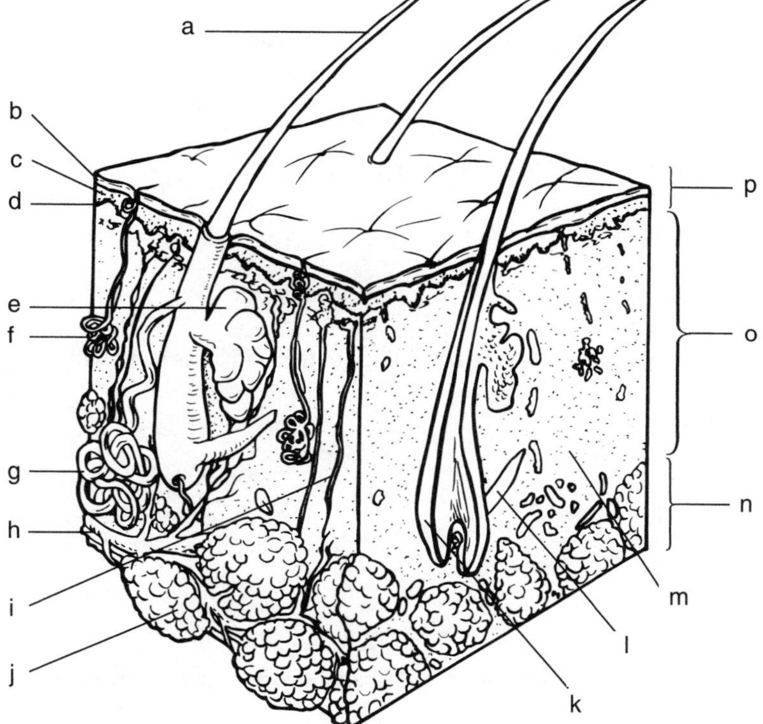

From Jarvis C: *Student Laboratory Manual for Physical Examination and Health Assrssment*, ed 4, Philadelphia, 2004, Saunders.

a. ______________________ i. ______________________

b. ______________________ j. ______________________

c. ______________________ k. ______________________

d. ______________________ l. ______________________

e. ______________________ m. ______________________

f. ______________________ n. ______________________

g. ______________________ o. ______________________

h. ______________________ p. ______________________

2. Match the following skin structures and substances with their descriptions (answers may be used more than once).

_____	a. Pigment-producing cells	1. Epidermis
_____	b. Attaches skin to muscle and bone	2. Dermis
_____	c. Site of vitamin D synthesis	3. Subcutaneous tissue
_____	d. Specialized protective protein	4. Keratinocytes
_____	e. Composed of collagen fibrils	5. Melanocytes
_____	f. Produce collagen and elastin in dermis	6. Keratin
_____	g. Form the basic cells of epidermis	7. Papillary layer
_____	h. Form the stratum corneum	8. Fibroblasts
_____	i. Dermal layer responsible for skin ridging	
_____	j. Location of skin glands and vessels	
_____	k. Location of skin-producing cells	

3. Identify the causes of the following assessment findings of the skin associated with aging.

   a. Wrinkling and skin laxity

   b. Dryness

   c. Easy bruising

   d. Thick, ridged, brittle nails

4. When obtaining important health information from a patient during assessment of the skin, it is important for the nurse to ask about

   a. a history of freckles as a child.
   b. patterns of weight gain and loss.
   c. communicable childhood illnesses.
   d. skin problems related to the use of medications.

5. Identify one specific finding identified by the nurse during assessment of each of the patient's functional health patterns that would indicate a risk factor for skin problems or a patient response to a skin problem.

   a. Health perception–health management

   b. Nutritional-metabolic

   c. Elimination

   d. Activity-exercise

   e. Sleep-rest

   f. Cognitive-perceptual

   g. Self-perception–self-concept

   h. Role-relationship

   i. Sexuality-reproductive

   j. Coping–stress tolerance

   k. Value-belief

6. When performing a physical assessment of the skin, the nurse

   a. palpates the temperature of the skin with the fingertips.
   b. assesses the degree of turgor by pinching the skin on the forearm.
   c. inspects specific lesions before performing a general examination of the skin.
   d. asks the patient to completely undress so all areas of the skin may be inspected.

7. The nurse observes that redness remains after palpation of a discolored lesion on the patient's leg. This finding is characteristic of

   a. varicosities.
   b. intradermal bleeding.
   c. dilated blood vessels.
   d. erythematous lesions.

8. A woman calls the health clinic and describes a rash that she has over the abdomen and chest. She tells the nurse it has raised, fluid-filled, small blisters that are distinct.

   a. Identify the type of primary skin lesion described by this patient.

   b. What is the distribution terminology for these lesions?

   c. What additional information does the nurse need to record the critical components of these lesions?

9. Match the following skin lesions with their descriptions.

_____	a. Angioma	1. Firm plaque caused by fluid in dermis
_____	b. Fissure	2. A defined collection of free fluid up to 0.5 cm in diameter
_____	c. Macule	3. Tiny purple spots resulting from tiny hemorrhage
_____	d. Papule	4. A circumscribed, flat discoloration
_____	e. Plaque	5. Linear loss of epidermis and dermis
_____	f. Scales	6. Circumscribed collection of leukocytes and free fluid
_____	g. Wheal	7. Elevated solid lesion up to 0.5 cm in diameter
_____	h. Ulcer	8. Excess dead epidermal cells
_____	i. Vesicle	9. Benign tumor of blood or lymph vessels
_____	j. Pustule	10. Circumscribed, elevated solid lesion formed by confluence of papules
_____	k. Petechiae	11. Irregular, crater-like loss of the epidermis and dermis

10. The primary difference between an excoriation and an ulcer is that

a. ulcers do not penetrate below the epidermal junction.
b. excoriations involve only thinning of the epidermis and dermis.
c. excoriations will form crusts or scabs whereas ulcers remain open.
d. an excoriation heals without scarring since the dermis is not involved.

11. When assessing for changes in skin color in an African-American person, the nurse should assess the

a. soles of the feet.
b. palms of the hands.
c. conjunctiva or sclera.
d. nailbeds or oral mucosa.

12. A patient has a plaque lesion on the dorsal forearm. The type of biopsy most likely to be used for diagnosis of the lesion is

a. a punch biopsy.
b. a shave biopsy.
c. an incisional biopsy.
d. an excisional biopsy.

13. The most common diagnostic test used to determine a causative agent of skin infections is

a. a culture.
b. the Tzanck test.
c. immunofluorescent studies.
d. potassium hydroxide slides.

14. Match the following assessment abnormalities with their descriptions.

_____	a. Intertrigo	1. Excavation of epidermis
_____	b. Hirsutism	2. Small, superficial dilated blood vessels
_____	c. Nevus	3. Loss of melanin
_____	d. Hematoma	4. Excessive scar tissue
_____	e. Excoriation	5. Abnormal hairiness in women
_____	f. Keloid	6. Thickening of skin
_____	g. Vitiligo	7. Mole
_____	h. Comedo	8. Swelling caused by bleeding
_____	i. Telangiectasia	9. Overlying skin surfaces
_____	j. Lichenification	10. Associated with acne vulgaris

CHAPTER 23 NURSING MANAGEMENT: INTEGUMENTARY PROBLEMS

1. Identify whether the following statements are true or false. If a statement is false, correct the bold word(s) to make the statement true.

_____ a. Exposure to **ultraviolet A (UVA) rays** is believed to be a major factor in the development of skin cancer.

_____ b. It is especially important for a patient taking a **loop** diuretic to prevent sun exposure.

_____ c. When purchasing a sunscreen to prevent exposure to both UVA and UVB rays, the consumer should look for the inclusion of **benzophenones**.

_____ d. The nurse should carefully question the patient with urticaria about the use of **medications**.

_____ e. Dermatologic symptoms of erythema, bullae, and seborrhea-like lesions are associated with deficiencies of **vitamin C**.

2. When teaching patients to prevent skin problems, the nurse stresses that the most important factor to avoid is overexposure to

a. sunlight.
b. radiation.
c. alkaline soaps.
d. over-the-counter skin preparations.

3. Match the following characteristics with the appropriate malignant skin conditions (answers may be used more than once).

_____ a. Skin cancer with highest mortality rate
_____ b. Slow-growing tumor with rare metastasis
_____ c. Neoplastic growth of melanocytes
_____ d. Precursor of squamous cell carcinoma
_____ e. Lesions keratitic and firm
_____ f. Treated with topical 5-FU
_____ g. Frequently occurs on previously damaged skin
_____ h. Irregular color and asymmetric shape
_____ i. Precursor of malignant melanoma
_____ j. Noduloulcerative type has "pearly" borders

1. Actinic keratosis
2. Dysplastic nevus syndrome
3. Basal cell carcinoma
4. Squamous cell carcinoma
5. Malignant melanoma

4. Describe what is indicated by the ABCDs of malignant melanoma.

A:

B:

C:

D:

5. The nurse plans care for a patient with a newly diagnosed malignant melanoma based on the knowledge that initial treatment most often involves

a. Mohs' surgery.
b. localized radiation.
c. wide surgical excision.
d. topical nitrogen mustard.

6. A patient is a 78-year-old woman who has had chronic respiratory disease for 30 years. She weighs 212 lb (96.4 kg) and is 5 ft 1 in (152.5 cm) tall. She has recently completed corticosteroid and antibiotic treatment for an exacerbation of her respiratory disease. Identify four specific predisposing factors for bacterial skin infection in this patient.

a.

b.

c.

d.

7. Match the following skin conditions with the appropriate descriptions.

_____	a. Deep inflammation of subcutaneous tissue	1. Tinea
_____	b. Associated with poor hygiene	2. Herpes simplex 1
_____	c. White, patchy yeast infection	3. Acne
_____	d. Varicella infection of dermatome	4. Pediculosis
_____	e. Warty, irregular papules or plaques	5. Furuncle
_____	f. Papillomavirus infection	6. Candidiasis
_____	g. Head, body, or pubic lice	7. Cellulitis
_____	h. Excessive turnover of epithelial cells	8. Seborrheic keratosis
_____	i. Dermatophyte fungal infection	9. Lentigo
_____	j. Streptococcal infection of dermis	10. Impetigo
_____	k. Sebaceous gland inflammation	11. Herpes zoster
_____	l. Increase in normal melanocytes	12. Psoriasis
_____	m. Viral oral vesicles	13. Scabies
_____	n. Deep follicular staphylococcal infection	14. Warts
_____	o. Allergic reaction to mite eggs	15. Erysipelas

8. Three conditions of the skin that more commonly occur in immunosuppressed patients are

_______________________, __________________, and ____________________.

9. The nurse should advise the patient with urticaria to

a. apply topical benzene hexachloride.
b. avoid contact with the causative agent.
c. gradually expose the area to increasing amounts of sunlight.
d. use over-the-counter antihistamines routinely to prevent the condition.

10. A nurse caring for an ill-kempt patient observes that the patient has small red lesions flush with the skin on the head and body. The patient complains of severe itching at the sites. The nurse should further assess the patient for

a. nits on the shafts of his head hair.
b. a history of sexually transmitted diseases.
c. the presence of ticks attached to the scalp.
d. the presence of burrows in the interdigital webs.

11. A patient with a contact dermatitis is treated with calamine lotion. The nurse knows that the base for this topical preparation includes

    a. a suspension of oil and water to lubricate and prevent drying.
    b. an emulsion of oil and water used for lubrication and protection.
    c. insoluble powders suspended in water that leave a residual powder on the skin.
    d. a mixture of a powder and ointment that causes drying when moisture is absorbed.

12. A patient with psoriasis is being treated with psoralen plus UVA light (PUVA) phototherapy. During the course of therapy, the nurse teaches the patient to wear protective eyewear that blocks all UV rays

    a. continuously for 6 hours after taking the medication.
    b. until the pupils are able to constrict on exposure to light.
    c. for 12 hours following treatment to prevent retinal damage.
    d. for 24 hours following treatment when indoors near a bright window.

13. Identify one instruction the nurse should provide to a patient receiving the following medications for dermatologic problems.

    a. Topical antibiotics

    b. Topical corticosteroids

    c. Systemic antihistamines

    d. Topical fluorouracil

14. Match the surgical interventions with conditions they are used to treat.

_____	a. Electrodesiccation/coagulation	1. Cutaneous malignancies
_____	b. Excision	2. Common and genital warts
_____	c. Mohs' micrographic surgery	3. Small basal and squamous cell carcinomas
_____	d. Curettage	4. Telangiectasias
_____	e. Cryosurgery	5. Lesions involving the dermis
		6. Seborrheic keratoses

15. The most appropriate dressings to use to promote comfort for a patient with an inflamed, pruritic dermatitis are

    a. cool tap water dressings.
    b. cool acetic acid dressings.
    c. warm sterile saline dressings.
    d. warm potassium permanganate dressings.

16. An appropriate intervention to promote debridement and removal of scales and crusts of skin lesions is

    a. warm oatmeal baths.
    b. warm saline dressings.
    c. cool sodium bicarbonate baths.
    d. cool magnesium sulfate dressings.

17. Identify the rationale for using the following interventions to control pruritus.

    a. Cool environment

    b. Topical corticosteroids

    c. Decrease irritants

    d. Soaks and baths

18. A female patient with chronic skin lesions of the face and arms tells the nurse that she cannot stand to look at herself in the mirror anymore because of her appearance. Based on this information, the nurse identifies the nursing diagnosis of

    a. anxiety related to personal appearance.
    b. disturbed body image related to perception of unsightly lesions.
    c. social isolation related to decreased activities secondary to poor self-image.
    d. ineffective therapeutic regimen management related to lack of knowledge of cover-up techniques.

19. To prevent lichenification related to chronic skin problems, the nurse encourages the patient to

    a. use measures to control itching.
    b. wear sterile gloves when touching the lesions.
    c. use careful hand washing and safe disposal of soiled dressings.
    d. use topical antibiotics with wet-to-dry dressings over the lesions.

20. A nursing intervention that is most helpful for a male patient with the nursing diagnosis of anxiety related to personal appearance is to

    a. encourage the patient to express feelings of anxiety.
    b. teach the patient use of cosmetics and cover-up techniques.
    c. refer the patient for counseling to help the patient accept the situation.
    d. touch the patient as appropriate to demonstrate acceptance of appearance.

21. The most common reason that elective cosmetic surgery is requested by patients is to

    a. improve self-image.
    b. remove deep acne scars.
    c. lighten the skin in pigmentation problems.
    d. prevent skin changes associated with aging.

22. Identify one cosmetic procedure indicated for each of the following problems.

    a. Redundant soft tissue conditions

    b. Obesity with subcutaneous fat accumulation

    c. Hypertrophic scars and wrinkled skin

    d. Actinic and seborrheic keratoses

    e. Lentigines and freckles

23. A skin graft that is used to transfer skin and subcutaneous tissue to large areas of deep tissue destruction is a

    a. skin flap.
    b. free graft.
    c. soft tissue extension.
    d. free graft with microscopic vascular anastomoses.

CASE STUDY

CELLULITIS

Patient Profile

Mr. J.B. cut his lower arm on a kitchen knife. At the time of the injury he did not seek medical attention. On the fourth day following the injury, he began to be concerned about the condition of the wound and the way he was feeling.

Subjective Data

- States he has a fever and has had a general feeling of malaise
- Has pain in the area of the cut and the entire lower arm

Objective Data

- 4-cm area around cut is hot, erythematous, and edematous
- Temperature: 100.8° F (38.2° C)

Critical Thinking Questions

1. What care of the wound could J.B. have taken to have possibly prevented the occurrence of cellulitis in the wound?

2. What are the usual etiologies of this type of infection?

3. What would you tell J.B. about the usual treatment of cellulitis?

4. What could result if treatment is not initiated and maintained?

5. Based on the assessment data presented, write one or more appropriate nursing diagnoses. Are there any collaborative problems?

CHAPTER 24 NURSING MANAGEMENT: BURNS

1. Match the following characteristics of burns with the types of burns (answers may be used more than once).

_____	a. Risk for cardiac arrhythmias or arrest	1. Thermal
_____	b. Hot cooking oil	2. Chemical
_____	c. Tissue adherence with protein hydrolysis	3. Smoke and inhalation
_____	d. Causes coagulation necrosis	4. Electrical
_____	e. Can be caused by explosive flare	
_____	f. May cause carbon monoxide poisoning	
_____	g. Indicated by facial burns and hoarseness	

2. Identify whether the following statements are true or false. If a statement is false, correct the bold word(s) to make the statement true.

_____ a. Inhalation injury below the glottis may occur with **exposure to toxic fumes**.

_____ b. **Acid substances** that cause chemical burns continue to cause tissue damage even after neutralized.

_____ c. Lavage with large amounts of water is important to stop the burning process in **scald** injuries.

_____ d. The visible skin injury seen with **an electrical burn** often does not represent the full extent of tissue damage.

_____ e. Metabolic acidosis occurs immediately following an **acid chemical burn**.

3. Indicate the burn classification (minor, moderate uncomplicated, major) indicated in the following situations.

_______________ a. A 25-year-old with a 5% full-thickness burn of the left hand

_______________ b. A 45-year-old with smoke inhalation and superficial partial-thickness injury of the face

_______________ c. A 58-year-old with 20% deep partial-thickness burns of the legs

_______________ d. A 32-year-old who has been struck by lightning

_______________ e. A 19-year-old with a superficial partial-thickness sunburn of the legs, arms, and back

4. When assessing a patient's full-thickness burn injury during the emergent phase, the nurse would expect to find

a. leathery, dry, hard skin.
b. red, fluid-filled vesicles.
c. massive edema at the injury site.
d. serous exudate on a shiny, dark-brown wound.

5. A patient has the following mixed deep partial-thickness and full-thickness burn injuries: face, anterior neck, right anterior trunk, and anterior surfaces of the right arm and lower leg.

   a. According to the Lund-Browder chart, what is the extent of the patient's burns? __________% TBSA

   b. According to the rule of nines chart, what is the extent of the patient's burns? __________% TBSA

   c. Is it possible to determine the actual extent and depth of burn injury during the emergent phase of the burn? Why or why not?

   d. What would be the American Burn Association classification of this injury?

6. The initial intervention in the emergency management of a burn of any type is

   a. establish and maintain an airway.
   b. assess for other associated injuries.
   c. establish an IV line with a large-gauge needle.
   d. remove the patient from the burn source and stop the burning process.

7. Describe the criteria for each of the phases of burn injury and the approximate time frame of each phase.

   a. Emergent

   b. Acute

   c. Rehabilitation

8. During the early emergent phase of burn injury, the patient's laboratory results would most likely include

   a. ↑ Hct, ↓ serum Na, ↑ serum K, ↓ urine Na.
   b. ↓ Hct, ↓ serum albumin, ↓ serum Na, ↑ serum K.
   c. ↓ Hct, ↑ serum Na, ↑ serum K, ↑ urine specific gravity.
   d. ↑ Hct, ↓ serum Na, ↓ serum K, ↓ urine specific gravity.

9. The initial cause of hypovolemia during the emergent phase of burn injury is

   a. increased capillary permeability.
   b. loss of sodium to the interstitium.
   c. decreased vascular oncotic pressure.
   d. fluid loss from denuded skin surfaces.

10. The response of the immune system to a burn injury includes

    a. decreased activity of neutrophils.
    b. an increase in T-helper lymphocytes.
    c. increased production of interleukin-1 and interleukin-2.
    d. becoming overwhelmed by microorganisms entering denuded tissue.

11. One clinical manifestation that the nurse would expect to find during the emergent phase in a patient with a full-thickness burn over the lower half of the body is

a. fever.
b. severe pain.
c. intense thirst.
d. unconsciousness.

12. A patient has a 20% TBSA deep partial-thickness and full-thickness burn to the right anterior chest and entire right arm. It is most important that the nurse assess the patient for

a. presence of pain.
b. swelling of the arm.
c. formation of eschar.
d. presence of pulses in the arms.

13. Nasotracheal or endotracheal intubation is instituted in burn patients who have

a. electrical burns causing cardiac arrhythmias.
b. thermal burn injuries to the face, neck, or airway.
c. symptoms of hypoxia secondary to carbon monoxide poisoning.
d. respiratory distress to inelastic eschar formation around the chest.

14. The physician orders IV mannitol (Osmitrol) and sodium bicarbonate to be given in addition to replacement fluids to a patient in the emergent phase of burn injury. The nurse understands that the rationale for these drugs is to help prevent

a. pulmonary edema.
b. metabolic acidosis.
c. hypovolemic shock.
d. acute tubular necrosis.

15. A patient is admitted to the emergency department at 1015 following a flame burn at 0930. The patient has major 40% TBSA burns and weighs 132 lb.

a. According to the Parkland formula, the type of fluid prescribed for the patient would be

__________________________, and the total amount to be administered during the first 24 hours would be

_____________ ml.

b. The schedule for the fluid administration would be _____ ml between __________ and __________ (time),

_____ ml between __________ and __________, and _____ ml between __________ and __________.

c. Dextrose and water is given the second 24 hours at a rate determined by the ______________________.

d. The three parameters used to determine the adequacy of the patient's fluid replacement are

__________________________, __________________, and ______________________________.

16. A patient's deep partial-thickness burns are treated with the open method. The nurse plans to

    a. ensure that sterile water is used in the debridement tank.
    b. apply topical silver sulfadiazine (Silvadene) with clean gloves.
    c. use clean gloves to remove the dressings and wash the wounds.
    d. wear a cap, mask, gown, and gloves when caring for the patient.

17. A patient with deep partial-thickness burns over 45% of his trunk and legs is going for debridement in a hydrotherapy tank 48 hours postburn. The drug of choice to control the patient's pain during this activity is

    a. IV morphine.
    b. midazolam (Versed).
    c. IM meperidine (Demerol).
    d. long-acting oral morphine.

18. The nurse assesses absent bowel sounds and abdominal distention in a patient 12 hours postburn. The nurse notifies the physician and prepares to

    a. withhold all oral intake except water.
    b. insert a nasogastric tube for decompression.
    c. administer a histamine-2 blocking agent such as cimetidine (Tagamet).
    d. administer nutritional supplements through a feeding tube placed in the duodenum.

19. The nurse positions the patient with ear, face, and neck burns

    a. prone.
    b. on the side.
    c. without pillows.
    d. with extra padding around the head.

20. Identify three factors that increase nutritional needs during the emergent and acute phases of burn injury.

    a.

    b.

    c.

21. At the end of the emergent phase and the initial acute phase of burn injury, a patient has a serum sodium of 152 mEq/L (152 mmol/L) and a serum potassium of 2.8 mEq/L (2.8 mmol/L). The nurse recognizes that these imbalances could occur as a result of

    a. free oral water intake.
    b. prolonged hydrotherapy.
    c. mobilization of fluid and electrolytes at the acute phase.
    d. excessive fluid replacement with dextrose in water without potassium supplementation.

22. A burn patient has a nursing diagnosis of impaired physical mobility related to a limited range of motion secondary to pain. An appropriate nursing intervention for this patient is to

    a. have the patient perform ROM exercises when pain is not present.
    b. teach the patient the importance of exercise to prevent contractures.
    c. provide analgesic medications before physical activity and exercise.
    d. arrange for the physical therapist to encourage exercise during hydrotherapy.

23. The nurse suspects the possibility of sepsis in the burn patient based on changes in

a. vital signs.
b. urinary output.
c. gastrointestinal function.
d. burn wound appearance.

24. Identify one major complication of burns that is believed to be stress related that may occur in each of the following systems during the acute burn phase.

a. Neurologic

b. Gastrointestinal

c. Endocrine

25. Complete the following sentences.

a. A permanent skin graft that may be available for the patient with large body surface area burns who has limited skin for donor harvesting is ______________________________.

b. Early excision and grafting of burn wounds involves excising ____________ down to clean viable tissue and applying __________________________.

c. Blebs can be removed from skin grafts by _________________________ or ______________________.

26. To help a burn patient who has developed an increasing dread of painful dressing changes, it would be most appropriate to ask the physician to prescribe

a. midazolam (Versed) to be used with morphine before dressing changes.
b. morphine in a dosage range so that more may be given before dressing changes.
c. buprenorphine (Buprenex) to be administered with morphine before dressing changes.
d. patient-controlled analgesia so that the patient may have control over analgesic administration.

27. During the rehabilitation phase of wound injury, the contour of scarring can be controlled with

a. pressure garments.
b. avoidance of sunlight.
c. splinting joints in extension.
d. application of emollient lotions.

CASE STUDY

BURN PATIENT IN REHABILITATION PHASE

Patient Profile

Kim is a 30-year-old woman who has been in the burn center for 1 month. She sustained partial- and full-thickness burns to both hands and forearms while cooking with grease. She has undergone three surgeries to date for escharotomies and split-thickness skin grafting. Kim is married and has three young children at home. Her physicians feel she is nearly ready for discharge, but she has been tearful and noncompliant with therapy. Kim and her husband refuse to look at her hand grafts, which continue to require light dressings. She has not seen her children since admission.

Critical Thinking Questions

1. When should discharge planning be initiated with Kim? Who should be involved in the planning and implementation of the educational process before discharge?

2. Describe the nutritional needs Kim will have after discharge and interventions to meet those needs.

3. Kim has been wearing hand and elbow splints at night while in the burn center. What instructions will Kim need regarding her splinting and exercise routine at home?

4. Kim complains of tightness in her hands, which restricts her motion. She uses this excuse to avoid exercise and independent performance of her activities of daily living. What activities and education would be beneficial to address this?

5. Kim and her husband have been extremely upset and anxious regarding Kim's discharge. They are not actively participating in the discharge planning process. What interventions should the staff implement to assist the couple?

6. What are some of the feelings Kim and her family may experience following her return home? What can the nurse do to prepare the family?

7. What are the needs that must be addressed with Kim and her husband regarding dressing changes and graft care before discharge from the burn center? Discuss how this should be managed.

8. Based on the assessment data presented, write one or more appropriate nursing diagnoses. Are there any collaborative problems?

CHAPTER 25 NURSING ASSESSMENT: RESPIRATORY SYSTEM

1. Identify the structures in the following illustration.

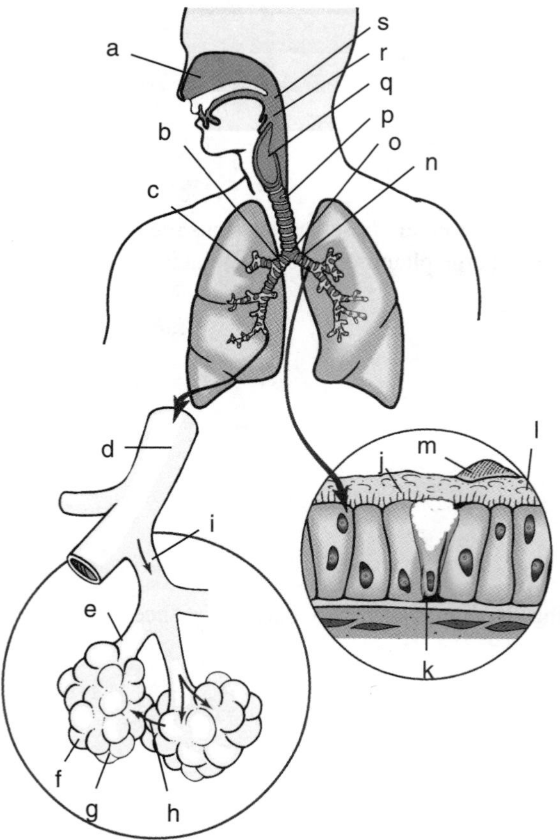

a. ______________________

b. ______________________

c. ______________________

d. ______________________

e. ______________________

f. ______________________

g. ______________________

h. ______________________

i. ______________________

j. ______________________

k. ______________________

l. ______________________

m. ______________________

n. ______________________

o. ______________________

p. ______________________

q. ______________________

r. ______________________

s. ______________________

2. Identify the structures and the landmarks of the chest wall in the following illustrations.

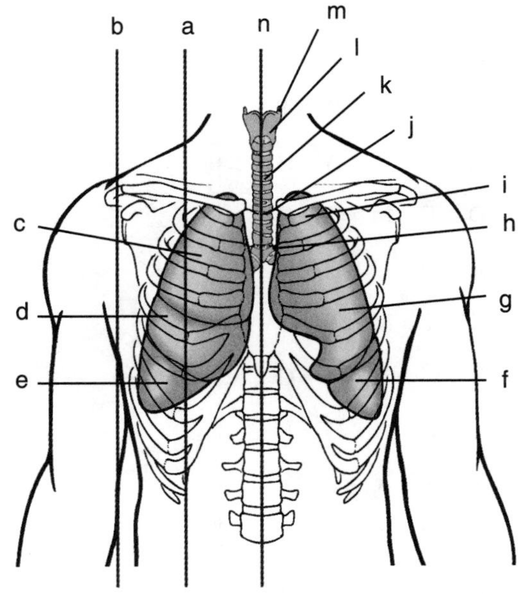

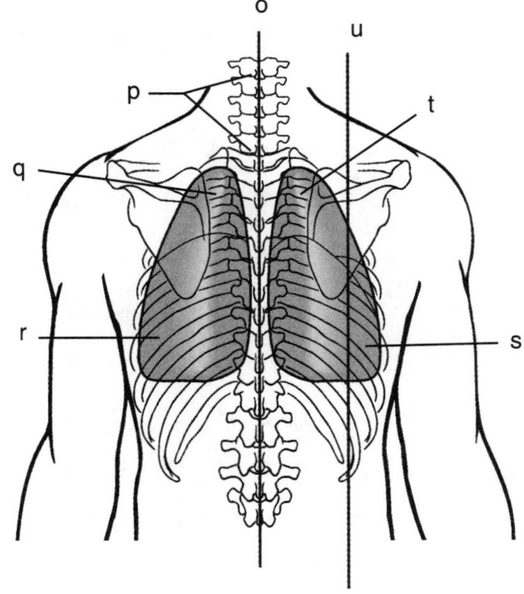

a. ______________________

b. ______________________

c. ______________________

d. ______________________

e. ______________________

f. ______________________

g. ______________________

h. ______________________

i. ______________________

j. ______________________

k. ______________________

l. ______________________

m. ______________________

n. ______________________

o. ______________________

p. ______________________

q. ______________________

r. ______________________

s. ______________________

t. ______________________

u. ______________________

3. Word Search: Find the words that are defined by the clues given below. The words may be located horizontally, vertically, or diagonally, and may be reversed.

E	D	T	N	A	T	C	A	F	R	U	S	T	A
S	E	M	P	Y	E	M	A	N	I	C	U	R	T
E	A	R	O	C	A	R	I	N	A	L	U	A	H
T	D	I	P	W	M	I	R	S	D	E	M	C	O
A	S	V	I	S	C	E	R	A	L	O	C	H	N
N	P	I	M	T	A	A	Y	P	S	I	M	E	G
I	A	S	O	I	L	A	L	M	L	G	B	A	O
B	C	T	H	O	R	A	C	I	C	C	A	G	E
R	E	F	E	S	T	L	A	R	Y	N	X	I	T
U	L	V	T	E	P	I	G	L	O	T	T	I	S
T	L	S	I	U	O	L	F	O	E	L	G	N	A
A	E	R	O	C	O	M	P	L	I	A	N	C	E
W	A	E	V	R	E	N	C	I	N	E	R	H	P
P	F	B	W	E	T	I	S	R	A	M	D	E	S

Clues

a. Shapes and supports the chest wall
b. Covers the larynx during swallowing
c. Separates the larynx and the bronchi
d. Point of bifurcation of trachea into bronchi
e. 150 ml of air in this area not available for gas exchange
f. Keeps the alveoli from collapsing
g. Terminal structures of the respiratory tract
h. Elasticity of the lungs and thorax
i. Location of the vocal cords
j. Warm and moisturize inhaled air
k. Manubriosternal junction at level of carina
l. Membrane lining the chest cavity
m. Innervates the diaphragm
n. Small hairs that move mucus up the respiratory tract
o. The _________ pleura lines the lungs
p. Collection of pus in thoracic cavity

4. Identify whether the following statements are true or false. If a statement is false, correct the bold word(s) to make the statement true.

_____ a. **Arterial oxygen tension (PaO_2)** is the amount of oxygen bound to hemoglobin in comparison with the amount of oxygen the hemoglobin can carry, and is expressed **in mm Hg**.

_____ b. **Arterial oxygen saturation (SaO_2)** is the amount of oxygen dissolved in plasma and is expressed **as a percent**.

_____ c. If hemoglobin is **desaturated of oxygen**, more oxygen is released from the hemoglobin and dissolved in the blood to provide oxygen to the tissues.

_____ d. The oxygen-hemoglobin dissociation curve indicates that a patient is adequately oxygenated when PaO_2 is above 60 mm Hg because hemoglobin saturation **remains above 90%**.

_____ e. A patient has an oxyhemoglobin saturation of 90%. On the normal oxygen-hemoglobin dissociation curve with this saturation, he would have an arterial oxygen tension of about **90 mm Hg**.

5. In a patient with a shift to the right in the oxygen-hemoglobin dissociation curve caused by an acidosis

a. low concentrations of oxygen are administered because more oxygen is delivered to the tissues.
b. high concentrations of oxygen are necessary because blood picks up less oxygen from the lungs.
c. low concentrations of oxygen are administered because blood picks up more oxygen from the lungs.
d. high concentrations of oxygen may be administered to compensate for decreased unloading of oxygen in tissues.

6. A patient with an SaO_2 of 85% has a PaO_2 of 50 mm Hg. This indicates a

a. shift to the left in the oxygen-hemoglobin dissociation curve that could be caused by acidosis.
b. shift to the right in the oxygen-hemoglobin dissociation curve that could be caused by alkalosis.
c. shift to the left in the oxygen-hemoglobin dissociation curve that could be caused by hypothermia.
d. shift to the right in the oxygen-hemoglobin dissociation curve that could be caused by hyperthermia.

7. A 75-year-old patient breathing room air has an analysis of arterial blood gases. Normal results the nurse would expect for the patient include

a. pH 7.32; PaO_2 90 mm Hg, $PaCO_2$ 50 mm Hg.
b. pH 7.40; PaO_2 72 mm Hg, $PaCO_2$ 40 mm Hg.
c. pH 7.44; PaO_2 84 mm Hg, $PaCO_2$ 33 mm Hg.
d. pH 7.51; PaO_2 68 mm Hg, $PaCO_2$ 28 mm Hg.

8. Differences between normal arterial blood gas values and normal mixed venous blood gas values

a. indicate impaired cardiac output.
b. indicate that the patient is hemodynamically unstable.
c. reflect the normal capillary oxygen–carbon dioxide exchange.
d. occur when the patient has inadequate delivery of oxygen to the tissues.

9. A pulse oximetry monitor indicates that the patient has a drop in SpO_2 from 95% to 85% over several hours. The first action the nurse should take is to

a. order stat ABGs to confirm the SpO_2 with a SaO_2.
b. notify the physician of the change in baseline PaO_2.
c. check the position of the probe on the finger or earlobe.
d. start oxygen administration by nasal cannula at 2L/min.

10. Pulse oximetry may not be a reliable indicator of oxygen saturation in the patient

    a. with a fever.
    b. who is anesthetized.
    c. in hypovolemic shock.
    d. receiving oxygen therapy.

11. A patient has an SpO_2 of 70%. What are four other assessments the nurse should consider in making a judgment about the adequacy of the patient's oxygenation?

    a.

    b.

    c.

    d.

12. Criteria for the use of continuous oxygen therapy include

    a. SpO_2 of 95%; PaO_2 of 70 mm Hg.
    b. SpO_2 of 90%; PaO_2 of 60 mm Hg.
    c. SpO_2 of 88%; PaO_2 of 55 mm Hg.
    d. SpO_2 of 75%; PaO_2 less than 40 mm Hg.

13. An excess of carbon dioxide causes an increased respiratory rate and volume because

    a. CO_2 displaces oxygen on hemoglobin leading to a decreased PaO_2.
    b. CO_2 causes an increase in the amount of hydrogen ions available in the body.
    c. CO_2 combines with water to form carbonic acid, lowering the pH of cerebrospinal fluid.
    d. CO_2 directly stimulates chemoreceptors in the medulla to increase respiratory rate and volume.

14. The respiratory defense mechanism that is most impaired by smoking is

    a. filtration of air.
    b. the cough reflex.
    c. mucociliary clearance.
    d. reflex bronchoconstriction.

15. Identify two specific causes of the following age-related changes in the respiratory system.

    a. Decreased PaO_2

    b. Barrel chest appearance

    c. Decreased secretion clearance

    d. Decreased resistance to infection

16. Identify one specific finding identified by the nurse during assessment of each of the patient's functional health patterns that indicates a risk factor for respiratory problems or a patient response to an actual respiratory problem.

a. Health perception–health management

b. Nutritional-metabolic

c. Elimination

d. Activity-exercise

e. Sleep-rest

f. Cognitive-perceptual

g. Self-perception–self-concept

h. Role-relationship

i. Sexuality-reproductive

j. Coping–stress tolerance

k. Value-belief

17. Match the following abnormal assessment findings with the assessment technique used to detect them (answers may be used more than once).

_____	a. Nasal polyps	1. Inspection
_____	b. Limited chest expansion	2. Palpation
_____	c. Hyperresonance	3. Percussion
_____	d. Increased tactile fremitus	4. Auscultation
_____	e. Finger clubbing	
_____	f. Tracheal deviation	
_____	g. Pleural friction rub	
_____	h. Wheeze	
_____	i. Use of accessory muscles	
_____	j. Barrel chest	

18. To assess the patient's chest expansion, the nurse places

a. the thumbs at the midline of the chest.
b. the palms of the hands against the chest wall.
c. the index fingers on either side of the trachea.
d. one hand on the lower anterior chest and one hand on the upper abdomen.

19. The nurse records the presence of an increased AP diameter of the chest when

    a. there is a prominent protrusion of the sternum.
    b. the width of the chest is equal to the depth of the chest.
    c. there is equal but diminished movement of the two sides of the chest.
    d. the patient cannot fully expand the lungs because of kyphosis of the spine.

20. The presence of bronchovesicular breath sounds in the peripheral lung fields is described as

    a. rhonchi.
    b. crackles.
    c. adventitious sounds.
    d. abnormal lung sounds.

21. Match the descriptions or possible etiologies with the appropriate abnormal assessment findings.

_____	a. Finger clubbing	1. Lung consolidation with fluid or exudate
_____	b. Stridor	2. Air trapping
_____	c. Wheezes	3. Atelectasis
_____	d. Pleural friction rub	4. Interstitial filling with fluid
_____	e. Increased tactile fremitus	5. Bronchoconstriction
_____	f. Hyperresonance	6. Partial obstruction of trachea or larynx
_____	g. Fine crackles	7. Chronic hypoxemia
_____	h. Absent breath sounds	8. Pleurisy

22. A nurse has been exposed to tuberculosis during care of a patient with TB and has TB skin testing performed. The nurse is considered uninfected if

    a. there is no redness or induration at the injection site.
    b. there is an induration of only 5 mm at the injection site.
    c. testing causes a 10 mm reddened flat area at the injection site.
    d. a negative skin test is followed by another negative skin test in 3 weeks.

23. A primary nursing responsibility after obtaining a blood specimen for ABGs is

    a. adding heparin to the blood specimen.
    b. applying pressure to the puncture site for 2 full minutes.
    c. taking the specimen immediately to the laboratory in an iced container.
    d. avoiding any changes in oxygen intervention for 20 minutes following the procedure.

24. When preparing a patient for a pulmonary angiogram scan, the nurse

    a. assesses the patient for iodine allergy.
    b. implements NPO orders for 6 to 12 hours before the test.
    c. ensures that informed consent has been obtained from the patient.
    d. informs the patient that radiation isolation for 24 hours after the test is necessary.

25. To prepare the patient for a thoracentesis, the nurse positions the patient

    a. side lying with the affected side up.
    b. flat in bed with the arms extended out to the side.
    c. sitting upright with the elbows on an overbed table.
    d. in a semi-Fowler's position with the arms above the head.

26. The nurse observes the patient for symptoms of a pneumothorax following a

    a. thoracentesis.
    b. ventilation-perfusion scan.
    c. bronchoscopic lung biopsy.
    d. positron emission tomography.

27. The physician orders a pulmonary angiogram for a patient admitted with dyspnea and hemoptysis. The nurse recognizes that this test is most commonly used to diagnose

    a. tuberculosis.
    b. cancer of the lung.
    c. airway obstruction.
    d. pulmonary embolism.

28. Match the following pulmonary capacities and function tests with their descriptions.

_____	a. VT	1. Amount of air exhaled in first second of forced vital capacity
_____	b. RV	2. Maximum amount of air lungs can contain
_____	c. TLC	3. Volume of air inhaled and exhaled with each breath
_____	d. VC	4. Maximum amount of air that can be exhaled after maximum inhalation
_____	e. FVC	5. Amount of air that can be quickly and forcefully exhaled after maximum inspiration
_____	f. PEFR	6. Maximum rate of airflow during forced expiration
_____	g. FEV_1	7. Amount of air remaining in lungs after forced expiration

CHAPTER 26 NURSING MANAGEMENT UPPER RESPIRATORY PROBLEMS

1. Identify whether the following statements are true or false. If a statement is false, correct the bold word(s) to make the statement true.

_____ a. A major deviation in the nasal septum that causes obstruction of nasal airflow is usually corrected by a **rhinoplasty**.

_____ b. In the patient who has suffered a major frontal blow with a nasal fracture, the nurse should monitor for **leakage of cerebrospinal fluid**.

_____ c. Preoperative teaching for the patient planning an elective rhinoplasty for cosmetic effects includes informing the patient to avoid **aspirin-containing products** for 2 weeks before and immediately following the surgery.

_____ d. **Perennial** rhinitis usually occurs as an allergic response when pollen counts are high in spring and fall.

_____ e. Nasal polyps are a complication of long-term **allergic rhinitis**.

2. A patient develops epistaxis upon removal of a nasogastric tube. The nurse should

a. pinch the soft part of the nose.
b. position the patient on the side.
c. apply an ice pack to the forehead.
d. have the patient hyperextend the neck.

3. When caring for a patient hospitalized with posterior nasal packing for control of epistaxis, the nurse

a. monitors for hypoxemia and hypercapnia.
b. cleans the nares and applies petroleum jelly.
c. expects the patient to have a low grade fever.
d. administers nonsteroidal antiinflammatory drugs for pain.

4. The nurse teaches the patient with allergic rhinitis that the most effective way to decrease allergic symptoms is to

a. undergo weekly immunotherapy.
b. identify and avoid triggers of the allergic reaction.
c. use cromolyn nasal spray prophylactically year-round.
d. use over-the-counter antihistamines and decongestants during an acute attack.

5. During assessment of the patient with a viral upper respiratory infection, the nurse recognizes that antibiotics may be indicated based on the finding of

a. fever.
b. cough and sore throat.
c. purulent nasal discharge.
d. dyspnea and purulent sputum.

6. A 36-year-old patient asks the nurse if an influenza vaccine is necessary every year. The best response by the nurse is

   a. "Only health care workers in contact with high-risk patients should be immunized each year."
   b. "Annual vaccination is not necessary because previous immunity will protect you for several years."
   c. "New antiviral drugs, such as zanamivir (Relenza), eliminate the need for vaccine except in the older adult."
   d. "You should get the vaccine if you have a chronic disease or want to reduce your chances of acquiring influenza."

7. A patient uses echinacea and goldenseal herbal therapy when experiencing symptoms of a common cold. The nurse correctly explains that

   a. there is no proof that these agents have any effect on colds.
   b. these products work best when combined with antibiotic therapy.
   c. both products have limitations on the length of time they should be used as immunostimulants.
   d. zinc is a more effective agent to stimulate the immune system and relieve symptoms of a cold.

8. The nurse identifies a nursing diagnosis of altered health maintenance related to lack of knowledge of therapeutic regimen for a patient with acute sinusitis who

   a. continues to take antibiotics for a week after symptoms are relieved.
   b. uses aspirin or aspirin-containing products to relieve headache and facial pain.
   c. uses over-the-counter antihistamines to relieve symptoms of congestion and drainage.
   d. reports a lack of improvement in symptoms after 3 days of taking broad-spectrum antibiotics.

9. A patient with an acute pharyngitis is seen at the clinic with fever and severe throat pain that affects swallowing. On inspection the throat is reddened and edematous with patchy yellow exudates. The nurse anticipates that management will include

   a. treatment with antibiotics.
   b. treatment with antifungal agents.
   c. a throat culture or rapid strep antigen test.
   d. treatment with medication only if the pharyngitis does not resolve in 3 to 4 days.

10. A patient's wife tells the nurse that she thinks her husband has sleep apnea because he snores so loudly. Additional information that should be collected by the nurse related to obstructive sleep apnea includes her husband's history of

    a. evening headaches.
    b. sleeping on a soft mattress.
    c. frequent awakening at night.
    d. frequent upper respiratory infections.

11. The physician prescribes nasal bilevel positive airway pressure (BiPAP) for the patient with sleep apnea. To help the patient tolerate this device, the nurse teaches the patient

    a. to sleep with the head of the bed elevated.
    b. to use the device only on nights when insomnia occurs.
    c. to use nighttime sedatives to relax the tone of the upper airway.
    d. that although it is uncomfortable, it is very effective in relieving sleep apnea.

12. While the nurse is feeding a patient, the patient appears to choke on the food. List four symptoms that indicate to the nurse that the patient has a partial airway obstruction.

    a.

    b.

    c.

    d.

13. An advantage of a tracheostomy over an endotracheal tube for long-term management of an upper airway obstruction is that a tracheostomy

    a. is safer to perform in an emergency.
    b. allows for more comfort and mobility.
    c. has a lower risk of tracheal pressure necrosis.
    d. is less likely to lead to lower respiratory tract infection.

14. Match the following descriptions with the types of tracheostomy tubes (answers may be used more than once).

_____ a. Patient can speak with attached air source with cuff inflated

_____ b. Patient can swallow without aspiration but requires suctioning of secretions

_____ c. Cuff pressure monitoring not required

_____ d. Two tubings, one opening just above the cuff

_____ e. Most likely to cause airway obstruction if exact steps are not followed to produce speech

_____ f. Pilot tubing is not capped

_____ g. Airflow around tube and through window allows speaking when cuff deflated and plug inserted

_____ h. Patient does not require mechanical ventilation and can protect airway

_____ i. Cuff fills passively with air

1. Cuffless tracheostomy tube
2. Speaking tracheostomy tube
3. Fenestrated tracheostomy tube
4. Tracheostomy tube with foam-filled cuff

15. If a tracheostomy tube has an inner cannula, it is designed to

    a. allow the patient to speak.
    b. facilitate suctioning of secretions from the tube.
    c. promote cleaning of mucus from the inside of the tube.
    d. increase the volume of air that can be delivered by mechanical ventilation.

16. List three precautions used to prevent dislodgement of a tracheostomy tube the first several days after its placement.

    a.

    b.

    c.

17. Nursing care of the patient with a cuffed tracheostomy tube in place includes

    a. changing the tube every 3 days.
    b. recording cuff pressure every 8 hours.
    c. performing mouth care every 12 hours.
    d. assessing arterial blood gases every 8 hours.

18. In the event that a tracheostomy tube becomes dislodged, the nurse should immediately

    a. notify the physician.
    b. attempt to replace the tube.
    c. place the patient in high Fowler's position.
    d. ventilate the patient with a manual resuscitation bag until the physician arrives.

19. To determine when the patient with a tracheostomy tube can effectively swallow, the nurse deflates the cuff and

    a. checks for a gag reflex at the back of the tongue with a tongue blade.
    b. asks the patient to drink 30 ml of milk and suctions the tube for colored secretions.
    c. has the patient swallow a small amount of water and observes for symptoms of respiratory distress.
    d. has the patient drink a small amount of blue-colored water, observing for coughing and colored secretions.

20. During the nursing assessment of the patient with cancer of the head and neck, the nurse would expect to find a history of

    a. long-term denture use.
    b. heavy tobacco and alcohol use.
    c. persistent swelling of the neck and face.
    d. chronic herpes simplex infections of the mouth and lips.

21. The management of early vocal cord malignancies usually includes

    a. radiation therapy that preserves the quality of the voice.
    b. a hemilaryngectomy that prevents the need for a tracheostomy.
    c. a radical neck dissection that removes possible sites of metastasis.
    d. a total laryngectomy to prevent development of second primary cancers.

22. During preoperative teaching for the patient scheduled for a total laryngectomy, the nurse includes information related to

    a. the postoperative use of nonverbal communication techniques.
    b. techniques that will be used to alleviate a dry mouth and prevent stomatitis.
    c. the need for frequent, vigorous coughing in the first 24 hours postoperatively.
    d. self-help groups and community resources for patients with cancer of the larynx.

23. When assessing the patient upon return to the surgical unit following a total laryngectomy and radical neck dissection, the nurse would expect to find

    a. a closed wound drainage system.
    b. a nasal endotracheal tube in place.
    c. a tracheostomy tube and mechanical ventilation.
    d. placement of a nasogastric tube with orders for tube feedings.

24. Following a supraglottic laryngectomy, the patient is taught how to use the supraglottic swallow to minimize the risk of aspiration. In teaching the patient about this technique, the nurse instructs the patient to

    a. perform Valsalva maneuver immediately after swallowing.
    b. breathe between each Valsalva maneuver and cough sequence.
    c. cough after swallowing to remove food from the top of the vocal cords.
    d. practice swallowing thin, watery fluids before attempting to swallow solid foods.

25. Discharge teaching by the nurse for the patient with a total laryngectomy includes

    a. how to use esophageal speech to communicate.
    b. how to use a mirror to suction the tracheostomy.
    c. the necessity of never covering the laryngectomy stoma.
    d. the need to use baths instead of showers for personal hygiene.

26. The most normal functioning method of speech restoration in the patient with a total laryngectomy is

    a. a voice prosthesis.
    b. esophageal speech.
    c. an electrolarynx held to the neck.
    d. an electrolarynx placed in the mouth.

CASE STUDY

RHINOPLASTY

Patient Profile

Mr. N. is a 28-year-old married accountant who sustained a bilateral fracture of the nose in an automobile accident 3 days ago. He had a rhinoplasty to reestablish an adequate airway and improve cosmetic appearance.

Subjective Data

- Upon return to his room following surgery, Mr. N. reports facial pain and mouth dryness
- Expresses concern about his "fat face" and appearance

Objective Data

- Respirations 24 and shallow
- Nasal packing present in both nares
- Mustache dressing in place with a small amount of serosanguineous drainage
- Steri-Strips are applied to the skin under a plastic splint molded to the nose
- Nose and upper cheeks are edematous

Critical Thinking Questions

1. What assessments should the nurse make of Mr. N. in the immediate postoperative period?

2. What interventions should the nurse implement to increase Mr. N.'s comfort?

3. What information should the nurse provide to Mr. N. regarding his appearance?

4. Mr. N.'s nasal packing is removed in 24 hours and he is to be discharged. What predischarge teaching should the nurse perform?

5. Based on the assessment data presented, write one or more appropriate nursing diagnoses. Are there any collaborative problems?

CHAPTER 27 NURSING MANAGEMENT: LOWER RESPIRATORY PROBLEMS

1. A patient has chronic bronchitis. To prevent the development of an acute exacerbation of chronic bronchitis (AECB), the nurse teaches the patient to take provided antibiotics with the onset of

   a. rhinitis and headache.
   b. diffuse rhonchi and wheezing.
   c. fever and increased productive cough.
   d. chest pain with a nonproductive cough.

2. List the three methods by which microorganisms that cause pneumonia reach the lungs.

   a.

   b.

   c.

3. The classification of pneumonia as community-acquired pneumonia (CAP) or hospital-acquired pneumonia (HAP) is clinically useful because

   a. atypical pneumonia syndrome is more likely to occur in HAP.
   b. diagnostic testing does not have to be used to identify causative agents.
   c. causative agents can be predicted and empirical treatment is often effective.
   d. intravenous antibiotic therapy is necessary for HAP while oral therapy is adequate for CAP.

4. Match the following microorganisms to the type of pneumonia they are most commonly associated with (answers may be used more than once).

_____	a. *Pneumocystis carinii*	1. Community-acquired pneumonia
_____	b. *Escherichia coli*	2. Hospital-acquired pneumonia
_____	c. *Pseudomonas aeruginosa*	3. Opportunistic pneumonia
_____	d. *Legionella pneumophila*	
_____	e. *Staphylococcus aureus*	
_____	f. *Streptococcus pneumoniae*	
_____	g. *Enterobacter*	
_____	h. *Klebsiella*	
_____	i. *Haemophilus influenzae*	
_____	j. Cytomegalovirus	
_____	k. *Mycoplasma pneumoniae*	

5. Identify the pathophysiologic stages of pneumococcal pneumonia.

   a. Massive dilation of capillaries with alveolar filling with organisms, neutrophils, and fibrin

   ____

   b. Exudate becomes lysed and processed by macrophages and normal lung tissue restored

   ____

   c. Outpouring of fluid into alveoli that supports microorganism growth and spread

   ____

   d. Blood flow decreases and leukocytes and fibrin consolidate in affected lung tissue

   ____

6. When obtaining a health history from the patient with suspected community-acquired pneumonia (CAP), the nurse expects the patient to report

   a. an insidious onset.
   b. a dry productive cough.
   c. a recent loss of consciousness.
   d. an abrupt onset of fever and chills.

7. Initial antibiotic treatment for pneumonia is usually based on

   a. the severity of symptoms.
   b. the presence of characteristic leukocytes.
   c. Gram's stains and cultures of sputum specimens.
   d. history and physical examination and characteristic chest x-ray findings.

8. An example of a metastatic infection that occurs as a complication of pneumococcal pneumonia is

   a. pleurisy.
   b. empyema.
   c. meningitis.
   d. pleural effusion.

9. Complete the following sentences related to antibiotic treatment for pneumonia.

   a. The class of antibiotics most commonly used to treat a Category 1 CAP is

   ____________________.

   b. The drug of choice for treatment of *Pneumocystis carinii* pneumonia is ____________________.

   c. A Group 3 HAP caused by *Pseudomonas aeruginosa* is most likely to be treated with an

   ____________________.

   d. A patient with a methicillin-resistant *Staphylococcus aureus* has a Group 3 HAP. Treatment would include

   the antibiotic ____________________.

   e. Group 1 HAPs caused by enteric gram-negative bacilli, such as *Klebsiella*, are treated with a

   ____________________.

10. Identify five clinical situations in which hospitalized patients are at risk for aspiration pneumonia and one nursing intervention for each situation that is indicated to prevent pneumonia.

	Situation	Intervention
a.		
b.		
c.		
d.		
e.		

11. A patient with pneumonia has a nursing diagnosis of ineffective airway clearance related to pain, fatigue, and thick secretions. An appropriate nursing intervention for this diagnosis is to

    a. encourage a fluid intake of at least 3 L/day.
    b. administer oxygen as prescribed to maintain optimal oxygenation.
    c. place the patient in semi-Fowler's position to maximize lung expansion.
    d. teach the patient to take three or four shallow breaths before coughing to minimize pain.

12. A patient is admitted to the hospital with fever, chills, productive cough with rusty sputum, and pleuritic chest pain. Pneumococcal pneumonia is suspected. An appropriate nursing diagnosis for the patient based on the systemic manifestations of pneumococcal pneumonia is

    a. diarrhea related to inflammatory process.
    b. hyperthermia related to acute infectious process.
    c. risk for injury related to disorientation and confusion.
    d. acute pain related to pleuritis and ineffective pain management.

13. The nurse advises a 75-year-old man that to prevent pneumonia, he should

    a. obtain the pneumococcal vaccine every 5 or 6 years.
    b. obtain the pneumococcal vaccine and an annual influenza vaccine.
    c. seek medical care and antibiotic therapy for all upper respiratory infections.
    d. obtain the pneumococcal vaccine if he is exposed to individuals with pneumonia.

14. The resurgence in tuberculosis due to emergence of multidrug-resistant strains of *M. tuberculosis* is primarily the result of

    a. a lack of effective means to diagnose TB.
    b. poor compliance with drug therapy in patients with TB.
    c. the increased population of immunosuppressed individuals with AIDS.
    d. indiscriminate use of antitubercular drugs in treatment of other infections.

15. One of the characteristic pathophysiologic responses to infection by the tubercular bacillus is

    a. metastases of osteocytes from the bone to the lung where they calcify lung tissue.
    b. necrotic abscesses formed from reactions of the tubercular bacilli with lymphocytes.
    c. deposition of antibody-antigen immune complexes in the alveoli of the affected lung.
    d. formation of epithelioid cell granulomas from activation of the cellular immune system.

16. A patient diagnosed with Class 3 TB 1 week ago is admitted to the hospital with symptoms of chest pain and a possible myocardial infarction. The nurse knows that

    a. the patient has a TB infection without clinical evidence of the disease.
    b. respiratory isolation may be required while the patient is hospitalized.
    c. the patient has a history of a previous episode of TB with no evidence of current disease.
    d. the patient is suspected of having TB but a definite diagnosis is pending the results of diagnostic studies.

17. Usual initial clinical manifestations of TB include

    a. chest pain, hemoptysis, and weight loss.
    b. fatigue, low grade fever, and night sweats.
    c. cough with purulent mucus and fever with chills.
    d. pleuritic pain, nonproductive cough, and temperature elevation at night.

18. Circle the appropriate words from the choices in parentheses to complete the following sentences related to classifications and treatment protocols for TB.

    a. A health care provider who has cared for a patient with TB has a 7-mm reaction to PPD skin testing. This individual has been (exposed to/infected with) TB.
    b. When a person who is taking corticosteroids for rheumatoid arthritis has a positive PPD skin test, treatment would include drugs for (clinical/latent) TB infection.
    c. A patient who has HIV and clinical TB should receive combination drug therapy for a minimum of (9/12) months and (6/9) months beyond culture conversion.
    d. Latent TB infection is treated with (INH/combination) therapy.
    e. The minimum treatment period for patient with active TB infection is (6/9) months.
    f. A diagnosis of TB is established with (chest x-ray/positive smear and culture).

19. Identify the recommended drug protocol for the *initial* treatment of clinically active TB.

20. A patient with active TB does not have negative sputum cultures after 6 months of treatment because she says she cannot remember to take the medication all the time. The best action by the nurse is to

    a. schedule the patient to come to the clinic every day to take the medication.
    b. have a patient who has recovered from TB tell the patient about his successful treatment.
    c. schedule more teaching sessions so the patient will understand the risks of noncompliance.
    d. arrange for directly observed therapy by a responsible family member or a public health nurse.

21. A patient receiving chemotherapy for breast cancer develops cryptococcoses and is treated with IV amphotericin B. The nurse monitors the patient for side effects of the amphotericin B with the knowledge that this patient is at risk for increased

  a. renal impairment.
  b. immunosuppression.
  c. nausea and vomiting.
  d. hypersensitivity reactions.

22. The nursing assessment of a patient with bronchiectasis is most likely to reveal a history of

  a. chest trauma.
  b. childhood asthma.
  c. smoking or oral tobacco use.
  d. recurrent lower respiratory tract infections.

23. In planning care for the patient with bronchiectasis, the nurse includes measures that will

  a. relieve or reduce pain.
  b. prevent paroxysmal coughing.
  c. prevent spread of the disease to others.
  d. promote drainage and removal of mucus.

24. The nurse uses protective measures with patients at risk for lung abscesses based on the knowledge that lung abscesses occur most frequently in patients with

  a. lung tumors.
  b. altered consciousness.
  c. altered immune response.
  d. pulmonary infarct infections.

25. The most important precaution in reducing the risk of most occupational lung diseases is

  a. maintaining smoke-free work environments for all employees.
  b. using masks and effective ventilation systems to reduce exposure to irritants.
  c. inspection and monitoring of workplaces by national occupational safety agencies.
  d. requiring periodic chest x-rays and pulmonary function tests for exposed employees.

26. During a health-promotion program, the nurse teaches the participants that the best way to prevent lung cancer is to

  a. stop smoking and avoid secondhand smoke.
  b. have an annual chest x-ray after the age of 50.
  c. wear masks when exposed to industrial carcinogens.
  d. seek medical care for a cough that persists for more than 2 to 3 weeks.

27. A patient is diagnosed with cancer of the lung after seeking medical treatment for symptoms of syndrome of inappropriate antidiuretic hormone (SIADH). The nurse recognizes that the lung malignancy most commonly related to this symptom

  a. can be successfully treated with radiation.
  b. metastasizes early and has the poorest prognosis.
  c. has a good prognosis if surgical resection is possible.
  d. is associated with lung scarring and chronic interstitial fibrosis.

28. A patient with a lung mass found on chest x-ray is undergoing further testing. A definitive diagnosis of cancer of the lung may be made with

 a. CT scans.
 b. lung tomograms.
 c. pulmonary angiography.
 d. identification of malignant cells in sputum.

29. Match the following treatments for lung cancer with their descriptions.

_____ Standard treatment for NSCLC		1. Surgical therapy
_____ Dye activated by laser light that destroys cancer cells		2. Radiation therapy
		3. Chemotherapy
_____ Freezes bronchial tumors with use of bronchoscope radiation		4. Prophylactic cranial
_____ Palliative treatment for airway collapse or compression therapy		5. Bronchoscopic laser
		6. Phototherapy
_____ Best procedure for cure of lung cancer		7. Airway stenting
_____ Palliative treatment by bronchoscope to remove obstructing bronchial tumors		8. Cryotherapy
_____ Improves survival when combined with chemotherapy and surgery		
_____ Used with chemotherapy to overcome effect of blood-brain barrier		

30. In assisting a patient to stop smoking, the nurse advises the patient that the most successful programs for smoking cessation include

 a. hypnosis and acupuncture.
 b. self-help programs with group therapy.
 c. aversion therapy and individual psychotherapy.
 d. behavior modification approach with nicotine replacement.

31. A patient with advanced lung cancer refuses pain medication, saying, "I deserve everything this cancer can give me." The nurse's best response to the patient is

 a. "Would you like to talk to a counselor?"
 b. "Can you tell me what the pain means to you?"
 c. "Are you using the pain as a punishment for your past behavior?"
 d. "Pain control will help you to deal more effectively with your feelings."

32. Complete the following statements.

  a. Collapse of the lung due to accumulation of air in the intrapleural space caused by a sucking chest wound is a ______________________________.

  b. Multiple fractured ribs causing paradoxic chest movement is known as ______________________________.

  c. Collapse of the lung due to accumulation of blood in the intrapleural space is a ______________________________.

  d. Collapse of the lung due to accumulation of air in the intrapleural space caused by an injury to the lungs from closed rib fractures is known as a ______________________________.

  e. When air in the intrapleural space progressively increases intrathoracic pressure because it cannot escape during expiration, a ______________________________ occurs.

  f. Accumulation of lymphatic fluid in the pleural space due to leak in the thoracic duct is known as ______________________________.

  g. The usual treatment for large pneumothorax or hemothorax of any cause is a ______________ connected to ______________________________.

33. Signs and symptoms that indicate to the nurse that a tension pneumothorax is developing in a patient with chest trauma include

  a. dull percussion sounds on the injured side.
  b. severe respiratory distress and tracheal deviation.
  c. muffled and distant heart sounds with decreasing blood pressure.
  d. decreased movement and diminished breath sounds on the affected side.

34. Indicate the function of each of the chambers in a three-chamber water-seal pleural drainage system.

  a. First chamber

  b. Second chamber

  c. Third chamber

35. The nurse should check for leaks in the chest tube and water-seal system when

a. there is constant bubbling of water in the suction-control chamber.
b. there is continuous bubbling from the tube in the water-seal chamber.
c. the water levels in the water-seal and suction-control chambers are decreased.
d. fluid in the tubing in the water-seal chamber fluctuates with the patient's breathing.

36. When caring for the patient with a chest tube, the nurse questions the practice of

a. looping the drainage tubing on the bed.
b. clamping the chest tube momentarily to check for leaks.
c. having the patient cough and deep breathe every 2 hours.
d. stripping or milking a chest tube used to treat a pneumothorax.

37. Match the following chest surgeries with their descriptions.

_____	a. Thoracotomy	1. Removal of a small lesion
_____	b. Lobectomy	2. Removal of a lung
_____	c. Wedge resection	3. Incision into the thorax
_____	d. Segmental resection	4. Stripping of a fibrous membrane
_____	e. Decortication	5. Removal of one lung lobe
_____	f. Pneumonectomy	6. Removal of lung segment

38. Following a thoracotomy, the patient has a nursing diagnosis of ineffective airway clearance related to inability to cough secondary to pain and positioning. The best nursing intervention for this patient is to

a. have the patient drink 16 ounces of water before attempting to deep breathe.
b. auscultate the lungs before and after deep-breathing and coughing regimens.
c. place the patient in the Trendelenburg position for 30 minutes before the coughing exercises.
d. medicate the patient with analgesics 20 to 30 minutes before assisting to cough and deep breathe.

39. Match the following restrictive lung conditions with the mechanisms that cause decreased vital capacity (VC) and decreased total lung capacity (TLC).

_____	a. Pleural effusion	1. Central depression of respiratory rate and depth
_____	b. Empyema	2. Lung expansion restricted by fluid in pleural space
_____	c. Pleurisy	3. Paralysis of respiratory muscles
_____	d. Atelectasis	4. Excess fat restricts chest wall and diaphragmatic excursion
_____	e. Idiopathic pulmonary fibrosis	5. Inflammation of the pleura restricting lung movement
_____	f. Kyphoscoliosis	6. Lung expansion restricted by pus in intrapleural space
_____	g. Narcotic and sedative overdose	7. Presence of collapsed, airless alveoli
_____	h. Muscular dystrophy	8. Spinal angulation restricting ventilation
_____	i. Pickwickian syndrome	9. Excessive connective tissue in lungs

40. Match the following conditions with their related mechanisms of pulmonary hypertension.

_____ a. Chronic obstructive pulmonary disease (COPD)

_____ b. Pulmonary fibrosis

_____ c. Pulmonary embolism

_____ d. Neuromuscular disorders

1. Stiffening of pulmonary vasculature
2. Obstruction of pulmonary blood flow
3. Pulmonary capillary/alveolar damage
4. Local vasoconstriction and shunting

41. While caring for a patient with primary pulmonary hypertension, the nurse observes that the patient has exertional dyspnea and chest pain, in addition to fatigue. The nurse knows that these symptoms are related to

a. decreased left ventricular output.
b. right ventricular hypertrophy and dilation.
c. increased systemic arterial blood pressure.
d. development of alveolar interstitial edema.

42. The primary treatment for cor pulmonale is directed toward

a. controlling arrhythmias.
b. dilating the pulmonary arteries.
c. strengthening the cardiac muscle.
d. treating the underlying pulmonary condition.

43. Six days after a heart-lung transplant patient develops a low-grade fever and a decreased SpO_2 with exercise. The nurse recognizes that this indicates

a. a normal response to extensive surgery.
b. a frequently fatal cytomegalovirus infection.
c. acute rejection that can be treated with corticosteroids.
d. obliterative bronchiolitis that plugs terminal bronchioles.

CASE STUDY

PULMONARY HYPERTENSION

Patient Profile

Ms. S. is a 46-year-old patient who was diagnosed with primary pulmonary hypertension at the age of 42. At that time she presented to her primary care physician with a history of increasing fatigue and recent onset of swelling in her feet and ankles. A chest x-ray revealed severe cardiomegaly with pulmonary congestion. She underwent a right cardiac catheterization, which showed very high pulmonary artery pressures. Since then she has been treated with several drugs, but her pulmonary hypertension has never been controlled and her peripheral edema has progressively worsened.

Subjective Data

- Short of breath at rest and exercise intolerant to the extent that she had to quit her job
- Recently divorced from her husband
- Has two children, a girl who is 10 years old and a son who is 4 years old

Objective Data

- 3+ pitting edema from her feet to her knees
- Respirations: 28 at rest
- Heart rate: 92 and bounding

Critical Thinking Questions

1. What drugs might Ms. S. have been given to treat her pulmonary hypertension?

2. Is Ms. S. a candidate for heart-lung or lung transplantation? Why or why not?

3. What transplantation procedure would be considered for Ms. S? What is the rationale?

4. What preoperative counseling would be necessary for Ms. S. to prepare for a transplantation procedure?

5. Based on the assessment data presented, write one or more appropriate nursing diagnoses. Are there any collaborative problems?

CHAPTER 28 NURSING MANAGEMENT: OBSTRUCTIVE PULMONARY DISEASES

1. Obstructive pulmonary disease is characterized by

   a. destruction of lung tissue.
   b. decreased total lung capacity.
   c. obstruction or narrowing of airways.
   d. constant limitations in expiratory airflow.

2. Number in sequence the processes that occur in the early- and late-phase responses of asthma.

   _____ a. Onset of bronchial smooth muscle constriction, vascular permeability, and increased mucus secretion

   _____ b. Inflammation causing mucosal edema and obstruction of airways

   _____ c. Allergen or irritant cross-links IgE receptors on mast cells in bronchial basement membrane

   _____ d. Eosinophils and neutrophils infiltrate airway releasing mediators that cause further mast cell degranulation

   _____ e. Monocytes and lymphocytes infiltrate airways

   _____ f. Epithelial damage causes heightened airway reactivity that worsens symptoms of future attacks

   _____ g. Activated mast cells release histamine, leukotrienes, bradykinin, prostaglandins, and chemotactic factors

3. In assisting a patient with asthma to identify specific triggers of the asthma, the nurse recognizes that

   a. food and drug allergies do not manifest in respiratory symptoms.
   b. exercise-induced asthma is seen only in individuals with sensitivity to cold air.
   c. asthma attacks are psychogenic in origin and can be controlled with relaxation techniques.
   d. viral upper respiratory infections are a common precipitating factor in acute asthma attacks.

4. On assessment the nurse determines that the patient has severe obstruction and impending respiratory failure based on the findings of

   a. markedly diminished breath sounds with no wheezing.
   b. inspiratory and expiratory wheezing with an unproductive cough.
   c. use of accessory muscles of respiration and a feeling of suffocation.
   d. a respiratory rate of 34 breaths per minutes and increased pulse and blood pressure.

5. Arterial blood gas results that would be expected in a patient early in an acute asthma attack include

   a. pH 7.20, $PaCO_2$ 52 mm Hg, PaO_2 60 mm Hg.
   b. pH 7.35, $PaCO_2$ 42 mm Hg, PaO_2 74 mm Hg.
   c. pH 7.40, $PaCO_2$ 50 mm Hg, PaO_2 80 mm Hg.
   d. pH 7.48, $PaCO_2$ 30 mm Hg, PaO_2 78 mm Hg.

6. One indication for intubation and mechanical ventilation for the patient in status asthmaticus is when

   a. $PaCO_2$ levels are at 60 mm Hg.
   b. PaO_2 levels decrease to 70 mm Hg.
   c. severe respiratory muscle fatigue occurs.
   d. the patient has extreme anxiety and fear of suffocation.

7. Marked bronchoconstriction with air trapping and hyperinflation of the lungs in the patient with asthma is indicated by

   a. SaO_2 of 85%.
   b. FEV_1 of 85% of predicted.
   c. PEFR of 100 to 150 L/min.
   d. chest x-ray showing a flattened diaphragm.

8. Match the following drugs, first with their use in promoting quick-relief of asthma symptoms or long-term control of symptoms and then with their primary mode of action (answers may be used more than once).

Use	Action	Drug	
_____	_____	a. Albuterol nebulizer	1. Long-term control
_____	_____	b. Oral prednisone	2. Quick-relief agent
_____	_____	c. Triamcinolone inhaler	3. Beta-adrenergic agonist
_____	_____	d. Ipratropium inhaler	4. Mast-cell stabilizer
_____	_____	e. Oral theophylline	5. Leukotriene inhibitor
_____	_____	f. Cromolyn inhaler	6. Steroid antiinflammatory
_____	_____	g. Budesonide inhaler	7. Methylxanthine bronchodilator
_____	_____	h. Intravenous aminophylline	8. Anticholinergic
_____	_____	i. Formoterol inhaler	
_____	_____	j. Zileuton	
_____	_____	k. Metaproterenol inhaler	
_____	_____	l. Beclomethasone inhaler	
_____	_____	m. Nedocromil inhaler	
_____	_____	n. Salmeterol inhaler	

9. Of the following instructions for patients about the use of asthma medications, check all those that are correct.

_____ a. When using pirbuterol (Maxair) and fluticasone (Flovent) inhalers, use the pirbuterol inhaler before using the fluticasone inhaler.

_____ b. Albuterol (Proventil) or cromolyn (Intal) inhalers should be used before exercise or when anticipating exposure to allergens known to cause asthma.

_____ c. The mouth should be rinsed thoroughly after using the ipratropium (Atrovent) inhaler to prevent oral candidiasis.

_____ d. The salmeterol (Serevent) inhaler should not be used more than every 12 hours.

_____ e. When you have increasing symptoms of asthma, you should use your metaproterenol (Alupent) inhaler as often as every 20 minutes until the symptoms are relieved.

_____ f. The best way to use a metered-dose inhaler is to hold it about 1 to 2 inches in front of your mouth before depressing the inhaler.

_____ g. You must use your flunisolide (Aerobid) inhaler every day as prescribed to prevent worsening of your asthma, even if you have no asthma symptoms.

_____ h. You should wait 5 minutes before taking a second puff of any inhaled medication.

_____ i. If you use a spacer with your inhaler, depress the inhaler before starting to inhale.

_____ j. You should take azfirlukast (Accolate) tablets on an empty stomach.

_____ k. To use your dry powder inhaler (DPI), empty your lungs of air, close your lips around the mouthpiece, and inhale quickly and deeply.

10. One of the best ways to decrease the patient's sense of panic during an acute asthma attack is for the nurse to

a. leave the patient alone to rest in a quiet, calm environment.
b. stay with the patient and encourage slow, pursed-lip breathing.
c. reassure the patient that the attack can be controlled with treatment.
d. let the patient know his or her status is being closely monitored with frequent measurement of vital signs and SpO_2.

11. When a patient with asthma is admitted to the emergency department in severe respiratory distress, the nurse anticipates that initial drug treatment will most likely include administration of

a. inhaled ipratropium.
b. aerosolized albuterol.
c. intravenous aminophylline.
d. intravenous hydrocortisone.

12. When teaching the patient with asthma about the use of the peak flow meter, the nurse instructs the patient to

a. carry the flow meter with the patient at all times in case an asthma attack occurs.
b. increase the use of quick-relief medications if the meter indicates the yellow zone.
c. use the flow meter to check the status of the patient's asthma every time the patient takes quick- relief medication.
d. use the flow meter by emptying the lungs, closing the mouth around the mouthpiece, and inhaling through the meter as fast as possible.

13. The nurse recognizes that additional teaching is needed when the patient with asthma says

a. "I should exercise every day if my symptoms are controlled."
b. "I may use over-the-counter bronchodilator drugs occasionally if I develop chest tightness."
c. "I should inform my spouse about my medications and how to get help if I have a severe asthma attack."
d. "A diary to record my medication use, symptoms, PEFRs, and activity level will help in adjusting my therapy."

14. Match the following effects of smoking with the related components of cigarette smoke (answers may be used more than once).

_____	a. Destruction of alveolar walls	1. Nicotine
_____	b. Hyperplasia of bronchial cells	2. Carbon monoxide
_____	c. Decreased ciliary action	3. Smoke gases
_____	d. Increased mucus production by goblet cells	4. Oxidants
_____	e. Peripheral vasoconstriction and increased BP	
_____	f. Inactivation of the protease inhibitor alpha$_1$-antitrypsin	
_____	g. Decreased oxygen-carrying capacity	
_____	h. Stimulate neutrophil and macrophage release of proteases	
_____	i. Psychomotor impairment and impaired judgment	
_____	j. Increased oxygen need of heart	

15. Use the given words to complete the following sentences (some words may be used more than once).

alpha$_1$-antitrypsin (AAT)	collagen	elastin
smoking	infection	hereditary AAT deficiency
inhaled irritants		

a. In the normal lung, the action of proteases and elastases released from macrophages and neutrophils is balanced by the presence of the protease inhibitor __________________.

b. In emphysema, three known factors that increase the release of proteases and elastases are ____________________, ____________________, and ______________.

c. The action of the proteases and elastases destroy ______________ and ______________ of the alveolar walls and the supporting structures of the lung.

d. The action of the proteases and elastases is inhibited by ________________.

e. Two factors that are known to cause a decrease in AAT levels or activity are ______________________ and ______________________________.

f. ___________________ is the one factor that both increases protease release and decreases AAT activity.

16. The effect of alveolar destruction in emphysema results in

    a. decreased lung compliance.
    b. air trapping in distal alveoli.
    c. dilation of small bronchioles.
    d. obstruction of airflow into alveoli.

17. The chronic inflammation of the bronchi characteristic of chronic bronchitis results in

    a. collapse of small bronchioles on expiration.
    b. permanent, abnormal dilation of the bronchi.
    c. hyperplasia of mucus-secreting cells and bronchial edema.
    d. destruction of the elastic and muscular structures of the bronchial wall.

18. Indicate whether the following clinical manifestations of COPD are most characteristics of emphysema (E), chronic bronchitis (CB), or both (B).

    _____ a. Barrel chest

    _____ b. Persistent cough

    _____ c. Flattened diaphragm

    _____ d. Early polycythemia

    _____ e. Decreased breath sounds

    _____ f. Cor pulmonale

    _____ g. Weight loss

    _____ h. Early onset

    _____ i. Finger clubbing

    _____ j. Early hypercapnia

    _____ k. Decreased diaphragmatic excursion

    _____ l. Copious mucus production

19. The pulmonary vasoconstriction leading to the development of cor pulmonale in the patient with COPD results from

    a. increased viscosity of the blood.
    b. alveolar hypoxia and hypercapnia.
    c. long-term low-flow oxygen therapy.
    d. administration of high concentrations of oxygen.

20. Explain how the following findings on pulmonary function testing relate to the pathophysiologic changes of COPD.

a. decreased FEV_1

b. decreased VC

c. increased RV

d. increased TLC

21. Arterial blood gas results that are characteristic of late stage COPD include

a. pH 7.26, $PaCO_2$ 58 mm Hg, PaO_2 60 mm Hg, HCO_3 30 mEq/L.
b. pH 7.30, $PaCO_2$ 45 mm Hg, PaO_2 55 mm Hg, HCO_3 18 mEq/L.
a. pH 7.40, $PaCO_2$ 40 mm Hg, PaO_2 70 mm Hg, HCO_3 25 mEq/L.
a. pH 7.52, $PaCO_2$ 30 mm Hg, PaO_2 80 mm Hg, HCO_3 35 mEq/L.

22. In addition to smoking cessation, treatment for COPD that is indicated to slow the progression of the disease includes

a. use of bronchodilating drugs.
b. use of inhaled corticosteroids.
c. lung volume reduction surgery.
d. prevention of respiratory tract infections.

23. Match the following characteristics with their methods of oxygen administration.

_____ a. Provides highest oxygen concentrations
_____ b. May cause aspiration of condensed fluid
_____ c. Safest system to use in patient with COPD
_____ d. Most comfortable and causes least restriction on activities
_____ e. Provides 40-60% oxygen concentration
_____ f. Invasive placement of catheter into trachea
_____ g. Used to give oxygen quickly for short time

1. Nasal cannula
2. Simple face mask
3. Partial rebreathing mask
4. Non-rebreathing mask
5. Venturi mask
6. Tracheostomy collar
7. Transtracheal catheter

24. Identify whether the following statements are true or false. If a statement is false, correct the bold word(s) to make the statement true.

_____ a. A decrease in mental status and hypoventilation that occurs after oxygen administration is started may indicate **oxygen toxicity**.

_____ b. The risk for oxygen toxicity is high in the patient receiving **more than 50% oxygen for more than 24 hours**.

_____ c. Absorption atelectasis occurs when high FIO_2 causes displacement of **carbon dioxide** from the alveoli.

_____ d. Patients at highest risk for CO_2 narcosis are those with chronic **high carbon dioxide** levels.

_____ e. Alterations in skin integrity with pressure ulcer formation during oxygen therapy is most likely to occur at the **top of the ears**.

_____ f. Medicare reimbursement criteria for long-term home oxygen therapy for patients with chronic hypoxemia is a PaO_2 **≤ 59 mm Hg** and an SaO_2 **≤ 89%**.

25. A patient is being discharged with plans for home oxygen therapy provided by a liquid oxygen reservoir with a refillable portable unit. In preparing the patient to use the equipment, the nurse teaches the patient that

a. the portable tank filled from the reservoir will last about 6 to 8 hours at 2L/min.
b. the unit concentrates oxygen from the air, providing a continuous oxygen supply.
c. the unit should be kept out of the bedroom and extension tubing used at night because of the noise.
d. weekly delivery of four or five large cylinders of oxygen will be necessary for a 7- to 10-day supply of oxygen.

26. A breathing technique the nurse should teach the patient with COPD to promote exhalation is

a. huff coughing.
b. thoracic breathing.
c. pursed-lip breathing.
d. diaphragmatic breathing.

27. In planning for postural drainage for the patient with COPD, the nurse

a. schedules the procedure 1 hour before and after meals.
b. has the patient cough before positioning to clear the lungs.
c. assesses the patient's tolerance for dependent (head-down) positions.
d. ensures that percussion and vibration are performed before positioning the patient.

28. A dietary modification that helps meet the nutritional needs of patients with COPD is

a. a high-carbohydrate, low-fat diet.
b. avoiding foods that require a lot of chewing.
c. preparing most foods of the diet to be eaten hot.
d. drinking fluids with meals to promote digestion.

29. During an acute exacerbation of COPD, the patient is severely short of breath and the nurse identifies a nursing diagnosis of ineffective breathing pattern related to obstruction of airflow and anxiety. The best action by the nurse is to

    a. prepare and administer bronchodilator medications.
    b. perform chest physiotherapy to promote removal of secretions.
    c. administer oxygen at 5 L/min until the shortness of breath is relieved.
    d. position the patient upright with the elbows resting on the overbed table.

30. The husband of a patient with COPD tells the nurse that they have not had any sexual activity since the patient was diagnosed with COPD because she becomes too short of breath. The best response by the nurse is

    a. "You need to discuss your feelings and needs with your wife so she knows what you expect of her."
    b. "There are other ways to maintain intimacy besides sexual intercourse that will not make her short of breath."
    c. "Would you like for me to talk to you and your wife about some modifications that can maintain sexual activity?"
    d. "You should explore other ways to meet your sexual needs since your wife is no longer capable of sexual activity."

31. In teaching the patient with COPD about the need for physical exercise, the nurse informs the patient that

    a. all patients with COPD should be able to gradually increase walking to 20 minutes a day.
    b. a bronchodilator inhaler should be used to relieve exercise-induced dyspnea immediately after the exercise.
    c. shortness of breath is expected during exercise but should return to baseline within 5 minutes after the exercise.
    d. monitoring the heart rate before and after exercise is the best way to determine how much exercise can be tolerated.

32. The pathophysiologic mechanism of cystic fibrosis leading to obstructive lung disease is

    a. fibrosis of mucous glands and destruction of bronchial walls.
    b. destruction of lung parenchyma from inflammation and scarring.
    c. production of abnormally thick, copious secretions from mucous glands.
    d. increased serum levels of pancreatic enzymes that are deposited in the bronchial mucosa.

33. The primary treatment for cystic fibrosis is

    a. heart-lung transplantation.
    b. administration of prophylactic antibiotics.
    c. administration of nebulized bronchodilators.
    d. vigorous and consistent chest physiotherapy.

34. Meeting the developmental tasks of young adulthood becomes a major problem for young adults with cystic fibrosis primarily because

    a. they have an expected shortened life span.
    b. any children they have will develop cystic fibrosis.
    c. they must also adapt to a newly diagnosed chronic disease.
    d. their illness keeps them from becoming financially independent.

CASE STUDY

CHRONIC OBSTRUCTIVE PULMONARY DISEASE

Patient Profile

Mr. D. has a history of emphysema and chronic bronchitis. He is a 73-year-old retired farmer who can no longer walk his farm without extreme breathlessness. He is treated at the outpatient medicine clinic today for increasing shortness of breath, even at rest.

Subjective Data

- Reports that his sputum production has increased over the past week and the color has changed to a greenish yellow
- Has more sputum in the morning that gradually reduces over the day
- Has been taking albuterol (Proventil, Ventolin) MDI and beclomethasone (Vanceril, Beclovent) MDI 2 puffs every 6 hours
- Takes no other medication at this time

Objective Data

- Appears to be a frail older adult on observation
- Labored breathing and use of accessory muscles of respiration
- Sitting in a tripod position and using pursed-lip breathing
- Chest assessment: crackles in left lower lobe and diffuse expiratory wheezing throughout his chest; left lower lobe dull to percussion
- Vital signs: BP normal; P 96; R 28; T 101.8° F (38.8° C)
- ABGs: pH 7.36
  PaO_2 55 mm Hg
  $PaCO_2$ 65 mm Hg

Treatment is initiated with an intravenous catheter and IV fluids at 50 ml/hr, nebulized albuterol, sputum for culture and sensitivity, IV antibiotics, antipyretics, and oral corticosteroids.

Critical Thinking Questions

1. Mr. D. is most likely experiencing an exacerbation of his COPD. What assessment data provided indicates the presence of pneumonia?

2. What are the nursing care priorities for Mr. D.?

3. What are possible causes of Mr. D.'s exacerbation of COPD?

4. What do his ABG values indicate?

5. What is the home care plan for this patient?

6. Based on the assessment data presented, write one or more appropriate nursing diagnoses. Are there any collaborative problems?

CHAPTER 29 NURSING ASSESSMENT: HEMATOLOGIC SYSTEM

1. Match the following characteristics with the appropriate blood cells (answers may be used more than once).

_____	a. May become tissue macrophages	1. Erythrocyte
_____	b. 30% of volume stored in spleen	2. Reticulocyte
_____	c. Primarily responsible for immune response	3. Neutrophil
_____	d. Make up 4%-8% of WBCs	4. Basophil
_____	e. Production stimulated by hypoxia	5. Eosinophil
_____	f. Make up 0%-2% of WBCs	6. Lymphocyte
_____	g. Immature cell is a band	7. Monocyte
_____	h. Increased in individuals with allergies	8. Platelet
_____	i. Responds first at injury site	
_____	j. Make up 20%-40% of WBCs	
_____	k. Releases granules that increase allergic and inflammatory responses	
_____	l. Arises from megakaryocyte	
_____	m. Make up 50%-70% of WBCs	
_____	n. Increases indicate an increased rate of erythropoiesis	
_____	o. Make up 2%-4% of WBCs	
_____	p. Also known as "segs"	

2. Complete the following statements.

   a. Granulocytic leukocytes include ____________________, ______________, and ________________.

   b. Red blood cell production is stimulated by the release of the hormone ________________ from the kidney.

   c. Nutrients essential for red blood cell production include ____________, ____________________, and ______________.

   d. Obstruction of the lymph flow results in accumulation of lymph fluid known as __________________.

   e. Organs of the hematologic system that have filtering functions include the ______________, ____________________, and ______________.

3. Match the following processes with the appropriate response of normal blood coagulation (answers may be used more than once).

_____	a. Thrombin converts fibrinogen to fibrin	1. Vascular response
_____	b. Release of adenosine diphosphate	2. Platelet response
_____	c. Release of tissue thromboplastin	3. Plasma clotting factors
_____	d. Release of PF3, serotonin, and epinephrine	
_____	e. Vasoconstriction	
_____	f. Prothrombin converted to thrombin	
_____	g. Damaged vascular surface	
_____	h. Serum calcium activity as factor IV	
_____	i. Platelet clumping and plugging	

4. Fibrinolysis involves the action of

a. heparin.
b. plasmin.
c. fibrinogen.
d. prothrombin.

5. The effects of fibrin split products (FSPs) include

a. clot stabilization.
b. increase in prothrombin.
c. impaired platelet aggregation.
d. decreased release of tissue thromboplastin.

6. In analyzing the results of a 83-year-old patient's CBC, the nurse would expect to find as a normal age-related change a decrease in

a. platelets.
b. total WBC.
c. hemoglobin.
d. red blood cells.

7. A patient's CBC indicates a pancytopenia. The nurse suspects that the patient has an impairment of the

a. liver.
b. spleen.
c. bone marrow.
d. lymph system.

8. During the nursing assessment of a patient with anemia, the nurse notes as significant the patient's history of

a. recurring infections.
b. a partial gastrectomy.
c. corticosteroid therapy.
d. oral contraceptive use.

9. Identify one specific finding identified by the nurse during assessment of each of the patient's functional health patterns that indicates a risk factor for hematologic problems or a patient response to an actual hematologic problem.

   a. Health perception–health management

   b. Nutritional-metabolic

   c. Elimination

   d. Activity-exercise

   e. Sleep-rest

   f. Cognitive-perceptual

   g. Self-perception–self-concept

   h. Role-relationship

   i. Sexuality-reproductive

   j. Coping–stress tolerance

   k. Value-belief

10. Using light pressure with the index and middle fingers, the nurse cannot palpate any of the patient's superficial lymph nodes. The nurse

    a. records this finding as normal.
    b. should reassess the lymph nodes using deeper pressure.
    c. asks the patient if there is a history of any radiation therapy.
    d. notifies the physician that x-rays of the nodes will be necessary.

11. During physical assessment of a patient with thrombocytopenia, the nurse would expect to find

    a. sternal tenderness.
    b. petechiae and purpura.
    c. jaundiced sclera and skin.
    d. tender, enlarged lymph nodes.

12. A patient with a hematologic disorder has a smooth, shiny red tongue. The nurse would expect the patient's laboratory results to include

    a. WBC 13500/μl.
    b. neutrophils 45%.
    c. RBC 6.4 x 106/μl.
    d. Hb 9.6 g/dl (96 g. L).

13. A patient is being treated with chemotherapeutic agents. The nurse revises the patient's care plan based on the CBC results of

    a. Hct 38%.
    b. MCV 85 fl.
    c. WBC 4000/μl.
    d. platelets 80,000/μl.

14. Identify the type of condition that is indicated by the following lab study results.

    a. Serum iron 40 μg/dl (7 μmol/L)

    b. Erythrocyte sedimentation rate (ESR) 30 mm/hr

    c. Increased band neutrophils

    d. Activated partial thromboplastin time 60 sec

    e. Indirect bilirubin 2.0 mg/dl (34 μmol/L)

    f. Urine Bence Jones protein

15. If a patient with blood type O Rh^+ is given AB Rh^- blood, the nurse would expect

    a. the patient's Rh factor to react with the red blood cells of the donor blood.
    b. no adverse reaction since the patient has no antibodies against the donor blood.
    c. the anti-A and anti-B antibodies in the patient's blood to hemolyze the donor blood.
    d. the anti-A and anti-B antibodies in the donor blood to hemolyze the patient's blood.

16. A patient is undergoing a contrast computed tomography (CT) of the spleen. Before this test is it important for the nurse to ask the patient about

    a. iodine sensitivity
    b. prior blood transfusions.
    c. phobia of confined spaces.
    d. internal metal implants or appliances.

17. The most common site for a bone marrow aspiration in an adult is the

    a. tibia.
    b. scapula.
    c. sternum.
    d. iliac crest.

18. When preparing the patient for a bone marrow examination, the nurse explains that

    a. the procedure will be done under general anesthesia because it is so painful.
    b. the patient will not have any pain after the area at the puncture site is anesthetized.
    c. the patient will experience a brief, very sharp pain during aspiration of the bone marrow.
    d. there will be no pain during the procedure but an ache will be present several days afterward.

19. A lymph node biopsy is most often performed to diagnose

    a. leukemias.
    b. hemorrhagic tendencies.
    c. the cause of lymphedema.
    d. neoplastic cells in the lymph nodes.

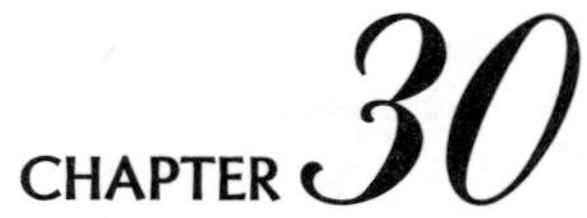

CHAPTER 30 NURSING MANAGEMENT: HEMATOLOGIC PROBLEMS

1. Match each of the anemic states with both etiologic and morphologic classification systems (answers may be used more than once).

_____	_____	a. Acute trauma	**Etiologic:**
_____	_____	b. Malaria	1. Decreased RBC production
_____	_____	c. Anemia of gastritis	2. Blood loss
_____	_____	d. Anemia of renal failure	3. Increased RBC destruction
_____	_____	e. Aplastic anemia	**Morphologic:**
_____	_____	f. G6PD	4. Normocytic, normochromic
_____	_____	g. Iron deficiency anemia	5. Macrocytic, normochromic
_____	_____	h. Thalassemia	6. Microcytic, hypochromic
_____	_____	i. Pernicious anemia	
_____	_____	j. Sickle cell anemia	
_____	_____	k. Anemia of leukemia	
_____	_____	l. Anemia associated with prosthetic heart valve	

2. A patient with a hemoglobin level of 7.8 g/dl (78 g/L) has cardiac palpations, a heart rate of 102, and an increased reticulocyte count. At this severity of anemia, the nurse would also expect the patient to manifest

   a. pallor.
   b. dyspnea.
   c. a smooth tongue.
   d. sensitivity to cold.

3. A 76-year-old woman has an Hb of 7.3 g/dl (73 g/L) and is experiencing ataxia and confusion. During assessment of the patient, it is most important for the nurse to ask about

   a. food and drug intake.
   b. a family history of anemia.
   c. any exposure to chemical toxins.
   d. the presence of postmenopausal bleeding.

4. On physical assessment of the patient with severe anemia, the nurse would expect to find

   a. nervousness and agitation.
   b. fever and tenting of the skin.
   c. systolic murmurs and tachycardia.
   d. bluish mucous membranes and reddened skin.

5. A nursing diagnosis that is appropriate for patients with moderate to severe anemia of any etiology is

   a. impaired skin integrity related to edema and pruritus.
   b. disturbed body image related to changes in appearance and body function.
   c. imbalanced nutrition: less than body requirements related to lack of knowledge of adequate nutrition.
   d. activity intolerance related to decreased hemoglobin and imbalance between oxygen supply and demand.

6. Match the following descriptions with their associated types of anemia (answers may be used more than once).

_____	a. Chronic bone marrow hyperplasia	1. Iron deficiency
_____	b. Hypoxia-induced change in RBCs	2. Thalassemia
_____	c. Responds to treatment with erythropoietin	3. Cobalamin deficiency
_____	d. Most common type of anemia	4. Folic acid deficiency
_____	e. Related to RBC metabolism of glucose	5. Anemia of chronic disease
_____	f. Megaloblastic cells without neurologic involvement	6. Aplastic anemia
		7. Sickle cell
_____	g. Autoimmune-related disease	8. G6PD anemia
_____	h. May occur with removal of the duodenum	
_____	i. May occur with removal of the stomach	
_____	j. Altered globin synthesis of hemoglobin	
_____	k. Lack of intrinsic factor	
_____	l. Associated with vascular occlusion and tissue infarction	
_____	m. Decrease in all blood cells	
_____	n. May be caused by adrenal hypofunction	
_____	o. Associated with chronic blood loss	
_____	p. Treatment causes chronic iron toxicity	
_____	q. Oral contraceptives a contributing factor	

7. Explain the following laboratory findings in anemia.

   a. Reticulocyte counts are increased in chronic blood loss but decreased in cobalamin (vitamin B_{12}) deficiency.

   b. Bilirubin levels are increased in sickle cell anemia but are normal in acute blood loss.

   c. MCV is increased in folic acid deficiency but is decreased in iron deficiency anemia.

8. To prevent a common side effect of oral iron supplements, the nurse teaches the patient to

   a. take the iron preparations with meals.
   b. increase fluid and dietary fiber intake.
   c. report the presence of black stools to the physician.
   d. use enteric-coated preparations taken with orange juice.

9. To administer iron intramuscularly, the nurse should

   a. use a short, fine needle to avoid pain.
   b. massage the site after the injection to promote absorption.
   c. include 0.5 ml of air in the syringe to clear the iron from the needle.
   d. administer the injection in the vastus lateralis to prevent nerve damage.

10. The nurse evaluates that teaching for the patient with iron deficiency anemia has been effective when the patient states

    a. "I will need to take the iron supplements the rest of my life."
    b. "I will increase my dietary intake of milk and milk products."
    c. "I should increase my activity to increase my aerobic capacity."
    d. "I should take the iron for several months after my blood is normal."

11. In teaching the patient with pernicious anemia about the disease, the nurse explains that it results from a lack of

    a. folic acid.
    b. intrinsic factor.
    c. extrinsic factor.
    d. cobalamine intake.

12. In addition to the general symptoms of anemia, the patient with pernicious anemia also manifests

    a. neurologic symptoms.
    b. coagulation deficiencies.
    c. cardiovascular disturbances.
    d. a decreased immunologic response.

13. The nurse explains to the patient with pernicious anemia that

    a. death can be prevented by cobalamin supplementation for the rest of the patient's life.
    b. the symptoms of the disease can be completely reversed with cobalamin (vitamin B_{12}) therapy.
    c. bone marrow transplantation to change the defective marrow cells is an alternative therapy for pernicious anemia.
    d. dietary intake of foods high in cobalamin is the most inexpensive and convenient treatment of pernicious anemia.

14. Laboratory and diagnostic test findings the nurse would expect in an anemic patient with chronic alcoholism include

    a. achlorhydria and macrocytic erythrocytes.
    b. decreased serum folate and increased MCHC.
    c. increased indirect bilirubin and increased reticulocytes.
    d. decreased total iron binding capacity and increased MCH.

15. The strict vegetarian is at highest risk for the development of

    a. thalassemias.
    b. iron deficiency anemia.
    c. folic acid deficiency anemia.
    d. cobalamin deficiency anemia.

16. A nursing diagnosis that is appropriate for the effects of the deficiency of all of the cells associated with aplastic anemia is

    a. risk for injury: falls.
    b. impaired physical mobility.
    c. risk for impaired skin integrity.
    d. risk for impaired oral mucous membrane.

17. Nursing interventions for the patient with aplastic anemia are directed toward the prevention of the complications of

    a. fatigue and dyspnea.
    b. hemorrhage and infection.
    c. thromboemboli and gangrene.
    d. cardiac arrhythmias and heart failure.

18. Identify whether the following statements are true or false. If a statement is false, correct the bold word(s) to make the statement true.

    _____ a. The most reliable way to evaluate the effect and degree of blood loss in a patient with hemorrhage is with **laboratory data**.

    _____ b. A patient with acute blood loss that has normal vital signs at rest but has increased heart rate and postural hypotension with exercise has lost approximately **30%** of the total blood volume.

    _____ c. The anemia that follows acute blood loss is most frequently treated with **increased dietary iron intake**.

    _____ d. In addition to the general symptoms of anemia, the patient with a hemolytic anemia also manifests **jaundice**.

    _____ e. A major concern in hemolytic anemias is maintenance of **liver** function.

    _____ f. An example of an intravascular extrinsic hemolytic anemia results from **blood transfusion reactions**.

19. The anemia of sickle cell disease is caused by

a. intravascular hemolysis of sickled RBCs.
b. accelerated breakdown of abnormal RBCs.
c. autoimmune antibody destruction of RBCs.
d. isoimmune antibody-antigen reactions with RBCs.

20. A patient with sickle cell anemia asks the nurse why the sickling crisis does not stop when oxygen therapy is started. The nurse explains that

a. sickling occurs in response to decreased blood viscosity, which is not affected by oxygen therapy.
b. when red cells sickle, they occlude small vessels, which causes more local hypoxia and more sickling.
c. the primary problem during a sickle cell crisis is destruction of the abnormal cells resulting in fewer RBCs to carry oxygen.
d. oxygen therapy does not alter the shape of the abnormal erythrocytes but only allows for increased oxygen concentration in hemoglobin.

21. A nursing intervention that is indicated for the patient during a sickle cell crisis is

a. frequent ambulation.
b. application of antiembolism hose.
c. restriction of sodium and oral fluids.
d. administration of large doses of continuous narcotic analgesics.

22. During discharge teaching with a patient with newly diagnosed sickle cell disease, the nurse teaches the patient to decrease the risk of a sickle cell crisis by

a. limiting fluid intake.
b. avoiding hot, humid weather.
c. eliminating exercise from the lifestyle.
d. seeking early medical intervention for upper respiratory infections.

23. Identify whether the following statements are true or false. If a statement is false, correct the bold word(s) to make the statement true.

_____ a. Genetic counseling and family planning is indicated for couples when one of them has **thalassemia**.

_____ b. Immune thrombocytopenic purpura is characterized by increased platelet destruction by the **spleen**.

_____ c. Alterations in platelet function are assessed with the use of **prothrombin** times.

_____ d. Thrombotic thrombocytopenic purpura is characterized by **decreased** platelets, **decreased** RBCs, and **decreased** agglutination function of platelets.

_____ e. A classic clinical manifestation of thrombocytopenia that the nurse would expect to find on physical examination of the patient is **ecchymosis**.

_____ f. Patients with platelet deficiencies usually bleed from **superficial sites** while those with diminished clotting factors experience **deep or internal** bleeding.

_____ g. Treatment of **hemachromatosis** involves weekly phlebotomy for 2 to 3 years.

_____ h. The nurse suspects heparin-induced thrombocytopenia and thrombosis syndrome when a patient receiving heparin requires **decreased** heparin to maintain therapeutic activated thromboplastin times.

24. In planning the care of a patient hospitalized with polycythemia vera, the nurse recognizes that a nursing intervention that is most likely to prevent organ damage or death is

    a. maintaining protective isolation.
    b. promoting leg exercises and ambulation.
    c. protecting the patient from injury or falls.
    d. promoting hydration with a large fluid intake.

25. A patient has a platelet count of 50,000/μl and is diagnosed with immune thrombocytopenic purpura. The nurse would expect initial treatment to include

    a. splenectomy.
    b. corticosteroids.
    c. administration of platelets.
    d. immunosuppressive therapy.

26. During the care of the patient with thrombocytopenia, the nurse

    a. takes frequent temperatures to assess for fever.
    b. maintains the patient on strict bed rest to prevent injury.
    c. monitors the patient for headaches, vertigo, or confusion.
    d. removes oral crusting and scabs with firm friction every 2 hours.

27. In analyzing the laboratory results of a patient with classic hemophilia, the nurse would expect to find

    a. an absence of factor IX.
    b. a decreased platelet count.
    c. a prolonged bleeding time.
    d. a prolonged partial thromboplastin time.

28. Treatment of hemophilia most often includes periodic administration of

    a. whole blood.
    b. thromboplastin.
    c. factor concentrates.
    d. fresh frozen plasma.

29. A patient with hemophilia is hospitalized with acute knee pain and swelling. Nursing interventions for the patient include

    a. wrapping the knee with an elastic bandage.
    b. placing the patient on bed rest and applying ice to the joint.
    c. gently performing ROM exercises to the knee to prevent adhesions.
    d. administering nonsteroidal antiinflammatory drugs as needed for pain.

30. Number in sequence the events that occur in disseminated intravascular coagulation (DIC).

_____ a. Activation of fibrinolytic system

_____ b. Uncompensated hemorrhage

_____ c. Widespread fibrin and platelet deposition in capillaries and arterioles

_____ d. Release of fibrin split products

_____ e. Fibrinogen converted to fibrin

_____ f. Inhibition of normal blood clotting

_____ g. Production of intravascular thrombin

_____ h. Depletion of platelets and coagulation factors

31. Early recognition of acute DIC by the nurse in a patient includes

a. providing appropriate care for managing the causative problem.
b. a knowledge of signs and symptoms of microvascular thrombosis.
c. administering necessary blood products and anticoagulants to susceptible patients.
d. astute, ongoing assessment with awareness of risk for DIC in patients with predisposing conditions.

32. A patient has a WBC of 2300/μl and a neutrophil percentage of 40%.

a. Does the patient have a leukopenia?

b. What is the patient's neutrophil count?

c. Does the patient have a neutropenia?

d. What is the patient's risk for developing a bacterial infection?

33. The most important method for identifying the presence of infection in a neutropenic patient is

a. frequent temperatures.
b. routine blood and sputum cultures.
c. assessing for redness and swelling.
d. monitoring white blood cell counts.

34. The major method of preventing infection in the patient with neutropenia is use of

a. HEPA filtration rooms.
b. prophylactic antibiotics.
c. private, laminar airflow rooms.
d. strict hand washing by all persons in contact with the patient.

35. Myelodysplastic syndrome (MDS) differs from acute leukemias in that MDS

 a. has a slower disease progression.
 b. does not result in bone marrow failure.
 c. is a clonal disorder of hematopoietic cells.
 d. only affects the production and function of platelets and WBCs.

36. Match the following characteristics with their related types of leukemia (answers may be used more than once).

_____	a. Neoplasm of activated B lymphocytes	1. AML
_____	b. Mature-appearing, but functionally inactive lymphocytes	2. ALL
		3. CML
_____	c. 85% of acute leukemia in adults	
		4. CLL
_____	d. Most common in children	
_____	e. Only cure is bone marrow transplant	
_____	f. Proliferation of immature lymphocytes in bone marrow	
_____	g. Increased incidence in atomic bomb survivors	
_____	h. Proliferation of precursors of granulocytes	
_____	i. Associated with Philadelphia chromosome	
_____	j. CNS manifestations common	
_____	k. Most common leukemia of adults	

37. A patient with acute myelogenous leukemia is to start chemotherapy. During the induction stage of chemotherapy, the nurse can expect the patient to

 a. experience mild side effects of the drugs.
 b. experience additive bone marrow suppression.
 c. receive high-dose treatment daily for several months.
 d. regain energy and become more resistant to infection.

38. Lymphadenopathy, splenomegaly, and hepatomegaly are common clinical manifestations of leukemia that are due to

 a. the development of infection at these sites.
 b. increased compensatory production of blood cells by these organs.
 c. infiltration of the organs by increased numbers of WBCs in the blood.
 d. normal hypertrophy of the organs in an attempt to destroy abnormal cells.

39. A patient with acute myelogenous leukemia is considering a bone marrow transplant and asks the nurse what is involved. The best response by the nurse is

   a. "Your bone marrow is destroyed by radiation and new bone marrow cells from a matched donor are injected into your bones."
   b. "A specimen of your bone marrow may be aspirated and treated to destroy any leukemic cells and then reinfused when your disease becomes worse."
   c. "During chemotherapy and total body radiation to destroy all your blood cells you are given transfusions of red cells and platelets to prevent complications."
   d. "All leukemic cells and bone marrow stem cells are eliminated with chemotherapy and total body radiation and new bone marrow cells from a donor are infused."

40. Nursing diagnoses that are appropriate for the patient with newly diagnosed chronic lymphocytic leukemia include

   a. pain and hopelessness.
   b. anxiety and risk for infection.
   c. self-care deficit and ineffective health maintenance.
   d. decisional conflict: treatment options and risk for injury.

41. Indicate whether the following characteristics are associated with Hodgkin's disease (HD), non-Hodgkin's lymphoma (NHL), or both (B).

   _____ a. Multiple histopathologic classifications

   _____ b. Presence of Reed-Sternberg cells

   _____ c. Treated with radiation and chemotherapy

   _____ d. Affects all ages

   _____ e. Originates in lymph nodes in most patients

   _____ f. Often widely disseminated at time of diagnosis

   _____ g. Alcohol-induced pain at site of disease

   _____ h. Primary initial clinical manifestation is painless lymph node enlargement

   _____ i. Over 90% cure rate in stage I disease

   _____ j. Associated with Epstein-Barr virus

42. The nurse prepares to administer IV GM-CSF (Leukine) to a patient with neutropenia resulting from chemotherapy for non-Hodgkin's lymphoma. The nurse explains to the patient that this preparation

   a. can stimulate the production and function of neutrophils and monocytes.
   b. is a type of interferon that may inhibit DNA and protein synthesis in tumor cells.
   c. is a chemotherapeutic agent that is less toxic to the bone marrow than other chemotherapeutic agents.
   d. is a monoclonal antibody linked to a radioactive isotope that will directly deliver radiation to malignant cells.

43. Identify whether the following statements are true or false. If a statement is false, correct the bold word(s) to make the statement true.

_____ a. Staging of lymphomas is important to **predict prognosis**.

_____ b. Nursing management of the patient undergoing treatment for Hodgkin's disease includes measures to prevent **infection**.

_____ c. Multiple myeloma is characterized by proliferation of malignant activated **T cells** that destroy the **kidneys**.

_____ d. Two important nursing interventions in the care of patients with multiple myeloma are increasing fluids to manage **hypercalcemia** and careful handling of the patient to prevent **pathologic fractures**.

44. When analyzing laboratory results of a patient with multiple myeloma, the nurse would expect to find

a. lymphopenia and myeloma protein.
b. neutrophilic leukocytosis and anemia.
c. decreased serum creatinine and BUN.
d. hyperuricemia and increased immunoglobulinemia.

45. Following a splenectomy for treatment of immune thrombocytopenic purpura, the nurse would expect the patient's lab results to reveal

a. decreased RBCs.
b. decreased WBCs.
c. increased platelets.
d. increased immunoglobulins.

46. While receiving a unit of packed red blood cells, the patient develops chills and a temperature of 102.2° F (39° C). The nurse

a. notifies the physician and the blood bank.
b. stops the transfusion and removes the IV catheter.
c. adds a leukocyte reduction filter to the blood administration set.
d. recognizes this as a mild allergic transfusion reaction and slows the transfusion.

47. A patient with thrombocytopenia with active bleeding has 2 units of platelets prescribed. To administer the platelets, the nurse

a. checks for ABO compatibility.
b. agitates the bag periodically during the transfusion.
c. takes vital signs every 15 minutes during the procedure.
d. refrigerates the second unit until the first unit has transfused.

48. Match the following characteristics with their related transfusion reactions (answers may be used more than once).

_____ a. May restart transfusion with antihistamine therapy in mild cases

_____ b. May be avoided by leukocyte reduction filters

_____ c. Acute renal failure may occur

_____ d. Destruction of donor RBCs

_____ e. Hypothermia common

_____ f. Leukocyte or plasma protein incompatibility

_____ g. ABO incompatibility

_____ h. Hypocalcemia and hyperkalemia

_____ i. Epinephrine used for severe reaction

_____ j. May occur in cardiac and renal insufficiency

1. Acute hemolytic reaction
2. Febrile reaction
3. Allergic reaction
4. Circulatory overload
5. Massive blood transfusion reaction

CASE STUDY

DISSEMINATED INTRAVASCULAR COAGULATION

Patient Profile

Mrs. G., a 35-year-old mother of two, is admitted in active labor to the labor and delivery department for delivery of her third child. She delivers a 9-lb boy following an unusually hard and prolonged labor.

Objective Data

- During her recovery period she continues to have heavy uterine bleeding and a boggy fundus.
- Her skin is pale and diaphoretic.
- BP 70/40; HR 150.
- Although the placenta appeared intact on exam, she is suspected of having retained placental fragments causing DIC.

Critical Thinking Questions

1. What is the pathologic mechanism that triggers DIC in this case?

2. What additional clinical findings would indicate the presence of DIC?

3. Describe the common laboratory findings that are indicative of DIC.

4. What therapeutic modalities are most appropriate for this patient and why?

5. Based on the assessment data presented, write one or more appropriate nursing diagnoses. Are there any collaborative problems?

CHAPTER 31 NURSING ASSESSMENT: CARDIOVASCULAR SYSTEM

1. Using the list of terms below, identify the structures in the following illustration.

List of Terms

Chordae tendineae	Papillary muscle
Cusp	Tricuspid valve
Mitral valve	Ventricular septum

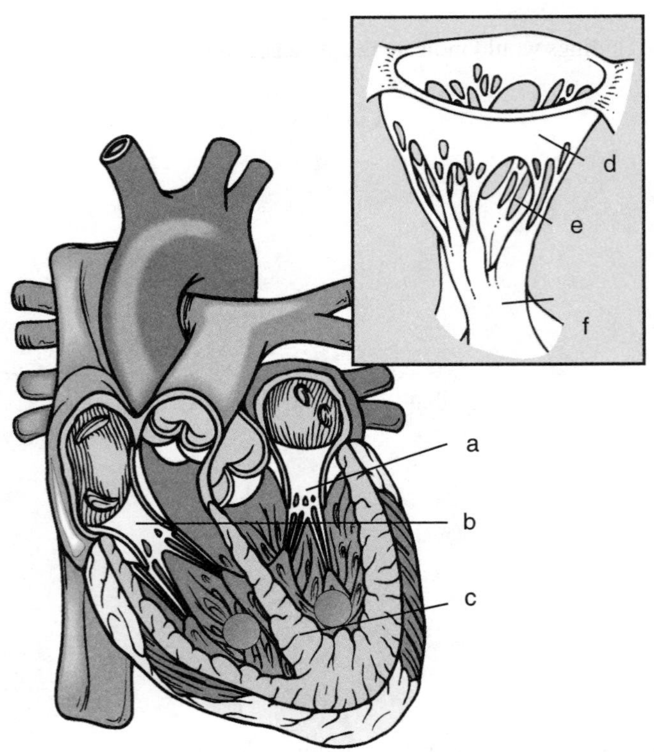

a. ____________________ d. ____________________

b. ____________________ e. ____________________

c. ____________________ f. ____________________

2. Identify the structures in the following illustrations by placing the correct term from the list below in the corresponding answer blank on the next page (some terms will be used more than once).

List of Terms

Anterior interventricular artery	Middle cardiac vein
Aorta	Posterior interventricular artery
Aortic semilunar valve	Posterior vein
Circumflex artery	Pulmonary trunk
Coronary sinus	Right atrium
Great cardiac vein	Right coronary artery
Left atrium	Right marginal artery
Left coronary artery	Right ventricle
Left marginal artery	Small cardiac vein
Left ventricle	Superior vena cava

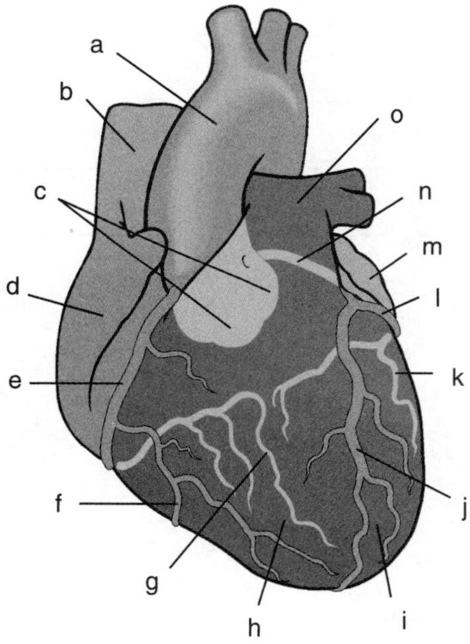

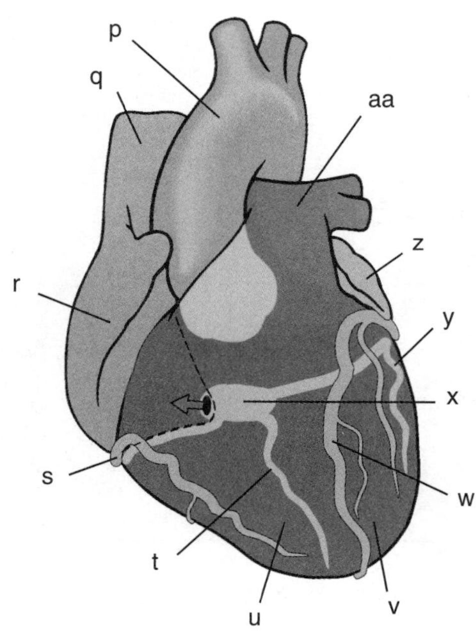

a. ____________________

b. ____________________

c. ____________________

d. ____________________

e. ____________________

f. ____________________

g. ____________________

h. ____________________

i. ____________________

j. ____________________

k. ____________________

l. ____________________

m. ____________________

n. ____________________

o. ____________________

p. ____________________

q. ____________________

r. ____________________

s. ____________________

t. ____________________

u. ____________________

v. ____________________

w. ____________________

x. ____________________

y. ____________________

z. ____________________

aa. ____________________

3. Complete the following statements.

   a. The three main coronary arteries are the ____________________, ____________________, and ____________________.

   b. In most people, the ____________________ artery supplies the AV node.

   c. Blood flow into the coronary arteries occurs primarily during the __________ phase of the cardiac cycle.

4. Number in sequence the path of the action potential along the conduction system of the heart.

_____ a. AV node

_____ b. Purkinje fibers

_____ c. Internodal pathways

_____ d. Bundle of His

_____ e. Ventricular cells

_____ f. SA node

_____ g. Right and left atrial cells

_____ h. Right and left bundle branches

5. Match the cardiac activity and time frames characteristic of the waveforms of the electrocardiogram (answers may be used more than once).

_____	a. Time of impulse spread from SA node to ventricles	1. P wave
_____	b. Repolarization of the ventricles	2. PR interval
_____	c. 0.12 to 0.20 sec	3. QRS interval
_____	d. Depolarization from SA node throughout atria	4. T wave
_____	e. 0.16 sec	5. QT interval
_____	f. Time of depolarization and repolarization of ventricles	
_____	g. 0.06 to 0.10 sec	
_____	h. Depolarization from AV node throughout ventricles	
_____	i. 0.06 to 0.12 sec	

6. Indicate what factor of stroke volume (i.e., preload, afterload, or contractility) is primarily affected by the following situations, and whether cardiac output is increased or decreased by the factor.

a. Valsalva maneuver _______________ CO _______________

b. Venous dilation _______________ CO _______________

c. Hypertension _______________ CO _______________

d. Administration of epinephrine _______________ CO _______________

e. Obstruction of pulmonary artery _______________ CO _______________

f. Hemorrhage _______________ CO _______________

7. Match the effects of the autonomic nervous system stimulation with the receptors responsible for the effects (answers may be used more than once).

_____	a. Increased force of cardiac contraction	1. α-Adrenergic stimulation
_____	b. Decreased rate of impulse conduction	2. β-Adrenergic stimulation
_____	c. Vasoconstriction	3. Parasympathetic stimulation
_____	d. Increased heart rate	
_____	e. Increased rate of impulse conduction	
_____	f. Decreased heart rate	

8. Complete the following statements.

   a. Since blood pressure is a factor of cardiac output (heart rate times stroke volume) times systemic vascular resistance, three effects of sympathetic nervous system stimulation responsible for increased blood pressure are ______________________, __________________, and ________________________.

   b. The one effect of parasympathetic nervous system stimulation that is responsible for decreased blood pressure is ___________________________.

   c. When a patient who has been in bed for a prolonged time is assisted to a standing position, the patient's heart rate increases by 20 beats per minute. The regulatory mechanism of the cardiovascular system that is responsible for this change is ______________________________.

   d. A patient has a BP of 136/76. The patient's pulse pressure is ____________, and the patient's mean arterial pressure (MAP) is ___________.

9. Identify the age-related physiologic changes that occur in the older adult that result in the following.

   a. Widened pulse pressure

   b. Decreased cardiac reserve

   c. Increased cardiac arrhythmias

   d. Decreased response to sympathetic stimulation

   e. Aortic systolic murmur

10. Information related to the patient's past health and medication history that the nurse identifies as significant during assessment of the cardiovascular system is a history of

    a. metastatic cancer.
    b. calcium supplementation.
    c. frequent viral pharyngitis.
    d. use of recreational/abused drugs.

11. Identify one specific finding identified by the nurse during assessment of each of the patient's functional health patterns that indicates a risk factor for cardiovascular disease or a patient response to an actual cardiovascular problem.

    a. Health perception–health management

    b. Nutritional-metabolic

    c. Elimination

    d. Activity-exercise

    e. Sleep-rest

    f. Cognitive-perceptual

    g. Self-perception–self-concept

    h. Role-relationship

    i. Sexuality-reproductive

    j. Coping–stress tolerance

    k. Value-belief

12. A normal positional blood pressure in lying, sitting, and standing positions is

    a. 106/70; 100/65; 90/62.
    b. 114/82; 110/76; 108/74.
    c. 120/82; 110/80; 100/78.
    d. 134/84; 130/80; 126/80.

13. When palpating the patient's popliteal pulse, the nurse feels a vibration at the site. This finding is recorded as a

    a. thready, weak pulse.
    b. bruit at the artery site.
    c. bounding pulse volume.
    d. thrill of the popliteal artery.

14. Match the points that are inspected and palpated on the chest wall with their locations (answers may be used more than once).

_____ a. Pulmonic area
_____ b. PMI
_____ c. Erb's point
_____ d. Tricuspid area
_____ e. Precordium
_____ f. Angle of Louis
_____ g. Aortic area
_____ h. Apex of heart
_____ i. Mitral area
_____ j. Base of the heart

1. Second ICS left of sternum
2. Manubrium and sternal junction at level of second rib
3. Second ICS right of sternum
4. Third ICS left of sternum
5. Fifth ICS left of sternum
6. Fifth ICS at left midclavicular line
7. Located between apex and sternum

15. Indicate whether the following are characteristic of the first heart sound (S_1) or the second heart sound (S_2).

_____ a. Indicates the onset of diastole
_____ b. Associated with closure of tricuspid and mitral valves
_____ c. Is loudest at pulmonic and aortic areas
_____ d. Soft lubb sound
_____ e. Heard when carotid pulse felt
_____ f. Indicates beginning of systole
_____ g. Associated with closure of semilunar valves
_____ h. Sharp dupp sound
_____ i. Is loudest at tricuspid and mitral areas

16. Match the following abnormal assessment findings with their descriptions or significance.

_____	a. Positive Homan's sign	1. Associated with increased right atrial pressure
_____	b. Heave	2. Flattening of angle of nail base and finger
_____	c. Central cyanosis	3. Decreased peripheral perfusion
_____	d. S_3	4. Lift of chest wall in precordial area
_____	e. Cardiac murmurs	5. Blue tinge around nose and ears
_____	f. Finger clubbing	6. Extra heart sound ending in late diastole
_____	g. Jugular vein distention	7. Calf pain on dorsiflexion of foot
_____	h. Delayed capillary filling time	8. Common with heart valve disorders
_____	i. S_4	9. Blue tinge around lips and conjunctiva
_____	j. Peripheral cyanosis	10. Extra heart sound ending in early diastole

17. A patient is scheduled for a Cardiolite scan with stress testing. The nurse explains to the patient that this test involves

   a. placement of electrodes inside the right heart chambers through a vein to directly record the electrical activity of the heart.
   b. exercising on a treadmill or stationary bicycle with continuous ECG monitoring to detect ischemic changes during exercise.
   c. the IV administration of a radioisotope of technetium-99 Sestimibi at the maximum heart rate during exercise to identify areas of cardiac damage.
   d. placement of a small transducer in four positions on the chest to record the direction and flow of blood through the heart by reflection of sound waves.

18. Evaluation of electrocardiographic responses to normal activity over a period of a day or two is performed with

   a. serial ECGs.
   b. Holter monitoring.
   c. electrophysiology studies.
   d. positron emission tomography.

19. Following a cardiac catheterization with coronary angiography, it is most important for the nurse to

   a. observe the catheter insertion site for swelling.
   b. assess for pain at the side of the catheter insertion.
   c. check the pulses distal to the catheter insertion site.
   d. monitor for symptoms of allergy to the constrast media.

20. A laboratory test that is a specific indicator of cardiac muscle damage is

   a. troponin T.
   b. apoproteins.
   c. lactic dehydrogenase (LDH)-3.
   d. serum aspartate aminotransferase (AST).

21. A female patient has a total cholesterol level of 232 mg/dl (6.0 mmol/L) and an HDL of 65 mg/dl (1.68 mmol/L). A male patient has a total cholesterol level of 210 and an HDL of 32. Based on these findings, the patient with the highest cardiac risk is

   a. the male, because his HDL is lower.
   b. the female, because her HDL is higher.
   c. the female, because her cholesterol is higher.
   d. the male, because his cholesterol-to-HDL ratio is higher.

CHAPTER 32 NURSING MANAGEMENT: HYPERTENSION

1. In the regulation of normal blood pressure, indicate whether the following mechanisms elevate blood pressure by increasing cardiac output (CO), increasing systemic vascular resistance (SVR), or increasing both (B), and identify how these mechanisms cause the increases indicated.

_____ a. β_1-Adrenergic stimulation ______________________________

_____ b. α_1-Adrenergic stimulation ______________________________

_____ c. α_2-Adrenergic stimulation ______________________________

_____ d. Enothelin release ______________________________

_____ e. Angiotensin II ______________________________

_____ f. Aldosterone release ______________________________

_____ g. ADH release ______________________________

2. A patient is given an α_1-adrenergic agonist and experiences a reflex bradycardia. What normal mechanism of blood pressure control is stimulated in this situation?

3. A patient uses a mixed β-adrenergic blocking agent for treatment of migraine headaches. What effect may this drug have on blood pressure and why?

4. A patient has blood pressures taken at an outpatient clinic. Blood pressure measurements that would indicate that the patient has hypertension include

a. an initial visit blood pressure of 156/96.
b. two different visit blood pressures of 142/92 and 136/86.
c. three different visit blood pressures of 144/94, 156/90, and 142/88.
d. three different visit blood pressures of 158/94, 136/88, and 146/92.

5. The nurse recognizes that the patient has stage 2 hypertension when the patient's average blood pressure is

a. 155/88 mm Hg.
b. 172/92 mm Hg.
c. 160/110 mm Hg.
d. 182/106 mm Hg.

6. Identify four risk factors for primary hypertension that are not related to lifestyle behaviors.

a.

b.

c.

d.

7. Secondary hypertension is differentiated from primary hypertension in that secondary hypertension

   a. has a more gradual onset than primary hypertension
   b. does not cause the target organ damage that occurs with primary hypertension.
   c. has a specific cause, such as renal disease, that often can be corrected by medicine or surgery.
   d. is caused by age-related changes in blood pressure regulatory mechanisms in those individuals over 65 years of age.

8. The patient with stage 2 hypertension is likely to report

   a. no symptoms.
   b. cardiac palpitations.
   c. dyspnea on exertion.
   d. dizziness and vertigo.

9. Most organ damage that occurs from hypertension is related to

   a. increased fluid pressure exerted against organ tissue.
   b. atherosclerotic changes in vessels that supply the organs.
   c. erosion and thinning of blood vessels from constant pressure.
   d. increased hydrostatic pressure causing leakage of plasma into organ interstitial spaces.

10. The organ that is damaged most directly as a result of high systemic vascular resistance is the

    a. brain.
    b. heart.
    c. retina.
    d. kidney.

11. Identify the significance of the following lab results found in patients with hypertension.

    a. BUN 48 mg/dl (17.1 mmol/L); creatinine 4.3 mg/dl (380 μmol/L)

    b. Serum K^+ 3.1 mEq/L (3.1 mmol/L)

    c. FBS 183 mg/dl (10.2 mmol/L)

    d. Serum uric acid 9.2 mg/dl (547 μmol/L)

    e. Low-density lipoproteins (LDL) 154 mg/dl (4.0 mmol/L)

12. A 42-year-old male patient has been diagnosed with essential hypertension with an average blood pressure of 162/92 on three consecutive clinic visits. What are four lifestyle modifications that may be indicated in the initial treatment of the patient?

a.

b.

c.

d.

13. A patient does not respond to treatment of stage 2 hypertension with lifestyle modifications within 1 year. Initial drug therapy that would be indicated for the patient includes

a. a thiazide diuretic.
b. a β-adrenergic blocker and an ACE inhibitor.
c. a loop diuretic and a direct-acting vasodilator.
d. a calcium channel blocker and an α-adrenergic blocker.

14. Match the following primary effects in reducing blood pressure with the classifications of drugs used to treat hypertension.

_____ a. Decrease extracellular fluid volume by decreasing Na^+ and water reabsorption in loop of Henle and distal tubule

_____ b. Decrease cardiac output by decreasing rate and strength of heart and decreasing renin secretion by kidney

_____ c. Act directly on smooth muscle of arterioles to cause vasodilation

_____ d. Cause vasodilation of arterioles by blocking movement of calcium into cells

_____ e. Decrease Na^+ and water reabsorption by blocking effect of aldosterone

_____ f. Block peripheral a-adrenergic receptors to cause arteriole and venous dilation

_____ g. Cause vasodilation by inhibiting sympathetic outflow from CNS

_____ h. Interfere with enzyme conversion necessary for production of angiotension II

1. Central adrenergic antagonists
2. Spironolactone
3. ACE inhibitors
4. Thiazide diuretics
5. β-adrenergic blockers
6. Calcium channel blockers
7. α-adrenergic blockers
8. Direct vasodilators

15. Teaching to include dietary sources of potassium is indicated for the hypertensive patient taking

a. enalapril (Vasotec).
b. labetalol (Normodyne).
c. spironolactone (Aldactone).
d. hydrochlorothiazide (HydroDiuril).

16. A patient with stage 3 hypertension taking hydrochlorothiazide (HydroDiuril) and lisinopril (Prinivil) has prazosin (Minipress) added to the medication regimen. It is most important for the nurse to teach the patient to

    a. weigh every morning to monitor for fluid retention.
    b. change position slowly and avoid prolonged standing.
    c. use sugarless gum or candy to help relieve dry mouth.
    d. take the pulse daily to note any slowing of the heart rate.

17. A 38-year-old man is treated for hypertension with amiloride/hydrochlorothiazide (Maxide) and metaprolol (Lopressor). Four months after his last clinic visit, his blood pressure returns to pretreatment levels and he admits he has not been taking his medication regularly. The best response by the nurse is

    a. "Try to always take your medication when you carry out another daily routine so you do not forget to take it."
    b. "If you would exercise more and stop smoking you probably would not need to be on medications for hypertension."
    c. "The drugs you are taking cause sexual dysfunction in many patients. Are you experiencing any problems in this area?"
    d. "You need to remember that hypertension can only be controlled with medication, not cured, and you must always take your medication."

18. When teaching a patient for whom clonidine (Catapres) has been prescribed, the nurse stresses that

    a. the drug should never be stopped abruptly.
    b. the drug should be taken early in the day to prevent nocturia.
    c. the first dose should be taken when the patient is in bed for the night.
    d. aspirin will decrease the drug's effectiveness and acetaminophen should be substituted for aspirin use.

19. The correct technique for blood pressure measurements includes

    a. always taking the blood pressure in both arms.
    b. releasing the pressure in the cuff at a rate of 1 mm Hg per second.
    c. inflating the cuff 10 mm Hg higher than the expected systolic pressure.
    d. taking additional readings if the first two readings differ more than 5 mm Hg.

20. A patient's blood pressure has not responded consistently to the prescribed medications for hypertension. The first cause of this lack of responsiveness the nurse should explore is

    a. progressive target organ damage.
    b. the possibility of drug interactions.
    c. the patient not adhering to therapy.
    d. the patient's possible use of recreational drugs.

21. A patient would be diagnosed with a hypertensive emergency when experiencing

    a. a systolic BP >200 mm Hg and a diastolic BP >120 mm Hg.
    b. a sudden rise in BP accompanied by neurologic impairment.
    c. symptoms of a cerebrovascular accident (CVA) with an elevated BP.
    d. a severe elevation of the blood pressure that occurs over several days or weeks.

22. Drugs that are most commonly used to treat hypertensive crises include

    a. labetalol (Normodyne) and diazoxide (Hyperstat).
    b. hydralazine (Apresoline) and captopril (Catapres).
    c. nitroglycerin (Tridil) and sodium nitroprusside (Nipride).
    d. intravenous enalaprilat (Vasotec) and minoxidil (Loniten).

23. During treatment of hypertensive emergencies with intravenous vasodilators, the initial goal of therapy is to

    a. lower the BP sufficiently to prevent target organ damage.
    b. decrease the BP to a normal level for the age of the patient.
    c. decrease the mean arterial pressure 10-20% in the first 1 to 2 hours.
    d. reduce the systolic BP to 150 mm Hg and the diastolic BP to 90 mm Hg as quickly as possible.

24. A nursing responsibility in the management of the patient with a hypertensive urgency often includes

    a. monitoring hourly urine output for drug effectiveness.
    b. providing for continuous ECG monitoring to detect side effects of the drugs.
    c. titrating intravenous drug dosages based on BP measurements every 2 to 3 minutes.
    d. instructing the patient to follow up with a health care professional 24 hours after outpatient treatment.

CASE STUDY

ISOLATED SYSTOLIC HYPERTENSION

Patient Profile

Mrs. J. is a 73-year-old white woman with no history of hypertension. She came to the doctor's office for a flu shot.

Subjective Data

- Says she has gained 20 pounds over the past year since her husband died
- Has never smoked and uses no alcohol
- Only medication is one multivitamin per day
- Eats a lot of canned food
- Does not exercise

Objective Data

- Height 64 in (162.6 cm); weight 170 lb (77.1 kg)
- BP 170/82 mm Hg
- Physical exam shows no abnormalities
- Serum potassium 3.3 mEq/L (3.3 mmol/L)

The physician diagnosed isolated systolic hypertension (ISH) and prescribed lifestyle modifications.

Critical Thinking Questions

1. What contributing factors to the development of ISH are present?

2. What additional risk factors are present?

3. What specific dietary changes would the nurse recommend for Mrs. J.?

4. What other teaching should be instituted by the nurse?

5. If drug therapy became necessary to treat Mrs. J.'s hypertension, what diuretic would be indicated on her laboratory results?

6. Based on the assessment data presented, write one or more appropriate nursing diagnoses. Are there any collaborative problems?

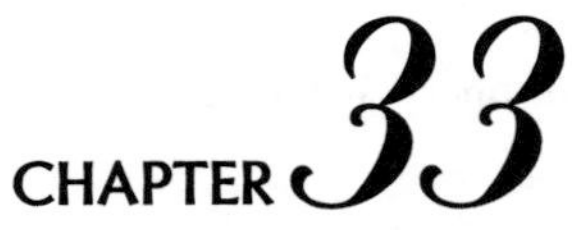

NURSING MANAGEMENT: CORONARY ARTERY DISEASE AND ACUTE CORONARY SYNDROME

1. Identify the three stages of lesions that occur in the development of coronary artery disease and the ages at which the stages are present.

	Stage	Age
a.		
b.		
c.		

2. Identify whether the following statements are true or false. If a statement is false, correct the bold word(s) to make the statement true.

_____ a. The leading theory of atherogenesis proposes that **aging** is the basic underlying cause of athero sclerosis.

_____ b. Endothelial alteration may be caused by chemical irritants such as **hyperlipidemia** or by **hypertension**.

_____ c. New findings indicate that certain **bacterial or viral infections** may damage the endothelium and contribute to the development of atherosclerosis.

_____ d. During development of the raised fibrous plaque, arterial wall changes may be initiated by **carbon monoxide produced by smoking**.

_____ e. Partial or total occlusion of the coronary artery occurs during the stage of **raised fibrous plaque**.

_____ f. Collateral circulation in the coronary circulation is more likely to be present in the **young** patient with CAD.

3. List the three most significant risk factors for atherosclerosis and indicate whether these risk factors are modifiable or unmodifiable.

a.

b.

c.

4. While taking nursing histories of patients, the nurse identifies that the patient with the highest risk for coronary artery disease is the patient who is

a. an African-American man, age 65, with obesity and a BP of 160/85.
b. a Caucasian man, age 54, who is a smoker and has a stressful lifestyle.
c. an Asian woman, age 45, with a cholesterol level of 240 mg/dl and a BP of 130/75.
d. a Caucasian woman, age 72, with a BP of 172/100 and who is physically inactive.

5. Match the following characteristics with their associated lipoproteins (answers may be used more than once).

_____ a. Contains most of the triglycerides
_____ b. Specific marker for cholesterol-depositing capacity of the blood
_____ c. Contains the most cholesterol
_____ d. The higher the level, the lower the risk for CAD
_____ e. Carries lipids away from arteries to liver
_____ f. Increases are associated with obesity
_____ g. Increases with exercise
_____ h. Genetically inherited lipoprotein that contributes to blood clot formation
_____ i. High levels correlate most closely with CAD
_____ j. Specific marker for cholesterol-clearing capacity of the blood
_____ k. Has an affinity for arterial walls

1. HDL
2. LDL
3. VLDL
4. Apolipoprotein A-1
5. Apolipoprotein B
6. Lipoprotein (a)

6. Identify the desirable levels of the following serum lipoproteins.

a. Total cholesterol ______________________________

b. Triglycerides ___________________________

c. LDL ___________________________

d. HDL ___________________________

7. The nurse is encouraging a sedentary patient with major risks for CAD to perform physical exercise on a regular basis. In addition to decreasing the risk factor of physical inactivity, the nurse tells the patient that exercise will also directly contribute to reducing the risk factors of

a. hyperlipidemia and obesity.
b. diabetes mellitus and hypertension.
c. elevated serum lipids and stressful lifestyle.
d. hypertension and elevated serum homocysteine.

8. Two risk factors for CAD that are considered to increase the workload of the heart and increase myocardial oxygen demand include

a. hypertension and elevated serum lipids.
b. cigarette smoking and diabetes mellitus.
c. cigarette smoking and physical inactivity.
d. type A behavior pattern and hypertension.

9. During a routine health examination, a 48-year-old man is found to have a total cholesterol level of 224 mg/dl (5.8 mmol/L) and an LDL level of 140 (3.6 mmol/L). The nurse teaches the patient that a Step 1 dietary change should include

   a. use of skim or 1% milk.
   b. elimination of red meat from the diet.
   c. elimination of alcohol and use of simple sugars.
   d. avoidance of all egg yolks and food prepared with whole eggs.

10. A 62-year-old woman has hypertension and smokes 1 pack of cigarettes per day. She has no symptoms of CAD, but a recent LDL level is 154 mg/dl (3.98 mmol/L). Based on these findings, the nurse would expect that treatment for the patient would include

    a. diet therapy only.
    b. drug therapy only.
    c. diet and drug therapy.
    d. exercise instruction only.

11. A patient with CAD has a total cholesterol of 280 mg/dl (7.24 mmol/L), LDL of 140 mg/dl (3.62 mmol/L), and a triglyceride level of 340 mg/dl (3.84 mmol/L). The nurse recognizes that an antilipemic drug that would be indicated for the patient is

    a. gemfibrozil (Lopid).
    b. lovastatin (Mevacor).
    c. nicotinic acid (niacin).
    d. cholestyramine (Questran).

12. Complete the following sentences.

    a. When myocardial ischemia is temporary and reversible, the condition is called

       ________________________________.

    b. The three conditions that are included as manifestations of acute coronary syndrome are

       ______________________, ______________________, and ________________________________.

    c. When myocardial cells die as a result of ischemia, the area of cellular necrosis is known as an

       ________________.

13. Use the following terms to complete the statements:

    increased oxygen demand
    decreased oxygen supply

    a. Myocardial ischemia occurs as a result of two factors: ______________________ and ______________________.

    b. Any factor that increases cardiac workload causes ______________________.

    c. Narrowing of coronary arteries by atherosclerosis is the primary reason for ______________________.

    d. Chronic dilation of coronary arteries below an obstruction area results in ______________________.

    e. Low blood volume or a decreased hemoglobin leads to ______________________.

    f. Left ventricular hypertrophy caused by chronic hypertension leads to ______________________.

    g. Sympathetic nervous system stimulation by drugs, emotions, or exertion constricts blood vessels and increases heart rate, resulting in ______________________.

    h. In the patient with atherosclerotic coronary arteries, anything that causes ______________________ may precipitate angina.

14. Angina pectoris, the pain, most likely occurs with myocardial ischemia as a result of

    a. death of myocardial tissue.
    b. arrhythmias caused by cellular irritability.
    c. lactic acid accumulation during anaerobic metabolism.
    d. elevated pressure in the ventricles and pulmonary vessels.

15. Tachycardia that is a response of the sympathetic nervous system to the pain of ischemia is detrimental because not only does it increase oxygen demand, but it

    a. decreases cardiac output.
    b. causes reflex hypotension.
    c. may lead to ventricular arrhythmias.
    d. impairs perfusion of the coronary arteries.

16. The patient's cardiac catheterization report reveals a 95% blockage of the left anterior descending artery. The patient is at greatest risk for an infarction of the

    a. lateral wall.
    b. inferior wall.
    c. anterior wall.
    d. posterior wall.

17. The point in the healing process of the myocardium following an infarct where early scar tissue results in an unstable heart wall is

a. 2 to 3 days after MI.
b. 4 to 10 days after MI.
c. 10 to 14 days after MI.
d. 6 weeks after MI.

18. Match the following types of angina with their characteristics (answers may be used more than once).

_____	a. Occurs only when the person is recumbent	1. Silent ischemia
_____	b. Usually precipitated by exertion	2. Prinzmetal's angina
_____	c. Unpredictable and unrelieved by rest	3. Stable angina
_____	d. Prevalent in persons with diabetes	4. Noctural angina
_____	e. Characterized by progressive severity	5. Unstable angina
_____	f. Occurs with same pattern of onset, duration, and intensity	6. Angina decubitus
_____	g. Asymptomatic myocardial ischemia	
_____	h. Usually occurs in response to coronary artery spasm	
_____	i. Occurs only at night	
_____	j. May occur in the absence of coronary artery disease	

19. As an acute coronary syndrome, unstable angina must be identified and treated because

a. the pain may be severe and disabling.
b. ECG changes and arrhythmias may occur during an attack.
c. atherosclerotic plaque deterioration may cause complete thrombus of the vessel lumen.
d. the spasm of a major coronary artery may cause total occlusion of the vessel with progression to MI.

20. The nurse stable suspects angina rather than myocardial infarction pain in the patient who reports chest pain that

a. is relieved by nitroglycerin.
b. is a sensation of tightness or squeezing.
c. does not radiate to the neck, back, or arms.
d. is precipitated by physical or emotional exertion.

21. A patient admitted to the hospital for evaluation of chest pain has normal cardiac enzyme values 4 hours after the onset of pain. A noninvasive diagnostic test that can differentiate angina from other types of chest pain is a(n)

a. ECG.
b. exercise stress test.
c. coronary angiogram.
d. transesophageal echocardiogram.

22. A 52-year-old man is admitted to the emergency department with severe chest pain. The nurse suspects an MI upon finding that the patient

    a. has pale, cool, clammy skin.
    b. reports nausea and vomited once at home.
    c. is anxious and has a feeling of impending doom.
    d. has had no relief of the pain with rest or position change.

23. To detect and treat the most common complication of MI, the nurse

    a. measures hourly urine output.
    b. auscultates the chest for crackles.
    c. uses continuous cardiac monitoring.
    d. takes vital signs q2hr for the first 8 hours.

24. Match the following complications of MI with the clinical manifestations that commonly indicate its occurrence.

4	a. Congestive heart failure	1. Intractable arrhythmias and CHF
5	b. Cardiogenic shock	2. Systolic murmur at the cardiac apex radiation toward the axilla
2	c. Papillary muscle dysfunction	3. Persistent or intermittent pericardial friction rub
1	d. Ventricular aneurysm	4. Crackles in lungs and S_3 or S_4 heart sound
3	e. Pericarditis	5. Decreased cardiac output with falling BP

25. In the patient with an acute MI, the nurse would expect diagnostic testing to reveal

    a. ECG changes at the onset of the pain.
    b. an enlarged heart with distended upper lobe veins.
    c. CK-MB enzyme elevations that peak 24 hours after the infarct.
    d. the appearance of troponin in the blood 48 hours after the infarct.

26. A second 12-lead ECG performed on a patient 4 hours after the onset of chest pain reveals ST-segment elevation. The nurse recognizes that this finding indicates a

    a. transient ischemia typical of unstable angina.
    b. lack of permanent damage to myocardial cells.
    c. myocardial infarction associated with prolonged and complete coronary thrombosis.
    d. myocardial infarction associated with transient or incomplete coronary artery occlusion.

27. The following are effects of drugs used to prevent and treat angina. Identify the classes of the drugs that are used to promote these effects.

    a. Decrease preload

    b. Dilate coronary arteries

    c. Prevent thrombosis of plaques

    d. Decrease heart rate

    e. Decrease afterload

    f. Decrease myocardial contractility

28. When teaching the patient with angina about taking nitroglycerin tablets, the nurse instructs the patient

    a. to take the tablet with a large amount of water so it will dissolve right away.
    b. to lie or sit down and place one tablet under the tongue when chest pain occurs.
    c. that if one tablet does not relieve the pain in 15 minutes the patient should go to the hospital.
    d. that if the tablet causes dizziness and a headache the medication should be stopped and the doctor notified.

29. A strategy used to prevent the development of tolerance to the effects of transdermal nitrates includes

    a. removing the patch during the night.
    b. changing the sites of the patch every day.
    c. using the patch only when chest pain occurs.
    d. applying the patch on an alternate-day schedule.

30. Match the following descriptions with the procedures used to treat CAD (answers may be used more than once).

	Description		Procedure
_____	a. Allows for dissolution of arterial plaques		1. Percutaneous transluminal coronary angioplasty (PTCA)
_____	b. Surgical construction of new vessels to carry blood beyond obstructed coronary artery		2. Stent placement
			3. Atherectomy
_____	c. Requires anticoagulation following the procedure		4. Laser angioplasty
_____	d. Most common alternative to CABG		5. Coronary artery bypass graft (CABG)
_____	e. Structure applied to hold vessels open		
_____	f. Use limited to lesions in proximal and middle portion of vessel		
_____	g. Laser-created channels between left ventricular		
_____	h. Recommended for patients with poor response to treatment of unstable angina		
_____	i. Removal of plaque with a rotating cutter		
_____	j. Compression of artherosclerotic plaque with a balloon		

31. The nurse explains to the patient who is to undergo a coronary artery bypass graft that the procedure may involve bypassing stenosed coronary arteries by

    a. using a synthetic graft as a conduit for blood flow from the aorta to a coronary artery distal to an obstruction.
    b. resecting a stenosed coronary artery and inserting a synthetic arterial tube graft to replace the diseased artery.
    c. removing the internal mammary artery and anastomosing it from the aorta to a coronary artery distal to a stenosis.
    d. anastomosing reversed segments of a saphenous vein from the aorta to the coronary artery distal to an obstruction.

32. A patient with a previous CABG operation is scheduled for a coronary revascularization using the inferior epigastric artery. The nurse recognizes that this surgery has a higher mortality risk than the usual revascularization procedure primarily because

    a. arterial grafts have a higher rate of restenosis and occlusion than vein grafts.
    b. the need for a laparotomy to access the artery increases the length of the surgery.
    c. this artery does not provide as great a blood supply to the myocardium as other grafts.
    d. use of cardiopulmonary bypass is necessary during arterial graft procedures but not for vein grafts.

33. Collaborative care of the patient with NSTEMI differs from that of a patient with STEMI in that NSTEMI is more frequently treated with

    a. acute intensive drug therapy.
    b. reperfusion therapy with fibrinolytics.
    c. a coronary artery bypass graft (CABG).
    d. percutaneous coronary intervention (PCI).

34. Fibrinolytic therapy is initiated for a patient with a STEMI. The nurse explains to the patient that this treatment is performed to

    a. prevent the development of life-threatening arrhythmias.
    b. prevent the development of further clotting in the coronary arteries.
    c. assist ventricular contraction and promote coronary artery perfusion.
    d. dissolve the clot in the coronary artery and prevent further cellular death.

35. The nurse recognizes that fibrinolytic therapy for the treatment of an MI has not been successful when the patient

    a. continues to have chest pain.
    b. develops major GI or GU bleeding during treatment.
    c. has a marked increase in CK enzyme levels within 3 hours of the therapy.
    d. develops premature ventricular contractions and ventricular tachycardia during treatment.

36. Match the following characteristics with the drugs used to treat myocardial infarction.

_____ a. Controls ventricular arrythmias
_____ b. Relieves pain by decreasing O_2 demand and increasing O_2 supply
_____ c. Helps prevent ventricular remodeling
_____ d. Relieves anxiety and cardiac workload
_____ e. Associated with decreased reinfarction and increased survival
_____ f. Minimizes bradycardia from vagal stimulation

1. Beta-adrenergic blockers
2. IV morphine
3. Stool softeners
4. IV amiodarone (Cordarone)
5. IV nitroglycerin
6. ACE inhibitors

37. Listed below are classes of drugs that may be used in a variety of situations and combinations to prevent or treat thrombus formation in the coronary arteries. Identify one specific use of each of the agents.

a. Aspirin

b. Glycoprotein (GP) IIB/IIIA inhibitors (abciximab, eptifibatide, tirofiban)

c. Direct thrombin inhibitors (bivalirudin, lepirudin, hirudin)

d. Adenosine diphosphate (ADP) receptor antagonists (ticlopidine, clopidogrel)

38. A patient with an MI has a nursing diagnosis of anxiety related to possible lifestyle changes and perceived threat of death. The nurse determines that outcome criteria have been met when the patient states

a. "I'm just going to take this recovery one step at a time."
b. "I feel much better and am ready to get on with my life."
c. "How soon do you think I will be able to go back to work?"
d. "I know you are doing everything possible to save my life."

39. A patient hospitalized for evaluation of unstable angina experiences severe chest pain and calls the nurse. List six interventions the nurse should implement in addressing the patient's pain.

a.

b.

c.

d.

e.

f.

40. Indicate what emotional responses (denial, anger, etc.) to acute MI are indicated by the following statements by patients.

    a. "I don't think I can take care of myself at home yet."

    b. "What's going to happen if I have another heart attack?"

    c. "I'll never be able to enjoy life again."

    d. "I hope my wife is happy now after harping at me about my eating habits all these years."

    e. "Yes, I'm having a little chest pain. It's no big deal."

41. The nurse and patient set a patient outcome that at the time of discharge after an MI the patient will be able to tolerate moderate-energy activities similar to

    a. golfing.
    b. walking at 5 mph.
    c. cycling at 13 mph.
    d. mowing the lawn by hand.

42. When teaching the patient who has had an MI about cardiac rehabilitation, the nurse recognizes that the phase of rehabilitation when a routine exercise program should be started is

    a. phase I.
    b. phase II.
    c. phase III.
    d. phase IV.

43. A 58-year-old patient is in a cardiac rehabilitation program. The nurse teaches the patient to stop exercising if

    a. the heart rate exceeds 150 beats/min.
    b. the patient develops pain or dyspnea.
    c. the respiratory rate increases to 30 beats/min.
    d. the heart rate is 30 beats over the resting heart rate.

44. In counseling the patient about sexual activity following an MI, the nurse

    a. should wait for the patient to ask about resuming sexual activity.
    b. may discuss sexual activity while teaching about other physical activity.
    c. should have the patient ask the physician when sexual activity can be resumed.
    d. should inform the patient that impotence is a common long-term complication following MI.

45. The nurse advises the patient who has had an MI that during sexual activity

    a. orogenital sex should be avoided.
    b. the patient should use the superior position.
    c. foreplay may cause too great an increase in heart rate.
    d. prophylactic nitroglycerin may be used if angina occurs.

46. Sudden cardiac death in persons with CAD occurs most often as a result of

    a. an acute MI.
    b. heart trauma.
    c. cardiac arrhythmias.
    d. primary left ventricular outflow obstruction.

47. Clinical manifestations in the older adult that would alert the nurse to the possibility of acute MI include

    a. diaphoresis and nausea.
    b. back and abdominal pain.
    c. tachycardia and elevated BP.
    d. dyspnea and profound weakness.

48. When teaching an older adult with CAD how to manage the treatment program for angina, the nurse instructs the patient

    a. to sit for 3 to 5 minutes before standing when getting out of bed.
    b. to exercise only twice a week to avoid unnecessary strain on the heart.
    c. that lifestyle changes are not as necessary as they would be in a younger person.
    d. that aspirin therapy is contraindicated in older adults because of the risk for bleeding.

49. While teaching women about the risks and incidence of CAD, the nurse stresses that

    a. women have an increased incidence of sudden death compared with men.
    b. smoking is not as significant a risk factor for CAD in women as it is in men.
    c. estrogen replacement therapy in postmenopausal women decreases the risk for CAD.
    d. CAD is the leading cause of death in women, with a higher mortality rate following MI than men.

CASE STUDY

CORONARY ARTERY DISEASE

Patient Profile

Mrs. C., a 47-year-old Navajo woman, comes to the clinic with a burning sensation in her epigastric area extending into her sternum.

Subjective Data

- Has had chest pain with activity that is relieved with rest for the past 3 months
- Has had type 2 diabetes mellitus since she was 35
- Has a 27 pack-year smoking history
- Is more than 30% over her ideal body weight
- Has no regular exercise program
- Expresses frustration with physical problems
- Is reluctant to get medical therapy because it will interfere with her life
- Has no health insurance

Objective Data

- Physical examination
  - Anxious, clutching fists
  - Appears overweight and withdrawn
- Diagnostic studies
  - Cholesterol 248 mg/dl (6.41mmol/L)
  - LDL 160 mg/dl (4.14 mmol/L)
  - Glucose 210 mg/dl (11.7 mmol/L)

Collaborative Care

- Nifedipine (Procardia) 10 mg tid
- Nitroglycerin 0.4 mg sublingual prn for chest pain
- Exercise treadmill testing

Critical Thinking Questions

1. What are Mrs. C.'s risk factors for CAD?

2. What nursing measures should be instituted to help her decrease her risk factors?

3. What symptoms would lead you to suspect the pain may be angina?

4. What kind of ECG changes would indicate myocardial ischemia?

5. What is the rationale for the use of the nifedipine?

6. What information should the nurse provide for Mrs. C. before the treadmill testing?

7. Based on the assessment data presented, write one or more appropriate nursing diagnoses. Are there any collaborative problems?

CHAPTER 34 NURSING MANAGEMENT: HEART FAILURE AND CARDIOMYOPATHY

1. Identify whether the following statements are true or false. If a statement is false, correct the bold word(s) to make the statement true.

_____ a. **Systolic failure** is characterized by abnormal resistance to ventricular filling.

_____ b. A primary risk factor for congestive heart failure is **coronary artery disease**.

_____ c. A common cause of diastolic failure is **left ventricular hypertrophy**.

_____ d. The mechanisms by which **hypervolemia** acts as a precipitating cause of heart failure include decreasing cardiac output and increasing the workload of oxygen requirements of the myocardium.

_____ e. Systolic heart failure results in a **normal** left ventricular ejection fraction.

2. Describe the primary ways in which each of the following compensatory mechanisms of congestive heart failure increases cardiac output, and identify at least one effect of the mechanism that is detrimental to cardiac function.

a. Cardiac dilation

↑ CO:

Detrimental effect:

b. Cardiac hypertrophy

↑ CO:

Detrimental effect:

c. Sympathetic nervous system stimulation

↑ CO:

Detrimental effect:

d. Neurohormonal response

(1) Renin-angiotensin system

↑ CO:

Detrimental effect:

(2) Atrial natriuretic peptide (ANP) and brain natriuretic peptide (BNP)

↑ CO:

Detrimental effect:

3. The following diagram illustrates the pathophysiology of left-sided heart failure that occurs from elevated systemic vascular resistance. Indicate the point in the process, by number, where the other causes of heart failure listed below the diagram (a–h) would most likely initiate the process.

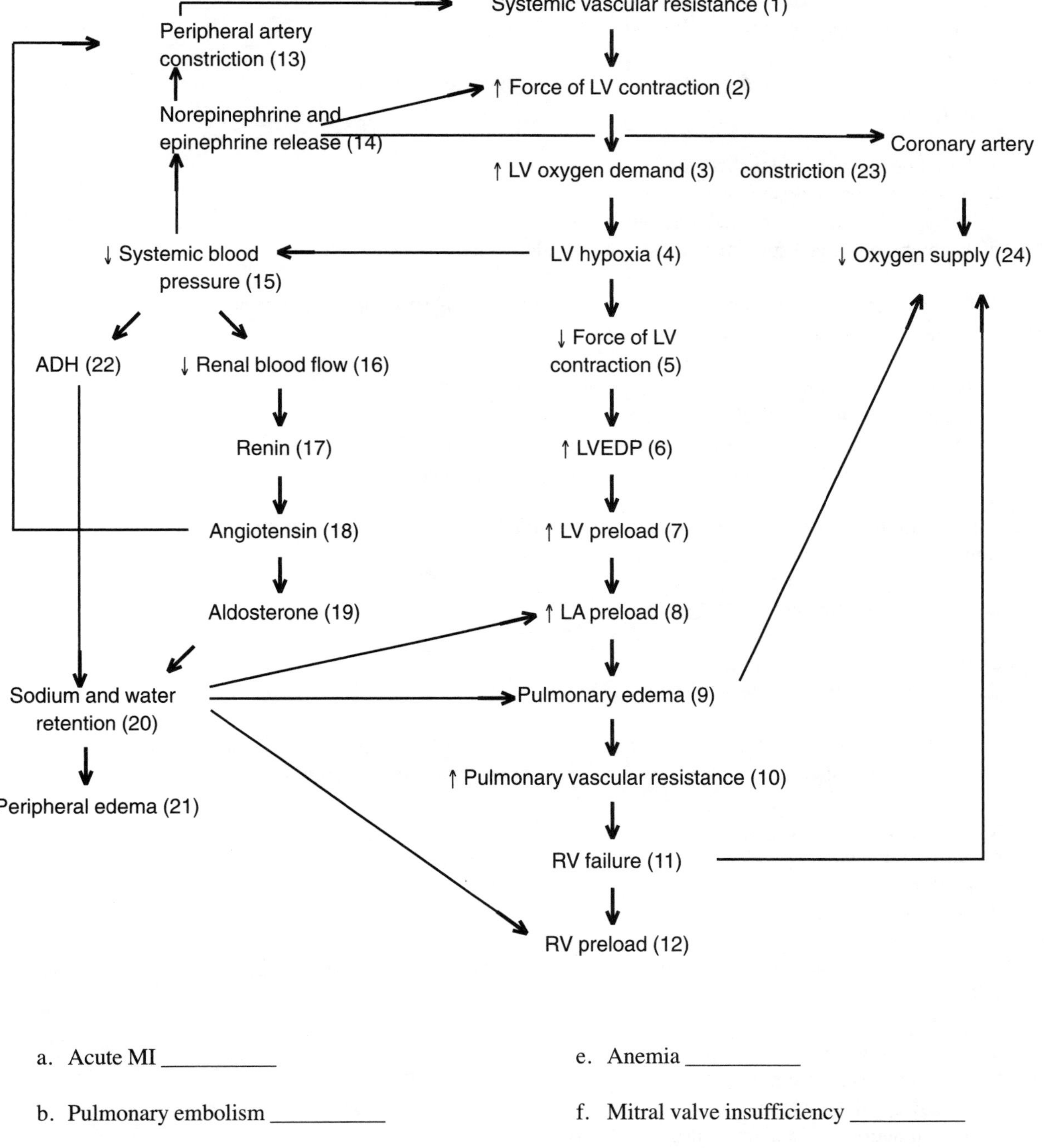

a. Acute MI __________

b. Pulmonary embolism __________

c. IV fluid overload __________

d. Severe hypothyroidism __________

e. Anemia __________

f. Mitral valve insufficiency __________

g. Cor pulmonale __________

h. Thyrotoxicosis __________

4. Using the diagram above, identify three points in the process, by number, where compensatory mechanisms enter the process: __________, __________, __________, __________.

5. The pathophysiologic mechanism that results in the pulmonary edema of left-sided heart failure is

   a. increased right ventricular preload.
   b. increased pulmonary hydrostatic pressure.
   c. impaired alveolar oxygen and carbon dioxide exchange.
   d. increased lymphatic flow of pulmonary extravascular fluid.

6. A physical assessment finding that the nurse would expect to be present in the patient with acute left-sided heart failure is

   a. bubbling crackles and tachycardia.
   b. hepatosplenomegaly and tachypnea.
   c. peripheral edema and cool, diaphoretic skin.
   d. frothy blood-tinged sputum and distended jugular veins.

7. The nurse assesses the patient with chronic biventricular congestive heart failure fo
   dyspnea by questioning the patient regarding

   a. frequent awakening to void during the night.
   b. the presence of a dry, hacking cough when resting.
   c. the presence of difficulty breathing when lying flat in bed.
   d. the use of two or more pillows to help breathing during sleep.

8. An indication that the patient with congestive heart failure is developing a complic
   failure is

   a. increased weight gain.
   b. development of ascites.
   c. restlessness and confusion.
   d. increased liver enzyme levels.

9. A patient with chronic congestive heart failure has atrial fibrillation and an LV eje
   decrease the risk of complications from these conditions, the nurse anticipates the

   a. diuretics.
   b. anticoagulants.
   c. β-adrenergic blockers.
   d. potassium supplements.

10. A diagnostic test that is most useful in assessing and monitoring the pulmonary effects of congestive heart failure is

    a. a chest x-ray.
    b. exercise stress testing.
    c. a cardiac catheterization.
    d. determination of blood urea nitrogen (BUN).

11. Using the diagram illustrated in question 4, indicate the point(s) in the process, by number, where the following treatment modalities are used to interrupt or reverse the pathophysiologic process of congestive heart failure.

a. Diuretics __________

b. IV nitroglycerin __________

c. IV nitroprusside __________

d. Oxygen therapy __________

e. ACE inhibitors __________

f. Digitalis __________

g. Amrinone (Inocor) __________

12. Match the following drugs used in the treatment of acute and chronic congestive heart failure with their therapeutic effects.

a. Spironolactone (Aldactone)
b. IV nitroglycerin
c. Digoxin (Lanoxin)
d. Furosemide (Lasix)
e. IV nitroprusside (Nipride)
f. Enalapril (Vasotec)
g. Dopamine (Intropin)
h. Milrinone (Primacor)
i. IV morphine
j. Carvedilol (Coreg)
k. Nesiritide (Natrecor)

1. Improves cardiac contractions, decreases afterload, and increases cardiac output
2. Dilates arterial and venous blood vessels in addition to relieving anxiety
3. Recombinant form of a natriuretic peptide that decreases preload and afterload
4. Primarily reduces preload and increases myocardial oxygen supply
5. Directly blocks sympathetic nervous system's negative effects on the failing heart
6. Potent vasodilator that decreases both preload and afterload, increasing cardiac contractility and output
7. Decreases afterload by reducing levels of angiotensin II and aldosterone
8. Primary effect is to decrease intravascular fluid volume, thus decreasing preload and improving left ventricular function
9. Increases cardiac contractility but may increase ventricular irritability
10. Increases cardiac contractility and output and slows heart rate
11. Blocks action of aldosterone, decreasing intravascular volume by sodium excretion, but retains potassium

13. A patient with chronic congestive heart failure is treated with hydrochlorothiazide, digoxin, and lisinopril (Prinivil). To prevent the risk of digitalis toxicity with these drugs, it is most important that the nurse monitor the patient's

    a. heart rate.
    b. blood pressure.
    c. potassium levels.
    d. gastrointestinal function.

14. The physician prescribes spironolactone (Aldactone) for the patient with chronic congestive heart failure. Diet modifications related to the use of this drug that the nurse includes in patient teaching include

    a. decreasing both sodium and potassium intake.
    b. increasing calcium intake and decreasing sodium intake.
    c. decreasing sodium intake and increasing potassium intake.
    d. decreasing sodium intake and using salt substitutes for seasoning.

15. The nurse monitors the patient receiving treatment for acute congestive heart failure with the knowledge that marked hypotension is most likely to occur with the intravenous administration of

    a. furosemide (Lasix).
    b. milrinone (Primacor).
    c. nitroglycerin (Tridil).
    d. nitroprusside (Nipride).

16. A 2,400 mg sodium diet is prescribed for a patient with chronic congestive heart failure. The nurse recognizes that additional teaching is necessary when the patient states

    a. "I should limit my milk intake to 2 cups a day."
    b. "I can eat fresh fruits and vegetables without worrying about sodium content."
    c. "I can eat most foods as long as I do not add salt when cooking or at the table."
    d. "I need to read the labels on prepared foods and medicines for their sodium content."

17. List four heart conditions that may lead to congestive heart failure and what can be done to prevent the development of congestive heart failure in each condition.

    a.

    b.

    c.

    d.

18. The nurse determines that treatment of congestive heart failure has been successful when the patient experiences

    a. weight loss and diuresis.
    b. warm skin and less fatigue.
    c. clear lung sounds and decreased heart rate.
    d. absence of chest pain and improved level of consciousness.

19. A patient with CHF has tachypnea, severe dyspnea and a SpO_2 of 84%. The nurse identifies a nursing diagnosis of impaired gas exchange related to increased preload and mechanical failure. An appropriate nursing intervention for this diagnosis is

    a. assist the patient to cough and deep breath q2h.
    b. assess intake and output q8hr and weigh patient daily.
    c. encourage alternate rest and activity periods to reduce cardiac workload.
    d. place the patient in a high Fowler's position with the feet dangling over the bedside.

20. The nurse determines that additional discharge teaching is needed when the patient with chronic congestive heart failure says,

    a. "I should hold my digitalis and call the doctor if I experience nausea and vomiting."
    b. "I will take my pulse every day and call the clinic if it is irregular or is less than 50."
    c. "I plan to organize my household tasks so I don't have to constantly go up and down the stairs."
    d. "I should weigh myself every morning and go on a diet if I gain more than 2 or 3 pounds in 2 days."

21. Indicate whether the following characteristics of cardiomyopathies are associated with dilated cardiomyopathy (D), hypertrophic cardiomyopathy (H), or restrictive cardiomyopathy (R).

    _____ a. The hyperdynamic systolic function creates a diastolic failure

    _____ b. Systemic embolization may occur because of stasis of blood in the ventricles

    _____ c. The most uncommon type of cardiomyopathy

    _____ d. Has a good prognosis with heart transplant

    _____ e. Autosomal dominant genetic relationship

    _____ f. Differs from chronic congestive heart failure in that there is no ventricular hypertrophy

    _____ g. Echocardiogram reveals cardiomegaly with thin ventricular walls

    _____ h. Often results in syncope during increased activity due to obstructed aortic valve outflow

    _____ i. Often follows an infective myocarditis or exposure to toxins or drugs

    _____ j. Surgery to remove myocardial tissue may be indicated for symptoms refractory to treatment

    _____ k. Characterized by ventricular stiffness

    _____ l. Characterized by massive thickening of intraventricular septum and ventricular wall

22. When performing discharge teaching for the patient with any type of cardiomyopathy, the nurse instructs the patient to

    a. abstain from all alcohol intake.
    b. avoid strenuous activity and allow for periods of rest.
    c. restrict fluids to prevent volume overload and to decrease cardiac workload.
    d. plan for periodic returns to the health care facility for intermittent dobutamine (Dobutrex) or milrinone (Primacor) infusions.

23. The evaluation team for cardiac transplantation determines that the patient who would most benefit from a new heart is

    a. a 24-year-old man with Down syndrome who has received excellent care from parents in their 60s.
    b. a 46-year-old single woman with a limited support system who has alcohol-induced cardiomyopathy.
    c. a 60-year-old man with inoperable coronary artery disease who has not been compliant with lifestyle changes and rehabilitation programs.
    d. a 52-year-old woman with end-stage coronary artery disease who has limited financial resources but is emotionally stable and has strong social support.

24. The nurse plans long-term goals for the patient who has had a heart transplant with the knowledge that the most common cause of death in heart transplant patients is

    a. rejection.
    b. infection.
    c. heart failure.
    d. embolization.

CASE STUDY

DILATED CARDIOMYOPATHY

Patient Profile

Mr. J. is a 43-year-old man who had an onset of flu with fever, pharyngitis, and malaise. Six days later he developed diffuse pericardial chest pain, jugular vein distention, dyspnea, and peripheral edema and was admitted to the hospital with a diagnosis of infectious myocarditis and possible dilated cardiomyopathy (CMP).

Subjective Data

- Has no history of cardiovascular disease
- Is very anxious and asks whether he is going to die
- Says his heart feels like it is "running away"
- Reports that he is so exhausted he can't eat or drink by himself

Objective Data

- Height 5 ft 10 in (175 cm); weight 180 lb (81.8 kg)
- Vital signs: T 99.6° F (37.6° C), HR 118 and irregular, RR 34, BP 90/58
- Cardiovascular: Distant S_1, S_2; S_3, S_4 present; PMI at sixth ICS and faint; all peripheral pulses are 1+; bilateral jugular vein distention; initial cardiac monitoring indicates a ventricular rate of 132 and atrial fibrillation
- Respiratory: Pulmonary crackles; decreased breath sounds right lower lobe; SpO_2 82%
- Gastrointestinal: BS present; hepatomegaly 4 cm below costal margin

Laboratory work and diagnostic testing are scheduled.

Critical Thinking Questions

1. What signs and symptoms of right and left heart failure is Mr. J. experiencing?

2. What difference in the ventricles is present in dilated cardiomyopathy as compared with congestive heart failure?

3. What diagnostic procedures and findings would help establish a diagnosis of dilated cardiomyopathy?

4. What nursing interventions are appropriate for Mr. J. at the time of his admission?

5. Drug therapy is started for Mr. J. to control his symptoms. What is the rationale for the administration of each of the following?

   a. digoxin (Lanoxin)

   b. furosemide (Lasix)

   c. milrinone (Primacor)

   d. enalapril (Vasotec)

   e. metoprolol (Lopressor)

6. Mr. J. does not respond well to treatment, and his condition deteriorates. Are there any alternative treatments for him?

7. Based on the assessment data presented, write one or more appropriate nursing diagnoses for Mr. J. Are there any collaborative problems?

CHAPTER 35 NURSING MANAGEMENT: ARRHYTHMIAS

1. Identify whether the following statements are true or false. If a statement is false, correct the bold word(s) to make the statement true.

_____ a. During **repolarization** of cardiac cells, sodium migrates rapidly into the cell, making the cell positive compared with the outside of the cell.

_____ b. Depolarization of the cells in the ventricles produces the **T wave** on the ECG.

_____ c. A patient with a regular heart rate has four QRS complexes between every 3-second marker on the ECG paper. The patient's heart rate is **40 beats/min**.

_____ d. The ECG pattern of a patient with a regular heart rate reveals 20 small squares between each R-R interval. The patient's heart rate is **75 beats/min**.

_____ e. For cardiac monitor with a lead II, the **positive** electrode is placed on the upper right chest and the **negative** electrode is placed on the lower left chest.

_____ f. Lead placement for MCL_1 monitoring is the positive electrode at the **fourth intercostal space at the right sternal border** and the negative electrode at the **left midclavicular line just below the clavicle**.

_____ g. If the SA node fails to discharge an impulse, or discharges very slowly, a secondary pacemaker in the AV node is able to discharge at a rate of **30 to 40** times a minute.

_____ h. **Reentrant excitation** causing premature beats may occur when areas of the heart do not repolarize at the same rate because of depressed conduction.

_____ i. An abnormal cardiac impulse that arises in the atria, ventricles, or AV junction that creates a premature beat is known as an **artifact**.

2. Match the following terms with their definitions.

_____ a. Contractibility

_____ b. Conductivity

_____ c. Excitability

_____ d. Automaticity

_____ e. Ectopic foci

_____ f. Refractoriness

1. Ability to spontaneously discharge an electrical impulse
2. Abnormal electrical impulses
3. Period in which heart tissue cannot be stimulated
4. Ability to respond mechanically to an impulse
5. Property of myocardial tissue that enables it to be depolarized by an impulse
6. Ability to transmit an impulse along a membrane

3. The patient's PR interval comprises six small boxes on the ECG graph. The nurse determines that this indicates

   a. a normal finding.
   b. a problem with ventricular depolarization.
   c. a disturbance in the repolarization of the atria.
   d. a problem with conduction from the SA node to the ventricular cells.

4. The nurse plans close monitoring for the patient who has undergone electrophysiologic testing because this test

   a. requires the use of dyes that irritate the myocardium.
   b. causes myocardial ischemia resulting in arrhythmias.
   c. induces arrhythmias that may require defibrillation to correct.
   d. involves the use anticoagulants to prevent thrombus and embolism.

5. Match the following arrhythmias with their descriptions.

_____ a. Premature atrial contractions
_____ b. Junctional escape rhythm
_____ c. Sinus tachycardia
_____ d. Asystole
_____ e. Paroxysmal supraventricular tachycardia (PSVT)
_____ f. First degree AV block
_____ g. Ventricular tachycardia
_____ h. Sinus bradycardia
_____ i. Atrial fibrillation
_____ j. Premature ventricular contraction (PVC)
_____ k. Type II AV block
_____ l. Ventricular fibrillation
_____ m. Third degree AV block

1. Absence of ventricular activity
2. Wide, distorted QRS
3. Usual spontaneous onset and termination
4. Associated with bundle branch blocks
5. Chaotic ventricular rhythm
6. Normal rhythm pattern with rate < 60
7. Heart rate of 40 to 60 beats/min
8. May precipitate supraventricular tachycardia
9. Atria and ventricles dissociated
10. A run of PVCs
11. Prolonged PR interval
12. Chaotic P wave
13. Sinus rate >100

6. Complete the following statements.

   a. A patient with an acute MI develops the following ECG pattern: atrial rate of 82 and regular; ventricular rate of 46 and regular; P wave and QRS complex are normal but there is no relationship between the P wave and the QRS complex. The nurse identifies the arrhythmia as ________________________, and the treatment indicated is ________________________.

   b. A common arrhythmia the nurse would expect to find in a patient with hypoxemia and hypovolemia is ________________________.

   c. Vagal stimulation induced by carotid massage may be used to treat the arrhythmia of ______________________.

   d. An arrhythmia that is characterized by progressive lengthening of the PR interval until an atrial impulse is not conducted and a QRS complex is dropped is known as ________________________.

   e. PVCs that occur on the T wave of a preceding contraction are always treated because they may precipitate ____________________ or ________________.

7. A patient with heart disease has a sinus bradycardia of 48 beats/min. The nurse recognizes that the patient is at greatest risk for

   a. asystole.
   b. heart block.
   c. sinus arrest.
   d. ectopic premature beats.

8. A patient with an acute MI has a sinus tachycardia of 126 beats/min. The nurse recognizes that if this arrhythmia is not treated, the patient is likely to experience

   a. hypertension.
   b. escape rhythms.
   c. ventricular tachycardia.
   d. an increase in infarct size.

9. A patient with no history of heart disease has a rhythm strip that shows an occasional distorted P wave followed by normal AV and ventricular conduction. The nurse questions the patient about

   a. the use of caffeine.
   b. the use of sedatives.
   c. any aerobic training.
   d. holding the breath during exertion.

10. A newly admitted patient has the following rhythm pattern: heart rate 84 beats/min; regular rhythm; absent P wave; normal QRS complex. The nurse asks the patient about the use of

    a. aspirin.
    b. digoxin.
    c. caffeine.
    d. metoprolol (Lopressor).

11. A patient's rhythm strip indicates a normal heart rate and rhythm with normal P wave and QRS complex, but the P-R interval is 0.26 second. The most appropriate action by the nurse is to

    a. continue to assess the patient.
    b. administer atropine per protocol.
    c. prepare the patient for synchronized cardioversion.
    d. prepare the patient for placement of a temporary pacemaker.

12. In the patient with an arrhythmia, the nurse identifies a nursing diagnosis of decreased cardiac output related to arrhythmias when the patient experiences

    a. hypertension and bradycardia.
    b. chest pain and decreased mentation.
    c. abdominal distention and hepatomegaly.
    d. bounding pulses and a ventricular heave.

13. A patient with an acute MI is having multifocal PVCs and ventricular couplets. He is alert and has a blood pressure of 118/78 with an irregular pulse of 86 beats/min. The most appropriate action by the nurse at this time is to

    a. continue to assess the patient.
    b. be prepared to administer CPR.
    c. administer antiarrhythmic drugs per protocol.
    d. ask the patient to perform Valsalva maneuver.

14. Premature ventricular contractions are indicated by a rhythm pattern finding of

    a. a QRS complex of > 0.12 second followed by a P wave.
    b. continuous wide QRS complexes with a ventricular rate of 160 beats/min.
    c. sawtooth P waves with no measurable PR interval and an irregular rhythm.
    d. P waves hidden in QRS complexes with a regular rhythm of 120 beats/min.

15. Following fibrinolytic therapy, the nurse monitors the patient for the common reperfusion arrhythmias of

    a. sinus tachycardia and atrial fibrillation.
    b. supraventricular and ventricular tachycardia.
    c. premature atrial and ventricular contractions.
    d. premature ventricular contractions and ventricular tachycardia.

16. A patient in the coronary care unit develops ventricular fibrillation. Within protocol guidelines, the first action the nurse should take is to

    a. initiate CPR.
    b. perform defibrillation.
    c. prepare for synchronized cardioversion.
    d. administer IV antiarrhythmic drugs per protocol.

17. Cardiac defibrillation

    a. enhances repolarization and relaxation of ventricular myocardial cells.
    b. provides an electrical impulse that stimulates normal myocardial contractions.
    c. depolarizes the cells of the myocardium to allow the SA node to resume pacemaker function.
    d. delivers an electrical impulse to the heart at the time of ventricular contraction to convert the heart to a sinus rhythm.

18. Initial treatment of asystole and pulseless electrical activity is

    a. CPR.
    b. defibrillation.
    c. administration of atropine.
    d. administration of epinephrine.

19. The nurse's responsibilities in preparing to administer defibrillation include

    a. applying gel pads to the patient's chest.
    b. setting the defibrillator to deliver 50 joules.
    c. setting the defibrillator to a synchronized mode.
    d. sedating the patient with midazolam (Versed) before defibrillation.

20. While providing discharge instructions to the patient who has had an implantable cardioverter-defibrillator (ICD) inserted, the nurse teaches the patient that if she is alone when the ICD fires, she should

    a. lie down.
    b. call the physician.
    c. push the reset button on the pulse generator.
    d. immediately take her antiarrhythmic medication.

21. A patient with a sinus node dysfunction has a permanent pacemaker inserted. Before discharge, the nurse teaches the patient to

    a. avoid cooking with microwave ovens.
    b. avoid high-voltage electrical generators.
    c. use mild analgesics to control the chest spasms caused by the pacing current.
    d. start lifting the arm above the shoulder right away to prevent a "frozen shoulder."

22. A patient with a newly implanted pacemaker refuses to move his involved arm and shoulder and will not participate in his care. An appropriate nursing diagnosis for the patient is

    a. decreased cardiac output related to arrhythmias.
    b. activity intolerance related to inadequate cardiac output.
    c. fear related to perceived vulnerability and reliance on pacemaker.
    d. impaired adjustment related to inability to modify lifestyle as needed.

23. The use of catheter ablation therapy to "burn" areas of the cardiac conduction system is indicated for treatment of

    a. sinus arrest.
    b. heart blocks.
    c. tachyarrhythmias.
    d. multifocal ectopic foci.

24. A 54-year-old patient who has no structural heart disease has an episode of syncope. Upright tilt-table testing is performed to rule out neurocardiogenic syncope. The nurse explains to the patient that if neurocardiogenic syncope is the problem, the patient will experience

 a. palpitations and dizziness.
 b. tachyarrhythmias and chest pain.
 c. marked bardycardia and hypotension.
 d. no change in heart rate or blood pressure.

25. The nurse finds a patient unresponsive in bed and determines that the patient is in cardiopulmonary arrest. From the time of cardiac arrest until CPR is started, the maximum time that should elapse is

 a. 35 seconds.
 b. 60 seconds.
 c. 3 to 4 minutes.
 d. 4 to 6 minutes.

26. Listed below are the steps required in establishing one-person CPR by a health professional in the hospital system. Number the steps in sequence.

 _____ a. Call a code and ask for the crash cart

 _____ b. Determine cessation of breathing

 _____ c. Begin chest compressions

 _____ d. Open the airway

 _____ e. Determine unresponsiveness

 _____ f. Position the victim on back

 _____ g. Determine absence of pulse

 _____ h. Ventilate twice

27. After chest compressions are initiated in CPR, reassessment to determine if spontaneous breathing and circulation have returned should be done after

 a. 2 cycles of compressions and ventilations.
 b. 4 cycles of compressions and ventilations.
 c. 8 cycles of compressions and ventilations.
 d. 5 minutes of compressions and ventilations.

28. The most significant factor in the positive outcome of a patient with a cardiac arrest is

 a. absence of underlying heart disease.
 b. rapid institution of emergency services and procedures.
 c. performance of perfect technique in resuscitation procedures.
 d. maintenance of 50% of normal cardiac output during resuscitation efforts.

29. While the nurse is feeding a patient who is sitting in a chair, the patient chokes, cannot speak, and turns blue. The nurse should

    a. place the patient on the floor and perform a finger-sweep maneuver to attempt to remove the obstruction.
    b. stand behind the chair, hug the patient, and deliver abdominal thrusts with the fist of one hand held by the other hand.
    c. leave the patient in the chair and attempt rescue breathing with mouth-to-mouth ventilation after hyperextending the head.
    d. move the patient to the floor, kneel astride the patient, and administer abdominal thrusts with the heel of one hand covered with the other hand.

30. Before administering drugs in cardiac emergencies as part of advanced cardiac life support (ACLS), it is important to first

    a. administer defibrillation.
    b. insert an endotracheal tube.
    c. check the patient for the presence of a pulse.
    d. establish ECG monitoring and identify arrhythmias.

31. Identify the following cardiac rhythms using the systematic approach to assessing cardiac rhythms found in Table 35-6 in the textbook. All rhythm strips are six seconds.

    a. 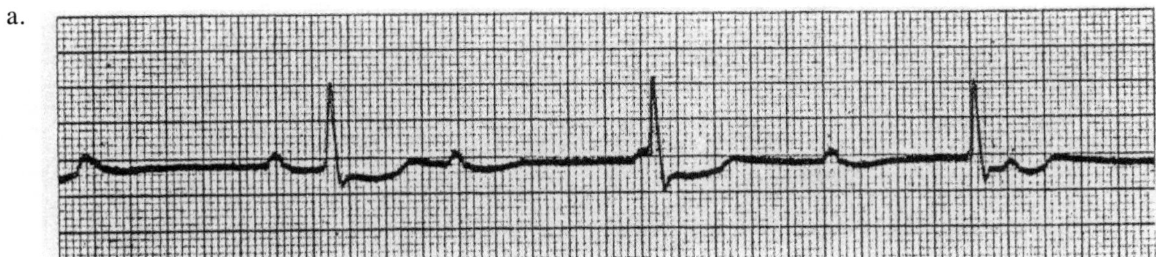

    b. 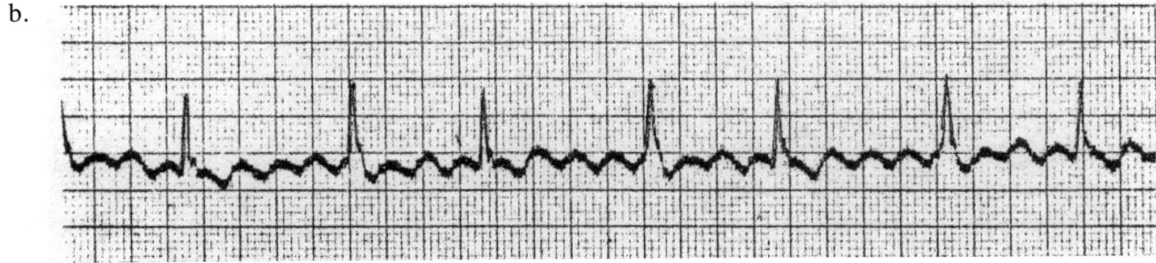

    c. 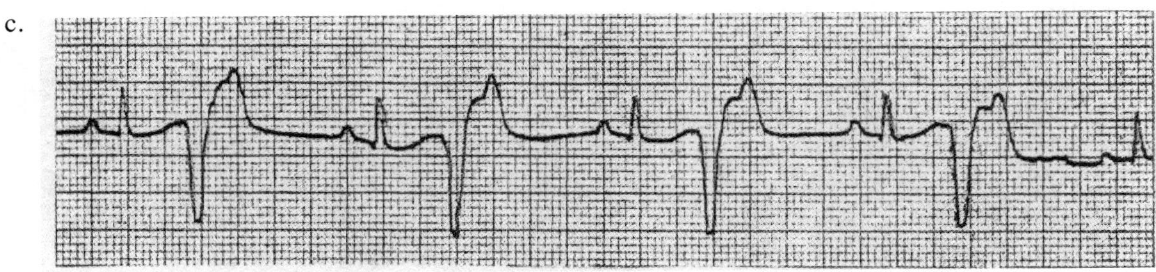

d.

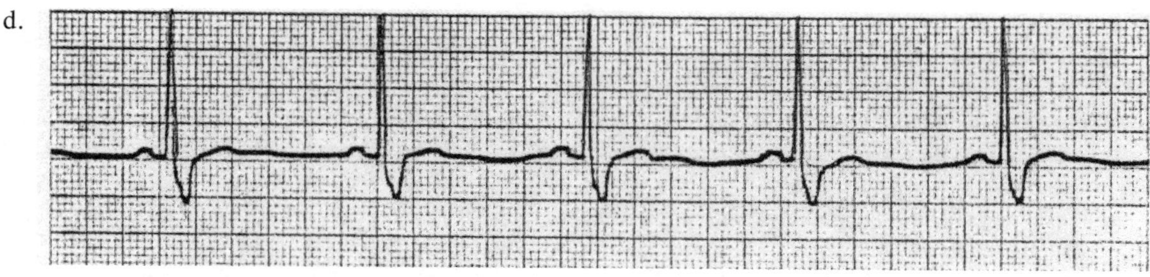

e.

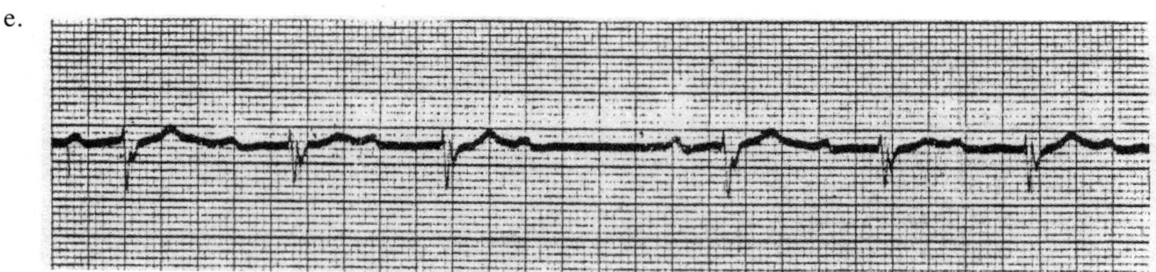

f.

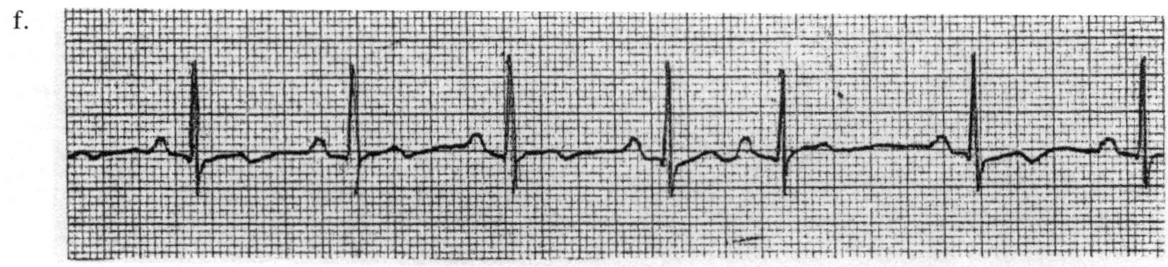

g.

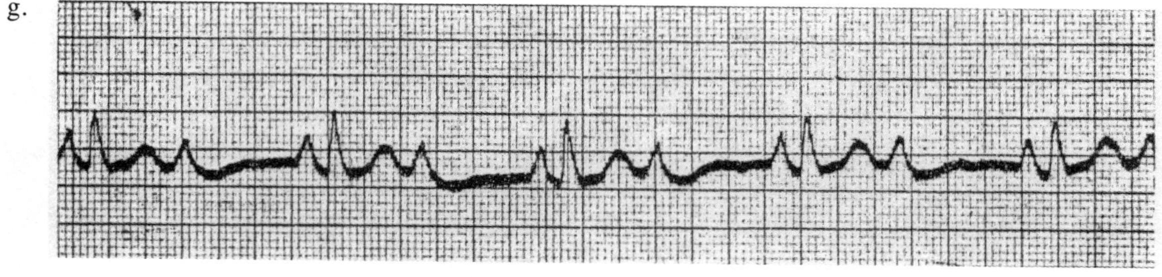

h.

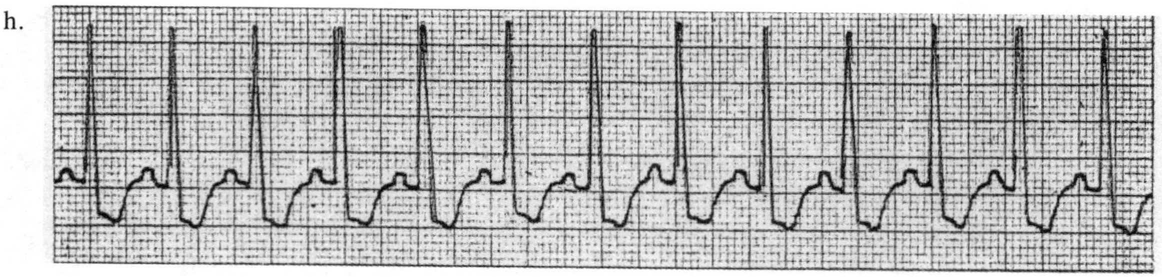

i.

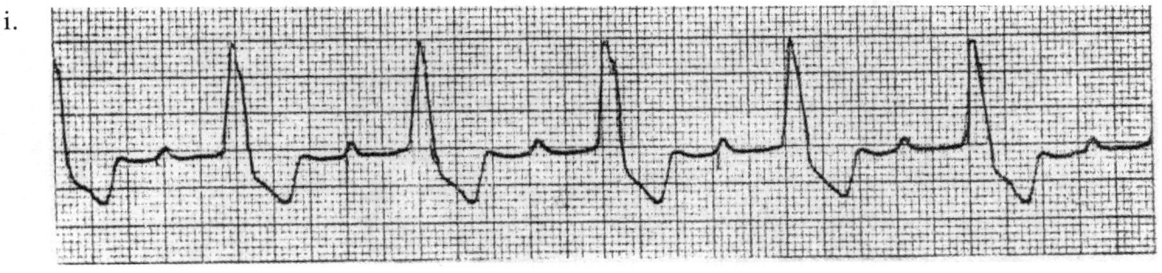

j.

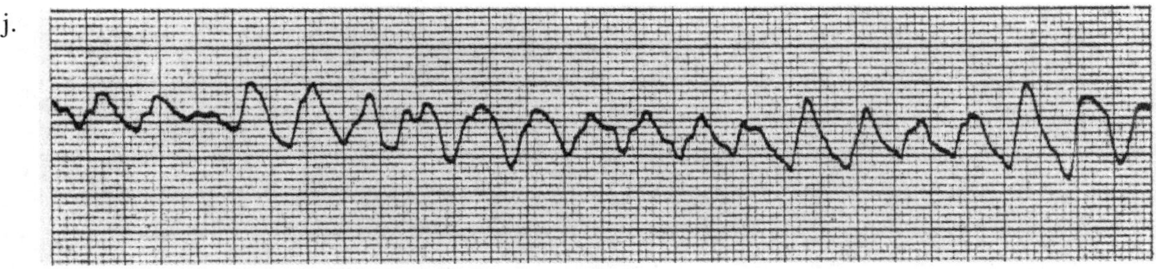

k.

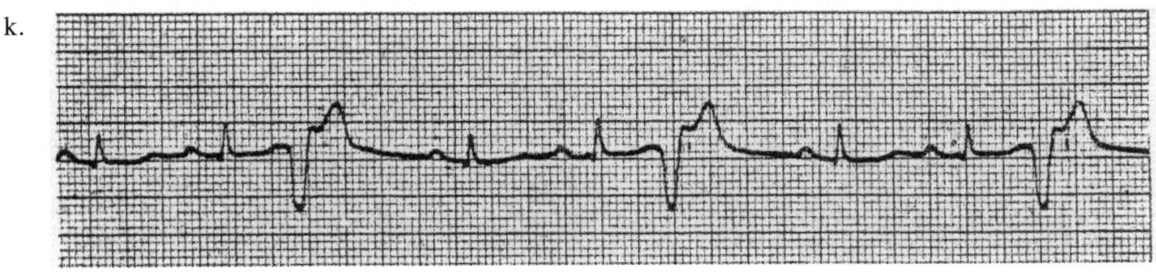

l.

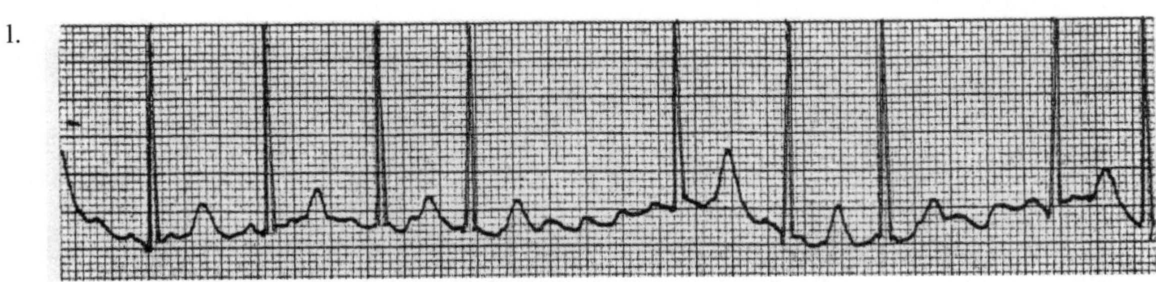

m.

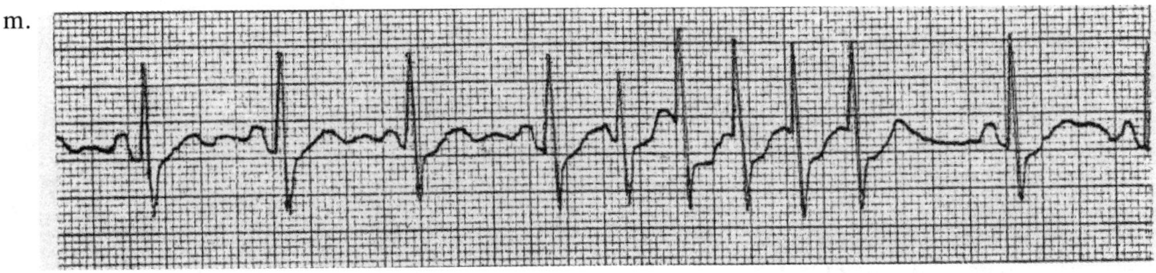

n.

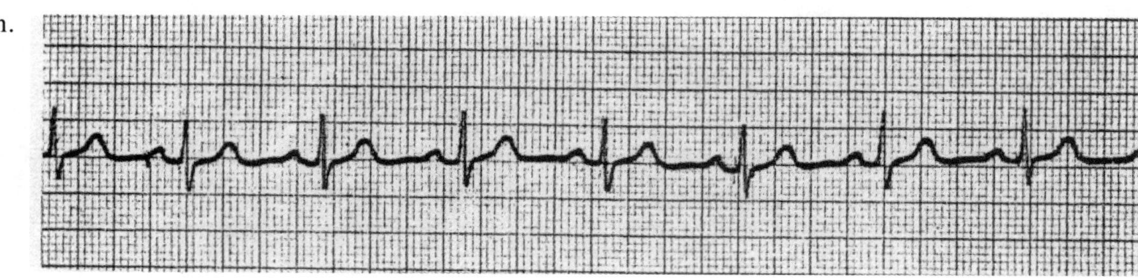

o.

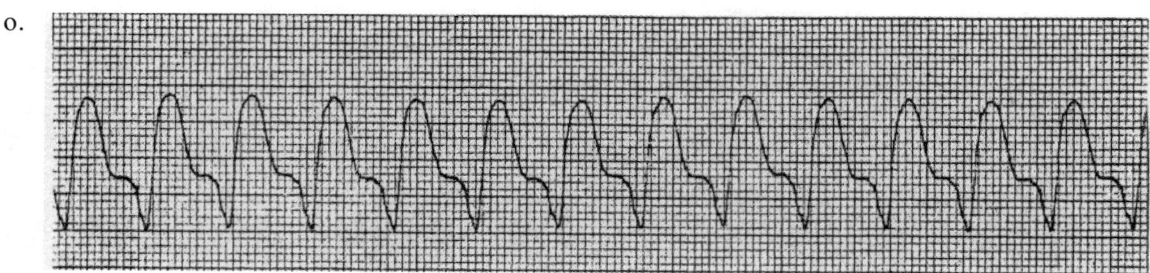

CASE STUDY

ARRHYTHMIA

Patient Profile

Mrs. S. is a 75-year-old woman admitted to the telemetry unit with a diagnosis of atrial fibrillation.

Subjective Data

- Has a history of hypothyroidism and hypertension
- Has no history of atrial fibrillation
- Is taking levothyroxin (Synthroid) 0.05 mg PO qd and enalapril (Vasotec) 5 mg PO bid
- Complains of palpitations, dizziness, shortness of breath, and mild chest pressure

Objective Data

- Physical examination
  - Alert, anxious, elderly woman
  - BP 100/70, HR 150/min, RR 32/min
  - Lungs: bibasilar crackles
  - Heart: S_1 and S_2, irregularly irregular
- Diagnostic study
  - ECG: atrial fibrillation

Collaborative Care

- Discontinue enalapril (Vasotec)
- Digoxin 0.25 mg PO qd
- Diltiazem (Cardizem) 60 mg PO q8h
- Warfarin (Coumadin) 5 mg PO qd

Critical Thinking Questions

1. What is the immediate goal of antiarrhythmic drug therapy for Mrs. S.?

2. What nonpharmacologic therapy may be used to treat the arrhythmia?

3. Explain the rationale for use of the medications ordered for Mrs. S.

4. Explain the pathophysiology of her symptoms on admission to the telemetry unit.

5. Describe the characteristics of her ECG wave form.

6. Based on the assessment data presented, write one or more appropriate nursing diagnoses. Are there any collaborative problems?

CHAPTER 36 NURSING MANAGEMENT: INFLAMMATORY AND VALVULAR HEART DISEASES

1. A 20-year-old patient has acute right-sided infective endocarditis. While obtaining a nursing history, the nurse recognizes as most significant the patient's history of

   a. intravenous drug abuse.
   b. a recent urinary tract infection.
   c. a recent professional teeth cleaning.
   d. rheumatic fever without a heart murmur.

2. A patient has an admitting diagnosis of acute left-sided infective endocarditis. The nurse explains to the patient that this diagnosis is best confirmed with

   a. blood cultures.
   b. a complete blood count.
   c. a cardiac catheterization.
   d. a transesophageal echocardiogram.

3. Match the following manifestations of infective endocarditis with their descriptions.

_____	a. Splinter hemorrhages	1. Hemorrhagic retinal lesions
_____	b. Janeways's lesions	2. Painful red or purple lesions on fingers or toes
_____	c. Osler's nodes	3. Black longitudinal streaks in nailbeds
_____	d. Roth's spots	4. Small hemorrhages in conjunctiva, lips, and buccal mucosa
_____	e. Petechiae	5. Flat, red, painless spots on palms and soles of feet

4. A patient with infective endocarditis of a prosthetic mitral valve develops a left hemiparesis and visual changes. The nurse expects that medical management of the patient will include

   a. an embolectomy.
   b. surgical valve replacement.
   c. administration of anticoagulants.
   d. higher than usual antibiotic dosages.

5. A patient with aortic valve endocarditis develops dyspnea, crackles in the lungs, and restlessness. The nurse suspects that the patient is experiencing

   a. vegetative embolization to the coronary arteries.
   b. pulmonary embolization from valve vegetations.
   c. nonspecific manifestations that accompany infectious diseases.
   d. valvular incompetence with possible infectious invasion of the myocardium.

6. A patient hospitalized for 1 week with subacute infective endocarditis is afebrile and has no signs of heart damage, and discharge with outpatient antibiotic therapy is planned. During discharge planning with the patient, it is most important for the nurse to

   a. plan how his needs will be met while he continues on bed rest.
   b. teach the patient to avoid crowds and exposure to upper respiratory infections.
   c. encourage the use of diversional activities to relieve boredom and restlessness.
   d. assess the patient's home environment in terms of family assistance and hospital access.

7. When teaching a patient with endocarditis how to prevent recurrence of the infection, the nurse instructs the patient to

   a. start on antibiotic therapy when exposed to persons with infections.
   b. take one aspirin a day to prevent vegetative lesions from forming around the valves.
   c. obtain prophylactic antibiotic therapy before any invasive medical or dental procedures.
   d. always maintain continuous antibiotic therapy to prevent the development of any systemic infection.

8. A patient is admitted to the hospital with a suspected acute pericarditis. To establish the presence of a pericardial friction rub, the nurse listens to the patient's chest

   a. while timing the sound with the respiratory pattern.
   b. with the bell of the stethoscope at the apex of the heart.
   c. with the diaphragm of the stethoscope at the lower left sternal border of the chest.
   d. with the diaphragm of the stethoscope to auscultate a high-pitched continuous rumbling sound.

9. A patient with acute pericarditis has markedly distended jugular veins, decreased blood pressure, tachycardia, tachypnea, and muffled heart sounds. The nurse recognizes that these symptoms occur when

   a. the pericardial space is obliterated with scar tissue and thickened pericardium.
   b. excess pericardial fluid compresses the heart and prevents adequate diastolic filling.
   c. the parietal and visceral pericardial membranes adhere to each other preventing normal myocardial contraction.
   d. fibrin accumulation on the visceral pericardium infiltrates into the myocardium creating generalized myocardial dysfunction.

10. Identify whether the following statements are true or false. If a statement is false, correct the bold word(s) to make the statement true.

    _____ a. To measure a pulsus paradoxus, the nurse determines the difference between the systolic pressure **at inspiration** and the systolic pressure **at expiration**.

    _____ b. A pulsus paradoxus of >10 mm Hg occurs with **cardiac tamponade**.

    _____ c. A pericardiocentesis is indicated for the patient with pericarditis when there is a **pericardial effusion of any amount**.

    _____ d. Acute pericarditis may be diagnosed with **specific ECG changes that evolve over time.**

    _____ e. Treatment of chronic constrictive pericarditis may include a **pericardiectomy.**

11. A patient with acute pericarditis has a nursing diagnosis of pain related to pericardial inflammation. An appropriate nursing intervention for the patient is

    a. administering narcotics as prescribed on an around-the-clock schedule.
    b. promoting progressive relaxation exercises with the use of deep, slow breathing.
    c. positioning the patient on the right side with the head of the bed elevated 15 degrees.
    d. positioning the patient in Fowler's position with a padded overbed table for the patient to lean on.

12. When obtaining a nursing history for a patient with myocarditis, the nurse specifically questions the patient about

    a. prior use of digoxin for treatment of cardiac problems.
    b. recent symptoms of a viral illness such as fever and malaise.
    c. a recent streptococcal infection requiring treatment with penicillin.
    d. a history of coronary artery disease with or without a myocardial infarction.

13. A 19-year-old patient with rheumatic heart disease is admitted to the hospital with a recurrence of acute rheumatic fever. In planning care for the patient, the nurse recognizes that an appropriate nursing diagnosis for the patient is

    a. ineffective coping related to refusal to carry out health promotion activities.
    b. risk for infection related to recent exposure to group A β-hemolytic streptococci.
    c. impaired adjustment related to unsuccessful life style modifications, goal setting, and problem solving.
    d. ineffective management of therapeutic regimen related to lack of knowledge of or compliance with prophylactic antibiotic therapy.

14. The most important role of the nurse in preventing rheumatic fever is to

    a. teach patients with infective endocarditis to adhere to antibiotic prophylaxis.
    b. identify patients with valvular heart disease who are at risk for rheumatic fever.
    c. encourage the use of antibiotics for treatment of all infections involving a sore throat.
    d. promote the early diagnosis and immediate treatment of group A β-hemolytic streptococcal pharyngitis.

15. A patient with rheumatic carditis asks the nurse if his heart is infected with streptococcal organisms. The best response by the nurse is

    a. "It is thought that antibodies produced in response to a streptococcal infection then attack normal body tissues."
    b. "Yes, it is a complication that may occur with any group A β-hemolytic streptococcal infection if it is not treated early."
    c. "The heart is not really infected, but toxins produced by streptococci infecting the throat can damage the heart and other tissues."
    d. "The relationship between streptococcal infections and rheumatic fever is not known, but penicillin is used in treatment just in case there is an infection."

16. The diagnosis of acute rheumatic fever is most strongly supported in the patient with

    a. organic heart murmurs, fever, and elevated ESR.
    b. polyarthritis, chorea, and increased antistreptolysin O titer.
    c. cardiac enlargement, polyarthritis, and erythema marginatum.
    d. positive C-reactive protein, elevated WBC, subcutaneous nodules.

17. Residual and chronic cardiac damage from acute rheumatic fever most often includes

    a. myocardial scarring.
    b. chronic constrictive pericarditis.
    c. blockade of the conduction system.
    d. scarring and contractures of the mitral valve.

18. Identify the rationale for the use of the following drugs in the treatment of acute rheumatic fever.

    a. Penicillin

    b. Aspirin

    c. Corticosteroids

19. To establish a balance of activity-rest to prevent hazards of immobility yet decrease cardiac workload in the patient with acute rheumatic carditis, the nurse

    a. allows full ambulation as soon as acute symptoms have subsided.
    b. promotes bed rest until antiinflammatory therapy has been discontinued.
    c. encourages nonstrenuous activities as soon as antibiotic therapy is initiated.
    d. maintains the patient on bed rest until symptoms of congestive heart failure are controlled.

20. The nurse teaches the adult patient recovering from rheumatic heart disease that antibiotic prophylaxis

    a. is required for only 5 years in adults with rheumatic heart disease.
    b. needs to be increased during invasive dental or surgical procedures.
    c. is only required if exposure to group A β-hemolytic streptococci is frequent.
    d. is not required if good nutrition, adequate rest, and stringent hygiene are maintained.

21. Identify whether the following statements are true or false. If a statement is false, correct the bold word(s) to make the statement true.

    _____ a. Valvular stenosis leads to **backward flow** of blood and **dilation** of the preceding chamber.

    _____ b. **Valvular regurgitation** causes a pressure gradient difference across an open valve.

    _____ c. The heart valve most commonly affected by stenosis or regurgitation is the **tricuspid** valve.

    _____ d. The most common form of valvular disease in the United States is **mitral stenosis**.

22. Number in sequence the pathophysiologic processes of mitral valve stenosis.

    _____ a. Fluid moves into the pulmonary extravascular space and alveoli.

    _____ b. Pulmonary artery pressure increases.

    _____ c. During diastole, a pressure gradient difference occurs between the left atrium and the left ventricle.

    _____ d. The left atrium dilates and pulmonary vessels hypertrophy.

    _____ e. The right ventricle fails.

    _____ f. Adhesions and contractures of valve leaflets and chordae tendineae occur, narrowing the valve opening.

    _____ g. The right ventricle hypertrophies in response to pressure overload in the pulmonary vasculature.

    _____ h. Pressure increases in left atrium, pulmonary veins, and pulmonary capillaries.

23. Match the following characteristics with the related type of valvular disease (answers may be used more than once).

_____ a. Sudden onset of cardiovascular collapse

_____ b. May be caused by pulmonary hypertension

_____ c. Rapid development of pulmonary edema and cardiogenic shock

_____ d. Dyspnea is prominent symptom

_____ e. Loud pansystolic or holosystolic murmur

_____ f. Ballooning of valve into left atrium during ventricular systole

_____ g. Characteristic systolic crescendo-decrescendo murmur

_____ h. Corrigan's (water-hammer) pulses

_____ i. Angina and syncope result from decreased cardiac output

_____ j. Embolization may result from chronic atrial fibrillation

_____ k. Major symptoms related to elevated systemic venous pressures

_____ l. Rapid onset prevents left chamber dilation

_____ m. Brisk carotid pulses present

1. Mitral stenosis
2. Acute mitral regurgitation
3. Chronic mitral regurgitation
4. Mitral valve prolapse
5. Aortic stenosis
6. Acute aortic regurgitation
7. Chronic aortic regurgitation
8. Tricuspid valve disease

24. Drugs that the nurse would expect to be prescribed for most any patient with valvular heart disease include

a. oral nitrates.
b. anticoagulants.
c. atrial antiarrhythmics.
d. beta-adrenergic blocking agents.

25. A patient with symptomatic mitral valve prolapse has atrial and ventricular arrhythmias. In addition to monitoring for decreased cardiac output related to the arrhythmias, an appropriate nursing diagnosis related to the arrhythmias identified by the nurse is

a. ineffective breathing pattern related to hypervolemia.
b. risk for injury related to dizziness and light-headedness.
c. disturbed sleep pattern related to paroxysmal nocturnal dyspnea.
d. ineffective therapeutic regimen management related to lack of knowledge of prevention and treatment strategies.

26. A patient is scheduled for a percutaneous transluminal balloon valvuloplasty. The nurse understands that this procedure is indicated for

    a. any patient with aortic regurgitation.
    b. older patients with tricuspid valve stenosis.
    c. young adult patients with mild mitral valve stenosis.
    d. patients with valvular stenosis that are poor surgical risks.

27. A patient is scheduled for an open surgical valvuloplasty of the mitral valve. In preparing the patient for surgery, the nurse recognizes that

    a. cardiopulmonary bypass is not required with this procedure.
    b. valve repair is a palliative measure while valve replacement is curative.
    c. the operative mortality rate is lower in valve repair than in valve replacement.
    d. patients with valve repair do not require postoperative anticoagulation as they do with valve replacement.

28. A mechanical prosthetic valve is most likely to be preferred over a biologic valve for valve replacement in a

    a. 41-year-old man with peptic ulcer disease.
    b. 22-year-old woman who desires to have children.
    c. 35-year-old man with a history of seasonal asthma.
    d. 62-year-old woman with early Alzheimer's disease.

29. When performing discharge teaching for the patient following a mechanical valve replacement, the nurse determines that further instruction is needed when the patient says

    a. "I may begin an exercise program to gradually increase my cardiac tolerance."
    b. "I will always need to have my blood checked once a month for its clotting function."
    c. "I should wear a Medic Alert bracelet to identify my valve and anticoagulant therapy."
    d. "The biggest risk I have during invasive health procedures is bleeding because of my anticoagulants."

CASE STUDY

INFECTIVE ENDOCARDITIS

Patient Profile

Mr. B. is a 60-year-old man who is hospitalized with a suspected cerebrovascular accident.

Subjective Data

- Had a laparoscopic cholecystectomy a few weeks ago

Objective Data

- Neurologic signs typical of a stroke
- Petechiae over chest
- Crescendo-decrescendo murmur present
- Rectal temperature 103° F (39.4° C)

Critical Thinking Questions

1. What places Mr. B. at high risk for infective endocarditis?

2. What asymptomatic underlying cardiac conditions may Mr. B. have had that contributed to his infectious endocarditis?

3. Explain the cause of Mr. B.'s assessment findings.

4. What is the relevance of the endoscopic surgery he had a few weeks before this hospital admission?

5. What treatment would the nurse anticipate for Mr. B.?

6. Discuss how Mr. B.'s infective endocarditis could have been prevented.

7. Based on the assessment data presented, write one or more appropriate nursing diagnoses. Are there any collaborative problems?

CHAPTER 37 NURSING MANAGEMENT: VASCULAR DISORDERS

1. When obtaining a health history from a 72-year-old man with peripheral arterial disease of the lower extremities, the nurse asks the patient about a history of other atherosclerotic manifestations such as

   a. venous thrombosis.
   b. venous stasis ulcers.
   c. pulmonary embolism.
   d. carotid artery disease.

2. Match the following descriptions with the related types of aneurysms.

_____	a. Pouchlike bulge of artery	1. Fusiform aneurysm
_____	b. Disruption of all layers of an artery with bleeding	2. Saccular aneurysm
		3. Pseudoaneurysm
_____	c. Uniform, circumferential dilation of artery	

3. A surgical repair is planned for a patient who has a 5-cm abdominal aortic aneurysm. On physical assessment of the patient, the nurse would expect to find

   a. hoarseness and dysphagia.
   b. severe back pain with flank ecchymosis.
   c. the presence of a bruit in the periumbilical area.
   d. weakness in the lower extremities progressing to paraplegia.

4. A thoracic aortic aneurysm is found when a patient has a routine chest x-ray. The nurse anticipates that additional diagnostic testing to determine the size and structure of the aneurysm will include

   a. a CT scan.
   b. angiography.
   c. echocardiography.
   d. ultrasoundography.

5. A patient with a small abdominal aortic aneurysm is not a good surgical candidate. The nurse teaches the patient that one of the best ways to prevent expansion of the lesion is to

   a. avoid strenuous physical exertion.
   b. control hypertension with prescribed therapy.
   c. comply with prescribed anticoagulant therapy.
   d. maintain a low-calcium diet to prevent calcification of the vessel.

6. During preoperative preparation of the patient scheduled for an abdominal aortic aneurysm the nurse establishes baseline data for the patient knowing that

   a. postoperatively all physiologic processes will be altered.
   b. the cause of the aneurysm is a systemic vascular disease.
   c. surgery will be canceled if any physiologic function is not normal.
   d. blood pressure and heart rate will be maintained below normal levels during the postoperative period.

7. Complete the following statements.

   a. A ________________ aneurysm may be surgically treated by excising only the weakened area and suturing the artery closed.

   b. During conventional aortic aneurysm repair, a ___________ ___________ is sutured to the aorta above and below the aneurysm, and the native aorta is replaced around the site.

   c. Repair of ____________ aneurysms requires cross-clamping of the aorta proximal and distal to the aneurysm.

   d. A synthetic bifurcation graft is used in aneurysm repair when an abdominal aortic aneurysm extends into the ___________ arteries.

   e. Repair of an aortic aneurysm by placing an aortic graft inside the aneurysm through the femoral artery is called the _____________ ___________ procedure.

   f. Major complications of aortic aneurysm repair are associated with involvement or obstruction of the ___________ arteries.

8. During the patient's acute postoperative period following repair of an aneurysm, the nurse should ensure that

   a. hypothermia is maintained to decrease oxygen need.
   b. the blood pressure and all peripheral pulses are evaluated at least every hour.
   c. IV fluids are administered at a rate to maintain an hourly urine output of 100 ml.
   d. the patient's blood pressure is kept lower than baseline to prevent leaking at the suture line.

9. Following an ascending aortic aneurysm repair, the nurse monitors for and immediately reports

   a. shallow respirations and poor coughing.
   b. decreased drainage from the chest tubes.
   c. a change in level of consciousness and ability to speak.
   d. lower extremity pulses that are decreased from preoperative baseline.

10. Identify at least one observation made by the nurse that would indicate the presence of the following complications of aortic aneurysm repair.

    a. Graft thrombosis

    b. Myocardial ischemia

    c. Bowel infarction

    d. Graft infection

    e. Impaired renal perfusion

    f. Spinal cord ischemia

11. Following discharge teaching with a male patient with an abdominal aortic aneurysm repair, the nurse determines that further instruction is needed when the patient says

    a. "I may have some permanent sexual dysfunction as a result of the surgery."
    b. "I may continue to have a poor appetite and irregular bowel patterns for a while."
    c. "I should take the pulses in my extremities and let the doctor know if they get too fast or too slow."
    d. "I must maintain a low-fat and low-cholesterol diet to help the new graft open."

12. During the nursing assessment of the patient with a distal descending aortic dissection, the nurse would expect the patient to manifest

    a. a cardiac murmur characteristic of aortic valve insufficiency.
    b. altered level of consciousness with dizziness and weak carotid pulses.
    c. severe hypertension and orthopnea and dyspnea of pulmonary edema.
    d. severe "ripping" back or abdominal pain with descending organ ischemia.

13. A patient with a dissection of the arch of the aorta has a decreased level of consciousness and weak carotid pulses. The nurse anticipates that initial treatment of the patient will include

    a. administration of packed RBCs to replace blood loss.
    b. immediate surgery to replace the torn area with a graft.
    c. administration of anticoagulants to prevent embolization.
    d. administration of antihypertensives to maintain a MAP of 70 to 80 mm Hg.

14. The nurse evaluates that treatment for the patient with an uncomplicated aortic dissection is successful when

    a. pain is relieved.
    b. surgical repair is completed.
    c. renal output is maintained at 30 ml/hr.
    d. blood pressure is within normal range.

15. Complete the following statements.

    a. The classic ischemic pain of peripheral arterial disease is known as ______________________________.

    b. Two serious complications of peripheral arterial disease that frequently lead to lower limb amputation are

       _________________ and ___________________.

    c. A patient with chronic arterial disease has a brachial systolic blood pressure of 132 mm Hg and an ankle

       systolic blood pressure of 102 mm Hg. The ankle-brachial index is _________ and indicates

       ______________ (mild/moderate/severe) arterial disease.

    d. Surgery for peripheral arterial disease is indicated when the patient has limb pain during ___________.

16. Drug therapy for peripheral arterial disease to increase blood flow and prevent intermittent claudication includes the administration of

    a. aspirin.
    b. cilostazol (Pletal).
    c. ticlopidine (Ticlid).
    d. clopidogrel (Plavix).

17. Match the following descriptions with the therapeutic procedures used for arterial occlusive disease.

_____	a. Removing obstructive plaques by opening the artery	1. Percutaneous transluminal balloon angioplasty
_____	b. Helps prevent restenosis following angioplasty	2. Peripheral arterial bypass
		3. Intravascular stent
_____	c. Often performed to reduce plaque size before angioplasty	4. Endarterectomy
_____	d. Surgical widening of the arterial lumen	5. Patch graft angioplasty
_____	e. Best results in localized iliac and femoral artery lesions	6. Atherectomy
_____	f. Autogenous vein or synthetic graft used to divert blood around occlusion	

18. A patient with peripheral arterial disease has a nursing diagnosis of ineffective peripheral tissue perfusion. Appropriate teaching for the patient includes instructions to

a. rest and sleep with the legs elevated.
b. soak the feet in warm water 30 minutes a day.
c. walk at least 30 minutes a day to the point of pain.
d. use nicotine replacement therapy as a substitute for smoking.

19. When teaching the patient with peripheral disease about modifying risk factors associated with the condition, the nurse emphasizes that

a. amputation is the ultimate outcome if the patient does not alter lifestyle behaviors.
b. risk-reducing behaviors initiated after angioplasty can stop the progression of the disease.
c. maintenance of normal body weight is the most important factor in controlling arterial disease.
d. modifications will reduce the risk of other atherosclerotic conditions such as coronary heart disease.

20. Indicate whether the following findings are characteristic of arterial disease (A) or venous disease (V).

_____ a. Paresthesia

_____ b. Heavy ulcer drainage

_____ c. Edema around the ankles

_____ d. Gangrene over bony prominences on toes and feet

_____ e. Decreased peripheral pulses

_____ f. Brown pigmentation of the legs

_____ g. Thickened, brittle nails

_____ h. Ulceration around the medial malleolus

_____ i. Pallor on elevation of the legs

_____ j. Dull ache in calf or thigh

_____ k. Pruritis

21. A patient with peripheral vascular disease has marked peripheral neuropathy. An appropriate nursing diagnosis for the patient is

    a. risk for injury related to decreased sensation.
    b. impaired skin integrity related to decreased peripheral circulation.
    c. ineffective peripheral tissue perfusion related to decreased arterial blood flow.
    d. activity intolerance related to imbalance between oxygen supply and demand.

22. During care of the patient following femoral bypass graft surgery, the nurse immediately notifies the physician if the patient experiences

    a. fever and redness at the incision site.
    b. 2+ edema of the extremity and pain at the incision site.
    c. a loss of palpable pulses and numbness and tingling of the feet.
    d. decreasing ankle-brachial indices and serous drainage from the incision.

23. A patient has chronic atrial fibrillation and develops an acute arterial occlusion at the iliac artery bifurcation. What are the six *P*s of acute arterial occlusion the nurse may find in the patient?

    a. ________________ c. ________________ e. ________________

    b. ________________ d. ________________ f. ________________

24. Indicate whether the following manifestations and treatments are characteristic of thromboangiitis obliterans (Buerger's disease) (B) or arteriospastic disease (Raynaud's phenomenon) (R).

    _____ a. Involves small cutaneous arteries of the fingers and toes

    _____ b. Inflammation of midsized arteries and veins

    _____ c. Treated with calcium-channel blockers, especially nifedipine (Procardia)

    _____ d. Strongly associated with smoking

    _____ e. Predominant in young females

    _____ f. Episodes involve white, blue, and red color changes of fingertips

    _____ g. Amputation of digits or legs below the knee may be necessary for ulceration and gangrene

    _____ h. Precipitated by exposure to cold, caffeine, and tobacco

    _____ i. Intermittent claudication of feet, arms, and hands may be present

    _____ j. Frequently associated with autoimmune disorders

25. Identify the factor(s) of Virchow's triad present in each of the following conditions associated with deep venous thrombosis (DVT).

   a. IV therapy

   b. Prolonged immobilization

   c. Estrogen therapy

   d. Abdominal surgery

   e. Smoking

   f. Pregnancy

26. Identify whether the following statements are true or false. If a statement is false, correct the bold word(s) to make the statement true.

   _____ a. The most common cause of superficial thrombophlebitis in the legs is **IV therapy**.

   _____ b. A tender, red, inflamed induration along the course of a subcutaneous vein is characteristic of a **deep venous thrombosis**.

   _____ c. A patient with deep venous thrombosis is scheduled for surgical treatment. The nurse recognizes that surgery is most commonly performed for this condition to **insert a vena cava interruption device** to prevent pulmonary embolism.

   _____ d. The method of prevention of deep venous thrombosis in hospitalized patients that addresses all three aspects of Virchow's triad is the use of **elastic compression stockings**.

27. To help prevent embolization of the thrombus in a patient with a DVT, the nurse teaches the patient to

   a. dangle the feet over the edge of the bed q2–3h.
   b. ambulate for short periods three to four times a day.
   c. keep the affected leg elevated above the level of the heart.
   d. maintain bed rest until edema is relieved and anticoagulation is established.

28. Match the following anticoagulant drugs with their characteristics (answers may be used more than once).

   _____ a. Is only administered IV
   _____ b. No antidote for anticoagulant effect
   _____ c. Vitamin K is antidote
   _____ d. Is only administered SC
   _____ e. Routine coagulation tests not usually required
   _____ f. Protamine sulfate is antidote
   _____ g. May be administered IV or SC
   _____ h. Is only administered orally
   _____ i. INH used to monitor anticoagulant effect

   1. Unfractionated heparin
   2. Low-molecular–weight heparin
   3. Hirudin derivatives
   4. Coumarin derivatives

29. The patient with DVT is receiving therapy with heparin and asks the nurse if the drug will dissolve the clot in her leg. The best response by the nurse is,

   a. "This drug will break up and dissolve the clot so that circulation in the vein can be restored."
   b. "The purpose of the heparin is to prevent growth of the clot or formation of new clots where the circulation is slowed."
   c. "Heparin won't dissolve the clot, but will inhibit the inflammation around the clot and delay the development of new clots."
   d. "The heparin will dilate the vein, preventing turbulence of blood flow around the clot that may cause it to break off and travel to the lungs."

30. A patient with DVT is to be discharged on long-term warfarin (Coumadin) therapy and is taught about prevention and continuing treatment of DVT. The nurse determines that discharge teaching for the patient has been effective when the patient states

   a. "I should expect that Coumadin will cause my stools to be somewhat black."
   b. "I should avoid all dark green and leafy vegetables while I am taking Coumadin."
   c. "Massaging my legs several times a day will help increase my venous circulation."
   d. "Swimming is a good activity to include in my exercise program to increase my circulation."

31. The nurse teaches the patient with any venous disorder that the best way to prevent venous stasis and increase venous return is to

   a. walk.
   b. sit with the legs elevated.
   c. frequently rotate the ankles.
   d. continuously wear compression gradient stockings.

32. Number in sequence the processes that occur as venous stasis precipitates varicose veins leading to venous stasis ulcers.

   _____ a. Venous blood flow reverses

   _____ b. Edema forms

   _____ c. Venous pressure increases

   _____ d. Additional venous distention occurs

   _____ e. Blood supply to local tissues decreases

   _____ f. Venous valves become incompetent

   _____ g. Ulceration occurs

   _____ h. Capillary pressure increases

   _____ i. Veins dilate

33. The most important measure in the treatment of venous stasis ulcers is

   a. elevation of the limb.
   b. extrinsic compression.
   c. application of moist dressings.
   d. application of topical antibiotics.

34. A postsurgical patient has an acute onset of dyspnea, tachycardia, and chest pain. While the physician is being notified, the nurse should

a. elevate the head of the bed.
b. administer oxygen at 6L/min.
c. elevate the lower extremities.
d. start an IV line with D_5W at a slow rate.

35. To determine the location of a pulmonary embolism, the nurse would expect the physician to order a(n)

a. ECG.
b. chest x-ray.
c. perfusion lung scan.
d. pulmonary angiogram.

CASE STUDY

ABDOMINAL AORTIC ANEURYSM (AAA)

Patient Profile

Mr. S. is a 73-year-old man who was brought to the local emergency department complaining of severe back pain.

Subjective Data

- Has a known AAA, which has been followed with yearly abdominal ultrasounds
- Has smoked one pack per day for 52 years
- Has had occasional bouts of angina for the past 3 years

Objective Data

- Has a pulsating abdominal mass
- BP 88/68 mm Hg
- Extremities are cool and clammy

Critical Thinking Questions

1. What are Mr. S.'s risk factors for AAA?

2. Define the etiology of an AAA.

3. Which signs or symptoms make the nurse suspect that Mr. S. has a ruptured AAA rather than a nonruptured AAA?

4. What is the first priority in this patient's care?

5. What is the nurse's role in assisting the family in this critical situation?

6. What steps, if any, could have been taken to prevent the rupture of the AAA?

7. Based on the assessment data presented, write one or more appropriate nursing diagnoses. Are there any collaborative problems?

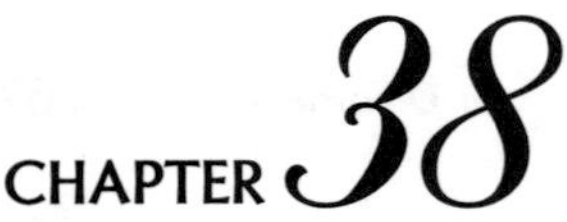

CHAPTER 38 NURSING ASSESSMENT: GASTROINTESTINAL SYSTEM

1. Identify the structures in the following illustrations.

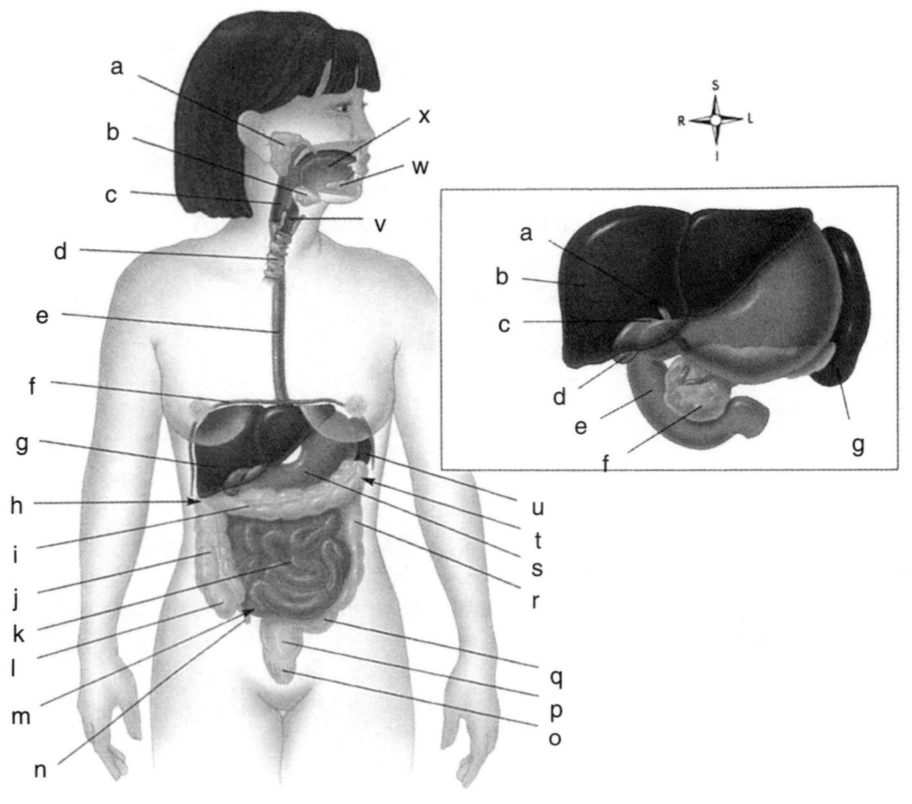

a. ______________________

b. ______________________

c. ______________________

d. ______________________

e. ______________________

f. ______________________

g. ______________________

h. ______________________

i. ______________________

j. ______________________

k. ______________________

l. ______________________

m. ______________________

n. ______________________

o. ______________________

p. ______________________

q. ______________________

r. ______________________

s. ______________________

t. ______________________

u. ______________________

v. ______________________

w. ______________________

x. ______________________

Inset:

a. ______________________

b. ______________________

c. ______________________

d. ______________________

e. ______________________

f. ______________________

g. ______________________

2. Identify the structures in the following illustration.

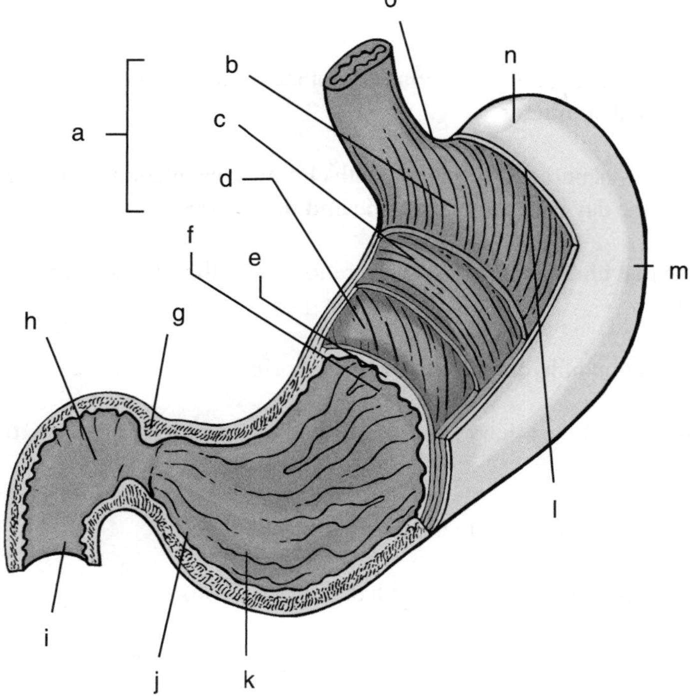

a. ______________________ f. ______________________ k. ______________________

b. ______________________ g. ______________________ l. ______________________

c. ______________________ h. ______________________ m. ______________________

d. ______________________ i. ______________________ n. ______________________

e. ______________________ j. ______________________ o. ______________________

3. A patient receives atropine, an anticholinergic drug, in preparation for surgery. The nurse expects this drug to affect the gastrointestinal tract by

   a. increasing gastric emptying.
   b. relaxing pyloric and ileocecal sphincters.
   c. decreasing secretions and peristaltic action.
   d. depressing the nervous system of the GI tract.

4. A patient with an inflamed gallbladder experiences pain after eating caused by contraction of the gallbladder. The mechanism responsive for this action is

   a. production of bile by the liver.
   b. production of secretin by the duodenum.
   c. release of gastrin from the stomach antrum.
   d. production of cholecystokinin by the duodenum.

5. A primary effect of removal of the stomach on nutritional status is

   a. iron deficiency.
   b. lactose intolerance.
   c. protein malnutrition.
   d. cobalamin (vitamin B_{12}) deficiency.

6. Identify whether the following statements are true or false. If a statement is false, correct the bold word(s) to make the statement true.

_____ a. The structure that prevents reflux of stomach contents into the esophagus is the **upper esophageal sphincter**.

_____ b. The nurse encourages the patient with chronic constipation to attempt defecation after the first meal of the day because **gastrocolic and duodenocolic reflexes** increase colon peristalsis.

_____ c. A drug that blocks the release of secretions from the stomach **chief cells** will decrease gastric acidity.

_____ d. The secretion of hydrochloric acid and pepsinogen is stimulated by the **sight and smell** of food.

_____ e. Obstruction of the biliary tract is indicated by increased **unconjugated (indirect)** bilirubin levels in the blood.

_____ f. The major blood supply to the liver is the **portal vein**.

7. Match the following digestive substances with their descriptions.

_____	a. Gastrin	1. Converted to pepsin by acidity
_____	b. Intrinsic factor	2. Converts maltose to glucose
_____	c. Secretin	3. Increases gastric motility and secretion
_____	d. Bile	4. Begins protein digestion
_____	e. Amylase	5. Responsible for absorption of cobalamin
_____	f. Enterokinase	6. Converts fats to fatty acids
_____	g. Pepsinogen	7. Stimulates pancreatic bicarbonate secretion
_____	h. Pepsin	8. Emulsifies fats
_____	i. Maltase	9. Converts trypsinogen to trypsin
_____	j. Lipase	10. Converts starch to disaccharides

8. The destruction of normal bowel bacteria by prolonged antibiotic therapy may cause

a. coagulation problems.
b. elevated serum ammonia levels.
c. impaired absorption of amino acids.
d. increased absorption of urobilinogen into the blood.

9. An obstruction at the sphincter of Oddi will affect the digestion of all nutrients because

a. bile is responsible for emulsification of all nutrients and vitamins.
b. intestinal digestive enzymes are released through the ampulla of Vater.
c. both bile and pancreatic enzymes enter the duodenum at the ampulla of Vater.
d. gastric contents can only pass to the duodenum when the sphincter of Oddi is open.

10. Identify the normal function of the liver that is impaired in the following findings in a patient with liver disease.

    a. Hyperaldosteronism

    b. Hypoalbuminemia

    c. Increased serum ammonia

    d. Increased serum unconjugated bilirubin

    e. Purpura and petechiae

    f. Decreased serum cholesterol

    g. Male gynecomastia

11. A patient experiences increased red blood cell destruction from a mechanical heart valve prosthesis. Describe what happens to the bilirubin that is released from the breakdown of hemoglobin from the red cells.

12. A clinical manifestation of age-related changes in the GI system the nurse would expect an older patient to report is

    a. gastric hyperacidity.
    b. intolerance to fatty foods.
    c. yellowish tinge to the skin.
    d. reflux of gastric contents into the esophagus.

13. Identify one specific finding identified by the nurse during assessment of each of the patient's functional health patterns that indicates a risk factor for gastrointestinal problems or the response of the patient to a gastrointestinal disorder.

    a. Health perception–health management

    b. Nutritional-metabolic

    c. Elimination

    d. Activity-exercise

    e. Sleep-rest

    f. Cognitive-perceptual

    g. Self-perception–self-concept

    h. Role-relationship

    i. Sexuality-reproductive

    j. Coping–stress tolerance

    k. Value-belief

14. A normal finding during physical assessment of the mouth is

    a. a red, slick appearance of the tongue.
    b. uvular deviation to the side on saying "Ahh."
    c. a thin, white coating of the dorsum of the tongue.
    d. scattered red, smooth areas on dorsum of tongue.

15. A normal finding on physical examination of the abdomen is

    a. auscultation of bruits.
    b. observation of visible pulsations.
    c. percussion of liver dullness in the left midclavicular line.
    d. palpation of the spleen 1 to 2 cm below the left costal margin.

16. A patient is admitted to the hospital with upper left quadrant pain. A possible source of the pain may be the

    a. liver.
    b. appendix.
    c. pancreas.
    d. gallbladder.

17. During auscultation of the abdomen

    a. the presence of borborygmi indicates hyperperistalsis.
    b. the bell of the stethoscope is used to auscultate high-pitched sounds.
    c. high-pitched, rushing, and tinkling bowel sounds are heard after eating.
    d. absence of bowel sounds for 3 minutes in each quadrant is reported as abnormal.

18. Complete the table below by indicating with check marks which of the following preparations are required for each of the diagnostic procedures listed.

    (1) NPO up to 8 or more hours
    (2) Bowel emptying with laxatives, enemas, or both
    (3) Informed consent
    (4) Allergy to iodine ascertained

	(1) NPO	**(2) Bowel**	**(3) Consent**	**(4) Allergy**
UGI series				
Barium enema				
IV cholangiogram				
Gallbladder ultrasound				
Hepatobiliary scintigraphy				
Upper GI endoscopy				
Colonoscopy				
Endoscopic retrograde cholangiopancreatography				

19. The diagnostic test that is most specific for acute pancreatitis is
    a. serum amylase.
    b. abdominal ultrasound.
    c. serum gamma-glutamyl transpeptidase (GGT).
    d. endoscopic retrograde cholangiopancreatography (ERCP).

20. A patient's serum liver enzyme tests reveal an elevated aspartate aminotransferase (AST). The nurse recognizes that the elevated AST

    a. eliminates infection as a cause of liver damage.
    b. is diagnostic for liver inflammation and damage.
    c. may reflect tissue damage in organs other than the liver.
    d. may cause nervous system symptoms related to hepatic encephalopathy.

21. Match the nursing responsibilities indicated for the diagnostic procedures (answers may be used more than once).

_____	a. Ensure no smoking morning of test	1. Barium swallow
_____	b. Monitor for LUQ pain and nausea/ vomiting	2. Gastric analysis
		3. Colonoscope
_____	c. Observe for white stools	4. Liver biopsy
_____	d. Monitor for rectal bleeding	5. Gastroduodenoscopy
_____	e. Position to right side after test	6. Endoscopic retrograde cholangiopancreatography
_____	f. Check for return of gag reflex	
_____	g. Monitor for internal bleeding	
_____	h. Check coagulation status before test	
_____	i. Insert nasogastric tube	
_____	j. Check temperature every 15 to 30 min for signs of perforation	

CHAPTER 39 NURSING MANAGEMENT: NUTRITIONAL PROBLEMS

1. A 30-year-old man's diet consists of 3000 calories with 120 g of protein, 160 g of fat, and 270 g of carbohydrate. He weighs 174 lb and is 5 ft 11 in tall.

   a. What percentage of total calories does each of the nutrients contribute to the man's diet?

      Protein

      Fat

      Carbohydrate

   b. According to the Food and Nutrition Board, how many grams of each of the nutrients is recommended for this man?

      Protein

      Fat

      Carbohydrate

   c. How many kcal would be recommended for him as an average adult?

   d. Using the food pyramid as a guide, what changes could the nurse suggest to bring the man's diet more in line with nutrition recommendations?

2. Identify whether the following statements are true or false. If a statement is false, correct the bold word(s) to make the statement true.

   _____ a. Overnutrition resulting in obesity is a type of **malnutrition**.

   _____ b. The two nutrients most often lacking in the diet of a vegan are **vitamin B_6** and **folic acid**.

   _____ c. The major nutritional problem in the U.S. today is the high intake of **carbohydrate** in the diet.

   _____ d. **Marasmus** is a type of malnutrition that results from a deficiency of protein intake superimposed on a catabolic stress event.

3. The most common cause of secondary protein-calorie malnutrition in the U.S. is

   a. the unavailability of foods high in protein.
   b. a lack of knowledge about nutritional needs.
   c. a lack of money to purchase high-protein foods.
   d. an alteration in ingestion, digestion, absorption, or metabolism.

4. Describe the metabolism of nutrients used for energy during starvation within the given approximate time frames.

   a. First 18 hours

   b. 18 hours to 5 to 9 days

   c. 9 days to 6 weeks

   d. Over 6 weeks

5. Failure of the sodium-potassium pump during severe protein depletion may lead to

   a. ascites.
   b. anemia.
   c. hyperkalemia.
   d. hypoalbuminemia.

6. Identify whether the following statements are true or false. If a statement is false, correct the bold word(s) to make the statement true.

   _____ a. A patient with a temperature of 101.6 will need approximately **20%** more calories to meet the increased basal metabolic rate (BMR) caused by the fever.

   _____ b. A patient who is nutritionally fit on admission may develop nutritional problems during hospitalization because of dietary restrictions imposed by **diagnostic testing**.

   _____ c. Vitamin deficiencies in adults most commonly are clinically manifested by disorders of the **skin**.

   _____ d. Prolonged **antibiotic therapy** may contribute to vitamin deficiencies because of loss of bowel bacteria activity.

7. Use the following drugs or drug classifications to complete the sentences below.

erythropoietin (Epoetin)	chlorpromazine (Thorazine)
amitriptyline (Elavil)	phenytoin (Dilantin)
barbiturates	warfarin (Coumadin)
monoamine oxidase inhibitors	xanthine bronchodilators
cholestyramine (Questran)	

a. Large amounts of caffeine may intensify the central nervous system–stimulant effects of

_______________________.

b. Deficiency of all fat-soluble vitamins may occur with prolonged use of _______________________.

c. Green leafy vegetables, dairy products, and meat may decrease the effect of ____________________.

d. Riboflavin deficiency may occur with the use of ___________________ and

_____________________.

e. Unless it is supplemented in the diet, folic acid deficiency may occur with the use of

___________________ and ___________________.

f. Aged cheese, fermented beverages, and smoked meats or poultry may cause a hypertensive crisis if taken

with _______________________.

g. Folic acid and cobalamin deficiencies may decrease the effectiveness of _______________________.

8. During assessment of the patient with protein-calorie malnutrition, the nurse would expect to find

a. a flat or concave abdomen.
b. increased sensitivity to cold.
c. increased pulse and respiratory rate.
d. increased reflexes and vibratory sense.

9. The nurse determines that the patient with the highest risk for the nursing diagnosis of imbalanced nutrition: less than body requirements related to decreased ingestion is the patient with

a. tuberculosis infection.
b. malabsorption syndrome.
c. draining decubitus ulcers.
d. severe anorexia secondary to radiation therapy.

10. The nurse monitors the lab results of the patient with protein-calorie malnutrition during treatment. An indication of improvement in the patient's condition is

a. decreased lymphocytes.
b. increased serum potassium.
c. increased serum transferrin.
d. decreased serum prealbumin.

11. When the nurse is concerned about the skeletal protein reserves of a patient who has been hospitalized during cancer chemotherapy, the assessment of the patient should include

    a. body mass index.
    b. height and weight.
    c. ideal body weight and frame size.
    d. mid-upper arm circumference and triceps skinfold.

12. The nurse evaluates that patient teaching about a high-calorie, high-protein diet has been effective when the patient selects for breakfast from the hospital menu

    a. 2 poached eggs, hash brown potatoes, and whole milk.
    b. 2 slices of toast with butter and jelly, orange juice, and skim milk.
    c. 3 pancakes with butter and syrup, 2 slices of bacon, and apple juice.
    d. cream of wheat with 2 tablespoons skim milk powder, one-half grapefruit, and a high- protein milkshake.

13. Upon admission to a long-term care facility, a 72-year-old woman with a small bone frame weighs 100 lb (45.5 kg) and is 5 ft 2 in (157.5 cm) tall. The nurse uses the Admission Nutrition Screening Tool (Table 39-12) to assess the patient's nutrition and determines that the patient

    a. is at nutritional risk because of her age.
    b. will require an increase in carbohydrate to maintain her weight.
    c. is at nutritional risk because she is <80% of her ideal body weight.
    d. should have her weight monitored frequently in the new environment.

14. When teaching the older adult about nutritional needs during aging, the nurse emphasizes that

    a. the need for all nutrients is decreased as one ages.
    b. fewer calories, but the same amount of protein, are required as one ages.
    c. fats, carbohydrates, and protein should be decreased, but vitamin and mineral intake should be increased.
    d. high-calorie oral supplements should be taken between meals to ensure that recommended nutrients are met.

15. When planning nutritional interventions for a healthy 83-year-old man, the nurse recognizes that the factor that is most likely to affect his nutritional status is

    a. living alone on a fixed income.
    b. changes in cardiovascular function.
    c. snacking between meals, resulting in obesity.
    d. an increase in gastrointestinal motility and absorption.

16. When considering tube feedings for a patient with severe protein-calorie malnutrition, the nurse knows that an advantage of a gastrostomy tube over a nasogastric tube is that

    a. there is less irritation to the nasal and esophageal mucosa.
    b. the patient experiences the sight and smells associated with eating.
    c. aspiration resulting from reflux of formulas into the esophagus is less common.
    d. routine checking for placement is not required because gastrostomy tubes do not become displaced.

17. Identify one nursing intervention that is indicated for each of the following desired outcomes of tube feeding.

    a. Prevention of aspiration

    b. Prevention of diarrhea

    c. Maintenance of tube patency

    d. Maintenance of tube placement

    e. Prevention of infection

18. Before administering a bolus of intermittent tube feeding to a patient with a percutaneous endoscopic gastrostomy (PEG), the nurse aspirates 220 ml of gastric contents. The nurse should

    a. return the aspirate to the stomach and recheck the volume of aspirate in an hour.
    b. return the aspirate to the stomach and continue with the tube feeding as planned.
    c. discard the aspirate to prevent overdistending the stomach when the new feeding is given.
    d. notify the physician that the feedings have been scheduled too frequently to allow for stomach emptying.

19. Indicate whether the following characteristics of total parenteral nutrition (TPN) apply more to central parenteral nutrition (CPN) or peripheral parenteral nutrition (PPN).

    _____ a. Limited to 20% glucose

    _____ b. Tonicity of 1600 mOsm/L

    _____ c. Small fluid volumes

    _____ d. Supplements oral feedings

    _____ e. Long-term nutritional support

    _____ f. Phlebitis more common

    _____ g. May use peripherally inserted catheter (PIC)

20. An indication for TPN that is not appropriate for enteral tube feedings is

    a. head and neck cancer.
    b. hypermetabolic states.
    c. malabsorption syndrome.
    d. protein-calorie malnutrition.

21. What nursing interventions are indicated during TPN to prevent the following complications?

    a. Infection

    b. Hyperglycemia

    c. Air embolism

22. The nurse is caring for a patient receiving 1000 ml of TPN solution over 24 hours. When it is time to change the solution, there is 150 ml remaining in the bottle. The most appropriate action by the nurse is to

    a. hang the new solution and discard the unused solution.
    b. notify the physician for instructions regarding the infusion rate.
    c. open the IV line and infuse the remaining solution as quickly as possible.
    d. wait to change the solution until the remaining solution infuses at the prescribed rate.

23. The physician inserts a central catheter for administration of parenteral nutrition and orders the solution to be started when x-ray confirms proper placement of the catheter. Following the x-ray, radiology notifies the nurse that the catheter tip is in the superior vena cava. The most appropriate action by the nurse is to

    a. start the solution at the prescribed introductory rate.
    b. notify the physician that the catheter needs readjustment.
    c. continue to infuse the isotonic solution until further orders from the physician.
    d. gently push the catheter in 2 to 3 inches to reposition the tip in the right atrium.

24. The physician orders a 10% fat emulsion solution to be administered to a patient who is currently receiving peripheral parenteral nutrition. The most appropriate action by the nurse is to

    a. administer the fat emulsion at the prescribed rate at a new, separate intravenous site.
    b. add the fat emulsion solution to the parenteral nutrition solution since they are compatible.
    c. refrigerate the fat solution until the current bottle of parenteral nutrition has infused and then start the fat emulsion.
    d. connect the tubing of the fat emulsion below the filter on the parenteral nutrition tubing at the injection site closest to the patient.

25. A patient receiving a fat emulsion solution develops nausea, vomiting, and fever. The nurse recognizes that these symptoms may indicate

    a. a fat embolism.
    b. a fatty acid deficiency.
    c. a too rapid infusion rate.
    d. an allergic reaction to the solution.

26. a. Use the nomogram in Figure 38-7 to determine the BMI for a patient who is 5 ft 5 in (165 cm) tall and weighs 202 lb (91.8 kg). ______________ What is the patient's weight classification? ________________

    b. Calculate the waist-to-hip ratio of a woman who has a waist measurement of 32 inches and hip measurement of 36 inches. ____________

    c. What does this value indicate? ________________

27. Explain the rationale for the following interventions in the management of obesity.

    a. 800- to 1200-calorie diet

    b. 1 to 2 pounds a week weight loss

    c. Keeping a diet diary

    d. Schedule several small meals a day

    e. Abstinence from alcohol

    f. Exercise program

    g. Behavioral-cognitive modification

28. Describe how the nurse would explain to the obese patient about the following.

    a. The rapid weight loss of first few days of dieting

    b. Why to weigh weekly rather than daily

    c. How gender influences weight loss

    d. Plateau periods

29. When medications are used in the treatment of obesity, it is important for the nurse to teach the patient that

    a. over-the-counter diet aids are safer than other agents and can be useful in controlling appetite.
    b. diet and exercise are the most important in weight control since drugs do not help change eating behaviors.
    c. all drugs used for weight control are capable of altering central nervous system function and should be used with caution.
    d. the primary effect of the medication is psychologic, controlling the urge to eat in response to stress or feelings of rejection.

30. Match the following characteristics with the appropriate surgical procedures used for treatment of morbid obesity (answers may be used more than once).

_____ a. Dumping syndrome common

_____ b. Staple-created pouch with restricted outlet

_____ c. A cosmetic procedure

_____ d. Removes folds of adipose tissue

_____ e. May require lifelong cobalamin supplementation

_____ f. Staple-created gastric pouch with jejunal outlet

_____ g. Distention of wall of pouch a complication

1. Vertical banded gastroplasty

2. Lipectomy

3. Roux-en-Y gastric bypass

31. Identify whether the following statements are true or false. If a statement is false, correct the bold word(s) to make the statement true.

_____ a. The **android** body fat distribution pattern is characterized by lower-body involvement and low waist-to-hip ratios and skinfold thickness.

_____ b. The highest risk for obesity associated with cardiovascular disease is seen in those individuals with **central** distribution of body fat.

_____ c. **Primary** obesity results from the consumption of more food than required for normal physiologic functions and growth.

32. The nurse plans care for the morbidly obese patient recognizing that complications of obesity necessitate the cautious use of

a. intravenous solutions.
b. hypoglycemic agents.
c. antihypertensive drugs.
d. sedative and hypnotics.

33. During care of the morbidly obese patient, it is important that the nurse

a. avoid reference to the patient's weight to avoid embarrassing the patient.
b. emphasize to the patient how important it is to lose weight to maintain health.
c. plan for necessary modifications in equipment and nursing techniques before initiating care.
d. recognize that a full assessment of each body system may not be possible because of numerous layers of skinfolds.

34. A postoperative nursing intervention for the obese patient who has undergone a verticle banded gastroplasty is

a. irrigating and repositioning the nasogastric tube as needed.
b. delaying ambulation until the patient has enough strength to support self.
c. keeping the patient positioned on the side to facilitate respiratory function.
d. using an extra-long or spinal needle to administer prescribed IM analgesics.

35. Dietary teaching for the patient following a Roux-en-Y gastric bypass includes information regarding the need to

a. gradually increase the amount of food ingested to preoperative levels.
b. maintain a long-term liquid diet to prevent damage to the surgical site.
c. avoid high-carbohydrate foods and limit fluids to prevent dumping syndrome.
d. consume foods high in complex carbohydrate, protein, and fiber to add bulk to intestinal contents.

36. Identify the following characteristics of eating disorders as associated with anorexia nervosa (A), bulimia (B), or both (AB).

_____ a. Morbid fear of obesity

_____ b. Treated with psychotherapy

_____ c. Ignores feelings of hunger

_____ d. Binge eating with purging

_____ e. Feels fat even when emaciated

_____ f. Conceals abnormal eating habits

_____ g. Concerned about body image

_____ h. Self-induced starvation

37. An 18-year-old female patient with anorexia nervosa is admitted to the hospital for treatment. On admission she weighs 82 lb (37 kg) and is 5 ft 3 in (134.6 cm) tall. Her lab results include the following: K^+ 2.8 mEq/L (2.8 mmol/L), Hg 8.9 g/dl (89 g/L), and BUN 64 mg/dl (22.8 mmol/L). In planning care for the patient, the nurse gives the highest priority to the nursing diagnosis of

a. risk for injury related to dizziness and weakness secondary to anemia.
b. imbalanced nutrition: less than body requirements related to inadequate food intake.
c. risk for decreased cardiac output related to arrhythmias secondary to hypokalemia.
d. risk for impaired urinary elimination related to elevated BUN secondary to renal failure.

CASE STUDY

MALNUTRITION

Patient Profile

Mrs. M., a 62-year-old widow, has recently undergone radiation and chemotherapy following surgery for breast cancer. On a follow-up visit to the clinic, the nurse notes that Mrs. M. appears more thin and tired than usual.

Subjective Data

- Says she has not had an appetite since the treatment for cancer was started
- Feels "weak" and "worn out"
- Thinks the treatment for cancer has not been effective
- Lives alone in an apartment in the inner city
- Is a nationalized citizen from Honduras
- Speaks English but only reads Spanish

Objective Data

- Height 62 in (155 cm); weight 92 lb (41.8 kg)
- BP 98/60, HR 60, RR 12
- Ulcerations of her buccal mucosal membranes and tongue
- Lab results: Serum albumin 2.8 g/dl (28 g/L)
  Hg 10 g/dl (100 g/L); Hct 32%

Critical Thinking Questions

1. What additional assessment data should the nurse obtain from Mrs. M. related to her nutritional status?

2. What physical and psychosocial factors have contributed to Mrs. M.'s malnutrition?

3. What additional symptoms would the nurse expect to see based on Mrs. M.'s laboratory test results?

4. What complications of malnutrition are most likely to occur in Mrs. M. because of her history and clinical manifestations?

5. What instructions could the nurse give Mrs. M. regarding her diet that would be most therapeutic?

6. Based on the assessment data presented, write one or more appropriate nursing diagnoses. Are there any collaborative problems?

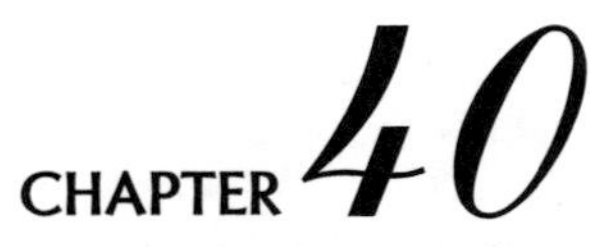

CHAPTER 40 NURSING MANAGEMENT: UPPER GASTROINTESTINAL PROBLEMS

1. Identify whether the following statements are true or false. If a statement is false, correct the bold word(s) to make the statement true.

_____ a. Immediately before the act of vomiting, activation of the **sympathetic nervous system** causes increased salivation, increased gastric mobility, and relaxation of the lower esophageal sphincter.

_____ b. Stimulation of the vomiting center by the chemoreceptor trigger zone (CTZ) is commonly caused by **stretch and distention of hollow organs**.

_____ c. Vomiting may occur in response to psychologic stress by stimulation of the vomiting center from **the cerebral cortex**.

_____ d. The acid-base imbalance most commonly associated with persistent vomiting is **metabolic acidosis** caused by loss of **bicarbonate**.

_____ e. **Regurgitation** is not accompanied by nausea and is associated with increased intracranial pressure.

2. Laboratory findings that the nurse would expect in the patient with persistent vomiting include

   a. ↓ pH, ↑ sodium, ↓ hematocrit.
   b. ↑ pH, ↓ chloride, ↓ hematocrit.
   c. ↑ pH, ↓ potassium, ↑ hematocrit.
   d. ↓ pH, ↓ potassium, ↑ hematocrit.

3. A patient's vomitus is dark brown and has a coffee-ground appearance. The nurse recognizes that this emesis is characteristic of

   a. stomach bleeding.
   b. an intestinal obstruction.
   c. bile reflux into the stomach.
   d. active bleeding of the lower esophagus.

4. A patient who has been vomiting for several days from an unknown cause is admitted to the hospital. The nurse anticipates collaborative care to include

   a. oral administration of broth and tea.
   b. administration of parenteral antiemetics.
   c. insertion of a nasogastric tube to suction.
   d. intravenous replacement of fluid and electrolytes.

5. A patient treated for vomiting is to begin oral intake when the symptoms have subsided. To promote rehydration, the nurse plans to administer

   a. hot tea.
   b. Gatorade.
   c. cool water.
   d. warm broth.

6. Ondansetron (Zofran) is prescribed for a patient with cancer chemotherapy-induced vomiting. The nurse understands that this drug

   a. is a derivative of cannabis and has a potential for abuse.
   b. has a strong antihistamine effect that provides sedation and induces sleep.
   c. is used only when other therapies are ineffective because of side effects of anxiety and hallucinations.
   d. relieves vomiting centrally by action in the vomiting center and peripherally by promoting gastric emptying.

7. Match the following characteristics of inflammations and infections of the mouth with their types (answers may be used more than once).

_____	a. Viral infection related to upper respiratory infections and sun sensitivity	1. Gingivitis
_____	b. Staphylococcal infection that may occur with prolonged NPO status	2. Vincent's infection
_____	c. Painful, bleeding gums with gingival necrosis and metallic-tasting saliva	3. Oral candidiasis
_____	d. Associated with prolonged high-dose antibiotic or corticosteroid therapy	4. Herpes simplex
_____	e. Formation of abscesses with loosening of teeth	5. Aphthous stomatitis
_____	f. Infectious ulcers of mouth and lips with a defined erythematous base	6. Parotitis
_____	g. White membranous lesions of mucosa of mouth and throat	7. Stomatitis
_____	h. Inflammation of mouth related to systemic disease and cancer chemotherapy	
_____	i. Shallow, painful vesicular ulcerations of lips and mouth	
_____	j. Results in decreased salivation and ear pain	
_____	k. Bacterial infection predisposed by fatigue, worry, and poor oral hygiene	

8. A patient is scheduled for a biopsy of a painful tongue ulcer. Based on knowledge of risk factors for oral cancer, the nurse specifically asks the patient about a history of

   a. excessive exposure to sunlight.
   b. recurrent herpes simplex infections.
   c. use of any type of tobacco products.
   d. difficulty swallowing and pain in the ear.

9. When caring for a patient following a glossectomy with dissection of the floor of the mouth and a radical neck dissection for cancer of the tongue, the nurse's primary concern is maintaining

   a. relief of pain.
   b. a patent airway.
   c. a positive body image.
   d. tube feedings to provide nutrition.

10. A patient with oral cancer has a history of heavy smoking, excessive alcohol intake, and personal neglect. During the patient's early postoperative course, the nurse anticipates that the patient may need

   a. oral nutritional supplements.
   b. drug therapy to prevent substance withdrawal symptoms.
   c. less pain medication because of cross-tolerance with CNS depressants.
   d. counseling about lifestyle changes to prevent recurrence of the tumor.

11. Identify four foods or beverages that decrease lower esophageal sphincter pressure that the nurse should teach the patient with gastroesophageal reflux disease (GERD) to avoid.

   a. alcohol
   b. Fatty foods
   c. Chocolate
   d. Coffee/tea

12. Bethanechol (Urecholine) is added to the step-up drug regimen of a patient with GERD. The nurse explains that the purpose of this drug is to

   a. act as a mechanical barrier to reflux.
   b. decrease the volume of gastric acid secretion.
   c. relieve heartburn by neutralizing hydrochloric acid.
   d. increase lower esophageal sphincter pressure and gastric emptying.

13. The nurse teaches the patient with a hiatal hernia or GERD to control symptoms by

   a. drinking 10 to 12 ounces of water with each meal.
   b. spacing six small meals a day between breakfast and bedtime.
   c. sleeping with the head of the bed elevated on 4- to 6-inch blocks.
   d. performing daily exercises of toe-touching, sit-ups, and weight lifting.

14. A patient is returned to the surgical unit following a laparoscopic fundoplication for repair of a hiatal hernia with an IV, NG tube to suction, and several small abdominal incisions. To prevent disruption of the surgical site, it is most important for the nurse to

   a. monitor for the return of peristalsis.
   b. position the patient on the right side.
   c. maintain the patency of the NG tube.
   d. assess the abdominal wounds for drainage.

15. A patient with esophageal cancer is scheduled for a partial esophagectomy. A nursing diagnosis that is likely to be of highest priority preoperatively is

    a. deficient fluid volume related to inadequate intake.
    b. impaired oral mucous membrane related to inadequate oral hygiene.
    c. imbalanced nutrition: less than body requirements related to dysphagia.
    d. ineffective therapeutic regimen maintenance related to lack of knowledge of disease process.

16. Following a patient's esophagogastrostomy for cancer of the esophagus, it is important for the nurse to

    a. report any bloody drainage from the nasogastric tube.
    b. maintain the patient in a semi-Fowler's or Fowler's position.
    c. monitor for abdominal distention that may disrupt the surgical site.
    d. expect to find decreased breath sounds bilaterally because of the surgical approach.

17. Match the following esophageal disorders with their descriptions.

_____	a. Esophagitis	1. Absence of peristalsis of lower two thirds of esophagus with nonrelaxing LES
_____	b. Esophageal diverticula	2. Inflammation of esophagus from irritants or gastric reflux
_____	c. Esophageal strictures	3. Narrowing of esophagus from scarring
_____	d. Achalasia	4. Precancerous esophageal metaplasia associated with GERD
_____	e. Barrett's esophagus	5. Common site is above the upper esophageal sphincter

18. Complete the following sentences.

    a. The self-limiting type of gastritis most likely to occur in a college student who has an isolated drinking binge is _______________ gastritis.

    b. _______________ gastritis is associated with an increased risk for stomach cancer.

    c. A definite diagnosis of gastritis is made with the use of ___________________.

    d. The microorganism that has a strong causative relationship with both diffuse antral and multifocal gastritis is _________________________.

    e. A complication of chronic gastritis that results from the destruction and atrophy of acid-secreting cells is the loss of _________________________, leading to pernicious anemia.

    f. Drugs that contain _______________ and _______________ can reduce the bleeding and promote healing of erosive gastritis.

19. Nursing management of the patient with chronic gastritis includes teaching the patient to

a. maintain a bland diet with six small meals a day.
b. take antacids before meals to decrease stomach acidity.
c. use NSAIDs instead of aspirin for any minor pain relief.
d. eliminate alcohol and caffeine from the diet when symptoms occur.

20. Identify what type of bleeding is indicated by the following findings.

a. Profuse bright-red hematemesis

b. Coffee-ground emesis

c. Melena

d. Hematemesis with negative stool guaiac

21. During the nursing assessment of a patient with upper GI bleeding, it is important to obtain a complete history of events leading to the bleeding episode. Match the following common causes of bleeding with the patient situations that may be discovered during a nursing assessment.

_____	a. Esophageal varices	1. Patient with GERD
_____	b. Stress ulcers	2. An older female patient with arthritis
_____	c. Esophagitis	3. Patient with no history of GI symptoms
_____	d. Mallory-Weiss syndrome	4. Patient with cirrhosis of the liver
_____	e. Hemorrhagic gastritis	5. Patient with history of chronic atrophic gastritis
_____	f. Drug-induced gastritis	6. Patient with excessive alcohol intake
_____	g. Cancer of the stomach	7. Patient with severe retching and vomiting
_____	h. Peptic ulcer	8. Patient with severe burns

22. A patient is admitted to the emergency department with profuse bright-red hematemesis. During the initial care of the patient, the nurse's first priority is to

a. perform a nursing assessment of the patient's status.
b. establish two intravenous sites with large-gauge catheters.
c. obtain a thorough health history to assist in determining the cause of the bleeding.
d. perform a gastric lavage with cool tap water in preparation for endoscopic examination and treatment.

23. A patient with upper GI bleeding is treated with several drugs. The nurse recognizes that an agent that is used to decrease bleeding and decrease gastric acid secretions is

a. ranitidine (Zantac).
b. omeprazole (Prilosec).
c. vasopressin (Pitressin).
d. octreotide (Sandostatin).

24. In teaching patients at risk for upper GI bleeding to prevent bleeding episodes, the nurse stresses that

    a. all stools and vomitus must be tested for the presence of blood.
    b. the use of over-the-counter medications of any kind should be avoided.
    c. antacids should be taken with all prescribed medications to prevent gastric irritation.
    d. misoprostol (Cytotec) should be used to protect the gastric mucosa in individuals with peptic ulcers.

25. The nurse evaluates that management of the patient with upper GI bleeding is effective when assessment and laboratory findings reveal a

    a. decreasing BUN.
    b. normal hematocrit.
    c. urinary output of 20 ml/hr.
    d. urine specific gravity of 1.030.

26. When reviewing the medication history of a patient with gastric bleeding the nurse consults with the physician about changing the use of

    a. famotidine (Pepcid) to nizatidine (Axid).
    b. naproxen (Naprosyn) to rofecoxib (Vioxx).
    c. aluminum hydroxide to sodium bicarbonate.
    d. diclofenac (Voltaren) to misoprostol (Cytotec).

27. Indicate whether the following characteristics are associated with gastric ulcers (G), duodenal ulcers (D), or both (B).

_____ a. Increased gastric secretion

_____ b. Superficial with smooth margins

_____ c. High recurrence rate

_____ d. Burning and cramping in midepigastric area

_____ e. Increased incidence with smoking, drug, and alcohol use

_____ f. Higher incidence in women in fifth and sixth decade

_____ g. Burning and gaseous pressure in high epigastrium

_____ h. Associated with psychologic stress

_____ i. May cause hemorrhage, perforation, and obstruction

_____ j. Possible seasonal trend in occurrence

_____ k. Pain 1 to 2 hours after meals

_____ l. Increased incidence in persons from lower socioeconomic class

_____ m. Associated with *H. pylori* infection

_____ n. Relief of pain with food

28. Match the following factors associated with the development of peptic ulcers with their probable pathophysiologic mechanisms.

_____ a. *Helicobacter pylori*

_____ b. Aspirin and NSAIDs

_____ c. Corticosteroids

_____ d. Vagal stimulation

_____ e. Severe physiologic stress

_____ f. Nicotine

1. Decrease rate of mucous cell turnover
2. Ischemia of gastric mucosa
3. Generate ammonia in mucous layer
4. Decrease pancreatic bicarbonate secretion
5. Inhibit synthesis of mucus and prostaglandins
6. Hypersecretion of hydrochloric acid

29. Regardless of the precipitating factor, the injury to mucosal cells in peptic ulcers is caused by

a. acid back-diffusion into the mucosa.
b. ammonia formation in the mucosal wall.
c. breakdown of the gastric mucosal barrier.
d. the release of histamine from gastrointestinal cells.

30. The nurse expects a patient with an ulcer of the posterior portion of the duodenum to experience

    a. pain that occurs after not eating all day.
    b. back pain that occurs 2 to 4 hours following meals.
    c. midepigastric pain that is unrelieved with antacids.
    d. high epigastric burning that is relieved with food intake.

31. Diagnostic testing is planned for a patient with a suspected peptic ulcer. The nurse explains to the patient that the most reliable test for determining the presence and location of an ulcer is a(n)

    a. endoscopy.
    b. gastric analysis.
    c. barium swallow.
    d. serologic test for *H. pylori*.

32. The nurse teaches a patient with newly diagnosed peptic ulcer disease to

    a. maintain a bland, soft, low-residue diet.
    b. use alcohol and caffeine in moderation and always with food.
    c. eat as normally as possible, eliminating foods that cause pain or discomfort.
    d. avoid milk and milk products because they stimulate gastric acid production.

33. Identify the rationale for treatment with nasogastric intubation for each of the following situations associated with peptic ulcer disease.

    a. Acute exacerbation

    b. Peritonitis

    c. Gastric outlet obstruction

34. A patient who has peptic ulcer disease has the following medications ordered:

    Magnesium hydroxide/aluminum hydroxide (Mylanta) 15 ml PO 1 hr ac and 3 hr pc and hs
    Ranitidine (Zantac) 300 mg PO hs
    Sucralfate (Carafate) 1.0 g 1 hr ac and hs

    The patient usually has meals at 7 AM, 12 noon, and 6 PM, and a bedtime snack at 10 PM.

    Plan an administration schedule that will be most therapeutic and acceptable to the patient.

Times

    a. Mylanta

    b. Ranitidine

    c. Sucralfate

35. Match the following characteristics with the drugs used to treat or prevent peptic ulcer disease (answers may be used more than once).

_____ a. Prevents conversion of pepsinogen to pepsin

_____ b. Used in patients with verified *H. pylori*

_____ c. Covers the ulcer, protecting it from hydroxide mixture erosion

_____ d. Decreases gastric acid secretion by blocking ATPase enzyme

_____ e. High incidence of side effects and contraindications

_____ f. High dose and frequency stimulate release of gastrin

_____ g. Reduce HCl acid secretion by blocking action of histamine

_____ h. Antisecretory effects in patients using antiprostaglandin drugs

_____ i. Has the greatest noncompliance

_____ j. Decrease HCl acid secretion and gastric motility

_____ k. Newer drugs in class more potent at reduced dosage

1. Famotidine (Pepcid)
2. Omeprazole (Prilosec)
3. Aluminum/magnesium hydroxide mixture
4. Sucralfate (Carafate)
5. Misoprostol (Cytotec)
6. Amoxicillin/clarithromycin/omeprazole
7. Anticholinergics

36. The nurse determines that teaching for the patient with peptic ulcer disease has been effective when the patient states

a. "I should stop all my medications if I develop any side effects."
b. "I should continue my treatment regimen as long as I have pain."
c. "I have learned some relaxation strategies that decrease my stress."
d. "I can buy whatever antacids are on sale because they all have the same effect."

37. A patient with a history of peptic ulcer disease is hospitalized with symptoms of a perforation. During the initial assessment, the nurse would expect the patient to report

a. vomiting of bright-red blood.
b. projectile vomiting of undigested food.
c. sudden, severe upper abdominal pain and shoulder pain.
d. hyperactive stomach sounds and upper abdominal swelling.

38. A patient with a gastric outlet obstruction has been treated with nasogastric decompression. After the first 24 hours, the patient develops nausea and increased upper abdominal bowel sounds. An appropriate action by the nurse is to

a. check the patency of the NG tube.
b. place the patient in a recumbent position.
c. assess the patient's vital signs and circulatory status.
d. encourage the patient to deep breathe and consciously relax.

39. When caring for a patient with an acute exacerbation of a peptic ulcer, the nurse finds the patient doubled up in bed with shallow, grunting respirations. The initial appropriate action by the nurse is to

a. notify the physician.
b. irrigate the patient's NG tube.
c. place the patient in a high Fowler's position.
d. assess the patient's abdomen and vital signs.

40. Match the descriptions with the following surgical procedures used to treat peptic ulcer disease.

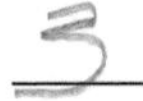
_____ a. Often performed with a vagotomy to increase gastric emptying

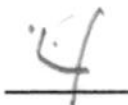
_____ b. Severing of a parasympathetic nerve to decrease gastric secretion

_____ c. Removal of distal two thirds of stomach with anastomosis to jejunum

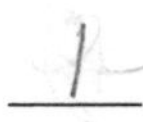
_____ d. Removal of distal two thirds of stomach with anastomosis to duodenum

1. Billroth I
2. Billroth II
3. Pyloroplasty
4. Vagotomy

41. Following a Billroth II procedure, a patient develops dumping syndrome. The nurse explains that the symptoms associated with this problem are caused by

a. distention of the smaller stomach by too much food and fluid intake.
b. hyperglycemia caused by uncontrolled gastric emptying into the small intestine.
c. irritation of the stomach lining by reflux of bile salts because the pylorus has been removed.
d. movement of fluid into the bowel because concentrated food and fluids move rapidly into the intestine.

42. The nurse determines that further dietary teaching is needed when a patient with dumping syndrome says

a. "I should eat bread with every meal."
b. "I should avoid drinking fluids with my meals."
c. "I should eat smaller meals about 6 times a day."
d. "I need to lie down for 30 to 60 minutes after my meals."

43. While caring for a patient following a subtotal gastrectomy with a gastroduodenostomy anastomosis, the nurse determines that the nasogastric tube is obstructed. The nurse should

a. replace the tube with a new one.
b. irrigate the tube until return can be aspirated.
c. reposition the tube and then attempt irrigation.
d. notify the surgeon to reposition or replace the tube.

44. In promoting early detection of cancer of the stomach, the nurse focuses on identification of patients who are at risk because of

a. achlorhydria.
b. acute gastritis.
c. heavy smoking.
d. peptic ulcer disease.

45. During assessment of the patient with gastric pain and discomfort, the nurse focuses on signs and symptoms that may differentiate cancer of the stomach from peptic ulcer disease. These findings include

   a. anorexia with weight loss.
   b. nausea, vomiting, and hematemesis.
   c. signs of anemia such as pallor, fatigue, and black tarry stools.
   d. pain that has previously been controlled with antacids becomes worse.

46. A patient with cancer of the stomach at the lesser curvature undergoes a total gastrectomy with an esophagojejunostomy. Postoperatively, the nurse teaches the patient to expect

   a. rapid healing of the surgical wound.
   b. to be able to return to normal dietary habits.
   c. close follow-up for development of peptic ulcers in the jejunum.
   d. lifelong intramuscular or intranasal administration of cobalamin.

47. A large number of children at a public school have developed profuse diarrhea and development of bloody stools. The school nurse suspects food poisoning from the school cafeteria and requests analysis and culture of

   a. chicken.
   b. ground beef.
   c. commercially canned fish.
   d. salads with mayonnaise dressing.

CASE STUDY

GASTRIC CANCER

Patient Profile

Mrs. E. is a 75-year-old retired garment worker who was diagnosed with gastric cancer 2 weeks ago. The home health nurse assigned to her case reads the following on her medical record:

Subjective Data

- Had a 6-month history of epigastric discomfort, anorexia, nausea, vomiting, and a 25 lb weight loss
- Stated she has had "stomach problems" for a long time, and was diagnosed with gastritis 20 years ago
- Stated she was told that they could not take out the tumor because it was too far gone
- Stated, "I've always been a strong person, but now I'm just too tired to eat or do anything."

Objective Data

- Physical exam: palpable mass in left upper quadrant of the abdomen
- Diagnostic tests: Barium swallow, gastroscopy, and biopsy/cytology all confirmed the presence of a well-advanced tumor in the fundus of the stomach
- Laboratory tests: Decreased hemoglobin and hematocrit
  Serum albumin 2.4 g/dl (24 g/L)
- Appears emaciated, with areas of skin discoloration on her forearms

When the nurse visits Mrs. E., she has just returned from a radiation treatment and is holding a plastic emesis basin and tissues in her lap.

Critical Thinking Questions

1. What pathophysiologic changes occur in gastric cancer that lead to the symptoms experienced by Mrs. E.?

2. What subjective and objective data indicate the presence of malnutrition in Mrs. E.?

3. What other factors might be contributing to Mrs. E.'s malnutrition besides those described?

4. What other complications may develop as a result of Mrs. E's malnutrition?

5. What treatment plan should the nurse provide for Mrs. E. and her family?

6. Mrs. E. asks the nurse if anyone with her stage of gastric cancer has ever recovered. What is the nurse's best response to Mrs. E.?

7. Based on the assessment data presented, write one or more appropriate nursing diagnoses. Are there any collaborative problems?

CHAPTER 41 NURSING MANAGMENT: LOWER GASTROINTESTINAL PROBLEMS

1. Match the causes and findings with the appropriate classes of diarrhea (answers may be used more than once).

_____	a. Irritable bowel syndrome	1. Decreased fluid absorption
_____	b. Bowel resection or bypass	2. Increased fluid secretion
_____	c. Stool positive for parasites	3. Motility disturbance
_____	d. Radiation mucosal damage	
_____	e. Dumping syndrome	
_____	f. Antibiotic-induced *C. difficile*	
_____	g. Lactase deficiency	
_____	h. High stool fat and undigested protein	
_____	i. Foods and drugs containing sorbitol	

2. The nurse identifies a need for additional teaching when a patient with acute infectious diarrhea states

   a. "I can use A&D ointment or Vaseline jelly around the anal area to protect my skin."
   b. "Gatorade is a good liquid to drink because it replaces the fluid and salts I have lost."
   c. "I must wash my hands after every bowel movement to prevent spreading the diarrhea to my family."
   d. "I may use over-the-counter loperamide (Imodium) or Parepectolin (paregoric, pectin, kaolin) as needed to control the diarrhea."

3. In instituting a bowel training program for a patient with fecal incontinence, the nurse plans to

   a. teach the patient to use a perianal pouch.
   b. place the patient on a bedpan 30 minutes before breakfast.
   c. insert a rectal suppository at the same time every morning.
   d. assist the patient to the bathroom at the time of the patient's normal defecation.

4. Explain the significance of the following information obtained from the patient with chronic constipation during the nursing assessment.

   a. Suppressing the urge to defecate while at work

   b. A history of diverticulosis

   c. Belief in necessity of daily bowel movement

   d. History of hemorrhoids and hypertension

   e. High dietary fiber with low fluid intake

5. The nurse teaches the patient with chronic constipation that of the following foods, dietary fiber is highest in

   a. bananas.
   b. popcorn.
   c. dried beans.
   d. shredded wheat.

6. The preferred immediate treatment for an acute episode of constipation is

   a. soapsuds enemas.
   b. stimulant cathartics.
   c. stool-softening cathartics.
   d. tap water or hypertonic enemas.

7. A patient is admitted to the emergency department with an acute abdomen. The nursing intervention that should be implemented first is

   a. measurement of vital signs to detect hypovolemic changes.
   b. administration of prescribed analgesics to promote patient comfort and relieve anxiety.
   c. a thorough assessment of the onset, location, intensity, duration, and character of the pain.
   d. a physical assessment of the abdomen for distention, masses, abnormal pulsations, bowel sounds, and pigmentation changes.

8. For the following causes of acute abdomen, indicate whether surgery is indicated.

   _____ a. Foreign body perforation

   _____ b. Pancreatitis

   _____ c. Ruptured abdominal aneurysm

   _____ d. Ruptured ectopic pregnancy

   _____ e. Pelvic inflammatory disease

   _____ f. Acute ischemic bowel

9. A patient returns to the surgical unit with a nasogastric tube to low intermittent suction, IV fluids, and a Jackson-Pratt drain at the surgical site following an exploratory laparotomy and repair of a bowel perforation. Four hours after admission, the patient experiences nausea and vomiting. An appropriate nursing intervention for the patient is to

   a. assess the abdomen for distention and bowel sounds.
   b. inspect the surgical site and drainage in the Jackson-Pratt.
   c. check the amount and character of gastric drainage and the patency of the NG tube.
   d. administer prescribed hydroxine (Vistaril) to control the nausea and vomiting.

10. On the second postoperative day, a patient who had an exploratory laparotomy complains of abdominal distention and gas pains. The patient asks the nurse if this indicates damage to the bowel during surgery. The nurse's best response to the patient is

    a. "Abdominal distention occurs as a normal response to inflammation and healing of the bowel."
    b. "Gas pains occur when a nasogastric tube is not used during surgery to remove air from the stomach."
    c. "This is a common complication of abdominal surgery but usually can be relieved by having a bowel movement."
    d. "This occurs because of bowel immobility caused by anesthesia and manipulation of abdominal contents during surgery."

11. A postoperative patient has a nursing diagnosis of pain related to immobility, medication, and decreased motility as evidenced by abdominal pain and distention and inability to pass flatus. An appropriate nursing intervention for the patient is to

    a. ambulate the patient more frequently.
    b. assess the abdomen for bowel sounds.
    c. place the patient in a high Fowler's position.
    d. withhold narcotics because they decrease bowel motility.

12. When caring for a patient with irritable bowel syndrome (IBS) the nurse recognizes that

    a. there is no definitive way to diagnose IBS.
    b. IBS is a psychogenic illness that requires psychologic interventions.
    c. new medications for IBS are available and effective for treatment of IBS.
    d. a diet high in dietary fiber is recommended for patient with IBS manifested by either diarrhea or constipation.

13. A 22-year-old patient calls the outpatient clinic complaining of nausea and vomiting and right lower abdominal pain. The nurse advises the patient to

    a. have the symptoms evaluated by a physician right away.
    b. use a heating pad to relax the muscles at the site of the pain.
    c. drink at least 2 quarts of juice to replace the fluid lost in vomiting.
    d. take a laxative to empty the bowel before examination at the clinic.

14. Identify whether the following statements are true or false. If a statement is false, correct the bold word(s) to make the statement true.

    _____ a. The nurse recognizes that surgery is indicated for the patient with abdominal trauma when positive findings are obtained with **peritoneal lavage**.

    _____ b. The major complication of appendicitis is **colitis**.

    _____ c. The site of pain localization in appendicitis is known as **Rovsing's sign**.

    _____ d. Regardless of the cause of peritonitis the nurse would anticipate that treatment of the patient would include **IV fluid replacement**.

    _____ e. The nurse advises the patient with gastroenteritis to start increasing fluid intake as soon as **vomiting subsides**.

15. A patient with a gunshot wound to the abdomen develops a bacterial peritonitis after surgery to repair the bowel. The nurse explains to the patient that this problem is caused primarily by

    a. immobility and loss of peristalsis of the bowel as a result of surgery.
    b. the penetration of unsterile foreign bodies into the abdominal cavity.
    c. spillage of bowel contents into the normally sterile abdominal cavity.
    d. accumulation of blood and fluid in the abdominal cavity as a result of the trauma.

16. Indicate whether the following characteristics of inflammatory bowel disease are most likely to be associated with ulcerative colitis (UC), Crohn's disease (CD), or both conditions (B).

_____ a. Presence of diarrhea

_____ b. Confined to large intestine

_____ c. Involves the entire thickness of the bowel wall

_____ d. Has periods of remission and exacerbation

_____ e. Can be cured with surgical colectomy

_____ f. Has segmented distribution

_____ g. Rectal bleeding

_____ h. Extraintestinal complications

_____ i. Risk of colon cancer

_____ j. Bowel perforation

_____ k. Formation of fistulas

_____ l. Unknown cause

_____ m. Abdominal pain

_____ n. Association with tumor necrosis factor-α

17. Indicate what lab findings are expected in ulcerative colitis as a result of the following:

a. Bloody diarrhea

b. Cellular mucosal breakdown

c. Diarrhea and vomiting

d. Toxic megacolon

18. Extraintestinal symptoms that are seen in both ulcerative colitis and Crohn's disease are

a. osteoporosis and conjunctivitis.
b. peptic ulcer disease and uveitis.
c. erythema nodosum and arthritis.
d. gluten intolerance and gallstones.

19. Match the following treatment modalities for inflammatory bowel disease with the appropriate rationale (answers may be used more than once).

_____	a. Corticosteroids	1. Promote bowel rest
_____	b. Parenteral nutrition	2. Control inflammation
_____	c. Cobalamin injections	3. Prevent secondary infection
_____	d. Antidiarrheal agents	4. Correct malnutrition
_____	e. Sulfasalazine (Azulfidine)	5. Alleviate stress
_____	f. IV fluids	6. Symptomatic relief of symptoms
_____	g. Sedatives	
_____	h. 6-Mercaptopurine	
_____	i. Nasogastric suction	
_____	j. Iron injections	
_____	k. NPO	

20. A patient with ulcerative colitis undergoes the first phase of a total colectomy with ileoanal anastomosis and formation of an ileal reservoir. On postoperative assessment of the patient, the nurse would expect to find

a. an unopened loop ileostomy.
b. a rectal tube set to low continuous suction.
c. an ileostomy stoma with a catheter in place to provide pouch irrigations.
d. a permanent ileostomy stoma in the right lower quadrant of the abdomen.

21. A patient with ulcerative colitis has a total colectomy with formation of a terminal ileum stoma. An important nursing intervention for this patient postoperatively is to

a. measure the ileostomy output to determine the status of the patient's fluid balance.
b. change the ileostomy appliance every 3 to 4 hours to prevent leakage of drainage onto the skin.
c. emphasize that the ostomy is temporary and the ileum will be reconnected when the large bowel heals.
d. teach the patient about the high-fiber, low-carbohydrate diet required to maintain normal ileostomy drainage.

22. A patient with Crohn's disease is hospitalized with an acute exacerbation. The physician orders an elemental diet for the patient. The nurse informs the patient that an advantage of this diet is that it is

a. high in fat, promoting an emollient effect on the bowel.
b. absorbed in the proximal small bowel, promoting distal bowel rest.
c. milk based, correcting protein, calcium, and other nutritional deficits.
d. administered parenterally, resting the bowel and providing nutrients and electrolytes.

23. A patient with inflammatory bowel disease has a nursing diagnosis of imbalanced nutrition: less than body requirements related to decreased nutritional intake and decreased intestinal absorption. Assessment data that support this nursing diagnosis are

a. pallor and hair loss.
b. frequent diarrhea stools.
c. anorectal excoriation and pain.
d. hypotension and urine output below 30 ml/hr.

24. Match the following intestinal obstructions with their descriptions.

_____ a. Adhesions
_____ b. Volvulus
_____ c. Intussusception
_____ d. Hernia
_____ e. Vascular obstruction
_____ f. Adynamic obstruction

1. Nervous paralysis of the bowel
2. Protrusion of bowel in weak or abnormal opening
3. Bands of scar tissue constrict the intestine
4. Closed loop twisting of bowel on itself
5. Bowel folding on itself
6. Emboli of arterial supply to the bowel

25. The fluid and electrolyte imbalances that occur with a low small bowel obstruction are a result of

a. decreased secretion of intestinal fluids.
b. loss of hydrochloric acid from persistent, copious vomiting.
c. bleeding from a strangulated obstruction resulting in necrosis.
d. movement of fluid and electrolytes from the bowel into the peritoneal cavity.

26. Identify whether the following statements are true or false. If a statement is false, correct the bold word(s) to make the statement true.

_____ a. A rapid onset of projectile vomiting occurs with a **large bowel obstruction**.

_____ b. Abdominal distention is the most apparent in an obstruction of the **large bowel**.

_____ c. Fecal vomiting is most likely to occur in a **low small** bowel obstruction.

_____ d. **Metabolic alkalosis** is most likely to occur with a low small bowel obstruction.

_____ e. Sudden, severe constant abdominal pain is indicative of an **upper small** bowel obstruction.

_____ f. Abdominal pain that is colicky and crampy, coming and going in waves, is characteristic of a **paralytic ileus**.

_____ g. Nasogastric and nasointestinal tubes are used to decompress the intestine in **large bowel** obstructions.

27. An important nursing intervention for the patient with a small bowel obstruction who has a nasointestinal tube is to

a. offer ice chips to suck prn.
b. provide mouth care every 1 to 2 hours.
c. irrigate the tube with normal saline every 8 hours.
d. keep the patient supine with the head of the bed elevated 30 degrees.

28. During a routine screening colonoscopy on a 56-year-old patient, a rectosigmoidal polyp was identified and removed. The patient asks the nurse if his risk for colon cancer is increased because of the polyp. The best response by the nurse is

    a. "It is very rare for polyps to become malignant, but you should continue to have routine colonscopies."
    b. "Individuals with polyps have a 100% lifetime risk of developing colorectal cancer, and at an earlier age than those without polyps."
    c. "All polyps are abnormal and should be removed, but the risk for cancer depends on the type and if malignant changes are present."
    d. "All polyps are premalignant and source of most colon cancer. You will need to have a colonoscopy every 6 months to check for new polyps."

29. Early screening for detection of cancers of the right side of the colon in individuals over 50 years of age that should be done every year include.

    a. serum CEA levels.
    b. flexible sigmoidoscopy.
    c. digital rectal examination.
    d. fecal testing for occult blood.

30. A knowledge of factors associated with colorectal cancer guides the nurse when obtaining a nursing history to ask specifically about

    a. usual diet.
    b. history of smoking.
    c. history of alcohol intake.
    d. environmental exposure to carcinogens.

31. Describe how the structures of the colon are altered during an abdominal-perineal resection.

32. Upon examining a patient 8 hours after formation of a colostomy, the nurse would expect to find

    a. hypoactive, high-pitched bowel sounds.
    b. a brick-red, puffy stoma that oozes blood.
    c. a purplish stoma, shiny and moist with mucus.
    d. a small amount of liquid fecal drainage from the stoma.

33. A male patient who has undergone an abdominal-perineal resection has a nursing diagnosis of risk for ineffective sexuality patterns. An appropriate nursing intervention for the patient is to

    a. have the patient's sexual partner reassure the patient that he is still desirable.
    b. reassure the patient that sexual function will return when healing is complete.
    c. remind the patient that affection can be expressed in other ways besides sexual intercourse.
    d. explain that physical and emotional factors can affect sexual function but not necessarily the patient's sexuality.

34. Describe the type of drainage expected from the stoma of each of the following.

 a. Ileostomy

 b. Descending colostomy

 c. Transverse loop colostomy

35. The nurse plans teaching for the patient with a colostomy, but the patient refuses to look at the nurse or the stoma, stating "I just can't see myself with this thing." An appropriate nursing diagnosis for the patient is

 a. self-care deficit related to refusal to care for colostomy.
 b. disturbed body image related to presence of colostomy stoma.
 c. ineffective coping related to feelings of helplessness and lack of coping skills.
 d. ineffective therapeutic regimen management related to lack of knowledge for care of colostomy.

36. In teaching a patient about colostomy irrigation, the nurse tells the patient to

 a. infuse 1500 to 2000 ml of warm tap water as irrigation fluid.
 b. allow 30 to 45 minutes for the solution and feces to be expelled.
 c. insert a firm plastic catheter 3 to 4 inches into the stoma opening.
 d. hang the irrigation bag on a hook about 36 inches above the stoma.

37. The nurse teaches the patient with diverticulosis to

 a. use anticholinergic drugs routinely to prevent bowel spasm.
 b. have an annual colonoscopy to detect malignant changes in the lesions.
 c. maintain a high-fiber diet and use bulk laxatives to increase fecal volume.
 d. exclude whole grain breads and cereals from the diet to prevent irritating the bowel.

38. During an acute attack of diverticulitis, the patient is

 a. monitored for signs of peritonitis.
 b. treated with daily medicated enemas.
 c. prepared for surgery to resect the involved colon.
 d. provided with a heating pad to apply to the left lower quadrant.

39. Match the types of hernias with their descriptions.

6	a. Reducible	1. Obstructed intestinal flow and blood supply
4	b. Incarcerated	2. Follows the spermatic cord or round ligament
1	c. Strangulated	3. Weakness at the site of previous incision
5	d. Femoral	4. Cannot be placed back into abdominal cavity
2	e. Inguinal	5. Protrusion into femoral canal
3	f. Ventral	6. Can be placed back into abdominal cavity

40. A nursing intervention that is indicated for a male patient following an inguinal herniorrhaphy is

    a. applying heat to the inguinal area.
    b. elevating the scrotum with a scrotal support.
    c. applying a truss to support the operative site.
    d. encouraging the patient to cough and deep breathe.

41. The most common form of malabsorption syndrome is treated with

    a. administration of antibiotics.
    b. avoidance of milk and milk products.
    c. supplementation with pancreatic enzymes.
    d. avoidance of gluten found in wheat, barley, oats, and rye.

42. Short bowel syndrome is most likely to occur in the patient with

    a. ulcerative colitis.
    b. irritable bowel syndrome.
    c. an extensive resection of the ileum.
    d. a colectomy performed for cancer of the bowel.

43. Match the following anorectal conditions with their descriptions.

_____	a. Pilonidal sinus	1. Engorged rectal vein around anal sphincter
_____	b. Anorectal abscess	2. Ulcer in anal wall
_____	c. Anal fissure	3. Tunnel leading from anus or rectum
_____	d. Hemorrhoid	4. Collection of perianal pus
_____	e. Anorectal fistula	5. Sacrococcygeal hairy tract

44. Following anal surgery, the nurse advises the patient to

    a. use daily laxatives to facilitate bowel emptying.
    b. use ice packs to the perineum to prevent swelling.
    c. avoid having a bowel movement for several days until healing occurs.
    d. take warm sitz baths several times a day to promote comfort and cleaning.

CASE STUDY

CANCER OF THE RECTUM

Patient Profile

Mr. D., a 63-year-old married insurance salesman, has undergone an abdominal-perineal resection for cancer of the rectum. He is one day postoperative on the general surgical unit.

Subjective Data

- Complains of pain in his abdominal and perineal incisions that is not well controlled even with his PCA machine
- Jokes about his stoma winking at him when the dressings are removed the first time and a temporary colostomy bag is applied
- Refers to his stoma as "Jake"
- Tells his wife that "Jake" will be watching her

Objective Data

- Stoma on left lower quadrant of abdomen, bright red, colostomy bag has small amount of pink mucus drainage
- Midline abdominal incision; no signs of infection; sutures intact
- Perineal incision partially closed, two Penrose drains with bulky dressings with large amount of serosanguineous drainage
- All vital signs normal
- PCA orders of 1 mg morphine sulfate every 10 minutes, with 17 attempts in the past hour

Critical Thinking Questions

1. What symptoms may have alerted Mr. D. to seek medical care for his cancer of the colon?

2. What care is indicated for Mr. D.'s perineal wound?

3. What are the primary goals of care for Mr. D.'s colostomy?

4. What would be the nurse's evaluation of Mr. D.'s adjustment to his colostomy?

5. What factors may be influencing the pain that Mr. D. is experiencing?

6. What teaching will need to be accomplished with Mr. D. before his discharge?

7. Based on the assessment data presented, write one or more appropriate nursing diagnoses. Are there any collaborative problems?

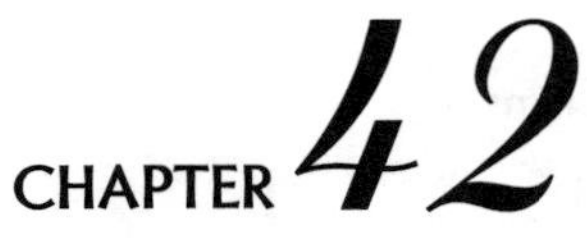

CHAPTER 42 NURSING MANAGEMENT: LIVER, BILIARY TRACT, AND PANCREAS PROBLEMS

1. Complete the following statements.

   a. The type of jaundice associated with gallstones is _______________ jaundice, and the type of serum bilirubin that is elevated is most likely _____________________.

   b. Hemolytic jaundice is caused by _______________________________, and the type of bilirubin elevated in the blood is _______________________.

   c. Jaundice resulting from failure of the liver to conjugate and excrete bilirubin is known as _______________ jaundice and causes serum elevations of _____________________ bilirubin.

2. Match the following characteristics of viral hepatitis with their related types (answers may be used more than once).

_____	a. IV drug use is method of greatest transmission	1. Hepatitis A (HAV)
_____	b. Uncommon in United States	2. Hepatitis B (HBV)
_____	c. Exists only with hepatitis B	3. Hepatitis C (HCV)
_____	d. Caused by a DNA virus	4. Hepatitis D (HDV)
_____	e. Most common cause of chronic hepatitis	5. Hepatitis E (HEV)
_____	f. Often causes asymptomatic anicteric hepatitis	
_____	g. Chronic carriers have increased risk for hepatocellular cancer	
_____	h. Has no chronic carrier state	
_____	i. No readily available diagnostic serology tests	
_____	j. Usual cause of hepatitis epidemics	

3. Serologic findings in viral hepatitis include both the presence of viral antigens and antibodies produced in response to the viruses. Identify the three antigens associated with active HBV and the corresponding antibodies for those antigens. (One of the antigens stimulates two antibodies.)

Antigen	**Antibodies**
a. (surface)__________________	__________________________
b. (e)______________________	__________________________
c. (core)____________________	__________________________
	__________________________

4. Complete the following sentences related to serologic findings in viral hepatitis.

   a. In addition to HBV antigens and antibodies, the best indicator of active, ongoing HBV replication is the presence of ________________ in the blood.

   b. The HBV antibody that is a marker of response to the HBV vaccine is ____________.

   c. The HBV antibody that does not appear after immunization is ____________.

   d. The HBV antigen that persists in chronic carrier states is ______________.

   e. HAV antigens are not tested in the blood, but like HBV, they stimulate specific IgM and IgG antibodies. Acute HVA infection is indicated by ___________ antibodies, whereas prior infection is indicated by _______________ antibodies.

   f. Co-infection of HDV with HBV can be detected by testing for the __________ antibody.

   g. Several tests are used to determine the presence of HCV. The initial screening for acute or chronic HVC includes testing for the _______________ antibody.

   h. A patient with anti-HVC antibodies can have active, chronic, or prior HCV infection. The test that best indicates active disease and can also detect HVC in an immunosuppressed patient is ____________.

   i. A more sensitive antibody test for HCV includes the use of the ________________________.

5. The systemic effects of viral hepatitis are caused primarily by

   a. cholestasis.
   b. impaired portal circulation.
   c. toxins produced by the infected liver.
   d. activation of the complement system by antigen-antibody complexes.

6. During the preicteric phase of viral hepatitis, the nurse would expect the patient to report

   a. pruritus and malaise.
   b. dark urine and easy fatigability.
   c. anorexia and right upper quadrant discomfort.
   d. constipation or diarrhea with light-colored stools.

7. Fulminant hepatic failure as a complication of viral hepatitis is highest in those individuals with

   a. hepatitis A.
   b. hepatitis C.
   c. hepatitis B accompanied with hepatitis C.
   d. hepatitis B accompanied with hepatitis D.

8. Identify the prophylactic immunologic agents that are used for the following.

   a. Preexposure protection to HBV

   b. Postexposure protection to HBV

9. The family members of a patient with hepatitis A ask if there is anything that will prevent them from developing the disease. The best response by the nurse is

   a. "No immunization is available for hepatitis A, nor are you likely to get the disease."
   b. "Only individuals who have had sexual contact with the patient should receive immunization."
   c. "All family members should receive the hepatitis A vaccine to prevent or modify the infection."
   d. "Those who have had household or close contact with the patient should receive immune globulin."

10. A patient newly diagnosed with acute hepatitis B asks if there is drug therapy to treat the disease. The most appropriate response by the nurse is informing the patient that

    a. there are no specific drug therapies that are effective for treating acute viral hepatitis.
    b. only chronic hepatitis C is treatable, primarily with antiviral agents and α-interferon.
    c. no drugs can be used for treatment of viral hepatitis because of the risk of additional liver damage.
    d. α-interferon combined with lamivudine (Epivir) will decrease viral load and liver damage if taken for 1 year.

11. The nurse identifies a need for further teaching when the patient with hepatitis B states

    a. "I should avoid alcohol completely for as long as a year."
    b. "I must avoid all physical contact with my family until the jaundice is gone."
    c. "I should use a condom to prevent spread of the disease to my sexual partner."
    d. "I will need to rest several times a day, gradually increasing my activity as I tolerate it."

12. One of the most challenging nursing interventions to promote healing in the patient with viral hepatitis is

    a. providing adequate nutritional intake.
    b. promoting strict bed rest during the icteric phase.
    c. providing pain relief without using liver-metabolized drugs.
    d. providing quiet diversional activities during periods of fatigue.

13. When caring for a patient with autoimmune hepatitis, the nurse recognizes that unlike viral hepatitis, the patient

    a. does not manifest hepatomegaly or jaundice.
    b. experiences less liver inflammation and damage.
    c. is treated with corticosteroids or other immunosuppressant agents.
    d. is usually an older adult who has used a wide variety of prescription and over-the-counter drugs.

14. Match the characteristics of cirrhosis with their related types (answers may be used more than once).

_____	a. Diffuse liver fibrosis	1. Alcoholic
_____	b. Vascular congestion of liver	2. Postnecrotic
_____	c. Malnutrition related	3. Biliary
_____	d. Associated with chemical toxicity	4. Cardiac
_____	e. Early fatty infiltration	
_____	f. Viral induced	
_____	g. Chronic biliary obstruction	

15. Match the following clinical manifestations with the pathophysiologic changes that occur in cirrhosis (answers may be used more than once).

_____	a. Jaundice	1. Decreased prothrombin production
_____	b. Testicular atrophy	2. Vascular congestion of spleen
_____	c. Anorexia and dyspepsia	3. Decreased estrogen metabolism
_____	d. Spider angiomas	4. Stretching of liver capsule
_____	e. Amenorrhea	5. Decreased bilirubin conjugation and excretion
_____	f. Peripheral neuropathy	6. Altered carbohydrate, protein, and fat metabolism
_____	g. Anemia, leukopenia, thrombocytopenia	7. Decreased testosterone metabolism
_____	h. Dull, heavy, RUQ pain	8. Vitamin B deficiencies
_____	i. Male gynecomastia	
_____	j. Petechia and purpura	

16. Describe the pathophysiologic changes of cirrhosis that cause the following:

a. Portal hypertension

b. Esophageal varices

17. Complete the following statements related to Figure 42-6 in the textbook.

a. Portal hypertension and the resulting increased blood hydrostatic pressure cause leakage of plasma into the abdominal cavity from three major sources. These sources are ______________________, ______________________, and ______________________.

b. Fluid also moves into the abdominal cavity, producing ascites because of decreased serum oncotic colloidal pressure. The decreased serum oncotic pressure is caused by ______________________.

c. Fluid sequestering in the peritoneal cavity results in (increased/decreased) ____________ vascular volume, (increased/decreased) ____________ blood return to the heart, and (increased/decreased) ____________ cardiac output.

d. The change in cardiac output results in (increased/decreased) ____________ kidney perfusion and secretion of ______________ and ______________, both of which increase fluid retention.

e. The retained fluid has low oncotic colloidal pressure, and it escapes into the interstitial spaces, causing ______________________.

f. Excessive fluid continues to be reabsorbed from the kidney because of the altered kidney perfusion and because ______________________ is not metabolized by the impaired liver.

g. The changes in laboratory test results that relate to this process are ______________________ and ______________________.

18. Laboratory test results that the nurse would expect to find in a patient with cirrhosis include

a. serum albumin: 7.0 g/dl (70 g/L).
b. bilirubin: total 3.2 mg/dl (54.7 μmol/L).
c. serum cholesterol: 260 mg/dl (6.7 mmol/L).
d. aspartate aminotransferase (AST): 6 U/L (0.1 μkat/L).

19. Identify the rationales for the following interventions in treating the cirrhotic patient with ascites.

a. Bed rest

b. Salt-poor albumin

c. Diuretic therapy

d. Low-sodium diet

e. Paracentesis

f. Peritoneovenous shunts

20. The nurse recognizes early signs of hepatic encephalopathy in the patient who

    a. manifests asterixis.
    b. becomes unconscious.
    c. has increasing oliguria.
    d. is irritable and lethargic.

21. Identify the rationales for the following interventions in treating the cirrhotic patient with hepatic encephalopathy.

    a. Low-protein diet

    b. Lactulose (Cephulac)

    c. Neomycin

    d. Eliminating blood from GI tract

22. A patient with cirrhosis has a nursing diagnosis of disturbed body image. Common etiologic factors for this diagnosis include

    a. jaundice and ascites.
    b. dyspnea and pruritus.
    c. alopecia and skin lesions.
    d. periorbital edema and decreased sensory perception.

23. A patient with advanced cirrhosis has a nursing diagnosis of imbalanced nutrition: less than body requirements related to anorexia and inadequate food intake. An appropriate midday snack for the patient would be

    a. peanut butter and salt-free crackers.
    b. popcorn with salt-free butter and herbal seasoning.
    c. canned chicken noodle soup with low-protein bread.
    d. a tomato sandwich with low-protein bread and salt-free butter.

24. A patient with ascites is short of breath and has an increased respiratory rate. The nurse should

    a. notify the physician so a paracentesis can be performed.
    b. initiate oxygen therapy at 2L/min to increase gas exchange.
    c. ask the patient to cough and deep breathe to clear respiratory secretions.
    d. place the patient in Fowler's position to relieve pressure on the diaphragm.

25. During the treatment of the patient with bleeding esophageal varices, it is most important that the nurse

    a. prepares the patient for immediate portal shunting surgery.
    b. performs guaiac testing on all stools to detect occult blood.
    c. maintains the patient's airway and prevents aspiration of blood.
    d. monitors for the cardiac stimulant effects of IV vasopressin and nitroglycerin.

26. A patient with cirrhosis that is refractory to other treatments for esophageal varicies undergoes a peritoneovenous shunt. As a result of this procedure, the nurse would expect the patient to experience

    a. an improved survival rate.
    b. decreased serum ammonia levels.
    c. improved metabolism of nutrients.
    d. improved hemodynamic function and renal perfusion.

27. In discussing long-term management with the patient with alcoholic cirrhosis, the nurse advises the patient that

    a. a daily exercise regimen is important to increase the blood flow through the liver.
    b. cirrhosis can be reversed if the patient follows a regimen of proper rest and nutrition.
    c. abstinence from alcohol is the most important factor in improvement of the patient's condition.
    d. the only over-the-counter analgesic that should be used for minor aches and pains is acetaminophen.

28. A patient is hospitalized with metastatic cancer of the liver. The nurse plans care for the patient based on the knowledge that

    a. chemotherapy is highly successful in the treatment of liver cancer.
    b. the patient will undergo surgery to remove the involved portions of the liver.
    c. supportive care that is appropriate for all patients with severe liver damage is indicated.
    d. metastatic cancer of the liver is more responsive to treatment than primary carcinoma of the liver.

29. A patient with cirrhosis asks the nurse about the possibility of a liver transplant. The best response by the nurse is

    a. "Liver transplants are only indicated in children with irreversible liver disease."
    b. "If you are interested in a transplant you really should talk to your doctor about it."
    c. "Rejection is such a problem in liver transplants that it is seldom attempted in patients with cirrhosis."
    d. "Cirrhosis is an indication for transplantation in some cases. Have you talked to your doctor about this?"

30. Match the complications of acute pancreatitis with the pathophysiologic mechanisms.

_____	a. Pseudocyst	1. Combining of calcium with fatty acids during fat necrosis
_____	b. Pancreatic abscess	2. Cavity continuous with pancreas filled with necrotic products and secretions
_____	c. Pleural effusion	3. Pancreatic enzymes pass from peritoneal cavity through diaphragmatic lymph channels
_____	d. Tetany	4. Exudation of blood and plasma into retroperitoneal space
_____	e. Hypovolemia	5. Extensive pancreatic necrosis with resultant fluid-filled cavity

31. When assessing a patient with acute pancreatitis, the nurse would expect to find

a. hyperactive bowel sounds.
b. hypertension and tachycardia.
c. severe midepigastric or LUQ pain.
d. a temperature greater than 102° F (38.9° C).

32. Combined with clinical manifestations, the lab finding that is most commonly used to diagnose acute pancreatitis is

a. increased serum lipase.
b. increased serum amylase.
c. increased urinary amylase.
d. decreased renal amylase-creatine clearance ratio.

33. Management of acute peritonitis related to alcohol abuse includes

a. surgery to remove the inflamed pancreas.
b. replacement of pancreatic enzymes with meals.
c. nasogastric suction to prevent gastric contents from entering the duodenum.
d. endoscopic pancreatic sphincterotomy using retrograde cholangiopancreatography (ERCP).

34. The most effective means of suppressing pancreatic secretion during an episode of pancreatitis is the use of

a. antibiotics.
b. NPO status.
c. antispasmotics.
d. H_2R blockers or proton pump inhibitors.

35. A patient with acute pancreatitis has a nursing diagnosis of pain related to distention of pancreas and peritoneal irritation. In addition to effective use of analgesics the nurse should

a. provide diversional activities to distract the patient from the pain.
b. provide small frequent meals to increase the patient's tolerance to food.
c. position the patient on the side with the head of the bed elevated 45 degrees.
d. ambulate the patient every 3 to 4 hours to increase circulation and decrease abdominal congestion.

36. The nurse determines that further discharge instruction is needed when the patient with acute pancreatitis states

    a. "I should observe for fat in my stools."
    b. "I must not use alcohol to prevent future attacks of pancreatitis."
    c. "I shouldn't eat salty foods or foods with high amounts of sodium."
    d. "I will need to continue to monitor my blood glucose levels until my pancreas is healed."

37. The patient with chronic pancreatitis is more likely than the patient with acute pancreatitis to

    a. need to abstain from alcohol.
    b. experience acute abdominal pain.
    c. have malabsorption and diabetes mellitus.
    d. require a high-carbohydrate, high-protein, low-fat diet.

38. A nursing intervention that is indicated in administration of pancreatic enzymes to the patient with chronic pancreatitis is to

    a. have the patient take the preparations with meals and snacks.
    b. dissolve the tablets in water before administration to activate the enzymes.
    c. monitor the patient's blood glucose levels to evaluate the effectiveness of the enzymes.
    d. administer liquid enzymes through a straw to eliminate contact with the oral mucous membrane.

39. A risk factor associated with cancer of the pancreas is

    a. alcohol intake.
    b. cigarette smoking.
    c. exposure to asbestos.
    d. increased dietary intake of milk and milk products.

40. In a radical pancreaticoduodenectomy (Whipple procedure) for treatment of cancer of the pancreas, what anatomic structures are completely resected?

    a.

    b.

    What anatomic structures are partially resected?

    c.

    d.

    What anastomoses are made?

    e.

    f.

    g.

41. Identify whether the following statements are true or false. If a statement is false, correct the bold word(s) to make the statement true.

_____ a. **Cholelithiasis** is the most common disorder of the biliary system.

_____ b. Most gallstones are composed primarily of **calcium and bile salts**.

_____ c. If a gallstone blocks the cystic duct, the patient will have brown stools and symptoms of **biliary colic**.

_____ d. Factors that cause stasis of bile flow lead to **cholecystitis**.

_____ e. Obstructive jaundice occurs when gallstones obstruct the **common bile duct**.

42. Of the following characteristics, identify those that are associated with cholelithiasis.

_____ a. Family history of gallbladder disease

_____ b. History of excessive alcohol intake

_____ c. Multiparous female

_____ d. Obesity

_____ e. High serum high-density lipoproteins

_____ f. African-American males

_____ g. Age over 40 years

_____ h. Use of estrogen or oral contraceptives

43. The patient with an obstruction of the common bile duct has the following signs and symptoms. Identify the pathophysiologic changes that cause these clinical manifestations.

a. Jaundice

b. Clay-colored stools

c. Dark urine

d. Steatorrhea

e. Pain with fatty food intake

44. The patient with suspected gallbladder disease is scheduled for an ultrasound of the gallbladder. The nurse explains to the patient that this test

a. is noninvasive and is a very reliable method of detecting gallstones.
b. is used only when other tests cannot be used due to allergy to contrast media.
c. is an adjunct to liver function tests to determine if the gallbladder is inflamed.
d. will outline the gallbladder and the ductal system to enable visualization of stones.

45. Identify the rationale for the treatment of acute cholecystitis with the following interventions.

a. NPO with nasogastric suction

b. Pain management with meperidine (Demerol)

c. Administration of antibiotics

d. Administration of antispasmodics

46. Match the following descriptions with the treatments used for cholelithiasis.

_____ a. External shock waves disintegrate stones

_____ b. Stones removed through sphincter of Oddi

______ c. Cholesterol solvent injected directly into gallbladder

______ d. Administered orally to dissolve stones and reduce cholesterol saturation

1. Endoscopic sphincterotomy
2. Lithotripsy
3. Methyl tertiary terbutal ether (MTBE)
4. Chenodeoxycholic acid (CDCA)

47. The surgical treatment of choice for the patient with symptomatic gallbladder disease is a

a. cholecystotomy.
b. choledocholithotomy.
c. cholecystoduodenostomy.
d. laparoscopic cholecystectomy.

48. Following a laparoscopic cholecystectomy, the nurse would expect the patient to

a. return to work in 2 to 3 weeks.
b. be hospitalized for 3 to 5 days postoperatively.
c. have four small abdominal incisions covered with small dressings.
d. have a T-tube placed in the common bile duct to provide bile drainage.

49. A patient with chronic cholecystitis asks the nurse if she will need to continue a low-fat diet after she has a cholecystectomy. The best response by the nurse is

a. "A low-fat diet will prevent the development of further gallstones and should be continued."
b. "Yes, because you will not have a gallbladder to store bile you will not be able to digest fats adequately."
c. "A low-fat diet is recommended for a few weeks after surgery until the intestine adjusts to receiving a continuous flow of bile."
d. "Removal of the gallbladder will eliminate the source of your pain associated with fat intake so you may eat whatever you like."

50. Postoperatively, a patient with an incisional cholecystectomy has a nursing diagnosis of ineffective breathing pattern related to splinted respirations secondary to a high abdominal incision. The nursing intervention that should be implemented first for this patient is to

a. assess lung sounds every 2 to 4 hours.
b. provide analgesics to relieve incisional pain.
c. assist the patient to cough and deep breathe every hour.
d. position the patient on the operative side to splint the incision.

51. To care for a T-tube in a patient following a cholecystectomy, the nurse

    a. keeps the tube supported and free of kinks.
    b. attaches the tube to low continuous suction.
    c. clamps the tube when ambulating the patient.
    d. irrigates the tube with 10 ml sterile saline every 2 to 4 hours.

52. During discharge instructions for a patient following a laparoscopic cholecystectomy, the nursing advises the patient to

    a. keep the incision areas clean and dry for at least a week.
    b. report the need to take pain medication for shoulder pain.
    c. report any bile-colored or purulent drainage from the incisions.
    d. expect some postoperative nausea and vomiting for a few days.

CASE STUDY

ACUTE PANCREATITIS

Patient Profile

Mr. A. is a 55-year-old man admitted to the hospital with acute pancreatitis.

Subjective Data

- Has severe abdominal pain in the LUQ, radiating to the back
- States he is nauseated and has been vomiting

Objective Data

- Vital signs: Temp 101° F (38.3° C); HR 114; RR 26; BP 92/58
- Jaundice noted in sclera
- Laboratory values: serum amylase 400 U/L (6.67 μkat/L)
  urinary amylase 3800 U/day
  WBC count 20,000/μl
  blood glucose 180 mg/dl (10 mmol/L)
  serum calcium 7 mg/dl (1.7 mmol/L)

Collaborative Care

- NPO status
- NG tube to low, intermittent suction
- IV therapy with lactated Ringer's solution
- Meperidine (Demerol) IVPB
- Ranitidine (Zantac) IVPB

Critical Thinking Questions

1. Explain the pathophysiology of acute pancreatitis.

2. What are the most common causes of acute pancreatitis?

3. How do the results of his laboratory values relate to the pathophysiology of acute pancreatitis?

4. What causes hypocalcemia in acute pancreatitis? How does the nurse assess for hypocalcemia?

5. Describe the characteristics of the pain that occurs in acute pancreatitis.

6. What complications can occur with acute pancreatitis?

7. Identify the purpose of each medication Mr. A. is taking.

8. Why is Mr. A. NPO? What is the purpose of the NG tube?

9. Based on the assessment data presented, write one or more appropriate nursing diagnoses. Are there any collaborative problems?

CHAPTER 43 NURSING ASSESSMENT: URINARY SYSTEM

1. Using the following list of terms, identify the structures in the illustrations below (some of the terms will be used in both illustrations).

List of Terms

adrenal gland
aort
bladder
cortex
fibrous capsule
kidney
major calyx
medulla
minor caly
papilla
pyramid
renal pelvis
right renal artery
right renal vein
ureter
urethra
vena cava

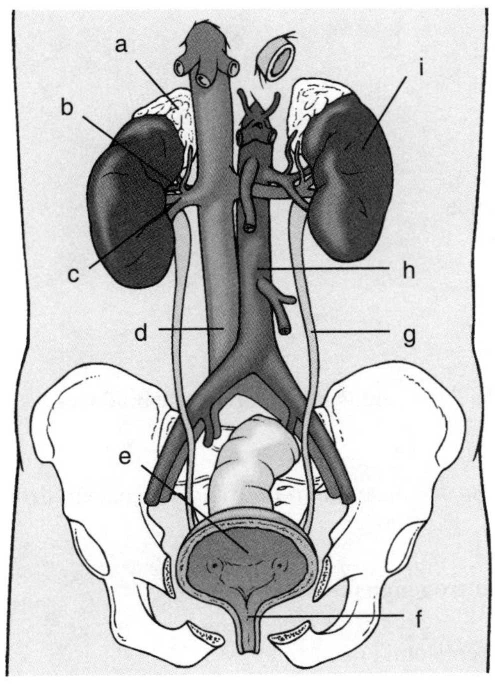

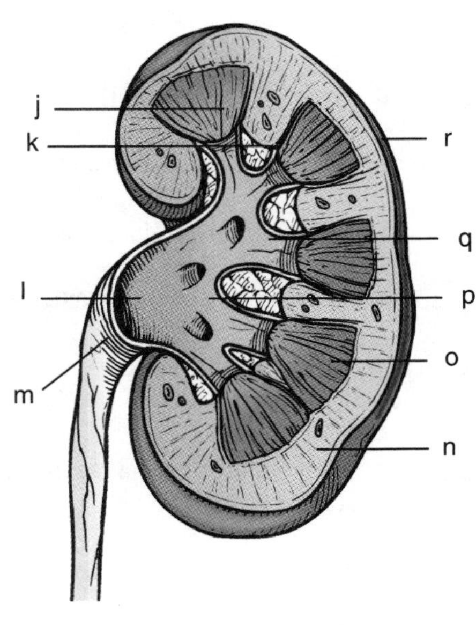

a. ______________ g. ______________ m. ______________

b. ______________ h. ______________ n. ______________

c. ______________ i. ______________ o. ______________

d. ______________ j. ______________ p. ______________

e. ______________ k. ______________ q. ______________

f. ______________ l. ______________ r. ______________

2. Match the following functions with the appropriate site in the nephron (answers may be used more than once).

_____	a. Active reabsorption of Cl^- and passive reabsorption of Na^+	1. Glomerulus
		2. Proximal convoluted tubule
_____	b. Formed from capillary network of afferent arterioles	3. Descending loop of Henle
_____	c. Secretion of H^+ into filtrate	4. Ascending loop of Henle
_____	d. Reabsorption of water without ADH	5. Distal convoluted tubule
_____	e. Blood filtered into Bowman's capsule	
_____	f. Reabsorption of Na^+ in exchange for K^+	
_____	g. Reabsorption of most of electrolytes	
_____	h. Reabsorption of bicarbonate	
_____	i. Reabsorption of Ca^{++} under parathormone influence	
_____	j. Reabsorption of glucose and amino acids	
_____	k. Reabsorption of water under ADH influence	

3. Identify whether the following statements are true or false. If a statement is false, correct the bold word(s) to make the statement true.

_____ a. Glomerular filtration rate is primarily dependent on adequate **blood flow** and adequate **hydro static pressure**.

_____ b. The primary function of the kidney is to **excrete nitrogenous waste products**.

_____ c. **Water** is the primary substance reabsorbed in the collecting duct.

_____ d. Atrial natriuretic factor (ANF) is secreted by the right atrium when atrial blood pressure is low, and it blocks the action of **aldosterone**.

_____ e. Increased permeability in the **glomerulus** causes loss of proteins into the urine.

4. A patient with an obstruction of the renal artery causing renal ischemia exhibits hypertension. One factor that may contribute to the hypertension is

a. increased renin release.
b. increased ADH secretion.
c. decreased aldosterone secretion.
d. increased synthesis and release of prostaglandins.

5. A clinical situation in which the increased release of erythropoietin would be expected is

a. hypoxemia.
b. hypotension.
c. hyperkalemia.
d. fluid overload.

6. Complete the following statements.

   a. The sites where urinary stones are most likely to obstruct the urinary system are at the

   ______________________ and the ________________________.

   b. The ureteral muscle fiber attachments into the bladder help prevent backflow of urine through the

   ________________________ junction.

   c. The volume of urine in the bladder that usually causes the urge to urinate is ___________ ml.

   d. Total bladder capacity ranges from ___________ ml to __________ ml.

   e. Absorption or leakage of urine wastes out of the urinary system is prevented by the cellular characteristics

   of the ________________________.

7. One factor that contributes to an increased incidence of urinary tract infections in women is

   a. the shorter length of the urethra.
   b. the larger capacity of the bladder.
   c. relaxation of pelvic floor muscles.
   d. the tight muscular support at the rhabdosphincter.

8. An age-related change in the kidney that leads to nocturia in an older adult is

   a. decreased renal mass.
   b. decreased detrusor muscle tone.
   c. decreased ability to conserve sodium.
   d. decreased ability to concentrate urine.

9. Identify one specific finding identified by the nurse during assessment of each of the patient's functional health patterns that indicates a risk factor for urinary problems or a patient response to a urinary disorder.

   a. Health perception–health management

   b. Nutritional-metabolic

   c. Elimination

   d. Activity-exercise

   e. Sleep-rest

   f. Cognitive-perceptual

   g. Self-perception–self-concept

   h. Role-relationship

   i. Sexuality-reproductive

   j. Coping–stress tolerance

   k. Value-belief

10. During physical assessment of the urinary system, the nurse

    a. auscultates the lower abdominal quadrants for fluid sounds.
    b. palpates an empty bladder at the level of the symphysis pubis.
    c. percusses the kidney with a firm blow at the posterior costovertebral angle.
    d. positions the patient prone to palpate the kidneys with a posterior approach.

11. Match the following abnormal assessment findings with their descriptions.

_____	a. Nocturia	1. Blood in the urine
_____	b. Dysuria	2. Scanty urine output
_____	c. Retention	3. Can be caused by sneezing
_____	d. Polyuria	4. Urine containing gas
_____	e. Enuresis	5. Incontinence during sleep
_____	f. Hematuria	6. Painful urination
_____	g. Oliguria	7. No urine formation
_____	h. Urgency	8. Frequent urination at night
_____	i. Anuria	9. Inability to void
_____	j. Hesitancy	10. Large amount of urine output
_____	k. Pneumaturia	11. Difficulty starting urine stream
_____	l. Stress incontinence	12. Strong desire to urinate

12. A urinalysis of a urine specimen that is not processed within 1 hour may result in erroneous measurement of

    a. glucose.
    b. bacteria.
    c. specific gravity.
    d. white blood cells.

13. Urinalysis results that most likely indicate a urinary tract infection include

    a. color yellow; protein 6 mg/dl; pH 6.8; 10^2 bacteria.
    b. cloudy, yellow; WBC 50/hpf; pH 8.2; numerous casts.
    c. cloudy, brown; ammonia odor; specific gravity 1.030; RBC 3/hpf.
    d. clear; colorless; glucose trace; ketones trace; osmolality 500 mOsm/kg (500 mmol/kg).

14. A patient who is being treated with diuretics for retained fluid would be expected to have a urine specific gravity of

    a. 1.002.
    b. 1.010.
    c. 1.025.
    d. 1.030.

15. Following a renal arteriogram, it is important that the nurse

    a. observe for gross bleeding in the urine.
    b. place the patient in high Fowler's position.
    c. monitor the patient for signs of allergy to the contrast medium.
    d. assess peripheral pulses in the involved leg every 30 to 60 minutes.

16. A patient with an elevated BUN

    a. has decreased urea in the urine.
    b. may have nonrenal tissue destruction.
    c. definitely has impaired renal function.
    d. will always have a rise in serum creatinine.

17. The test that is most specific for renal function is the

    a. renal scan.
    b. serum creatinine.
    c. blood urea nitrogen.
    d. creatinine clearance.

18. Identify the kidney function that is impaired in the following lab findings in a patient with kidney disease.

    a. serum Ca^{++}: 7.2 mg/dl (1.8 mmol/L)

    b. Hg: 9.6 g/dl (96 g/L)

    c. serum creatinine: 3.2 mg/dl (283 μmol/L)

19. Following a renal biopsy, it is important that the nurse

    a. offer warm sitz baths to relieve discomfort.
    b. test urine for microscopic bleeding with a dipstick.
    c. expect the patient to experience burning on urination.
    d. monitor the patient for symptoms of a urinary infection.

20. Match the following nursing responsibilities with the appropriate diagnostic test (answers may be used more than once).

_____	a. Use dipstick and read results with color chart	1. Urinalysis
		2. Creatinine clearance
_____	b. Ensure informed consent obtained	
		3. Clean catch urine specimen
_____	c. Explain that bladder will be filled with water to measure tone and stability	4. Residual urine
_____	d. Must start test with full bladder	5. Protein determination
_____	e. Keep patient NPO 8 hr before test	6. Cystoscopy
_____	f. Insert catheter immediately after voiding	7. Intravenous pyelogram
		8. Cystometrogram
_____	g. Clean meatus before voiding	
		9. Urinary flow study
_____	h. First morning specimen is best	
_____	i. Explain postprocedure pink urine normal	
_____	j. Have patient void, stop, void in container	
_____	k. Discard first specimen at start; include voided specimen 24 hours later	
_____	l. Use sterile container	
_____	m. Assess for iodine sensitivity	

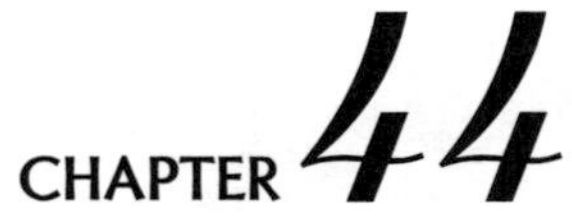

CHAPTER 44 NURSING MANAGEMENT: RENAL AND UROLOGIC PROBLEMS

1. Match the following characteristics with the appropriate classifications of urinary tract infection (UTI).

_____	a. Occurs in otherwise normal urinary tract	1. Upper UTI
_____	b. Initially resistant to antibiotics	2. Lower UTI
_____	c. Bacterial colonization of bladder without symptoms	3. Complicated UTI
		4. Uncomplicated UTI
_____	d. Exists in presence of obstruction or stones	5. Recurrent UTI
_____	e. Infection of kidney and/or kidney pelvis	6. Unresolved bacteriuria
_____	f. Infection of bladder and/or urethra	7. Bacterial persistence
_____	g. Continuing infection because of development resistance	8. Asymptomatic of resistance bacteriuria
_____	h. Reinfection following successful treatment of prior UTI	

2. The nurse identifies the patient with the greatest risk for a urinary tract infection as a

   a. 37-year-old man with renal colic associated with kidney stones.
   b. 26-year-old pregnant woman who has a history of urinary tract infections.
   c. 69-year-old man who has urinary retention caused by benign prostatic hyperplasia.
   d. 72-year-old woman hospitalized with a stroke who has a Foley catheter because of urinary incontinence.

3. While caring for a 77-year-old woman who has a Foley catheter, the nurse monitors the patient for the development of a UTI. The clinical manifestations the patient is most likely to experience include

   a. cloudy urine and fever.
   b. urethral burning and bloody urine.
   c. vague abdominal pain and disorientation.
   d. superpubic pain and slight decline in body temperature.

4. A woman with no history of UTIs who is experiencing urgency, frequency, and dysuria comes to the clinic, where a dipstick and microscopic urinalysis indicates a bacteriuria. The nurse anticipates that the patient will

   a. need to have a blood specimen drawn for a CBC and kidney function tests.
   b. not be treated with medication unless she develops fever, chills, and flank pain.
   c. be requested to obtain a clean-catch midstream urine specimen for culture and sensitivity.
   d. be treated empirically with trimethoprim-sulfamethasoxazole (TMP-SMX) for 3 days.

5. A female patient with a UTI has a nursing diagnosis of risk for infection related to lack of knowledge regarding prevention of recurrence. The nurse includes in the teaching plan instructions to

   a. empty the bladder at least 4 times a day.
   b. urinate before and after sexual intercourse.
   c. drink at least 3 quarts of any kind of liquid every day.
   d. clean the urinary meatus with an antiinfective agent after voiding.

6. Acute pyelonephritis resulting from an ascending infection from the lower urinary tract occurs most often when

   a. the kidney is scarred and fibrotic.
   b. the organism is resistant to antibiotics.
   c. there is a preexisting abnormality of the urinary tract.
   d. the patient does not take all of the antibiotics for treatment of a UTI.

7. The patient with acute pyelonephritis is more likely than the patient with a lower UTI to have a nursing diagnosis of

   a. hyperthermia related to infection.
   b. acute pain related to dysuria and bladder spasms.
   c. impaired urinary elimination related to infection.
   d. risk for infection related to lack of knowledge regarding prevention of recurrence.

8. Identify whether the following statements are true or false. If a statement is false, correct the bold word(s) to make the statement true.

   _____ a. **Acute** pyelonephritis causes progressive destruction of nephrons resulting in chronic renal insufficiency.

   _____ b. In a patient with acute pyelonephritis, an **IVP** may be performed **after** the infection is resolved to evaluate the urinary system for abnormalities.

   _____ c. Diagnosis of acute pyelonephritis always requires a **urine culture and sensitivity test.**

   _____ d. Following initial treatment of acute pyelonephritis, the patient must have a follow-up **CBC**.

   _____ e. The most common cause of urethritis in men is **sexually transmitted diseases**.

9. A patient with suprapubic pain and symptoms of urinary frequency and urgency has two negative urine cultures. One assessment finding that would indicate interstitial cystitis is

   a. a residual urine of greater than 200 ml.
   b. a large, atonic bladder on urodynamic testing.
   c. a voiding pattern that indicates psychogenic urinary retention.
   d. pain with bladder filling that is transiently relieved by urination.

10. When caring for the patient with interstitial cystitis, the nurse teaches the patient to

   a. avoid foods that make the urine more alkaline.
   b. use the dietary supplement calcium glycerophosphate (Prelief) to decrease bladder irritation.
   c. always keep a voiding diary to document pain, voiding frequencies, and patterns of nocturia.
   d. use high-potency vitamin therapy to decrease the autoimmune effects of the disorder.

11. Glomerulonephritis is characterized by glomerular damage caused by

   a. growth of microorganisms in the glomeruli.
   b. release of bacterial substances toxic to the glomeruli.
   c. hemolysis of red blood cells circulating through the glomeruli.
   d. accumulation of immune complexes and complement in the glomeruli.

12. Indicate whether the following clinical manifestations of acute poststreptococcal glomerulonephritis (APSGN) are related to decreased glomerular filtration rate (GFR) or injury to the glomerular basement membrane (GBM).

_____ a. Periorbital edema

_____ b. Smoky urine

_____ c. Proteinuria

_____ d. Hypertension

_____ e. Increased BUN and creatinine

_____ f. Oliguria

13. Restriction of dietary protein may be indicated in management of acute poststreptococcal glomerulonephritis when the patient has

a. hematuria.
b. proteinuria.
c. hypertension.
d. elevated BUN.

14. The nurse plans care for the patient with acute poststreptococcal glomerulonephritis (APSGN) based on the knowledge that

a. most patients with APSGN recover completely or rapidly improve with conservative management.
b. chronic glomerulonephritis leading to renal failure is a common sequela to acute glomerulonephritis.
c. pulmonary hemorrhage may occur as a result of antibodies also attacking the alveolar basement membrane.
d. a large percentage of patients with APSGN develop rapidly progressive glomerulonephritis resulting in kidney failure.

15. The edema associated with nephrotic syndrome occurs as a result of

a. hypercoagulability.
b. hyperalbuminemia.
c. decreased plasma oncotic pressure.
d. decreased glomerular filtration rate.

16. An appropriate nursing diagnosis for the patient with nephrotic syndrome is

a. risk for injury related to decreased clotting function.
b. risk for impaired skin integrity related to immobility.
c. risk for infection related to altered immune responses.
d. imbalanced nutrition: more than body requirements, related to high cholesterol intake.

17. Identify three HIV-associated renal syndromes.

a.

b.

c.

18. Number in sequence the following ascending pathologic changes that occur in the urinary tract in the presence of a bladder outlet obstruction.

_____ a. Hydronephrosis

_____ b. Reflux of urine into ureter

_____ c. Bladder detrusor muscle hypertrophy

_____ d. Ureteral dilation

_____ e. Renal atrophy

_____ f. Trabeculation of muscle cells

_____ g. Hydroureter

_____ h. Diverticula formation

_____ i. Chronic pyelonephritis

19. Patients at risk for renal lithiasis can prevent the stones in many cases by

a. leading an active lifestyle.
b. limiting protein and acid foods in the diet.
c. drinking enough fluids to produce a urine output of 2 L/day.
d. taking prophylactic antibiotics to control urinary tract infections.

20. Match the following characteristics with their associated urinary tract calculi (answers may be used more than once).

_____ a. More common in women

_____ b. Genetic autosomal recessive defect

_____ c. Often mixed with struvite and oxalate stones

_____ d. Frequently obstruct the ureter

_____ e. Always associated with UTI and urea-splitting bacteria

_____ f. Associated with gout

_____ g. Defective GI and kidney absorption

_____ h. Most common type of stone

_____ i. Often staghorn formation in kidney pelvis

_____ j. Most common in Jewish men

1. Calcium oxalate
2. Calcium phosphate
3. Struvite
4. Uric acid
5. Cystine

21. On assessment of the patient with a renal calculi passing down the ureter, the nurse would expect the patient to report

    a. dull, costovertebral flank pain.
    b. a history of chronic urinary tract infections.
    c. severe, colicky back pain radiating to the groin.
    d. a feeling of bladder fullness with urgency and frequency.

22. Prevention of calcium oxalate stones would include dietary restriction of

    a. milk and milk products.
    b. dried beans and dried fruits.
    c. liver, kidney, and sweetbreads.
    d. spinach, cabbage, and tomatoes.

23. Following lithotripsy for treatment of renal calculi, the patient has a nursing diagnosis of risk for infection related to introduction of bacteria following manipulation of the urinary tract. An appropriate nursing intervention for the patient is to

    a. monitor for hematuria.
    b. encourage high fluid intake.
    c. apply moist heat to the flank area.
    d. strain all urine through gauze or a special strainer.

24. Identify whether the following statements are true or false. If a statement is false, correct the bold word(s) to make the statement true.

    _____ a. Kidney injury should be suspected when a patient suffering a sports injury has **gross hematuria**.

    _____ b. Benign and accelerated nephrosclerosis cause necrosis of the renal parenchyma and are treated with **anticoagulants**.

    _____ c. The most common manifestations of renal artery stenosis include **flank pain and hematuria**.

    _____ d. Renal vein thrombosis is most commonly treated with **surgical revascularization**.

    _____ e. Patients with urethral strictures may be taught to dilate the urethra by **self-catheterization** every few days.

25. In providing care for the patient with adult-onset polycystic kidney disease, the nurse

    a. helps the patient cope with the rapid progression of the disease.
    b. suggests genetic counseling resources for the children of the patient.
    c. expects the patient to have polyuria and poor concentration ability of the kidneys.
    d. implements appropriate measures for the patient's deafness and blindness in addition to the renal problems.

26. Match the following metabolic and connective tissue diseases with the pathologic renal changes that occur in the diseases.

_____ a. Diabetes mellitus

_____ b. Gout

_____ c. Amyloidosis

_____ d. Systemic lupus erythematosus

_____ e. Scleroderma

1. Connective tissue changes affecting the glomerulus
2. Diffuse and nodular glomerulosclerosis
3. Deposition of sodium urate crystals in interstitium and tubules
4. Vascular lesions with fibrosis
5. Deposition of hyaline substance in kidney

27. When obtaining a nursing history from a patient with cancer of the urinary system, the nurse recognizes that a risk factor associated with cancer of both the kidney and the bladder is

a. smoking.
b. a family history of cancer.
c. chronic use of phenacetin.
d. chronic, recurrent nephrolithiasis.

28. The 5-year survival rate for cancer of the kidney is usually low primarily because

a. the only treatment modalities for the disease are palliative.
b. diagnostic tests are not available to detect tumors before they metastasize.
c. the classic symptoms of hematuria and palpable mass do not occur until the disease is advanced.
d. early metastasis to the brain impairs the patient's ability to recognize the seriousness of symptoms.

29. A 60-year-old man with cancer of the bladder has laser photocoagulation for treatment of the tumor. Following the procedure, the nurse plans to

a. assess the patient for symptoms of cystitis.
b. encourage the patient to use warm sitz baths.
c. monitor the patient for irritative bladder symptoms.
d. monitor urine output from the urinary catheter for hematuria.

30. Match the following characteristics with their associated types of urinary incontinence (answers may be used more than once).

_____ a. Caused by overactivity of the detrusor muscle

_____ b. Found following prostatectomy

_____ c. Treated with Kegel exercises

_____ d. Occurs with spinal cord lesions above S2

_____ e. Involuntary urination with minimal warning

_____ f. Common in postmenopausal women

_____ g. Loss of urine caused by problems of mobility

_____ h. Caused by outlet obstruction

_____ i. Occurs without warning or stress equally during day and night

_____ j. Bladder contracts reflexly, overriding central inhibition

_____ k. Leakage of urine from overfull bladder

_____ l. Involuntary urination with increased intraabdominal pressure

1. Stress incontinence
2. Urge incontinence
3. Overflow incontinence
4. Reflex incontinence
5. Functional incontinence

31. Indicate the type of incontinence the following drugs are used to treat and the rationale for their use.

a. Estrogen replacement

b. Anticholinergic drugs

c. Alpha-adrenergic blockers

d. Alpha-adrenergic agonists

32. To assist the patient with stress incontinence, the nurse teaches the patient to

a. void every 2 hours to prevent leakage.
b. use absorptive perineal pads to contain urine.
c. perform pelvic floor muscle exercises 4 to 5 times a day.
d. increase intraabdominal pressure during voiding to fully empty the bladder.

33. Nursing care that applies to the management of all urinary catheters in hospitalized patients includes

a. measuring urine output every 1 to 2 hours to ensure patency.
b. turning the patient frequently from side to side to promote drainage.
c. using strict sterile technique during irrigation or opening of the collecting system.
d. daily cleaning of the catheter insertion site with soap and water and application of an antimicrobial ointment.

34. A patient has a right ureteral catheter placed following a lithotripsy for a stone in the ureter. In caring for the patient after the procedure, the nurse

    a. milks or strips the catheter every 2 hours.
    b. measures ureteral urinary drainage every 1 to 2 hours.
    c. irrigates with catheter with 30 ml sterile saline q4h.
    d. encourages ambulation to promote urinary peristaltic action.

35. During assessment of the patient who has a nephrectomy, the nurse would expect to find

    a. shallow, slow respirations.
    b. clear breath sounds in all lung fields.
    c. decreased breath sounds in the lower left lobe.
    d. decreased breath sounds in the right and left lower lobes.

36. Match the following urinary diversions with their descriptions.

_____	a. Ileal conduit	1. Continent diversion created by formation of ileal pouch with stoma requiring catheterization
_____	b. Cutaneous ureterostomy	2. Abdominal stoma formed from resected ileum into which ureters are implanted
_____	c. Kock pouch	3. Stoma created from ureter(s) brought to abdominal wall
_____	d. Ureteroileosigmoidostomy	4. Continent diversion in which ureters are attached to resected segment of ileum implanted into sigmoid colon

37. A patient with bladder cancer undergoes cystectomy with formation of an ileal conduit. During the patient's first postoperative day, the nurse plans to

    a. measure and fit the stoma for a permanent appliance.
    b. teach the patient to self-catheterize the stoma every 4 to 6 hours.
    c. encourage high oral intake to flush mucus from the conduit.
    d. empty the drainage bag every 2 to 3 hours and measure the urinary output.

38. A teaching plan developed by the nurse for the patient with a new ileal conduit or ureterostomy stoma includes instructions to

    a. clean the skin around the stoma with alcohol every day.
    b. use a wick to keep the skin dry during appliance changes.
    c. use sterile supplies and technique during care of the stoma.
    d. change the appliance every day and wash it with soap and warm water.

CASE STUDY

BLADDER CANCER

Patient Profile

Mr. G. is a 55-year-old mechanic who has been healthy all of his life until he passed some blood in his urine and saw a urologist at his wife's insistence. A urine specimen for cytology revealed atypical cells, and a diagnosis of cancer of the bladder was made following a cystoscopy with biopsy of bladder tissue. Intravesical therapy with Bacille Calmette-Guérin (BCG) is planned.

Subjective Data

- Has smoked a pack of cigarettes a day since he was a teenager
- Says he dreads having the chemotherapy because he has heard cancer drugs cause such severe side effects

Objective Data

- Cystoscopy and biopsy results: moderately differentiated Jewett-Strong-Marshall stage A tumor on the left lateral bladder wall, with $T_2N_0M_0$ pathologic stage; fulguration performed during cystoscopy
- Continues to have gross hematuria

Critical Thinking Questions

1. What does staging of bladder tumors indicate?

2. What information and instructions would the nurse provide for Mr. G. about his intravesical therapy?

3. How can Mr. G. help prevent future bladder tumors from occurring?

4. How should the nurse explain the importance of follow-up cystoscopies?

5. What surgery may be indicated if the chemotherapy is not effective?

6. Based on the assessment data presented, write one or more appropriate nursing diagnoses. Are there any collaborative problems?

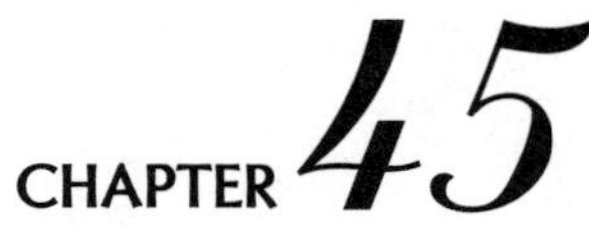

NURSING MANAGEMENT: ACUTE RENAL FAILURE AND CHRONIC KIDNEY DISEASE

1. Match the following conditions and characteristics with their associated etiologies of acute renal failure (answers may be used more than once).

_____ a. Decreased cardiac output

_____ b. Mechanical outflow obstruction

_____ c. Initial cause of most acute renal failure

_____ d. Prostate cancer

_____ e. Tubular obstruction by myoglobin

_____ f. Hypovolemia

_____ g. Renal stones

_____ h. Nephrotoxic drugs

_____ i. Bladder cancer

_____ j. Renal vascular obstruction

_____ k. Acute glomerulonephritis

_____ l. Anaphylaxis

1. Prerenal
2. Intrarenal
3. Postrenal

2. Complete the following statements related to acute tubular necrosis.

a. Acute tubular necrosis is a type of acute renal failure that results primarily from ________________ and ____________________.

b. Renal ischemia leads to acute tubular necrosis by disrupting the _____________ and causing patchy destruction of the _________________________.

c. Nephrotoxic agents cause necrosis of the ______________________ that sloughs off and blocks the ______________________.

d. Acute tubular necrosis from nephrotoxic injury is more likely to be reversible because the ________________________ is usually not initially destroyed.

3. Diagram the processes that occur when hypovolemia and decreased renal blood flow lead to decreased glomerular filtration rate (GFR) and tubular dysfunction with ultimate oliguria by filling in the blanks with the following terms.

Angiotensin-aldosterone system
Decreased glomerular capillary pressure
Decreased renal blood flow
Renal artery vasoconstriction
Renin

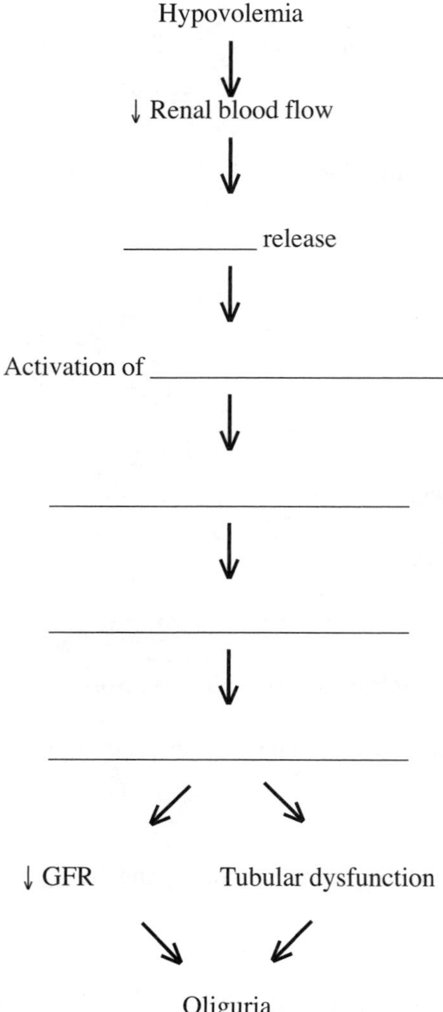

4. Diagram the processes that occur during kidney ischemia that continue to further decrease glomerular filtration rate and injured kidney cells by filling in the blanks with the following terms.

Tubular dysfunction/damage
Decreased glomerular filtration rate
Decreased tubular blood flow
Increased tissue pressure

Ischemia

↓

Injured glomerular epithelial cells

↓

↓ Glomerular capillary permeability

↓

____

↓

____

↓

____

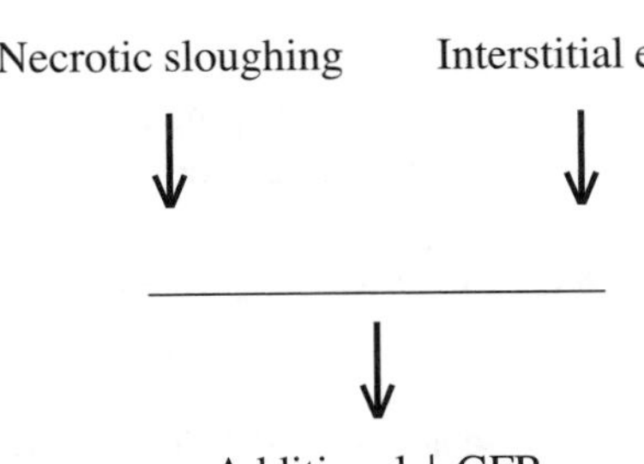

5. The nurse determines that a patient with oliguria has prerenal oliguria when

a. urine testing reveals a low specific gravity.
b. the causative factor is malignant hypertension.
c. urine testing reveals a high sodium concentration.
d. reversal of the oliguria occurs with fluid replacement.

6. Tubular damage is indicated in the patient with acute renal failure by a urinalysis finding of

a. hematuria.
b. specific gravity fixed at 1.010.
c. urine sodium of 12 mEq/L (12 mmol/L).
d. osmolality of 1000 mOsm/kg (1000 mmol/kg).

7. Metabolic acidosis occurs in the oliguric phase of acute renal failure as a result of impaired

   a. ammonia synthesis.
   b. excretion of sodium.
   c. excretion of bicarbonate.
   d. conservation of potassium.

8. Although both BUN and serum creatinine levels are increased in renal failure, a BUN of 85 mg/dl (30.3 mmol/L) and a serum creatinine of 3.8 mg/dl (336 μmol/L) would most likely occur in a patient with acute renal failure caused by

   a. massive trauma.
   b. bladder obstruction.
   c. congestive heart failure.
   d. acute glomerulonephritis.

9. The nurse determines that a patient with acute renal failure is in the recovery phase when the patient experiences

   a. a return to normal weight.
   b. a urine output of 3,700 ml/day.
   c. decreasing BUN and creatinine levels.
   d. decreasing sodium and potassium levels.

10. While caring for the patient in the oliguric phase of acute renal failure, the nurse monitors the patient for associated collaborative problems, notifying the physician when

    a. urine output is 300 ml/24 hr.
    b. edema occurs in the feet, legs, and sacral area.
    c. the cardiac monitor reveals a depressed T wave and a sagging ST segment.
    d. the patient experiences increasing muscle weakness and abdominal cramping.

11. Identify whether the following statements are true or false. If a statement is false, correct the bold word(s) to make the statement true.

    _____ a. The most common cause of death in acute renal failure is **irreversible metabolic acidosis**.

    _____ b. Serum **potassium** and **urea** are increased during catabolism of body protein.

    _____ c. During the oliguric phase of acute renal failure daily fluid intake is limited to **1000** ml plus the prior day's measurable fluid loss.

    _____ d. Dietary sodium and potassium during the oliguric phase of acute renal failure are managed according to the patient's **urinary output**.

    _____ e. One of the most important nursing measures in managing fluid balance in the patient in acute renal failure is **accurate daily weights**.

12. A 68-year-old man with a history of congestive heart failure secondary to hypertension has acute renal failure resulting from the effects of nephrotoxic diuretics. Currently his serum potassium is 6.2 mEq/L (6.2 mmol/L) with cardiac changes, his BUN is 108 mg/dl (38.6 mmol/L), his creatinine is 4.1 mg/dl (362 μmol/L), and his serum HCO_3^- is 14 mEq/L (14 mmol/L). He is somnolent and disoriented. What three criteria for treatment with dialysis does he meet?

a.

b.

c.

13. A patient with acute renal failure has a serum potassium level of 6.8 mEq/L (6.8 mmol/L) and the following arterial blood gas results: pH 7.28, $PaCO_2$ 30 mm Hg, PaO_2 86 mm Hg, HCO_3^- 18 mEq/L (18 mmol/L). The nurse recognizes that treatment of the acid-base problem would cause a decrease in the

a. pH.
b. potassium level.
c. bicarbonate level.
d. the carbon dioxide level.

14. In replying to a patient's questions about the seriousness of her chronic kidney disease, the nurse knows that the stage of chronic kidney disease is based on

a. the total daily urine output.
b. the glomerular filtration rate.
c. serum creatinine and urea levels.
d. the degree of altered mental status.

15. A patient with a creatinine clearance test of 30 ml/minute would have a glomerular filtration rate of _____ and stage _____ chronic kidney disease.

a. 3 ml/min/17.3 m^2; 5
b. 10 ml/min/17.3 m^2; 4
c. 30 ml/min/17.3 m^2; 3
d. 60 ml/min/17.3 m^2; 2

16. List two clinical manifestations and their pathophysiologic causes that can be noted by the nurse when performing physical assessment of the following systems on the patient with chronic renal disease.

	Findings	**Cause**
a. Skin		
b. Cardiovascular		
c. Respiratory		
d. GI		
e. Neurologic		

17. List the alterations that occur in at least 10 serum laboratory values in chronic renal disease.

a.

b.

c.

d.

e.

f.

g.

h.

i.

j.

18. The nurse identifies a nursing diagnosis of risk for injury: fracture related to alterations in calcium and phosphorus metabolism for a patient with chronic renal disease. The pathologic process directly related to the risk for fractures is

a. loss of aluminum through the impaired kidneys.
b. deposition of calcium phosphate in soft tissues of the body.
c. impaired vitamin D activation resulting in decreased GI absorption of calcium.
d. increased release of parathyroid hormone in response to decreased calcium levels.

19. A patient with chronic renal insufficiency weighs 70 kg and has the following lab results: creatinine clearance 18 ml/min; potassium 6.2 mEq/L (6.2 mmol/L); BUN 75 mg/dl (26.8 mmol/L), serum creatinine 6.3 mg/dl (557 μmol/L). An appropriate dietary modification for the patient is

a. a protein restriction of 70 g/day.
b. a potassium restriction of 2-3 g/day.
c. a sodium restriction of 1000 mg/day.
d. unlimited intake of breads and cereals.

20. In implementing care for the patient on peritoneal dialysis, the nurse recognizes that dietary needs include an increased amount of

a. fats.
b. protein.
c. calories.
d. carbohydrates.

21. The most appropriate snack for the nurse to offer the patient with chronic renal disease is

a. raisins.
b. ice cream.
c. dill pickles.
d. hard candy.

22. Match the following drugs with their use in chronic kidney disease (answers may be used more than once).

_____	a. Erythropoietin	1. Treatment of hyperkalemia
_____	b. IV glucose and insulin	2. Treatment of hyperphosphatemia
_____	c. Nifedipine (Procardia)	3. Treatment of anemia
_____	d. Sevelamer (Remagel)	4. Treatment of hypertension
_____	e. Sodium polystyrene sulfonate (Kayexalate)	
_____	f. Furosemide (Lasix)	
_____	g. Calcium acetate (PhosLo)	
_____	h. 10% calcium gluconate IV	

23. Identify whether the following statements are true or false. If a statement is false, correct the bold word(s) to make the statement true.

_____ a. A nutrient that is commonly supplemented for the patient on dialysis because it is dialyzable is **iron**.

_____ b. The syndrome that includes all the signs and symptoms seen in the various body systems in chronic kidney disease is **azotemia**.

_____ c. The use of calcium-based phosphate binders in the patient with chronic kidney disease is contraindicated when serum **phosphate** levels are increased.

_____ d. The use of **morphine** is contraindicated in the patient with chronic kidney disease because accumulation of its metabolites may cause seizures.

24. During the nursing assessment of the patient with renal insufficiency, the nurse asks the patient specifically about a history of

a. angina.
b. asthma.
c. hypertension.
d. rheumatoid arthritis.

25. When teaching a patient with chronic kidney disease about prevention of complications, the nurse instructs the patient to

a. monitor for proteinuria daily with a urine dipstick.
b. weigh daily and report a gain of greater than 4 pounds.
c. take calcium-based phosphate binders on an empty stomach.
d. perform self-catheterization every 4 hours to accurately measure I&O.

26. The patient with end-stage renal disease tells the nurse that she hates the thought of being tied to the machine, but is also glad to start dialysis because she will be able to eat and drink what she wants. Based on this information, the nurse identifies the nursing diagnosis of

a. self-esteem disturbance related to dependence on dialysis.
b. anxiety related to perceived threat to health status and role functioning.
c. ineffective management of therapeutic regimen related to lack of knowledge of treatment plan.
d. risk for imbalanced nutrition: more than body requirements, related to increased dietary intake.

27. Indicate whether the following characteristics are associated with peritoneal dialysis (PD) or hemodialysis (HD).

_____ a. Requires vascular access

_____ b. Increased hyperlipidemia

_____ c. Lowers serum triglycerides

_____ d. Portable system

_____ e. Less cardiovascular stress

_____ f. More protein loss

_____ g. Intensifies anemia

_____ h. Rapid fluid and creatinine loss

_____ i. Requires fewer dietary restrictions

28. The dialysate for peritoneal dialysis contains

a. electrolytes in an equal concentration to the blood.
b. calcium in a lower concentration than in the blood.
c. sodium in a higher concentration than in the blood.
d. glucose in a higher concentration than in the blood.

29. Complete the following statements.

a. An exchange in peritoneal dialysis includes the phases of _______________, ______________________,

and ______________________.

b. The amount of peritoneal dialysate used for one exchange is usually ______ liter(s).

c. The patient using ______________ peritoneal dialysis usually dialyzes during sleep and leaves the fluid in the abdomen during the day.

30. To prevent the most common serious complication of peritoneal dialysis, it is important for the nurse to

a. infuse the dialysate slowly.
b. use strict aseptic technique in the dialysis procedures.
c. have the patient empty the bowel before the inflow phase.
d. reposition the patient frequently and promote deep breathing.

31. The composition of the periotoneal dialysate solution requires careful monitoring of the patient who also has

a. diabetes.
b. liver disease.
c. congestive heart failure.
d. chronic obstructive pulmonary disease.

32. Match the characteristics with the type of vascular access sites (answers may be used more than once).

_____ a. 2 to 4 weeks required for healing

_____ b. Least likely to thrombose

_____ c. Usually used for temporary access for continuous renal replacement theory

_____ d. May lead to distal ischemia

_____ e. Most prone to infection

_____ f. 4 to 6 weeks required for healing

1. External AV shunt
2. AV fistula
3. AV graft

33. A patient on hemodialysis develops a thrombus of a subcutaneous AV graft requiring its removal. While waiting for a replacement graft or fistula, the patient is most likely to have

a. an external access shunt.
b. a percutaneous femoral vein cannula.
c. a percutaneous subclavian vein cannula.
d. a Silastic catheter tunneled subcutaneously to the jugular vein.

34. A patient with end-stage renal failure is scheduled for hemodialysis following healing of an AV fistula. The nurse explains that during dialysis

a. he will be able to visit, read, sleep, or watch TV while reclining in a chair.
b. he will be placed on a cardiac monitor to detect any adverse effects that might occur.
c. the dialyzer will remove and hold part of his blood for 20 to 30 minutes to remove the waste products.
d. a large catheter with two lumens will be inserted into the fistula to send blood to and return it from the dialyzer.

35. The nurse evaluates the patency of an AV graft by

a. palpating for pulses distal to the graft site.
b. auscultating for the presence of a bruit at the site.
c. evaluating the color and temperature of the extremity.
d. assessing for the presence of numbness and tingling distal to the site.

36. A patient returns from her initial hemodialysis treatment with nausea, confusion, twitching, and jerking. The pathophysiologic mechanism of dialysis responsible for these signs and symptoms is a

a. loss of blood into the dialyzer caused by heparin use.
b. rapid removal of vascular volume causing hypovolemia.
c. high osmotic gradient in the brain causing cerebral edema.
d. neuromuscular hypersensitivity resulting from fluid and sodium loss.

37. A patient in acute renal failure is a candidate for continuous renal replacement therapy (CRRT). The most common indication for use of CRRT is

a. azotemia.
b. pericarditis.
c. hyperkalemia.
d. fluid overload.

38. A patient rapidly progressing toward end-stage renal disease asks about the possibility of a kidney transplant. In responding to the patient, the nurse knows that contraindications to kidney transplantation include

    a. hepatitis C infection.
    b. coronary artery disease.
    c. refractory hypertension.
    d. extensive vascular disease.

39. A patient in end-stage renal disease is being evaluated for a kidney transplant from a live related donor. Results of histocompatibility testing that would indicate the best match of the patient and the donor include

    a. ABO compatibility and no HLA match.
    b. ABO compatibility and six-HLA match.
    c. ABO compatibility and negative antibody crossmatch.
    d. HLA-identical match and positive antibody crossmatch.

40. During the immediate postoperative care of the recipient of a kidney transplant, the nurse expects to

    a. regulate fluid intake hourly based on urine output.
    b. find urine-tinged drainage on the abdominal dressing.
    c. medicate the patient frequently for incisional flank pain.
    d. remove the Foley catheter to evaluate the ureteral implant.

41. Signs and symptoms of chronic rejection of the kidney are caused by

    a. recurrence of the original kidney disease.
    b. gradual occlusion of the renal blood vessels.
    c. T-cytotoxic cell attack on the foreign kidney.
    d. destruction of kidney tissue by sensitized antibodies.

42. Signs and symptoms of acute rejection that the nurse should teach the patient to observe for include

    a. tachycardia and headache.
    b. fever and painful transplant site.
    c. severe hypotension and weight loss.
    d. recurrent urinary tract infections and oral yeast infections.

CASE STUDY

KIDNEY TRANSPLANT

Patient Profile

Ms. B. had end-stage renal disease secondary to hypertension. She underwent hemodialysis for 2 years and then received a cadaveric renal transplant 1 year ago. She had one episode of acute rejection 3 months after transplant. Her baseline creatinine has been 1.2 to 1.3 mg/dl (106 to 115 mmol/L). She came to the clinic complaining of decreased urinary output, fever, and tenderness at the transplant site. She is admitted to the hospital for a kidney biopsy.

Subjective Data

- Tells the nurse if she loses this kidney she does not think she can stand to go back on dialysis

Objective Data

- Laboratory findings: serum creatinine 3.0 mg/dl (265 μmol/L)
  BUN 70 mg/dl (25 mmol/L)
  glucose 404 mg/dl (22.4 mmol/L)
  K^+ 5.1 mEq/L (5.1 mmol/L)
  HCO_3^- 18 mEq/L (18 mmol/L)
- Blood pressure 150/90 mm Hg

Collaborative Care

- Muromonab-CD3 (Orthoclone OKT3) therapy initiated for 10 days
- Mycophenolate mofetil (Cellcept)
- Methylprednisolone (Solu-Medrol)
- Furosemide (Lasix)
- Nifedipine (Procardia)
- Sodium bicarbonate
- Tacrolimus (Prograf)
- Insulin

Critical Thinking Questions

1. Explain the physiology of acute rejection.

2. Identify the abnormal diagnostic study results and why each would occur. What significance do the abnormal results have for nursing care?

3. Explain the rationale for Ms. B.'s collaborative care. How does each immunosuppressive medication work? (See Chapter 13.)

4. What clinical manifestations may develop as a result of immunosuppressive therapy? What nursing care is indicated?

5. Explain the long-term problems of a patient with a kidney transplant.

6. Based on the assessment data presented, write one or more appropriate nursing diagnoses. Are there any collaborative problems?

CHAPTER 46 NURSING ASSESSMENT: ENDOCRINE SYSTEM

1. Identify the glands in the following illustration.

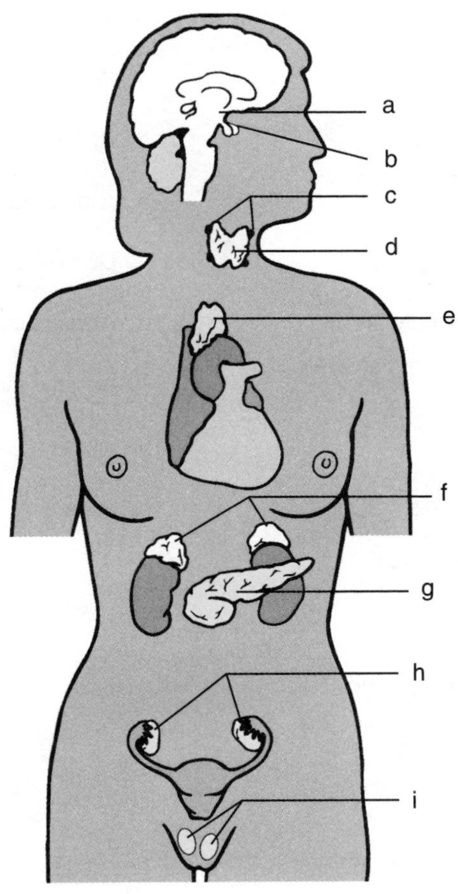

a. ______________________

b. ______________________

c. ______________________

d. ______________________

e. ______________________

f. ______________________

g. ______________________

h. ______________________

i. ______________________

2. Match the following hormones with their secretory gland (answers may be used more than once).

_____ a. Thyroxin (T_4)
_____ b. Cortisol
_____ c. Glucagon
_____ d. Prolactin
_____ e. Progesterone
_____ f. Growth hormone
_____ g. Triiodothyronine (T_3)
_____ h. Melanocyte-stimulating hormone
_____ i. Insulin
_____ j. TSH
_____ k. Calcitonin
_____ l. Gonadotropic hormones
_____ m. Somatostatin
_____ n. Epinephrine/norepinephrine
_____ o. ACTH
_____ p. ADH

1. Anterior pituitary
2. Posterior pituitary
3. Thyroid
4. Parathyroid
5. Beta cells of islets of Langerhans
6. Alpha cells of islet of Langerhans
7. Delta cells of islet of Langerhans
8. Adrenal cortex
9. Adrenal medulla
10. Ovaries

3. Identify whether the following statements are true or false. If a statement is false, correct the bold word(s) to make the statement true.

_____ a. Overproduction of the **adrenal cortex** may cause masculinization in women.

_____ b. Two hormones that have all cells as target tissue include **growth hormone** and **TSH**.

_____ c. Epinephrine and norepinephrine are considered **hormones** when they are secreted by the adrenal medulla and are considered **neurotransmitters** when they are secreted by nerve cells.

_____ d. In a person who normally works a night shift from 11:00 PM to 7:00 AM and sleeps from 8:00 AM to 3:00 PM, a serum analysis of cortisol taken at 7:30 AM would reveal a **false high** cortisol level.

_____ e. An example of a complex negative feedback system is the regulation of **insulin**.

_____ f. Hormones that act on the anterior pituitary gland to stimulate tropic hormone secretion are known as **releasing hormones**.

_____ g. Endocrine glands that have negative feedback systems to the hypothalamus include the **pancreas** and the **parathyroid gland**.

_____ h. **Androgens** secreted by the adrenal cortex are responsible for sex drive in women.

_____ i. The mechanism for the action of **protein hormones** is binding to receptors inside the cell.

4. Match each hormone with the primary factor that stimulates its secretion and the primary factor that inhibits its secretion (factors may be used more than once).

Stimulate	Inhibit	Hormone	Primary Factor
____	____	a. THS or thyrotropin	1. Increased stress
____	____	b. Corticotropin-releasing hormone	2. Increased serum thyroxin
____	____	c. ADH	3. Decreased serum T_3
____	____	d. FSH	4. Increased serum cortisol
____	____	e. Calcitonin	5. Increased serum estrogen
____	____	f. Aldosterone	6. Decreased serum estrogen
____	____	g. Glucagon	7. Increased serum glucose
____	____	h. Parathyroid hormone	8. Decreased serum glucose
____	____	i. Insulin	9. Increased serum calcium
			10. Decreased serum calcium
			11. Decreased arterial BP
			12. Increased arterial BP
			13. Increased plasma osmolality
			14. Decreased plasma osmolality

5. The normal response to increased serum osmolality is release of

a. aldosterone from the adrenal cortex, which stimulates sodium excretion by the kidney.
b. ADH from the posterior pituitary gland, which stimulates the kidney to reabsorb water.
c. mineralocorticoids from the adrenal gland, which stimulate the kidney to excrete potassium.
d. calcitonin from the thyroid gland, which increases bone resorption and decreases serum calcium levels.

6. The hormone that increases calcium resorption form the bones and kidney and increases absorption for the intestine is

a. TSH.
b. calcitonin.
d. aldosterone.
d. parathyroid hormone.

7. Hormones of one gland influence the function of hormones of another gland. This is demonstrated by the fact that

a. increased insulin levels inhibit the secretion of glucagon.
b. increased testosterone levels inhibit the release of estrogen.
c. increased cortisol levels stimulate the secretion of insulin.
d. increased atrial natriuretic hormone levels inhibit the secretion of aldosterone.

8. Following the ingestion of a high-protein, carbohydrate-free meal

   a. both insulin and glucagon are inhibited because blood glucose levels are unchanged.
   b. insulin is released to facilitate breakdown of amino acids into glucose and glucagon is inhibited.
   c. insulin is inhibited by low glucose levels and glucagon is released to promote gluconeogenesis.
   d. glucagon is released to promote gluconeogenesis and insulin is released to facilitate movement of amino acids into muscle cells.

9. In a patient with an elevated serum cortisol, the nurse would expect other laboratory findings to reveal

   a. hyponatremia.
   b. hyperkalemia.
   c. hypoglycemia.
   d. decreased serum triglycerides.

10. Two effects of hypokalemia on the endocrine system are

    a. decreased insulin and aldosterone release.
    b. decreased glucagon and increased cortisol release.
    c. decreased release of atrial natriuretic factor and increased ADH release.
    d. decreased release of parathyroid hormone and increased calcitonin release.

11. Manifestations of endocrine problems in the older adult that are commonly attributed the aging process are

    a. tremors and parathesias.
    b. fatigue and mental impairment.
    c. fluid retention and hypertension.
    d. hyperpigmentation and oily skin.

12. Common nonspecific manifestations that may alert the nurse to endocrine dysfunction include

    a. goiter and alopecia.
    b. exophthalmos and tremors.
    c. weight loss, fatigue, and depression.
    d. polyuria, polydipsia, and polyphagia.

13. Identify one specific finding identified by the nurse during assessment of each of the patient's functional health patterns that indicates a risk factor for endocrine problems or a patient response to an actual endocrine problem.

    a. Health perception–health management

    b. Nutritional-metabolic

    c. Elimination

    d. Activity-exercise

    e. Sleep-rest

    f. Cognitive-perceptual

    g. Self-perception–self-concept

    h. Role-relationship

    i. Sexuality-reproductive

    j. Coping–stress tolerance

    k. Value-belief

14. A potential adverse effect of palpation of the thyroid gland is

    a. carotid artery obstruction.
    b. damage to the cricoid cartilage.
    c. release of excessive thyroid hormone into circulation.
    d. hoarseness from pressure on the recurrent laryngeal nerve.

15. Complete the following sentences related to abnormal assessment findings of the endocrine system.

    a. Tetanic muscle spasms are associated with hypofunction of the ____________________ gland.

    b. Hyperpigmentation is associated with hypofunction of the ____________________ gland.

    c. Exophthalmos is associated with excessive secretion of the ____________________ gland.

    d. Moon face is associated with ________________ secretion of the adrenal gland.

    e. A goiter is associated with either hyper- or hypofunction of the ________________ gland.

    f. An increase in hand and foot size is associated with excessive secretion of ____________________ hormone.

    g. Striae are associated with excessive secretion of the ________________ gland.

    h. Heat intolerance is associated with ____________________ secretion of the thyroid gland.

16. A patient has a low serum T_3 level, and the physician orders a TSH level. If the TSH level is elevated, this indicates that

 a. the cause of the low T_3 is most likely primary hypothyroidism.
 b. the negative feedback system is failing to stimulate the anterior pituitary gland.
 c. the patient has an underactive thyroid gland that is not receiving TSH stimulation.
 d. there is most likely a tumor of the anterior pituitary gland that is causing increased production of TSH.

17. To ensure accurate results of a fasting blood glucose analysis, the nurse has the patient fast for at least

 a. 2 hours.
 b. 4 hours.
 c. 8 hours.
 d. 12 hours.

18. Match the following diagnostic studies with the descriptions.

_____	a. 5-hour glucose tolerance test	1. Normal response is drop in blood glucose to <40 mg/dl
_____	b. Growth hormone stimulation test	2. Normal response is decreased cortisol
_____	c. Serum phosphate	3. Normal response is increased plasma cortisol
_____	d. 17-ketosteroids	4. Evaluates hypoglycemia
_____	e. ACTH stimulation test	5. Decreases indicate hyperparathyroidism
_____	f. Glycosylated hemoglobin	6. Differentiates causes of polyuria
_____	g. Water deprivation test	7. Evaluates glucose control over time
_____	h. ACTH (Dexamethasone) suppression test	8. Evaluates steroid hormone function

CHAPTER 47 NURSING MANAGEMENT: DIABETES MELLITUS

1. Although the primary function of insulin is to promote glucose transport from the blood into the cell, insulin also

   a. enhances breakdown of adipose tissue for energy.
   b. stimulates hepatic glycogenolysis and gluconeogenesis.
   c. prevents the transport of triglycerides into adipose tissue.
   d. accelerates the transport of amino acids into cells and their synthesis into protein.

2. Complete the following statements:

   a. Tissues that require insulin for glucose transport are _______________ and _____________ tissues.

   b. During the development of type 1 diabetes, the β cell response to the hyperglycemia can be identified in the blood and urine by the presence of ______________________________.

   c. Two hormones released during physical and emotional stress that are counterregulatory to insulin are _______________ and _______________.

   d. The type of diabetes that is strongly related to human leukocyte antigen types is __________________.

3. Indicate whether the following mechanisms of diabetes are characteristic of the pathophysiology of type 1 (1) or type 2 (2) diabetes.

   _____ a. Insulin resistance

   _____ b. β cell secretory exhaustion

   _____ c. Inherited defect in insulin receptors

   _____ d. Production of islet cell antibodies

   _____ e. Genetic susceptibility for antibody production

   _____ f. Inappropriate glucose production by the liver

   _____ g. β cell destruction

   _____ h. Impaired glucose tolerance occurs gradually

   _____ i. Compensatory increased insulin production

4. Describe the process that occurs to cause the following classic diabetes symptoms.

   a. Polyuria

   b. Polydipsia

   c. Polyphagia

5. The nurse identifies that the risk for developing diabetes is highest in

   a. a 62-year-old obese Caucasian man.
   b. an obese, 50-year-old Hispanic woman.
   c. a child whose father has type 1 diabetes.
   d. a 34-year-old woman whose parents both have type 2 diabetes.

6. When caring for a patient with insulin resistance syndrome, the nurse plans teaching to decrease the patient's risk for

   a. hypertension.
   b. hypoglycemia.
   c. cardiovascular disease.
   d. hyperglycemic hyperosmolar nonketosis.

7. A 52-year-old patient admitted to the hospital with vomiting and diarrhea has a fasting blood sugar (FBS) of 512 mg/dl (28.4 mmol/L) and an arterial pH of 7.38. He is diagnosed with diabetes mellitus and treated with insulin and IV fluids. The nurse recognizes that it is most likely that this patient

   a. will require insulin treatment only during stress.
   b. is demonstrating the abrupt onset of type 1 diabetes.
   c. will require long-term insulin therapy to control the diabetes.
   d. has enough endogenous insulin to prevent diabetic ketoacidosis with the hyperglycemia.

8. During routine health screening a patient is found to have a fasting plasma glucose (FPG) of 132 mg/dl (7.33 mmol/L). At a following visit, a diagnosis of diabetes would be made based on

   a. glucosuria of 3+.
   b. an FPG of 126 mg/dl (7.0 mmol/L).
   c. a random plasma glucose of 210 mg/dl (11.7 mmol/L).
   d. a 2-hour oral glucose tolerance test (OGTT) of 190 mg/dl (10.5 mmol/L).

9. The nurse determines that a patient with a 2-hour OGTT of 152 mg/dl has

   a. diabetes.
   b. impaired fasting glucose.
   c. impaired glucose tolerance.
   d. elevated glycosolated hemoglobin.

10. When teaching the patient with diabetes about insulin administration, the nurse instructs the patient to

   a. pull back on the plunger after inserting the needle to check for blood.
   b. clean the skin at the injection site with an alcohol swab before each injection.
   c. consistently use the same size of the appropriate strength insulin syringe to avoid dosing errors.
   d. rotate injection sites from arms to thighs to abdomen with each injection to prevent lipodystrophies.

11. A patient with type 1 diabetes uses 20U of 70/30 (NPH/regular) in the morning and at 6:00 p.m. When teaching the patient about this regimen, the nurse stresses that

   a. hypoglycemia is most likely to occur before the noon meal.
   b. flexibility in food intake is possible since there is 24-hour insulin availability.
   c. a set meal pattern with a bedtime snack is necessary to prevent hypoglycemia.
   d. premeal glucose checks are required to determine needed changes in daily dosing.

12. Lispro insulin (Humalog) with NPH insulin is ordered for a patient with newly diagnosed type 1 diabetes. The nurse knows that when lispro insulin is used, it should be administered

    a. only once a day.
    b. 1 hour before meals.
    c. 30 to 45 minutes before meals.
    d. at mealtime or within 15 minutes of meals.

13. A diabetic patient is learning to mix regular insulin and NPH insulin in the same syringe. The nurse determines that additional teaching is needed when the patient

    a. withdraws the NPH dose into the syringe first.
    b. injects air equal to the NPH dose into the NPH vial first.
    c. removes any air bubbles after withdrawing the first insulin.
    d. adds air equal to the insulin dose into the regular vial and withdraws the dose.

14. The home care nurse should intervene to correct a patient whose insulin administration includes

    a. warming a prefilled refrigerated syringe in the hands before administration.
    b. storing syringes prefilled with lente and regular insulin needle-upward in the refrigerator.
    c. placing the insulin bottle currently in use in a small container on the bathroom countertop.
    d. mixing an evening dose of regular insulin with insulin glargine in one syringe for administration.

15. The major advantage of using an insulin pump or intensive insulin therapy is that

    a. tight glycemic control can be maintained.
    b. errors in insulin dosing are less likely to occur.
    c. complications of insulin therapy are prevented.
    d. frequent blood glucose monitoring is unnecessary.

16. A patient taking insulin has a glucose level of 214 mg/dl (11.9 mmol/L) on awakening in the morning. The nurse advises the patient to

    a. increase the evening insulin dose to prevent the dawn phenomenon.
    b. use a single-dose insulin regimen with an intermediate-acting insulin.
    c. monitor the glucose level at bedtime, between 2 and 4 a.m., and on arising.
    d. decrease the evening insulin dosage to prevent night hypoglycemia and the Somogyi effect.

17. Match the following oral glucose-lowering agents with their descriptions (answers may be used more than once).

_____	a. Decreases endogenous glucose production	1. Sulfonylurea
_____	b. Should be taken within 30 minutes of each meal	2. Meglitinide
_____	c. Decreases glycogenolysis	3. Biguanide
_____	d. Fewer adverse effects with second-generation agents	4. α-glucosidase inhibitor
_____	e. Rapid and short-acting release of insulin from pancreas	5. Thiazolidinedione
_____	f. Delays glucose absorption from the GI tract	
_____	g. Stimulates production and release of insulin and enhances cellular sensitivity to insulin	
_____	h. Increases glucose uptake, especially in muscles	
_____	i. Primary effect is decreased glucose production by liver	
_____	j. Not effective against fasting hyperglycemia	
_____	k. Taken with first bite of each meal	

18. One of the disadvantages of the use of oral antidiabetic agents in comparison with the use of insulin is that

a. hypoglycemic episodes are more common and prolonged than with the use of insulin.
b. more frequent blood glucose monitoring is necessary to evaluate the effect of oral antidiabetic agents.
c. patients may assume that their diabetes is not serious and that dietary modifications and meal scheduling are not important.
d. the use of other medications may cause interactions, potentiating the glucose-lowering effect of oral antidiabetic agents.

19. In nutritional management of all types of diabetes, it is important for the patient to

a. eat regular meals at regular times.
b. restrict calories to promote moderate weight loss.
c. eliminate sucrose and other simple sugars from the diet.
d. limit saturated fat intake to 30% of dietary calorie intake.

20. Goals of nutritional therapy for the patient with type 2 diabetes includes maintenance of

a. ideal body weight.
b. normal serum glucose and lipid levels.
c. a special diabetic diet using dietetic foods.
d. five small meals per day with a bedtime snack.

21. To prevent hyperglycemia or hypoglycemia with exercise, the nurse teaches the patient using glucose-lowering agents that exercise should be undertaken

a. only after a 10- to 15-g carbohydrate snack is eaten.
b. about 1 hour after eating when blood glucose levels are rising.
c. when glucose monitoring reveals that the blood glucose is in the normal range.
d. when blood glucose levels are high, because exercise always has a hypoglycemic effect.

22. The nurse assesses the diabetic patient's technique of self-monitoring of blood glucose (SMBG) 3 months after initial instruction. An error in the performance of SMBG noted by the nurse that requires intervention is

a. doing the SMBG before and after exercising.
b. puncturing the finger on the side of the finger pad.
c. cleaning the puncture site with alcohol before the puncture.
d. holding the hand down for a few minutes before the puncture.

23. Ideally, the goal of patient diabetes education is to

a. make all patients responsible for the management of their disease.
b. involve the patient's family and significant others in the care of the patient.
c. enable the patient to become the most active participant in the management of the diabetes.
d. to provide the patient with as much information as soon as possible to prevent complications of diabetes.

24. A nurse working in an outpatient clinic plans a screening program for diabetes. Recommendations for screening would include

a. OGTT for all minority populations every year.
b. FPG for all individuals at age 45 and then every 3 years.
c. testing all people before the age of 21 for islet cell antibodies.
d. testing for type 2 diabetes only in overweight or obese individuals.

25. A patient with diabetes calls the clinic because she is experiencing nausea and flulike symptoms. The nurse advises the patient to

a. administer the usual insulin dosage.
b. hold fluid intake until the nausea subsides.
c. come to the clinic immediately for evaluation and treatment.
d. monitor the blood glucose q1-2hr and call if the glucose rises over 150 mg/dl (8.3 mmol/L).

26. Ketoacidosis occurs as a complication of diabetes when

a. illnesses causing nausea and vomiting lead to bicarbonate loss with body fluids.
b. the glucose level becomes so high that osmotic diuresis promotes fluid and electrolyte loss.
c. an insulin deficit causes the body to metabolize large amounts of fatty acids rather than glucose for energy.
d. the patient skips meals after taking insulin leading to rapid metabolism of glucose and breakdown of fats for energy.

27. Number in sequence from 1 to 8 the processes of potassium imbalance in diabetic ketoacidosis (DKA).

_____ a. Treatment with insulin increases glucose metabolism and decreases fat metabolism

_____ b. Decreased H^+ ions in the blood

_____ c. K^+ from the cells moves into blood in exchange for H^+ ions

_____ d. Movement of K^+ back into cells

_____ e. K^+ excreted in urine with osmotic diuresis

_____ f. Increased serum K^+ concentration

_____ g. Total body K^+ deficit

_____ h. Increased H^+ ions present in form of acidic ketones and acetone

28. List five signs and symptoms that are present in DKA that are not seen in hyperglycemic hyperosmolar nonketotic syndrome (HHNS).

a.

b.

c.

d.

e.

29. The treatment for diabetic ketoacidosis (DKA) and hyperglycemic hyperosmolar nonketotic syndrome (HHNS) differ primarily in that

a. DKA requires administration of bicarbonate to correct acidosis.
b. potassium replacement is not necessary in management of HHNS.
c. HHNS requires greater fluid replacement to correct the dehydration.
d. administration of glucose is withheld in HHNS until the blood glucose reaches a normal level.

30. The nurse is alerted to the possibility of hypovolemic shock occurring in the patient with HHNS by the presence of

a. an increase in CVP.
b. deep, rapid respirations.
c. a change from polyuria to oliguria.
d. depressed ST segment and T waves on cardiac monitoring.

31. Indicate whether the following characteristics are associated with hypoglycemia (1), hyperglycemia (2), or both (3).

_____ a. Slurred speech and irritability

_____ b. Headache

_____ c. Nausea and vomiting

_____ d. Too much exercise without food

_____ e. Increased dietary intake

_____ f. Cold, clammy skin

_____ g. Precipitated by stress

_____ h. Changes in vision

32. A diabetic patient is found unconscious at home and a family member calls the clinic. After determining that no glucometer is available, the nurse advises the family member to

a. administer 10U regular insulin SC.
b. administer glucagon 1 mg IM or SC.
c. try to arouse the patient to drink some orange juice.
d. call for an ambulance to transport the patient to a medical facility.

33. Two days following a self-managed hypoglycemic episode at home, the patient tells the nurse that his blood glucose levels since the episode have been between 80 and 90 mg/dl. The best response by the nurse is,

   a. "That is a good range for your glucose levels."
   b. "You should call your physician because you need to have your insulin increased."
   c. "That level is too low in view of your recent hypoglycemia, and you should increase your food intake."
   d. "You should only take half your insulin dosage for the next few days to get your glucose level back to normal."

34. In diabetes, atherosclerotic disease affecting the cerebrovascular, cardiovascular, and peripheral vascular systems

   a. can be prevented by tight glucose control.
   b. occurs with a higher frequency and earlier onset than in the nondiabetic population.
   c. is caused by the hyperinsulinemia related to insulin resistance common in type 2 diabetes.
   d. cannot be modified by reduction of risk factors such as smoking, obesity, and high fat intake.

35. Match the following characteristics as they relate to complications of diabetes (answers may be used more than once).

_____	a. Male impotence	1. Microangiopathy
_____	b. Diffuse and nodular glomerulosclerosis	2. Macroangiopathy
_____	c. Related to altered lipid metabolism of diabetes	3. Autonomic neuropathy
		4. Sensory neuropathy
_____	d. Microaneurysms and destruction of retinal capillaries	
_____	e. Atrophy of small muscles of the hands	
_____	f. Capillary and arteriole basement membrane thickening specific to diabetes	
_____	g. Pain and paresthesia of legs	
_____	h. Ulceration and amputation of lower extremities	
_____	i. Shin spots	
_____	j. Delayed gastric emptying	
_____	k. Ischemic heart disease	

36. Following the teaching of foot care to a diabetic patient, the nurse determines that additional instruction is needed when the patient says

   a. "I should wash my feet daily with soap and warm water."
   b. "I should always wear shoes to protect my feet from injury."
   c. "If my feet are cold I should wear socks instead of using a heating pad."
   d. "I'll know if I have a sores or lesions on my feet because they will be painful."

37. A 72-year-old woman is diagnosed with diabetes. The nurse recognizes that management of diabetes in the older adult

    a. does not require as tight glucose control as in younger diabetics.
    b. is usually not treated unless the patient becomes severely hyperglycemic.
    c. does not include treatment with insulin because of limited dexterity and vision.
    d. usually requires that a younger family member be responsible for care of the patient.

CASE STUDY

HYPOGLYCEMIA

Patient Profile

Ms. W. was brought to the first aid tent provided for participants in a charity marathon. She is a 24-year-old type I diabetic well maintained on a regimen of self-monitoring of blood glucose, insulin, and diet.

Subjective Data

- States she feels cold, has a headache, and her fingers feel numb
- Took her usual insulin dose this morning but was unable to eat her entire breakfast due to lack of time
- Completed the entire marathon in a personal-best time

Objective Data

- Has slurred speech and unsteady gait
- Pulse 120 beats/min
- Appears confused
- Capillary blood glucose level 48 mg/dl (2.7 mmol/L)

Critical Thinking Questions

1. Describe what Ms. W. could have done to prevent this hypoglycemic event.

2. What is the etiology of the signs and symptoms displayed by Ms. W.?

3. How would you expect to treat her hypoglycemia?

4. What teaching is appropriate for this patient once her condition has been stabilized?

5. What adjustments in her diabetic regimen could Ms. W. make to allow her to continue with her exercise habits?

6. Based on the assessment data presented, write one or more appropriate nursing diagnoses. Are there any collaborative problems?

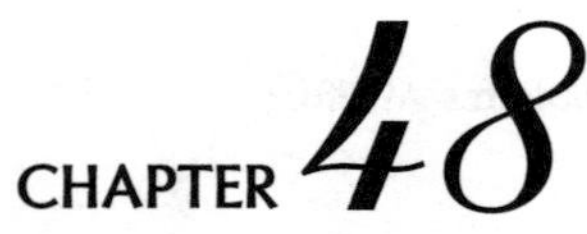

CHAPTER 48 NURSING MANAGEMENT: ENDOCRINE PROBLEMS

1. A patient suspected of having acromegaly has an elevated plasma growth hormone level. In acromegaly, the nurse would also expect the patient's diagnostic results to include

   a. hyperinsulinemia.
   b. a plasma glucose of less than 70 mg/dl (3.9 mmol/L).
   c. decreased growth hormone levels with an oral glucose challenge test.
   d. a serum somatomedin C (insulin-like growth factor-1) of more than 300 ng/ml.

2. During assessment of the patient with acromegaly, the nurse would expect the patient to report

   a. infertility.
   b. dry, irritated skin.
   c. undesirable changes in appearance.
   d. an increase in height of 2 to 3 inches a year.

3. A patient with acromegaly is treated with a transsphenoidal hypophysectomy. Postoperatively, the nurse

   a. ensures that any clear nasal drainage is tested for glucose.
   b. maintains the patient flat in bed to prevent cerebrospinal fluid leakage.
   c. assists the patient with toothbrushing q4h to keep the surgical area clean.
   d. encourages deep breathing and coughing to prevent respiratory complications.

4. Identify whether the following statements are true or false. If a statement is false, correct the bold word(s) to make the statement true.

   _____ a. Drugs used in the primary treatment of acromegaly are effective because they **block the action** of growth hormone.

   _____ b. A patient with diabetes mellitus who undergoes a hypophysectomy will require a **larger** dose of insulin than preoperatively.

   _____ c. Pituitary tumors causing either hyperpituitarism or hypopituitarism may cause **visual changes and disturbances**.

   _____ d. **Hyposecretion** of FSH is associated with the onset of menopause.

   _____ e. Early hypofunction of the pituitary gland usually results in nonspecific symptoms primarily because there are no obvious manifestations of **growth hormone** deficiencies in adults.

5. Identify five hormones that are replaced when panhypopituitarism results from radiation therapy or total hypophysectomy as treatment for pituitary tumors.

   a.

   b.

   c.

   d.

   e.

6. In the following diagram of the pathophysiology of antidiuretic hormone (ADH) problems, indicate in the appropriate blanks whether the processes are increased (↑) or decreased (↓) in syndrome of inappropriate ADH (SIADH) and diabetes insipidus (DI).

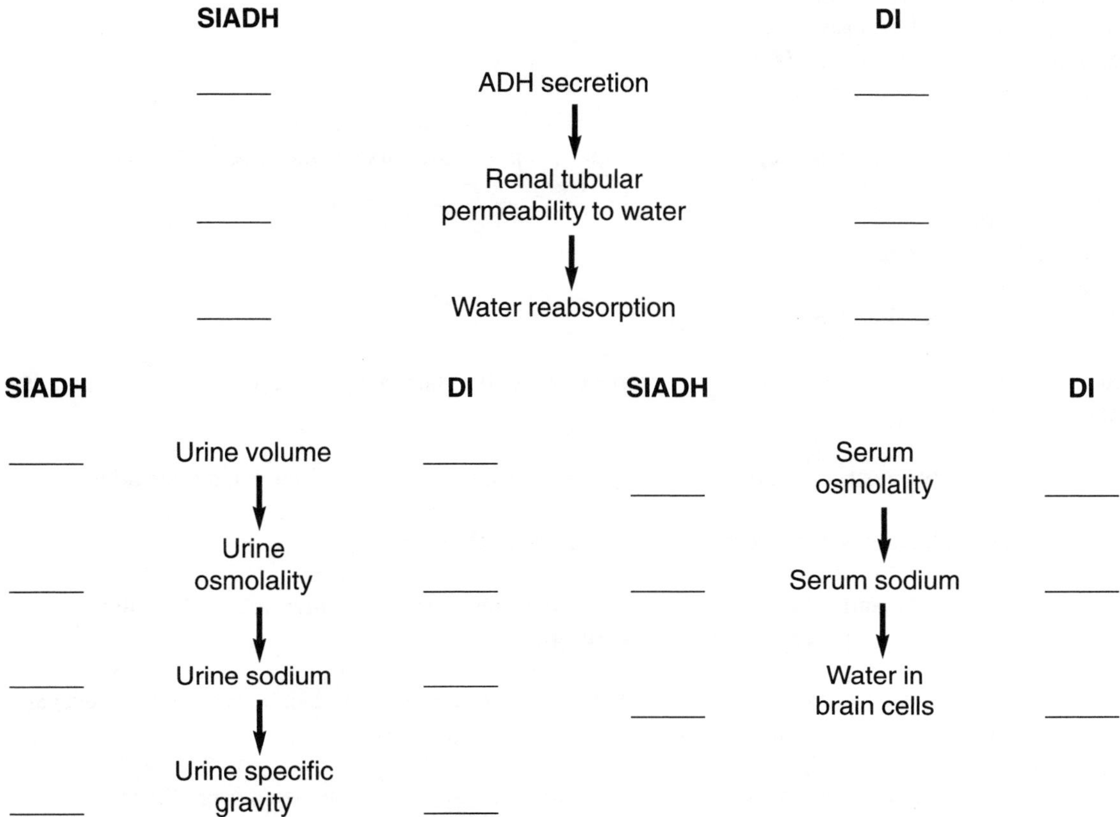

7. During care of the patient with syndrome of inappropriate ADH (SIADH), the nurse should

   a. monitor neurologic status q2hr or more often if needed.
   b. keep the head of the bed elevated to prevent ADH release.
   c. teach the patient receiving treatment with diuretics to restrict sodium intake.
   d. notify the physician if the patient's blood pressure decreases more than 20 mm Hg from baseline.

8. A patient with SIADH is treated with water restriction and administration of IV fluids. The nurse evaluates that treatment has been effective when the patient experiences

   a. increased urine output, decreased serum sodium, and increased urine specific gravity.
   b. increased urine output, increased serum sodium, and decreased urine specific gravity.
   c. decreased urine output, increased serum sodium, and decreased urine specific gravity.
   d. decreased urine output, decreased serum sodium, and increased urine specific gravity.

9. In a patient with central diabetes insipidus, administration of aqueous vasopressin during a water deprivation test will result in a

   a. decrease in body weight.
   b. increase in urinary output.
   c. decrease in blood pressure.
   d. increase in urine osmolality.

10. A patient with diabetes insipidus is treated with nasal desmopressin. The nurse recognizes that the drug is not having an adequate therapeutic effect when the patient experiences

   a. headache and weight gain.
   b. nasal irritation and nausea.
   c. a urine specific gravity of 1.002.
   d. an oral intake greater than urinary output.

11. When caring for a patient with nephrogenic diabetes insipidus, the nurse would expect treatment to include

   a. fluid restriction.
   b. thiazide diuretics.
   c. a high-sodium diet.
   d. chlorpropamide (Diabinese).

12. Identify whether the following statements are true or false. If a statement is false, correct the bold word(s) to make the statement true.

   _____ a. The two most common forms of hyperthyroidism are **Graves' disease** and **toxic adenoma**.

   _____ b. Exophthalmos may occur in **any form of hyperthyroidism**.

   _____ c. Clinical manifestations of hyperthyroidism occur as a result of **increased metabolic rate** and **an increased number of β-adrenergic receptors**.

   _____ d. Diagnostic testing in the patient with Graves' disease will reveal an **increased TSH level** and a radioactive iodine uptake of **<5%**.

   _____ e. Goitrogens are substances that **promote** thyroid function and are **encouraged** for patients with hypothyroidism.

13. A patient with Graves' disease asks the nurse what caused the disorder. The best response by the nurse is

   a. "The cause of Graves' disease is not known, although it is thought to be genetic."
   b. "It is usually associated with goiter formation from an iodine deficiency over a long period of time."
   c. "Antibodies develop against thyroid tissue and destroy it, causing a deficiency of thyroid hormones."
   d. "In genetically susceptible persons antibodies form that attack thyroid tissue and stimulate overproduction of thyroid hormones."

14. A patient is admitted to the hospital in thyrotoxic crisis. On physical assessment of the patient, the nurse would expect to find

   a. hoarseness and laryngeal stridor.
   b. bulging eyeballs and arrhythmias.
   c. elevated temperature and signs of heart failure.
   d. lethargy progressing suddenly to impairment of consciousness.

15. Match the following characteristics and rationales for the uses of the drugs used in treatment of hyperthyroidism (answers may be used more than once).

_____ a. Should be taken with a straw to avoid staining the teeth

_____ b. Is not used in patients of childbearing age

_____ c. Decreases release of thyroid hormones

_____ d. Often used with iodine to produce euthyroid before surgery

_____ e. May cause agranulocytosis

_____ f. Used to decrease size and vascularity of thyroid gland preoperatively

_____ g. Used to control sympathetic symptoms

_____ h. Blocks peripheral conversion of T_4 to T_3

_____ i. Decreases thyroid secretion by damaging thyroid gland

_____ j. Indications of toxicity are excessive salivation and skin reactions

_____ k. Often causes hypothyroidism over time

1. Propylthiouracil (PTU)
2. Potassium iodide
3. Propranolol (Inderal)
4. Radioactive iodine (^{131}I)

16. Identify one nursing diagnosis that is appropriate for the patient with the following manifestations of hyperthyroidism.

a. Exophthalmos

b. Weight loss and hunger

c. Hair loss and vitiligo

d. Exhaustion and dyspnea

17. Preoperative instructions for the patient scheduled for a subtotal thyroidectomy includes teaching the patient

a. how to support the head with the hands when moving.
b. that coughing should be avoided to prevent pressure on the incision.
c. that the head and neck will need to remain immobile until the incision heals.
d. that any tingling around the lips or in the fingers after surgery is expected and temporary.

18. Identify the rationale for having the following items immediately available in the patient's room following a thyroidectomy.

    a. Tracheostomy tray

    b. Calcium salts for IV administration

    c. Oxygen equipment

19. When providing discharge instructions to a patient following a subtotal thyroidectomy, the nurse advises the patient to

    a. never miss a daily dose of thyroid replacement therapy.
    b. avoid regular exercise until thyroid function is normalized.
    c. avoid eating foods such as soybeans, turnips, and rutabagas.
    d. use warm salt water gargles several times a day to relieve throat pain.

20. Match the following characteristics with their related disorders.

_____	a. Viral-induced hyperthyroidism	1. Goiter
_____	b. Autoimmune fibrous and lymphocytic replacement of thyroid gland	2. Thyroid nodules
		3. Hashimoto's thyroiditis
_____	c. Enlarged thyroid gland	
		4. Subacute granulomatous thyroiditis
_____	d. Lymphocytic infiltration of thyroid gland that may occur postpartum	5. Silent thyroiditis
_____	e. Bacterial or fungal infection of thyroid gland	6. Acute thyroiditis
_____	f. Malignant or benign deformity of the thyroid gland	

21. Causes of primary hypothyroidism in adults include

    a. malignant or benign thyroid nodules.
    b. surgical removal or failure of the pituitary gland.
    c. surgical removal or radiation of the thyroid gland.
    d. autoimmune-induced atrophy of the thyroid gland.

22. The nurse has identified the following nursing diagnoses for a patient who is hypothyroid. For each nursing diagnoses, identify an appropriate etiology for the diagnosis and at least two common signs or symptoms of hypothyroidism that support the diagnosis.

    a. Disturbed sleep pattern related to ______________________________ as manifested by

       ______________________ and ______________________________.

    b. Imbalanced nutrition: more than body requirements related to ______________________________ as

       manifested by ______________________ and ______________________________.

    c. Disturbed thought processes related to ______________________________ as manifested by

       ______________________ and ______________________________.

    d. Activity intolerance related to ______________________________ as manifested by

       ______________________ and ______________________________.

23. Physical changes of hypothyroidism that must be monitored when replacement therapy is started include

    a. achlorhydria and constipation.
    b. slowed mental processes and lethargy.
    c. anemia and increased capillary fragility.
    d. decreased cardiac contractility and coronary atherosclerosis.

24. A patient with hypothyroidism is treated with levothyroxin (Synthroid). When teaching the patient about the therapy, the nurse

    a. explains that caloric intake must be reduced when drug therapy is started.
    b. provides written instruction for all information related to the medication therapy.
    c. assures the patient that a return to normal function will occur with replacement therapy.
    d. informs the patient that medications must be taken until hormone balance is reestablished.

25. Indicate whether the following clinical manifestations are characteristic of hyperparathyroidism (1) or hypoparathyroidism (2).

    _____ a. Decreased bone density

    _____ b. Muscle spasms and stiffness

    _____ c. Psychomotor retardation

    _____ d. Calcium nephrolithiasis

    _____ e. Anorexia and abdominal pain

    _____ f. Decreased contractility of myocardium

    _____ g. Laryngeal spasm

    _____ h. Skeletal pain

    _____ i. Abdominal cramping

    _____ j. Cardiac irritability

26. An appropriate nursing intervention for the patient with hyperparathyroidism is to

    a. pad side rails as a seizure precaution.
    b. increase fluid intake to 3000 to 4000 ml/day.
    c. maintain bed rest to prevent pathologic fractures.
    d. monitor the patient for Trousseau's phenomenon and Chvostek's sign.

27. When the patient with parathyroid disease experiences symptoms of hypocalcemia, a measure that can be used to temporarily raise serum calcium levels is to

    a. administer IV normal saline.
    b. have the patient rebreathe in a paper bag.
    c. administer furosemide (Lasix) as ordered.
    d. administer oral phosphorous supplements.

28. A patient with hypoparathyroidism as a result of surgical treatment of hyperparathyroidism is preparing for discharge. The nurse teaches the patient that

    a. milk and milk products should be increased in the diet.
    b. parenteral replacement of PTH will be required for life.
    c. calcium supplements with vitamin D can effectively maintain calcium balance.
    d. bran and whole grain foods should be used to prevent GI effects of replacement therapy.

29. A patient is admitted to the hospital with a diagnosis of Cushing syndrome. On physical assessment of the patient, the nurse would expect to find

    a. hypertension, peripheral edema, and petechiae.
    b. weight loss, buffalo hump, and moon face with acne.
    c. abdominal and buttock striae, truncal obesity, and hypotension.
    d. anorexia, signs of dehydration, and hyperpigmentation of the skin.

30. To prevent complications in the patient with Cushing syndrome, the nurse monitors the patient for

    a. hypotension.
    b. hypoglycemia.
    c. cardiac arrhythmias.
    d. decreased cardiac output.

31. A patient is scheduled for a bilateral adrenalectomy. During the postoperative period, the nurse would expect administration of corticosteroids to be

    a. reduced to promote wound healing.
    b. withheld until symptoms of hypocortisolism appear.
    c. increased to promote an adequate response to the stress of surgery.
    d. reduced because excessive hormones are released during surgical manipulation of the glands.

32. A patient with Addison's disease comes to the emergency department with complaints of nausea, vomiting, diarrhea, and fever. The nurse would expect collaborative care to include

    a. parenteral injections of ACTH.
    b. IV administration of vasopressors.
    c. IV administration of hydrocortisone.
    d. IV administration of D_5W with 20 mEq KCl.

33. The nurse determines that the patient in acute adrenal insufficiency is responding favorably to treatment when

    a. the patient appears alert and oriented.
    b. the patient's urinary output has increased.
    c. pulmonary edema is reduced as evidenced by clear lung sounds.
    d. laboratory tests reveal serum elevations of potassium and glucose and a decrease in sodium.

34. During discharge teaching for the patient with Addison's disease, the nurse identifies a need for additional instruction when the patient says

    a. "I should always call the doctor if I develop vomiting or diarrhea."
    b. "If my weight goes down, my dosage of steroid is probably too high."
    c. "I should double or triple my steroid dose if I undergo rigorous physical exercise."
    d. "I need to carry an emergency kit with injectable hydrocortisone in case I can't take my medication by mouth."

35. A patient who is on corticosteroid therapy for treatment of an autoimmune disorder has the following additional drugs ordered. How is the need for these drugs related to the effects of glucocorticosteroids?

    a. Furosemide (Lasix)

    b. Ranitidine (Zantac)

    c. Alendronate (Fosamax)

    d. Insulin

    e. Potassium

    f. Isoniazid (INH)

36. A patient with mild iatrogenic Cushing syndrome is on an alternate-day regimen of corticosteroid therapy. The nurse explains to the patient that this regimen

    a. maintains normal adrenal hormone balance.
    b. prevents ACTH release from the pituitary gland.
    c. minimizes hypothalamic-pituitary-adrenal suppression.
    d. provides a more effective therapeutic effect of the drug.

37. When caring for a patient with primary hyperaldosteronism, the nurse would question a physician's order for the use of

    a. furosemide (Lasix).
    b. amiloride (Midamor).
    c. spironolactone (Aldactone).
    d. aminoglutethimide (Cytadren).

38. The most important nursing intervention during the medical and surgical treatment of the patient with a pheochromocytoma is

    a. administering IV fluids.
    b. monitoring blood pressure.
    c. monitoring I&O and daily weights.
    d. administering β-adrenergic blocking agents.

CASE STUDY

CUSHING SYNDROME

Patient Profile

Mr. H. is a 26-year-old elementary school teacher. He seeks the advice of his physician because of changes in his appearance over the past year.

Subjective Data

- Complains of weight gain, particularly through his midsection, easy bruising, and edema of his feet, lower legs, and hands
- Has been having increasing insomnia

Objective Data

- Physical exam: BP 150/110; 2+ edema of lower extremities; purplish striae on abdomen; thin extremities with thin, friable skin; severe acne of the face and neck
- Blood analysis: glucose 167 mg/dl (9.3 mmol/L), WBC 13,600/μl, lymphocytes 12%, RBC 6.6×10^6 μl, K^+ 3.2 mEq/L (3.2 mmol/L)

Critical Thinking Questions

1. Discuss the probable causes of the alterations in Mr. H.'s blood values.

2. Explain the pathophysiology of Cushing syndrome.

3. What diagnostic testing would identify the cause of Mr. H.'s Cushing syndrome?

4. What is the usual treatment of Cushing syndrome?

5. What is meant by a "medical adrenalectomy"?

6. What are the major nursing responsibilities in the care of this patient?

7. Based on the assessment data presented, write one or more appropriate nursing diagnoses. Are there any collaborative problems?

CHAPTER 49 NURSING ASSESSMENT: REPRODUCTIVE SYSTEM

1. Identify the structures in the following illustrations by filling in the blanks on the next page with the correct answers from the list of terms below (some terms will be used in both illustrations).

List of Terms

anterior cul-de-sac
anus
body (corpus) of uterus
Cowper's gland
cervix
clitoris
corpus cavernosum
corpus spongiosum
ductus deferens
ejaculatory duct
epididymis
fallopian tube
fornix of vagina
fundus of uterus
glans
labia majora
labia minora
penis
posterior cul-de-sac
prostate gland
rectum
round ligament
scrotum
seminal vesicle
symphysis pubis
testis
ureter
urethra
urinary bladder
vagina

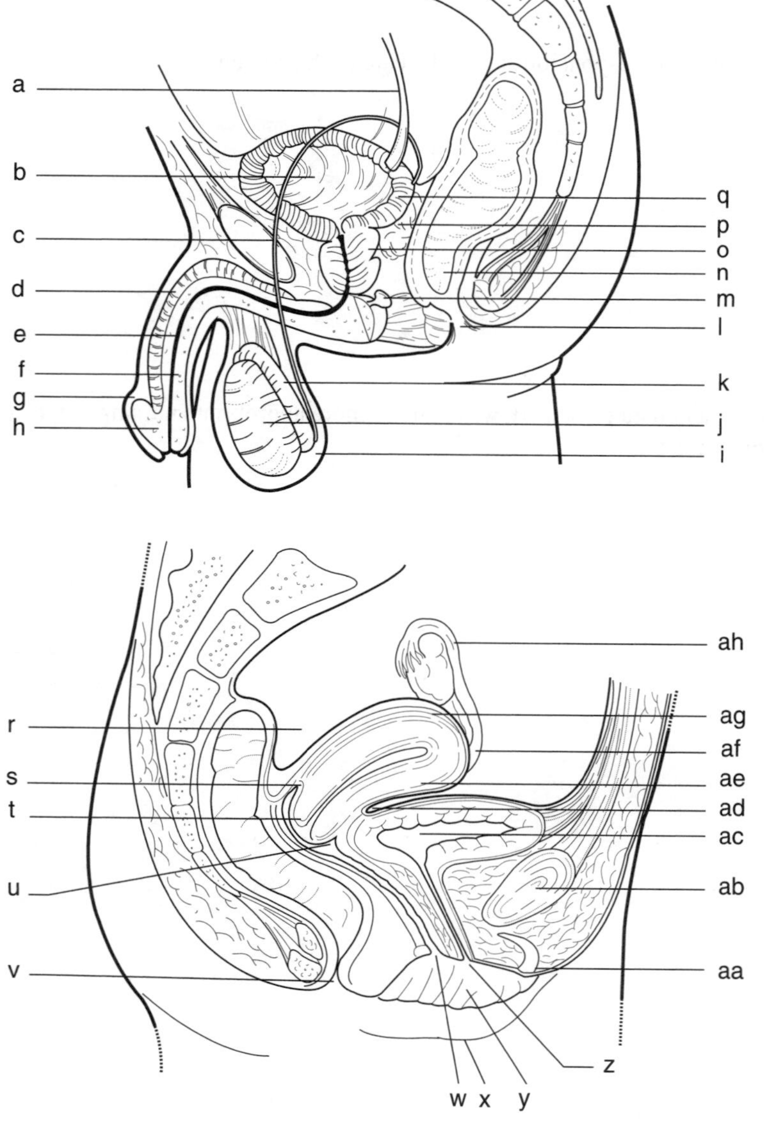

a. ____________________
b. ____________________
c. ____________________
d. ____________________
e. ____________________
f. ____________________
g. ____________________
h. ____________________
i. ____________________
j. ____________________
k. ____________________
l. ____________________
m. ____________________
n. ____________________
o. ____________________
p. ____________________
q. ____________________
r. ____________________
s. ____________________
t. ____________________
u. ____________________
v. ____________________
w. ____________________
x. ____________________
y. ____________________
z. ____________________
aa. ____________________
bb. ____________________
cc. ____________________
dd. ____________________
ee. ____________________
ff. ____________________
gg. ____________________
hh. ____________________

2. Using the list of terms below, identify the structures in the following illustrations.

List of Terms

alveoli	nipple
anus	pectoralis major muscle
areola	perineum
clitoris	prepuce
labia majora	urethra
labia minora	vagina
mons pubis	vestibule

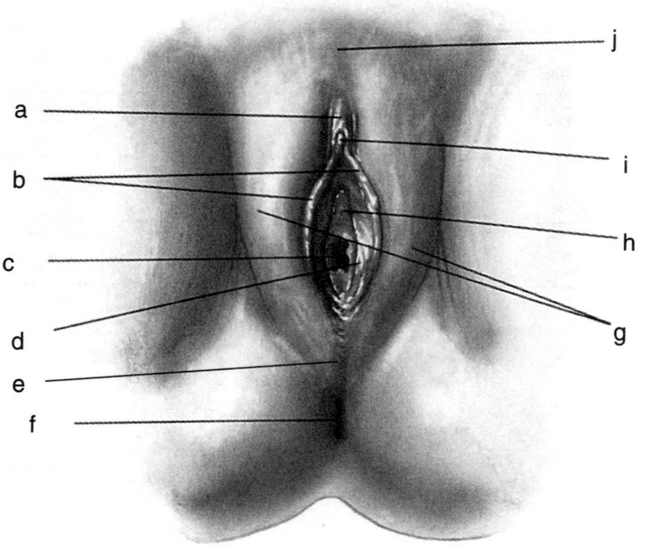

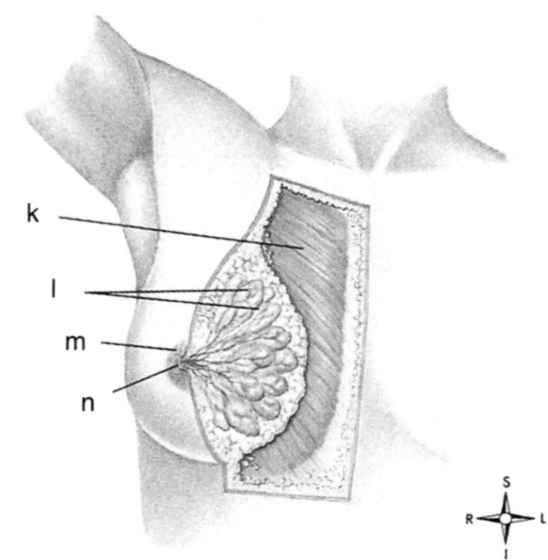

a. ______________________ h. ______________________

b. ______________________ i. ______________________

c. ______________________ j. ______________________

d. ______________________ k. ______________________

e. ______________________ l. ______________________

f. ______________________ m. ______________________

g. ______________________ n. ______________________

3. Number in sequence from 1 to 8 the passage of sperm through, and the formation of semen in, the structures of the male reproductive system.

_____ a. Ductus deferens

_____ b. Urethra

_____ c. Epididymis

_____ d. Prostate gland

_____ e. Seminiferous tubules

_____ f. Cowper's glands

_____ g. Seminal vesicles

_____ h. Ejaculatory duct

4. Match the following descriptions with the structures of the female breast.

_____	a. Pigmented center of breast	1. Alveoli
_____	b. Erectile tissue containing pores	2. Montgomery's tubercles
_____	c. Carry milk from alveoli to lactiferous sinuses	3. Lactiferous sinuses
		4. Areola
_____	d. Major composition of nonlactating breast	5. Ligaments of Cooper
_____	e. Store milk during lactation	6. Ducts
_____	f. Sebaceous-like gland on areola	7. Adipose tissue
_____	g. Secrete milk during lactation	8. Nipple
_____	h. Anchor glandular tissue, skin, and muscles	

5. Identify whether the following statements are true or false. If a statement is false, correct the bold word(s) to make the statement true.

_____ a. The normal process of destruction of oocytes throughout the female life span is known as **atresia**.

_____ b. Fertilization of an ovum by a sperm occurs in the **uterus**.

_____ c. A Pap smear should include cells from the **ectocervix**.

_____ d. Mobility of sperm into the uterus is promoted by **thin, watery cervical mucus** at the time of ovulation.

_____ e. A middle-aged woman is considered to be in menopause when she has not had a menstrual period for **2 years**.

6. Match the descriptions with the reproductive hormones (answers may be used more than once).

_____	a. Called ICSH in males	1. FSH
_____	b. Stimulated by elevated estrogen levels	2. LH
_____	c. Produced by testes	3. Prolactin
_____	d. Elevated at onset of menopause	4. Estrogen
_____	e. Produced by corpus luteum	5. Progesterone
_____	f. Stimulates testosterone production	6. Testosterone
_____	g. Required for female sex characteristics	7. ICSH
_____	h. Needed for growth of mammary glands	8. GnRH
_____	i. Needed for male sex characteristics	
_____	j. Decreased by increased testosterone levels	
_____	k. Responsible for ovarian follicle maturation	
_____	l. Responsible for spermatogenesis	
_____	m. Maintains implanted egg	
_____	n. Completes follicle maturation	

7. Match the events of the menstrual cycle with their associated phases (answers may be used more than once).

_____	a. Corpus luteum secretes estrogen	1. Follicular phase
_____	b. Estrogen secreted by follicles	2. Luteal phase
_____	c. FSH secretion suppressed	3. Menstrual phase
_____	d. GnRH secreted	
_____	e. Ischemia of the endometrium	
_____	f. LH released	
_____	g. Release of mature ovum	
_____	h. FSH released	

8. A 52-year-old woman tells the nurse that she thinks she has started menopause and asks what changes she can expect. The nurse explains that

   a. she is at increased risk for dyspareunia because of changes in the vaginal epithelium.
   b. after menopause she will only stop menstruating; there are no other significant changes that she should worry about.
   c. postmenopausal women are likely to have difficulty with sexual pleasure because of drastic changes in the female sexual response.
   d. she should use hormone replacement therapy to prevent the many uncomfortable and pathologic effects of ovarian failure.

9. A 72-year-old male patient asks the nurse whether it is normal for him to become impotent at his age. The best response by the nurse includes the information that

   a. most decreased sexual function in older adults is due to psychologic stress.
   b. physiologic changes of aging may require increased stimulation for an erection to occur.
   c. although the penis decreases in size in older males, there should be no change in sexual function.
   d. benign changes in the prostate gland that occur with aging can cause a decreased ability to attain an erection.

10. When obtaining information related to reproductive function from a female patient, the nurse knows that sensitive issues may best be discussed by first asking about

    a. sexual practices.
    b. obstetric history.
    c. menstrual history.
    d. use of recreational drugs.

11. List one problem associated with each of the following that may be identified during assessment of the reproductive system.

    a. Rubella

    b. Mumps

    c. Diabetes mellitus

    d. Antihypertensive agents

12. Identify one specific finding identified by the nurse during assessment of each of the patient's functional health patterns that indicates a risk factor for reproductive problems or a patient response to an actual reproductive problem.

    a. Health perception–health management

    b. Nutritional-metabolic

    c. Elimination

    d. Activity-exercise

    e. Sleep-rest

    f. Cognitive-perceptual

    g. Self-perception–self-concept

    h. Role-relationship

    i. Sexuality-reproductive

    j. Coping–stress tolerance

    k. Value-belief

13. A 58-year-old man has difficulty starting a urinary stream, and benign prostatic hyperplasia (BPH) is suspected. Assessment of the patient for the presence of BPH involves

    a. palpation of the scrotum and testes for a mass.
    b. palpating the base of the penis for enlargement.
    c. palpating the inguinal ring while the patient bears down.
    d. a digital rectal examination to palpate the prostate gland.

14. When assessing an aging adult male, the nurse notes as normal the finding of

    a. decreased penis size.
    b. decreased pubic hair.
    c. a decrease in scrotal color.
    d. unilateral breast enlargement.

15. During examination of the breast, the nurse establishes the presence of nipple and skin retraction by

    a. compressing the nipple.
    b. lying the patient supine with her hand above and behind her head.
    c. systematically palpating the breast tissue in a circular or spoke pattern.
    d. asking the patient to lift her hands above her head and then press her hands on her hips while seated.

16. During examination of the female reproductive system, the nurse notes as abnormal the finding of

    a. clear vaginal discharge.
    b. perineal episiotomy scars.
    c. nonpalpable Skene's ducts.
    d. diamond pubic hair distribution.

17. A 36-year-old woman calls the clinic to schedule a pelvic exam and Pap smear. The nurse informs the patient that

    a. she should douche the day before the test.
    b. the exam should be scheduled in the middle of her menstrual cycle.
    c. she should not have sexual intercourse for 48 hours before the examination.
    d. the exam must be performed during the secretory phase of the menstrual cycle, after ovulation.

18. Match the following laboratory tests with their purpose.

_____	a. Urine HCG	1. Identifies secondary gonadal failure
_____	b. Serum estradiol	2. Used for rapid diagnosis of gonorrhea
_____	c. Serum FSH	3. Specific antibody test for syphilis
_____	d. VDRL	4. Measures ovarian function
_____	e. Fluorescent treponemal antibody absorption (FTAAbs)	5. Detects pregnancy
		6. Used to detect prostate cancer
_____	f. Urine FSH assay	7. Nonspecific antibody test for syphilis screening
_____	g. Gram's stain	
_____	h. Alpha-fetoprotein (AFP)	8. Tumor marker for testicular cancer
_____	i. PSA	9. Used to validate menopause

19. Following a dilation and curettage (D&C), it is important for the nurse to assess the patient for the complication of

    a. infection.
    b. hemorrhage.
    c. urinary retention.
    d. perforation of the bladder.

20. Diagnostic tests of the reproductive system that are operative procedures requiring surgical anesthesia include

    a. culdoscopy and conization.
    b. colposcopy and breast biopsy.
    c. laparoscopy and endometrial biopsy.
    d. dilation with curettage and contrast mammography.

21. The fertility test that requires the couple to have sexual intercourse at the time of ovulation and come for testing 2 to 8 hours after intercourse is the

    a. Huhner test.
    b. semen analysis.
    c. endometrial biopsy.
    d. hysterosalpingogram.

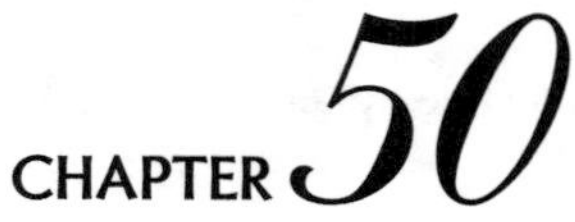

CHAPTER 50 NURSING MANAGEMENT: BREAST DISORDERS

1. The nurse encourages all women to perform breast self-examination (BSE) primarily because

   a. most breast lesions are discovered by women themselves.
   b. breast lesions can be felt before they are evident on a mammogram.
   c. BSE has been shown to reduce mortality in breast cancer in women under age 50.
   d. early detection and treatment of breast cancer is the most significant factor in survival rates.

2. Identify three guidelines for breast surveillance practices accepted by organizations involved with breast cancer.

   a.

   b.

   c.

3. When planning teaching of BSE, the nurse knows that a woman is more likely to perform regular breast self-examination when

   a. the perceived risk for breast cancer is high.
   b. she knows what to do if a lesion is detected.
   c. active practice by the woman increases her confidence in her skill.
   d. she is aware of the statistics related to breast cancer survival and mortality.

4. The diagnostic test that is most accurate and advantageous in terms of time and expense in diagnosing malignant breast disorders is

   a. mammography.
   b. open surgical biopsy.
   c. fine-needle aspiration.
   d. stereotactic core biopsy.

5. While examining a patient's breasts, the nurse notes multiple, bilateral mobile lumps. To assess the patient further, the most appropriate question by the nurse is

   a. "Do you have a high caffeine intake?"
   b. "When did you last have a mammogram?"
   c. "Is there a history of breast cancer in your mother or sisters?"
   d. "Do the size and tenderness of the lumps change with your menstrual cycle?"

6. While teaching the patient with fibrocystic changes in the breast, the nurse explains to the patient that this condition is significant because fibrocystic changes

   a. commonly become malignant over time.
   b. make it more difficult to examine the breasts.
   c. will eventually cause atrophy of breast tissue.
   d. can be controlled with hormone replacement therapy.

7. Match the following descriptions with their related benign breast disorder (answers may be used more than once).

_____	a. Almost always self-limiting and disappears	1. Fibroadenoma
_____	b. Peaks at age 40	2. Mastitis
_____	c. Most common between ages 21 and 25	3. Intraductal papilloma
_____	d. Occurs most often during lactation	4. Ductal ectasia
_____	e. Associated with increased conversion of androgens to estrogen	5. Fat necrosis
_____	f. Associated with breast trauma	6. Prepubescent gynecomastia
_____	g. Multicolored, sticky nipple discharge	7. Senescent gynecomastia
_____	h. Caused by increased estrogen production in those 13 to 17 years old	
_____	i. Common cause is *S. aureus*	
_____	j. Involves ducts in subareolar area	
_____	k. Usually resolves in 6 to 12 months	
_____	l. Wartlike growth in mammary ducts near nipple	
_____	m. Well-delineated, very mobile tumors	

8. The risk for breast cancer is highest in women who

   a. are obese.
   b. are over the age of 60.
   c. have fibrocystic breast changes.
   d. have an inherited aberration of the BRCA1 or 2 gene.

9. The nurse would be most concerned when examination of a patient's breasts revealed

   a. a large, tender, moveable mass in the upper inner quadrant.
   b. an immobile, hard, nontender lesion in the upper outer quadrant.
   c. a 2 to 3 cm, firm, defined, mobile mass in the lower outer quadrant.
   d. a painful, immobile mass with reddened skin in the upper outer quadrant.

10. The best prognosis is indicated in the patient with breast cancer when diagnostic studies reveal

    a. negative axillary lymph nodes.
    b. aneuploid DNA tumor content.
    c. cells with high S-phase fractions.
    d. an estrogen and progesterone receptor–negative tumor.

11. Recurrence or metastasis of breast cancer occurs

    a. most often at sites distant from the breast.
    b. only through the lymphatic chains draining the breast.
    c. most commonly to the bowel and reproductive organs.
    d. in patients who have small tumors with negative axillary lymph nodes.

12. The physician of a patient with a positive biopsy of a 2 cm breast tumor has recommended a lumpectomy with radiation therapy or a modified radical mastectomy as treatment. The patient says she doesn't know how to choose and asks the female nurse what she would do if she had to make the choice. The best response by the nurse is

    a. "It doesn't matter what I would do. It is a decision you have to make for yourself."
    b. "There are advantages and disadvantages of both procedures. What do you know about these procedures?"
    c. "I would choose the modified radical mastectomy because it would ensure the entire tumor was removed."
    d. "The lumpectomy maintains a nearly normal breast but the survival rate is not as good as it is with a mastectomy."

13. A patient undergoing either a mastectomy or a lumpectomy for treatment of breast cancer can usually also expect to undergo

    a. chemotherapy.
    b. radiation therapy.
    c. hormonal therapy.
    d. axillary node dissection.

14. Identify the type of radiation therapy (primary, adjunctive to surgery, high-dose brachytherapy, or palliative) related to the following situations.

    a. Used to treat possible local residual cancer cells postmastectomy

    b. Used to reduce tumor size and stabilize metastatic lesions for pain relief

    c. Alternative to traditional radiation therapy for early stage breast cancer

    d. Follows local excision of tumor

    e. Used to reduce the size of a tumor before other therapy

    f. May be completed in 5 days

15. Systemic chemotherapy is indicated in treatment of patients with breast cancer

    a. only for estrogen receptor–negative tumors.
    b. only when there is evidence of node involvement.
    c. only for postmenopausal patients with nodal involvement.
    d. in premenopausal women even when no nodal involvement is present.

16. A patient with a positive breast biopsy tells the nurse that she has read about tamoxifen (Nolvadex) in magazines and asks about its use. The best response by the nurse includes the information that

    a. tamoxifen is used only to prevent the development of new primary tumors.
    b. tamoxifen is the primary treatment for breast cancer if axillary lymph nodes are positive for cancer.
    c. tamoxifen is the treatment of choice after surgery if the tumor has receptors for estrogen on its cells.
    d. because tamoxifen has been shown to increase the risk for uterine cancer, it is used only when other treatment has not been successful.

17. During the immediate postoperative period following a mastectomy, the nurse initially institutes exercises for the affected arm by

    a. performing full passive ROM exercises to the affected arm.
    b. having the patient brush or comb her hair with the affected arm.
    c. asking the patient to flex and extend the fingers and wrist of the operative side.
    d. having the patient crawl her fingers up the wall, raising her arm above her head.

18. Following a modified radical mastectomy, a patient develops lymphedema of the affected arm. The nurse teaches the patient to

    a. avoid skin softening agents on the arm.
    b. protect the arm from any type of trauma.
    c. abduct and adduct the arm at the shoulder hourly.
    d. keep the arm positioned so that it is in straight and dependent alignment.

19. A patient undergoing surgery and radiation for treatment of breast cancer has a nursing diagnosis of disturbed body image related to absence of the breast. An appropriate nursing intervention for the patient is to

    a. provide the patient with information about surgical breast reconstruction.
    b. restrict visitors and phone calls until the patient feels better about herself.
    c. arrange for a Reach to Recovery visitor or similar resource available in the community.
    d. encourage the patient to obtain a permanent breast prosthesis as soon as she is discharged from the hospital.

20. A 56-year-old patient is undergoing a mammoplasty for breast reconstruction following a mastectomy 1 year ago. During the preoperative preparation of the patient, it is important that the nurse

    a. determine why the patient is choosing reconstruction surgery rather than the use of an external prosthesis.
    b. ensure that the patient has realistic expectations about the outcome and possible complications of the surgery.
    c. inform the patient that implants used for breast reconstruction have been shown to cause immune-related diseases.
    d. let the patient know that although the shape will be different from the other breast the nipple can be reconstructed from other erectile tissue.

21. A patient undergoing a modified radical mastectomy for cancer of the breast is going to use tissue expansion and an implant for breast reconstruction. The nurse knows that

    a. weekly injections of water or saline into the expander will be required.
    b. the expander cannot be placed until healing from the mastectomy is complete.
    c. this method of breast reconstruction uses the patient's own tissue to replace breast tissue.
    d. the nipple from the affected breast will be saved to be grafted onto the reconstructed breast.

CASE STUDY

METASTATIC BREAST CANCER

Patient Profile

Mrs. T., a 57-year-old married lawyer, was found to have a 4 cm by 6 cm firm, fixed mass in the upper, outer quadrant of the right breast during a routine physical examination, and a stereotactic core biopsy indicated a malignant tumor. Although the surgeon recommended a mastectomy because of the size of the tumor, Mrs. T. chose to have a lumpectomy. Now 3 weeks postoperative, she is scheduled for chemotherapy.

Subjective Data

- Never had a routine mammogram
- Never practiced breast self-examination
- States she deserves to have breast cancer for being so careless about her health
- Chose to have a lumpectomy to remove the tumor in spite of the large size because she felt her breasts are critical in her relationship with her husband

Objective Data

- Physical examination
  - Right breast: healed lumpectomy breast incision and right axillary incision
  - Limited ROM of right arm
  - Port of Groshong catheter in place on left upper chest

- Diagnostic studies
  - Pathology: estrogen receptor–positive infiltrating ductal carcinoma; 8 of 12 lymph nodes positive for malignant cells
  - Staging: stage IIIB carcinoma of the right breast

- Clinical course
  - Lumpectomy performed to remove tumor 3 weeks ago
  - Chemotherapy with CAF protocol planned—cyclophosphamide (Cytoxan), doxorubicin (Adriamycin), and 5-fluorouracil (5-FU)

Critical Thinking Questions

1. Why is chemotherapy indicated for Mrs. T.?

2. Compare the three chemotherapeutic agents planned for Mrs. T. with respect to classification type, cell specificity, and common side effects.

3. What can the nurse do to help Mrs. T. reduce or manage the common physical effects of the chemotherapy?

4. What does the finding that Mrs. T.'s tumor is estrogen receptor-positive mean? What additional treatment modalities might this suggest?

5. How could the nurse help Mrs. T. cope with her feelings of guilt and maintain a positive relationship with her husband?

6. What are some possible reasons that Mrs. T. did not perform BSE or have mammography performed?

7. What teaching by the nurse is indicated for Mrs. T. regarding follow-up care related to recurrence of the breast cancer?

8. Based on the assessment data presented, write one or more appropriate nursing diagnoses. Are there any collaborative problems?

CHAPTER 51 NURSING MANAGEMENT: SEXUALLY TRANSMITTED DISEASES

1. The current incidence of sexually transmitted diseases (STDs) is related in part to

   a. increased virulence of organisms causing STDs.
   b. an increase in the recognition of homosexuality.
   c. the use of oral agents and intrauterine devices as contraceptives.
   d. development of resistance of microorganisms to common antibiotics.

2. Match the following microorganisms with the disease they cause.

_____	a. *Treponema pallidum*	1. Gonorrhea
_____	b. *Chlamydia trachomatis*	2. Genital herpes
_____	c. *Neisseria gonorrhoeae*	3. Syphilis
_____	d. Human papillomavirus	4. Nongonococcal urethritis
_____	e. Herpes simplex virus	5. Genital warts

3. A female patient with a purulent vaginal discharge is seen at an outpatient clinic. The nurse would expect a diagnosis of gonorrhea to

   a. be treated with benzathine penicillin G.
   b. indicate the presence of pelvic inflammatory disease.
   c. be confirmed with a Gram's stain smear of the exudate.
   d. be treated with ceftriaxone (Rocephin) and doxycycline (Vibramycin).

4. A 22-year-old woman with multiple sexual partners seeks care after several weeks of experiencing painful and frequent urination and vaginal discharge. Although the results of a culture of cervical secretions are not yet available, the nurse explains to the patient that she will be treated as if she has gonorrhea and chlamydia in order to prevent

   a. obstruction of the fallopian tubes.
   b. endocarditis and aortic aneurysms.
   c. disseminated gonococcal infection.
   d. polyarthritis and generalized adenopathy.

5. Indicate whether the following clinical manifestations of syphilis are characteristic of primary (P), secondary (S), latent (L), or tertiary (T) syphilis.

_____ a. Condyloma lata

_____ b. Aortic valve insufficiency

_____ c. Destructive skin, bone, and soft tissue lesions

_____ d. Chancre

_____ e. Mental deterioration

_____ f. Generalized adenopathy

_____ g. Absence of symptoms with a positive fluorescent treponemal antibody (FTAAbs) test

_____ h. Tabes dorsalis

_____ i. Generalized cutaneous rash

_____ j. Saccular aneurysms

6. A premarital blood test for syphilis reveals that a woman has a positive VDRL test. The nurse advises the patient that

a. a single dose of penicillin will cure the syphilis.
b. she should question her fiancé about prior sexual contacts.
c. additional testing to detect specific antitreponomal antibodies is necessary.
d. a lumbar puncture to evaluate cerebrospinal fluid is necessary to rule out active syphilis.

7. The nurse encourages serologic testing for HIV in the patient with syphilis primarily because

a. syphilis is more difficult to treat in patients with HIV infection.
b. the presence of HIV infection increases the risk of contacting syphilis.
c. CNS involvement is more common in patients with HIV infection and syphilis.
d. the incidence of syphilis is highest in those with high rates of sexual promiscuity and drug abuse.

8. In establishing screening programs for populations at high risk for chlamydial infections, the nurse recognizes that in women, *C. trachomatis* infection most often results in

a. cervicitis.
b. no symptoms.
c. acute urethritis.
d. liver inflammation.

9. A male patient returns to the clinic with a recurrent urethral discharge after being treated for a chlamydial infection 2 weeks ago. Which statement by the patient indicates the most likely cause of the recurrence of his infection?

a. "I took the vibramycin twice a day for a week."
b. "I haven't told my girlfriend about my infection yet."
c. "I had a couple of beers while I was taking the medication."
d. "I've only had sexual intercourse once since my medication was finished."

10. A diagnosis of chlamydial infection is made in a male patient with a purulent urethral discharge when

a. cultures for chlamydial organisms are positive.
b. direct fluorescent antibody (DFA) tests are positive.
c. Gram's stain smears and cultures are negative for gonorrhea.
d. signs and symptoms of epididymitis or proctitis are also present.

11. Identify whether the following statements are true or false. If a statement is false, correct the bold word(s) to make the statement true.

_____ a. Herpes simplex virus type 2 (HSV-2) is capable of causing **only genital lesions**.

_____ b. The primary symptoms of genital herpes include painful **vesicular lesions that rupture and ulcerate.**

_____ c. Treatment with acyclovir can **cure** genital herpes.

_____ d. To prevent transmission of genital herpes, **condoms should be used** when lesions are present.

_____ e. Recurrent symptomatic genital herpes may be precipitated by **sexual activity** and **stress**.

12. During the physical assessment of a female patient with human papillomavirus infection, the nurse would expect to find

a. purulent vaginal discharge.
b. a painless, indurated lesion on the vulva.
c. painful perineal vesicles and ulcerations.
d. multiple, coalescing gray warts in the perineal area.

13. It is most important for the nurse to teach the female patient with genital warts to

a. have an annual Pap smear.
b. apply topical acyclovir faithfully as directed.
c. have her sexual partner treated for the condition.
d. use a contraceptive to prevent pregnancy that may exacerbate the disease.

14. Based on the incidence of sexually transmitted diseases (STDs) in the United States, the nurse informs individuals who have unprotected sexual activity with multiple partners that they are at highest risk for contracting

a. syphilis.
b. gonorrhea.
c. chlamydia.
d. genital warts.

15. Indicate what treatment or precautions should be taken during pregnancy or delivery when the patient has active

a. Syphilis

b. Gonorrhea

c. Genital herpes

d. Chlamydia

e. Genital warts

16. The nurse counsels the sexually active individual that the best prevention of STDs includes

    a. using condoms with a spermicidal jelly.
    b. voiding immediately following intercourse.
    c. substituting oral-anal for vaginal intercourse.
    d. thorough hand washing after contact with genitals.

17. The patient who is most likely to have a nursing diagnosis of risk for noncompliance is the patient with

    a. syphilis.
    b. gonorrhea.
    c. genital herpes.
    d. HPV infection.

CASE STUDY

GONORRHEA

Patient Profile

Jack, a 20-year-old college student, had intercourse with a prostitute while on vacation. He returns home 3 days later and has intercourse with his fiancée, Ann. The next day he begins to experience symptoms of a sexually transmitted disease.

Subjective Data

- Experiences pain and burning on urination
- Has a yellowish-white discharge from his penis
- Expresses concern over the possibility of having gonorrhea and what this diagnosis would mean in his relationship with his fiancée

Objective Data

- Positive Gram's stain for *N. gonorrhoeae*

Critical Thinking Questions

1. Jack asks the nurse's advice on how to tell his fiancée about the diagnosis. What should the nurse's advice be?

2. What symptoms will Ann have if she becomes infected?

3. What physical examinations and laboratory procedures are required to establish a diagnosis of gonorrhea in Jack and Ann?

4. What measures can be used to assist the couple in coping with the psychologic implications of the infection?

5. What treatment will be prescribed for Jack and Ann?

6. What are the possible complications of untreated gonorrhea in men and in women?

7. Based on the assessment data presented, write one or more appropriate nursing diagnoses. Are there any collaborative problems?

CHAPTER 52 NURSING MANAGEMENT: FEMALE REPRODUCTIVE PROBLEMS

1. A couple seeks assistance from an infertility specialist for evaluation of their infertility. The nurse informs the couple that during the initial visit they can expect

   a. physical examinations and review of menstrual history.
   b. assessment of tubal patency with a hysterosalpingogram.
   c. pelvic ultrasound for the woman and semen analysis for the man.
   d. postcoital testing to evaluate sperm numbers and motility in cervical and vaginal secretions.

2. An infertile couple is instructed in at-home ovulation testing using basal body temperature. The nurse explains that this testing

   a. can identify the need for intrauterine insemination as a result of anovulation.
   b. requires that the temperature be taken by the same route every morning on awakening before any activity.
   c. is an easy, nonstressful way to determine when ovulation occurs and when to have intercourse if pregnancy is desired.
   d. indicates when ovulation occurs by revealing a sharp rise in temperature followed by a drop in basal body temperature.

3. In working with couples with infertility, it is important for the nurse to

   a. inform the couple that most infertility can be successfully treated.
   b. warn the couple that treatment may exceed their financial resources.
   c. explain that most infertility results from causative factors in the woman.
   d. encourage the couple to participate in a support group for infertile couples.

4. A patient with a 10-week pregnancy is admitted to the emergency department with vaginal bleeding and abdominal cramping. The nurse recognizes that

   a. the patient will be scheduled for an immediate D&C.
   b. the patient will recover quickly when the bleeding stops.
   c. the patient is most likely experiencing a spontaneous abortion.
   d. treatment of the patient with bed rest is usually successful in preventing further bleeding.

5. Mifepristone (Mifeprex) is prescribed for a perimenopasual woman who has an unexpected and unwanted pregnancy. The nurse informs the patient that this drug

   a. is toxic to trophoblastic tissue and destroys embryonic cells.
   b. causes uterine contractions that expel the products of conception.
   c. is only effective in terminating a pregnancy during the first 4 weeks.
   d. will block the action of progesterone, which is needed to support pregnancy.

6. Premenstrual syndrome (PMS) is most likely to be diagnosed in a woman

   a. who has symptoms only when oral contraceptives are used.
   b. whose symptoms can be controlled with the use of progesterone.
   c. whose symptoms can be correlated with altered serum levels of estrogen and progesterone.
   d. who has the same symptom pattern following ovulation for 2 to 3 consecutive menstrual cycles.

7. When teaching a patient with PMS about management of the disorder, the nurse focuses on the need to

   a. supplement the diet with vitamins C and E.
   b. use estrogen supplements during the luteal phase.
   c. limit dietary intake of caffeine, salt, and refined sugar.
   d. limit exercise and physical activity when symptoms are present.

8. The rationale for the regular use of nonsteroidal antinflammatory drugs (NSAIDs) during the first several days of the menstrual period for women who have primary dysmenorrhea is that these drugs

   a. suppress ovulation and the production of prostaglandins that occur with ovulation.
   b. cause uterine relaxation and small vessel constriction, preventing cramping and abdominal congestion.
   c. inhibit the production of prostaglandins believed to be responsible for menstrual pain and associated symptoms.
   d. block the release of luteinizing hormone, preventing the increase in progesterone associated with maturation of the corpus luteum.

9. Match the following characteristics with their related menstrual irregularities (answers may be used more than once).

	Characteristic	Irregularity
_____	a. Common cause is use of hormonal contraceptives	1. Amenorrhea
		2. Menorrhagia
_____	b. May be caused by strenuous exercise or severe dieting	3. Metrorrhagia
_____	c. Bleeding or spotting between menstrual periods	4. Menometrorragia
_____	d. Associated with endometrial cancer	
_____	e. Increased duration or amount of menstrual bleeding	
_____	f. Excessive bleeding at irregular intervals	
_____	g. Absence of menses	

10. A young woman who runs vigorously as a form of exercise has not had a menstrual period in more than 6 months. The nurse advises her that

    a. normal periods will return when she stops running.
    b. uterine balloon therapy may be necessary to promote uterine sloughing of the overgrown endometrium.
    c. progesterone or birth control pills should be used to prevent persistent overgrowth of the endometrium.
    d. unopposed progestone production causes an overgrowth of the endometrium that increases her risk for endometrial cancer.

11. A patient with abdominal pain and irregular vaginal bleeding is admitted to the hospital with a suspected ectopic pregnancy. The most appropriate nursing intervention for the patient is to

    a. provide analgesics for pain relief.
    b. monitor her vital signs and pain frequently.
    c. explain the need for frequent blood samples for β-hCG monitoring.
    d. offer support for the patient's emotional response to the loss of the pregnancy.

12. Identify whether the following statements are true or false. If a statement is false, correct the bold word(s) to make the statement true.

_____ a. During the **perimenopausal** period a woman experiences cessation of menses.

_____ b. Menopause occurs in response to decreasing levels of **FSH**.

_____ c. Physical responses directly related to decreased estrogen during menopause include **hot flashes** and **atrophic vaginitis**.

_____ d. If estrogen replacement is used by a postmenopausal woman with a uterus, it is important that progesterone be taken to decrease the risk for **endometrial cancer**.

_____ e. Research contributing to evidence-based practice indicates that hormone replacement with estrogen and progesterone increases the risk for **cardiovascular disease**.

13. Identify four beneficial effects and four potential risks related to HRT that should be discussed with a woman during perimenopause.

Benefits	**Risks**
a. ______________________	e. ______________________
b. ______________________	f. ______________________
c. ______________________	g. ______________________
d. ______________________	h. ______________________

14. A menopausal woman decides not to use hormone replacement therapy (HRT). To decrease the serious effect of menopause, the nurse teaches the patient to

a. supplement the diet with vitamin E.
b. maintain a high-protein, low-fat diet.
c. maintain a calcium intake of 800 mg daily.
d. engage in regular aerobic, weight-bearing exercise.

15. A woman with manifestations of menopause does not want to use hormone replacement and asks the nurse about the use of alternative and complementary therapies. The nurse suggests that the phytoestrogen that appears to be the most effective and least toxic is

a. valerian.
b. dong quai.
c. soy products.
d. black cohosh.

16. On admission of a victim of sexual assault to the emergency department, the first priority of the nurse is to

a. contact a rape support person for the patient.
b. assess the patient for urgent medical problems.
c. question the patient about the details of the assault.
d. inform the patient what procedures and treatments will be performed.

17. To prepare a woman who has been raped for physical examination, the nurse first

    a. ensures that a signed informed consent is obtained from the patient.
    b. provides a private place for the patient to talk about what happened to her.
    c. administers prophylaxis for sexually transmitted diseases and tetanus.
    d. instructs the patient not to wash, eat, drink, or urinate before the examination.

18. Match the following characteristics with the related infections (answers may be used more than once).

_____	a. Pruritic, frothy greenish or gray discharge	1. Vulvovaginal candidiasis
_____	b. May be treated with OTC antifungal agents	2. Trichomoniasis
		3. Bacterial vaginosis
_____	c. Thick, white, cottage cheese–like discharge	
		4. Cervicitis
_____	d. Treated with regimens for chlamydia	
_____	e. Fishy-smelling watery discharge	
_____	f. Intense itching and dysuria	
_____	g. Hemorrhagic cervix and vagina	
_____	h. Severe recurrent infections associated with HIV infection	
_____	i. Mucopurulent discharge and postcoital spotting	

19. A patient is diagnosed and treated for a *Gardnerella vaginalis* infection at a clinic. For her treatment to be effective, the nurse tells the patient that

    a. her sexual partner must also be examined and treated.
    b. her sexual partner must use a condom during intercourse.
    c. she should wear minipads to prevent reinfection as long as she has vaginal drainage.
    d. the vaginal cream must be used at bedtime when she lies down to prevent loss from the vagina.

20. A young woman is admitted to the hospital with acute pelvic inflammatory disease (PID). During the nursing history, the nurse notes as a significant risk factor the patient's

    a. lack of any method of birth control.
    b. sexual activity with multiple partners.
    c. use of a vaginal sponge for contraception.
    d. recent antibiotic-induced monilial vaginitis.

21. In implementing care for the patient with acute PID, the nurse

    a. performs vaginal irrigations every 4 hours.
    b. promotes bed rest in a semi-Fowler's position.
    c. instructs the patient to use tampons to control vaginal drainage.
    d. ambulates the patient frequently to promote drainage of exudate.

22. A 20-year-old patient with PID is crying and tells the nurse that she is afraid she will not be able to have children as a result of the infection. The nurse's best response to the patient is

    a. "I would not worry about that right now. Our immediate concern is to cure the infection you have."
    b. "The possibility of infertility following PID is high. Would you like to talk about what it means to you?"
    c. "Sterility following PID is possible, but not common, and it is too soon to know what the effects will be."
    d. "The infection can cause more serious complications such as abscesses and shock that you should be more concerned about."

23. Identify whether the following statements are true or false. If a statement is false, correct the bold word(s) to make the statement true.

    _____ a. The presence of ectopic uterine tissue that bleeds and causes pelvic and abdominal adhesions and cysts is known as **uterine leiomyoma**.

    _____ b. Two gynecologic conditions that subside with the onset of menopause are **endometriosis** and **cervical polyps**.

    _____ c. Polycystic ovary syndrome results when eggs are not released monthly from the ovaries as a result of increased production of **LH** and decreased production of **FSH**.

    _____ d. Treatment of endometriosis and leiomyomas depends on the severity of the symptoms and **the woman's desire to maintain fertility**.

    _____ e. Danazol (Danacrine) and Lupron (gonadotropin-releasing hormone analog) are used to treat endometriosis and leiomyomas to create a **pseudopregnancy**.

    _____ f. The most common symptom of cervical polyps is **menorrhagia**.

    _____ g. An **ovarian cyst** may cause severe pain if twisting of the pedicle occurs.

24. A patient with a stage 0 cervical cancer identified from a Pap smear asks the nurse what this finding means. The nurse's response includes the information that

    a. malignant cells have extended beyond the cervix but not to the pelvic wall.
    b. abnormal cells are present but are confined to the epithelial layer of the cervix.
    c. atypical cells characteristic of inflammation, but not necessarily malignancy, are present.
    d. this is a common finding on Pap testing and she will be examined frequently to see if the abnormal cells spread beyond the cervix.

25. Fertility and normal reproductive function can be maintained when a cancer of the cervix is treated with

    a. external radiation therapy.
    b. internal radiation implants.
    c. conization or laser surgery.
    d. cryotherapy or subtotal hysterectomy.

26. A postmenopausal woman of 10 years calls the clinic because of vaginal bleeding. The nurse schedules a visit for the patient and informs her to expect to have

    a. an abdominal x-ray.
    b. an endometrial biopsy.
    c. a laser treatment to the cervix.
    d. only a routine pelvic examination and Pap smear.

27. A patient has been diagnosed with cancer of the ovary. In planning care for the patient, the nurse recognizes that treatment indicated for the patient depends on

   a. results of a direct-needle biopsy of the ovary.
   b. results of a laparoscopy with multiple biopsies.
   c. whether the patient desires to maintain fertility.
   d. the findings of metastasis by ultrasound or CT scan.

28. Indicate whether the following factors are associated with an increased risk for cervical cancer (C), endometrial cancer (E), ovarian cancer (O), or vaginal cancer (V).

   _____ a. Obesity

   _____ b. BRCA gene mutations

   _____ c. Smoking

   _____ d. Early sexual activity

   _____ e. Intrauterine exposure to estrogen (DES)

   _____ f. Unopposed estrogen-only replacement therapy

   _____ g. Human papillomavirus infection

   _____ h. Early menarche and late menopause

   _____ i. Low socioeconomic status

   _____ j. Family history

29. During assessment of the patient with vulvar cancer, the nurse would expect to find

   a. soreness and itching of the vulva.
   b. labial lesions with purulent exudate.
   c. severe excoriation of the labia and perineum.
   d. painless, firm nodules embedded in the labia.

30. A 44-year-old woman undergoing a total abdominal hysterectomy asks if she will need to take estrogen until she reaches the age of menopause. The best response by the nurse is

   a. "You are close enough to normal menopause that you probably won't need additional estrogen."
   b. "Yes, it will help prevent the more intense symptoms caused by surgically induced menopause."
   c. "Since your ovaries won't be removed, they will continue to secrete estrogen until your normal menopause."
   d. "There are so many risks associated with estrogen replacement therapy that it is best to begin menopause now."

31. While caring for a patient on her second postoperative day following an abdominal panhysterectomy, the nurse would be most concerned if the patient

   a. complains of abdominal distention and gas pains.
   b. complains of pain in her calf when her leg is extended.
   c. says she feels depressed and has periodic crying spells.
   d. has not voided for 4 hours following removal of the indwelling catheter.

32. A nursing diagnosis of disturbed body image is likely to be most appropriate for the patient undergoing a

a. vaginectomy
b. hemivulvectomy.
c. pelvic exenteration.
d. radical hysterectomy.

33. During treatment with an intrauterine radioactive implant, the patient

a. may ambulate in the room as desired.
b. should have all care provided by the same nurse.
c. can have unlimited duration and number of visitors.
d. is restricted to bed rest with turning from side to side.

34. When teaching a patient with problems of pelvic support to perform Kegel exercises, the nurse tells the patient to

a. contract her muscles as if trying to stop the flow of urine.
b. tighten the lower abdominal muscles over the bladder area.
c. squeeze all the perineal muscles as if trying to close the vagina.
d. lie on the floor and do leg lifts to strengthen the abdominal muscles.

35. Match the following uterine structure abnormalities with their descriptions.

_____	a. Uterine prolapse	1. Opening between vagina and bladder
_____	b. Cystocele	2. Protrusion of rectum through vaginal wall
_____	c. Rectocele	3. Protrusion of bladder through vaginal wall
_____	d. Vesicovaginal fistula	4. Opening between rectum and vagina
_____	e. Rectovaginal fistula	5. Displacement of uterus through vagina

36. An appropriate outcome for a patient who undergoes an anterior colporrhaphy is that the patient will

a. maintain normal bowel patterns.
b. adjust to temporary ileal conduit.
c. urinate within 8 hours postoperatively.
d. will experience healing of excoriated vaginal and vulvar tissue.

CASE STUDY

ACUTE PELVIC INFLAMMATORY DISEASE

Patient Profile

Ms. R., a 23-year-old unmarried woman, has a recent history of gonorrhea. For the past 2 weeks she has had a heavy purulent vaginal discharge and general malaise. Concerned that her symptoms appear to be worsening, Ms. R. makes an appointment at the gynecologic clinic.

Subjective Data

- Experiences an increase in lower abdominal pain during vaginal examination
- Expresses concern over worsening of her condition and the effect this will have on future childbearing ability

Objective Data

- Vital signs: T 101° F (38.3° C), HR 90, RR 18, BP 110/58
- Physical examination: heavy, purulent vaginal discharge
- Diagnostic studies: vaginal discharge positive for *N. gonorrhoeae*
- Admitted to the hospital for monitoring, IV fluids, and antibiotic therapy

Critical Thinking Questions

1. What route does the gonococcus take in the development of PID?

2. What are the clinical manifestations of acute PID?

3. How would Ms. R.'s infection be managed if it was decided to treat her as an outpatient? What instructions should she receive?

4. How does chronic PID compare with acute PID?

5. What measures should the nurse take to prevent extension of the infection?

6. How should the nurse respond to Ms. R.'s concern over the effect of this infection on her future childbearing ability?

7. Based on the assessment data presented, write one or more appropriate nursing diagnoses. Are there any collaborative problems?

CHAPTER 53 NURSING MANAGEMENT: MALE REPRODUCTIVE PROBLEMS

1. A patient asks the nurse what the difference between benign prostatic hyperplasia (BPH) and cancer of the prostate is. The best response by the nurse includes the information that BPH is

   a. a benign tumor that does not spread beyond the prostate gland.
   b. a precursor to prostate cancer but does not yet show any malignant changes.
   c. an enlargement of the gland caused by an increase in the size of existing cells.
   d. a benign enlargement of the gland due to an increase in the number of normal cells.

2. When taking a nursing history from a patient with BPH, the nurse would expect the patient to report

   a. nocturia, dysuria, and bladder spasms.
   b. urinary frequency, hematuria, and perineal pain.
   c. urinary hesitancy, postvoid dribbling, and weak urinary stream.
   d. urinary urgency with a forceful urinary stream and cloudy urine.

3. The extent of urinary obstruction caused by BPH can be determined by

   a. a cystometrogram.
   b. transrectal ultrasound.
   c. urodynamic flow studies.
   d. postvoiding catheterization.

4. The effect of finasteride (Proscar) in the treatment of BPH is

   a. reduction in the size of the prostate gland.
   b. relaxation of the smooth muscle of the urethra.
   c. increased bladder tone that promotes bladder emptying.
   d. relaxation of the bladder detrusor musculature promoting urine flow.

5. On admission to the ambulatory surgical center, a patient with BPH informs the nurse that he is going to have a steel tube placed in his urethra to hold it open. The nurse recognizes that the patient will need

   a. monitoring for postoperative urinary retention.
   b. teaching about the effects of general anesthesia.
   c. to be informed of the possibility of short-term incontinence.
   d. instruction about home management of an indwelling catheter.

6. Match the following therapies used for BPH with their characteristics (answers may be used more than once).

_____ a. Involves an external incision
_____ b. Results in delayed sloughing of tissue
_____ c. Most common surgical procedure to treat BPH
____ d. Use of low-wave radiofrequency to precisely destroy prostate tissue
_____ e. Resectoscopic excision and cauterization of prostate tissue
_____ f. Incisions made into prostate around bladder neck
_____ g. Most effective long-term treatment of BPH
_____ h. Use of microwave heat to destroy prostate tissue
_____ i. Can be used on patients taking anticoagulants
_____ j. Indicated for very large prostate gland
_____ k. Temporary solution to obstructive problems
_____ l. Inappropriate for men with rectal problems

1. Transurethral resection prostatectomy (TURP)
2. Transurethral incision of the prostate (TUIP)
3. Simple open prostatectomy
4. Transurethral microwave thermotherapy (TUMT)
5. Laser prostatectomy
6. Transurethral needle ablation (TUNA)

7. A health promotion intervention for detecting BPH in men over 50 is an annual

a. urinalysis.
b. PSA level.
c. cystoscopy.
d. digital rectal examination.

8. Before undergoing prostate surgery, the patient should be informed that

a. some degree of urinary incontinence will occur with all prostatectomies.
b. all prostatectomies except TUIP result in some degree of retrograde ejaculation.
c. erectile dysfunction will result if a vasectomy is performed with the prostatectomy.
d. he will be discharged with an indwelling catheter to maintain urinary output until healing is complete.

9. Following a TURP, a patient has a continuous bladder irrigation. Four hours after surgery, the catheter drainage contains thick, bright red clots and tissue. The nurse should

a. release the traction on the catheter.
b. manually irrigate the catheter until the drainage is clear.
c. clamp the drainage tube and notify the patient's physician.
d. increase the rate of the irrigation and take the patient's vital signs.

10. A patient with continuous bladder irrigation following a prostatectomy tells the nurse he has bladder spasms and leaking of urine around the catheter. The nurse should first

   a. slow the rate of the irrigation.
   b. assess the catheter and drainage tube for clots.
   c. encourage the patient to try to urinate around the catheter.
   d. administer a belladonna and opium suppository as prescribed.

11. The nurse provides discharge teaching to a patient following a TURP and determines that the patient understands the instructions when he says

   a. "I should use daily enemas to avoid straining until healing is complete."
   b. "At least I don't have to worry about developing cancer of the prostate now."
   c. "I should avoid heaving lifting, climbing, and driving until my follow-up visit."
   d. "Every day I should drink 10 to 12 glasses of liquids such as coffee, tea, or soft drinks."

12. Identify three findings in the following areas that are present in the patient with prostatic cancer that differ from findings in BPH.

   a. Prostatic palpation

   b. Blood tests

   c. Extraurinary symptoms

13. A patient with prostate cancer is scheduled for a radical prostatectomy with a perineal approach. The nurse assesses the patient's knowledge about the complications resulting from this surgery, primarily because of the high postoperative incidence of

   a. urinary retention.
   b. incisional infection.
   c. erectile dysfunction.
   d. loss of libido and gynecomastia.

14. Identify whether the following statements are true or false. If a statement is false, correct the bold word(s) to make the statement true.

_____ a. A **radical prostatectomy** is a treatment option for all patients with prostatic cancer except those with stage D tumors.

_____ b. The preferred hormonal therapy for treatment of prostate cancer includes **estrogen** and **androgen-receptor blockers**.

_____ c. Early detection of cancer of the prostate is increased with annual rectal examinations and **serum prostatic acid phosphatase (PAP) measurements**.

_____ d. Because of the variety of treatment options available for cancer of the prostate, it is common for a patient to have a nursing diagnosis of **decisional conflict**.

_____ e. An annual prostate examination is recommended starting at **age 45** for **Hispanic** men because of the increased mortality rate from prostatic cancer in this population.

_____ f. **Chronic bacterial prostatitis** manifests with symptoms of an urinary tract infection with a swollen, very tender prostate gland.

_____ g. Drainage of the prostate through intercourse, masturbation, and prostatic massage is indicated for management of **chronic prostatitis**.

15. Match the following terms with their descriptions.

_____	a. Testicular torsion	1. Painful, prolonged erection
_____	b. Hydrocele	2. Ventral urinary meatus
_____	c. Phimosis	3. Complication of mumps
_____	d. Epispadias	4. Twisted spermatic cord
_____	e. Cryptorchidism	5. Removal of penile foreskin
_____	f. Varicocele	6. Inflammation of the prepuce
_____	g. Epididymitis	7. Sperm-filled cyst of epididymis
_____	h. Priapism	8. Scrotal lymphedema
_____	i. Orchitis	9. Inflammation of the epididymis
_____	j. Hypospadias	10. Dorsal urinary meatus
_____	k. Spermatocele	11. Testicular vein dilation
_____	l. Circumcision	12. Undescended testicle

16. Serum tumor markers that may be elevated on diagnosis of cancer of the testicle and used to monitor the response to therapy include

a. tumor necrosis factor (TNF) and C-reactive protein (CRP).
b. alpha-fetoprotein (AFP) and human chorionic gonadotropin (HCG).
c. prostate-specific antigen (PSA) and prostate acid phosphatase (PAP).
d. carcinoembryonic antigens (CEA) and antinuclear antibodies (ANA).

17. When teaching a patient testicular self-examination, the nurse instructs the patient to report a finding of

a. an irregular-feeling epididymis.
b. one testis that is larger than the other.
c. the spermatic cord within the testicle.
d. a firm, nontender nodule on the testis.

18. The nurse teaches the patient having a vasectomy that following the procedure

a. the amount of ejaculate will be noticeably decreased.
b. he may have difficulty maintaining an erection for several months.
c. an alternative form of contraception must be used for 6 to 8 weeks.
d. the testes will gradually decrease production of sperm and testosterone.

19. A patient seeking medical intervention for erectile dysfunction should be thoroughly evaluated primarily because

a. treatment of erectile dysfunction is based on the cause of the problem.
b. psychologic counseling can reverse the problem in 80-90% of the cases.
c. new invasive and experimental techniques currently used have unknown risks.
d. most treatments for erectile dysfunction are contraindicated in patients with systemic diseases.

20. A functional erection requires desire, adequate blood supply, nerve innervation, and hormone balance. Identify two conditions or factors that may alter these requirements.

   a. Desire

   b. Blood supply

   c. Innervation

   d. Hormones

21. Match the following treatment modalities for erectile dysfunction with their characteristics (answers may be used more than once).

_____ a. Blood drawn into corporeal bodies and held with a ring

_____ b. Indicated for hypogonadism

_____ c. Relaxes smooth muscle in penis

_____ d. Direct application of drugs that increase blood flow in penis

_____ e. Devices implanted into corporeal bodies to firm the penis

_____ f. Should be avoided in those using nitrates

_____ g. Contraindicated in prostate cancer

_____ h. May cause priapism

1. Parenteral testosterone
2. Intracavernosal self-inection of vasoactive drugs
3. Vacuum constriction device (VCD)
4. Penile implants
5. Sildenafil (Viagra)

CASE STUDY

TESTICULAR CANCER

Patient Profile

Following a shower last evening, 19-year-old Jerry was performing his routine testicular self-examination when he discovered a firm lump on his left testis. After a medical examination, he was admitted to the hospital for a left orchiectomy and lymph node resection.

Subjective Data

- Has a history of an undescended left testis, which was surgically corrected at age 4
- Expresses concern about surgery and how it will affect him
- Asks about his prognosis and chances for recovery after the surgery
- Denies back pain

Objective Data

- Very firm, nontender nodule on left testis
- Local lymph node enlargement
- No gynecomastia noted
- Biopsy revealed seminoma germ cell tumor

Critical Thinking Questions

1. Explain the development and risk factors for cancer of the testes.

2. How does cancer of the testis differ from a spermatocele on examination?

3. What is Jerry's prognosis if the malignancy is in early stages?

4. What blood tests for tumor markers should be done preoperatively and are indicated for long-term follow-up care, and why?

5. How can the nurse help Jerry deal with the psychologic components of his illness?

6. What effect will this surgery have on Jerry's sexual functioning?

7. Based on the assessment data presented, write one or more appropriate nursing diagnoses. Are there any collaborative problems?

CHAPTER 54 NURSING ASSESSMENT: NERVOUS SYSTEM

1. Using the list of terms below, identify the structures in the following illustration.

List of Terms

axon
axon hillock
collateral axon
dendrites
gemmule
golgi apparatus
mitochrondrion
myelin sheath
neuron cell body
nissl bodies
node of Ranvier
nucleolus
nucleus
Schwann cell
synaptic knobs
telodendria

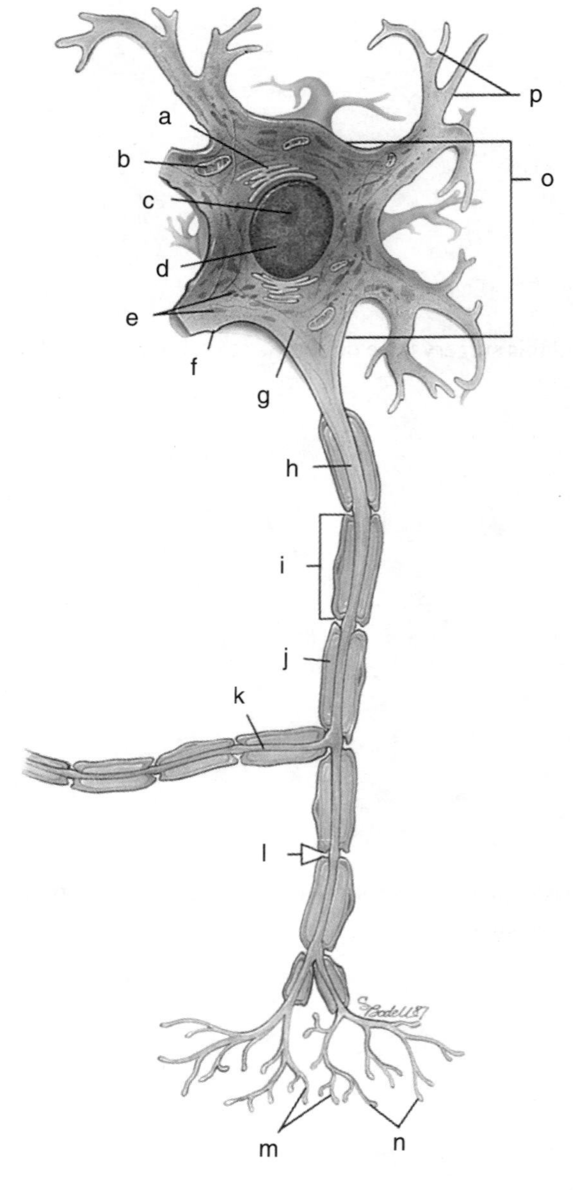

a. ______________________ g. ______________________ m. ______________________

b. ______________________ h. ______________________ n. ______________________

c. ______________________ i. ______________________ o. ______________________

d. ______________________ j. ______________________ p. ______________________

e. ______________________ k. ______________________

f. ______________________ l. ______________________

2. Using the following list of terms, identify the structures in the illustration below.

List of Terms

anterior corticospinal tract	fasciculus gracilis
anterior horn	lateral corticospinal tract
anterior spinocerebellar tract	lateral spinothalamic tract
anterior spinothalamic tract	posterior horn
central canal	posterior spinocerebellar tract
fasciculus cuneatus	posterolateral tract of Lissauer

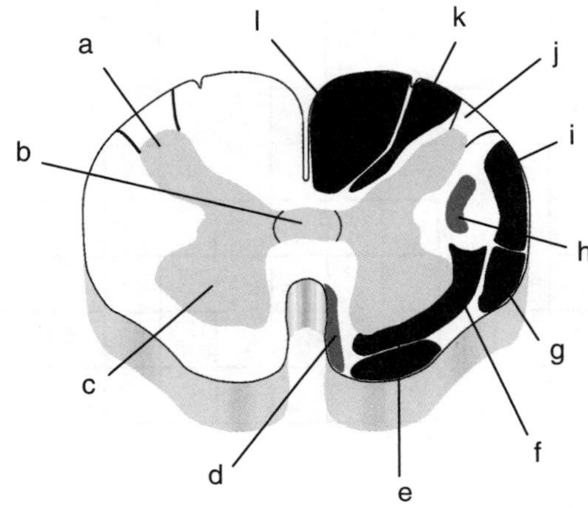

a. ______________________ g. ______________________

b. ______________________ h. ______________________

c. ______________________ i. ______________________

d. ______________________ j. ______________________

e. ______________________ k. ______________________

f. ______________________ l. ______________________

3. Crossword Puzzle

Across

3. Synaptic ______; spaces where neurotransmitters cross from neuron to neuron
6. Junction between two neurons
9. Produces myelin sheath of nerve fibers in CNS
11. Component of white matter
12. Part of the cell body of a neuron
14. Action _____; event that causes depolarization
15. Innermost meningeal mater
16. Site where cranial nerve V arises
17. Assessed in part with orientation and memory
18. Basic unit of the nervous system

Down

1. Gaps in peripheral nerve axons
2. Help form blood-brain barrier
3. Protective fluid of CNS
4. Lower extremity (abb.)
5. Produces myelin sheath of peripheral nerves
7. Carry impulses from nerve cell body
8. May occur with damage to peripheral axons
10. Carry impulses to nerve cell body
13. Area of brain concerned with emotions and aggression
14. Common symptom of disease
15. By mouth
16. Orally

4. Identify whether the following statements are true or false. If a statement is false, correct the bold word(s) to make the statement true.

_____ a. Neuroglial cells that line the ventricles and assist in production of cerebral spinal fluid (CSF) are called **microglia**.

_____ b. During depolarization of a nerve cell **sodium** moves into the cell, creating a **positive** intracellular environment relative to the outside.

_____ c. Breakdown of ATP for the sodium-potassium pump is required to move sodium **into the cell** and potassium **out of the cell** during repolarization.

_____ d. When an action potential reaches the end of an axon and releases an **excitatory** neurotransmitter, the permeability of K^+ and Cl^- at the receptor site is increased.

_____ e. The transmission of an action potential at a synapse depends on the **number** of presynaptic cells releasing neurotransmitters and the **frequency** of the release of neurotransmitters.

5. A patient has a lesion involving the fasciculus gracilis/cuneatus of the spinal cord. The nurse would expect the patient to experience loss of

a. pain and temperature sensations.
b. touch, deep pressure, vibration, and position sense.
c. unconscious information about body position and muscle tension.
d. voluntary muscle control from the cerebral cortex to the peripheral nerves.

6. Lower motor neurons differ from upper motor neurons primarily in that lesions of the lower motor neurons

a. cause hyporeflexia and flaccidity.
b. affect motor control of the lower body.
c. arise in structures above the spinal cord.
d. interfere with reflex arcs in the spinal cord.

7. Match the following functions with the associated area of the brain.

	Function		Area
_____	a. Major relay center for sensory and motor input to cerebrum	1.	Anterior frontal lobe
_____	b. Responsible for arousal	2.	Temporal lobe
_____	c. Controls initiation, execution, and completion of voluntary and automatic movements	3.	Parietal lobe
_____	d. Controls judgment, insight, and reasoning	4.	Occipital lobe
_____	e. Regulates respiratory, vasomotor, and cardiac function	5.	Limbic system
_____	f. Sound and visual interpretation	6.	Broca's area
_____	g. Maintains trunk stability and equilibrium	7.	Basal ganglia
_____	h. Registers visual images	8.	Thalamus
_____	i. Integrates somatic and special sensory inputs	9.	Hypothalamus
_____	j. Related to emotion and sexual response	10.	Reticular activating system
_____	k. Regulates endocrine and autonomic functions	11.	Medulla
_____	l. Responsible for verbal expression	12.	Cerebellum

8. Spinal nerves of the peripheral nervous system differ from cranial nerves in that

   a. only spinal nerves occur in pairs.
   b. cranial nerves affect only the sensory and motor function of the head and neck.
   c. the cell bodies of all cranial nerves are located in the brain while cell bodies of spinal nerves are located in the spinal cord.
   d. all spinal nerves contain both afferent sensory and efferent motor fibers while cranial nerves contain one or the other or both.

9. Indicate whether the following descriptions are characteristic of the sympathetic nervous system (S) or the parasympathetic nervous system (P).

_____ a. Preganglionic cells bodies are located in spinal segments T1-L2

_____ b. Norepinephrine released by most postganglionic fibers

_____ c. Responsible for conservation and restoration of energy stores

_____ d. Cause pupillary constriction and accommodation for near vision

_____ e. Necessary for male ejaculation

_____ f. Acetylcholine released at both preganglionic and postganglionic nerve endings

_____ g. Increase heart rate and dilate coronary arteries

_____ h. Relax sphincters of the GI and GU tract

_____ i. Necessary for male erection

_____ j. Preganglionic cells bodies located in brainstem and sacral spinal segment

_____ k. Responsible for some effects of cranial nerves III and X

10. A patient has an atherosclerotic plaque in the middle cerebral artery. The nurse recognizes that

a. assessment will reveal distended jugular veins.
b. cerebral circulation may be maintained through the circle of Willis.
c. the patient may develop a loss of temporal and parietal lobe function.
d. increased pressure in the middle cerebral artery will back up into the vertebral arteries.

11. Match the supportive and protective structures of the nervous system with their characteristics.

_____ a. Skull

_____ b. Vertebral column

_____ c. Cerebrospinal fluid (CSF)

_____ d. Blood-brain barrier

_____ e. Ventricles

_____ f. Falx cerebri

_____ g. Arachnoid layer

_____ h. Pia mater

_____ i. Tentorium cerebelli

1. Produce and circulate CSF
2. Forms a space with pia mater through which blood vessels and nerves pass
3. Separates cerebrum from the posterior fossa
4. Provides for flexibility while protecting spinal cord
5. Inner layer of meninges
6. Protects brain from external trauma
7. Protects against harmful blood-borne agents
8. Prevents expansion of brain tissue into adjacent hemisphere
9. Cushions the brain and spinal cord and provides nutrients

12. During neurologic assessment of the older adult, the nurse would expect to find

    a. absent deep tendon reflexes.
    b. below-average intelligence score.
    c. decreased sensation of touch and temperature.
    d. decreased frequency of spontaneous awakening.

13. Identify three factors that should be considered when taking the history of a patient with a neurologic problem.

    a.

    b.

    c.

14. During the nursing history of a patient with a neurologic problem, the nurse notes as significant the patient's report of

    a. kidney stones.
    b. a recent cholecystectomy.
    c. the use of aspirin for control of headache.
    d. a fainting episode associated with a severe menopausal hot flash.

15. Identify one specific finding identified by the nurse during assessment of each of the patient's functional health patterns that indicates a risk factor for neurologic problems or a patient response to an actual neurologic problem.

    a. Health perception–health management

    b. Nutritional-metabolic

    c. Elimination

    d. Activity-exercise

    e. Sleep-rest

    f. Cognitive-perceptual

    g. Self-perception–self-concept

    h. Role-relationship

    i. Sexuality-reproductive

    j. Coping–stress tolerance

    k. Value-belief

16. During a neurologic assessment, the nurse obtains most of the data related to mental status

    a. during the nursing history.
    b. by asking the patient specific problem-solving questions.
    c. noting behaviors while the patient is unaware of the nurse's presence.
    d. by asking the patient to complete a written standardized mental examination.

17. Match the following cranial nerves with their methods of evaluation (evaluation methods may be used more than once, and some nerves may be tested with more than one method).

_____	a. Olfactory (I)	1. Resistive shoulder shrug
_____	b. Optic (II)	2. Smile, frown, and close eyes
_____	c. Oculomotor (III)	3. Light touch to face
_____	d. Trochlear (IV)	4. Confrontation
_____	e. Trigeminal (V)	5. Tongue protrusion
_____	f. Abducens (VI)	6. Corneal reflex test
_____	g. Facial (VII)	7. Identify odors
_____	h. Cochlear branch of acoustic (VIII)	8. Pupillary response
_____	i. Glossopharyngeal (IX)	9. Oblique eye movement
_____	j. Vagus (X)	10. Salt and sugar discrimination
_____	k. Spinal accessory (XI)	11. Gag reflex
_____	l. Hypoglossal (XII)	12. Lateral eye movement
		13. Ticking watch

18. During an assessment of the motor system, the nurse finds that the patient has a staggering gait and an abnormal arm swing. The nurse uses this information to

a. protect the patient from injury due to falls.
b. assist the patient to cope with the disability.
c. plan a rehabilitation program for the patient.
d. help establish a diagnosis of cerebellar dysfunction.

19. Match the assessment methods that may elicit the following abnormal findings.

_____	a. Cotton wisp	1. Hypertonia
_____	b. Plantar stimulation	2. Loss of position sense
_____	c. Sharp end of pin	3. Lack of vibratory sense
_____	d. Heel-to-shin test	4. Absence of two-point discrimination
_____	e. Hold arms forward at shoulder with palms up	5. Analgesia
		6. Absence of light touch
_____	f. Passive ROM to limbs	7. Sensory extinction
_____	g. Applying dual stimulus a few mm apart on tips of fingers	8. Extension of the toes
_____	h. Simultaneously stimulating opposite sides of the body	9. Lack of coordination
		10. Pronator drift
_____	i. Have patient stand with feet close together and close eyes	
_____	j. Tuning fork to bony prominences	

20. The normal response to striking the triceps tendon with a reflex hammer is

a. forearm pronation.
b. extension of the arm.
c. flexion of the arm at the elbow.
d. flexion and supination of the elbow.

21. Normal deep tendon reflexes are graded

a. 1/5.
b. 2/5.
c. 3/5.
d. 4/5.

22. To prepare a patient for a lumbar puncture, the nurse

a. sedates the patient with medication before the test.
b. withholds beverages containing caffeine for 8 hours.
c. has the patient sit on the side of the bed, leaning on a padded overbed table.
d. positions the patient in a lateral recumbent position with the hips, knees, and neck flexed.

23. Following a lumbar puncture, the nurse assesses the patient for

a. headache.
b. lower limb paralysis.
c. allergic reactions to the dye.
d. hemorrhage from the puncture site.

24. Nursing care of the patient following a myelogram includes

    a. restricting fluids until the patient is ambulatory.
    b. keeping the patient positioned flat in bed for at least several hours.
    c. positioning the patient with the head of the bed elevated 30 degrees.
    d. providing mild analgesics for pain associated with the insertion of needles.

25. The neurologic diagnostic test that has the highest risk of complications and requires frequent monitoring of neurologic and vital signs following the procedure is

    a. myelogram.
    b. cerebral angiography.
    c. electroencephalogram.
    d. transcranial Doppler sonography.

26. In noting the results of an analysis of cerebrospinal fluid, the nurse identifies as an abnormal finding

    a. a pH of 7.35.
    b. WBCs of 6/μl (0.006/L).
    c. clear, colorless appearance.
    d. glucose of 30 mg/dl (1.7 mmol/L).

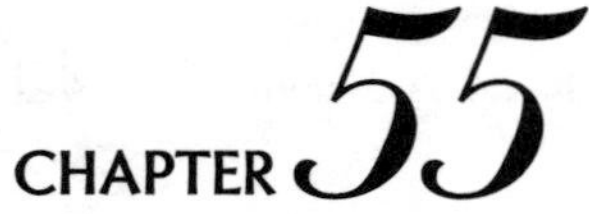

CHAPTER 55 NURSING MANAGEMENT: ACUTE INTRACRANIAL PROBLEMS

1. Identify two ways the following three volume components of intracranial pressure (ICP) can be changed to adapt to small increases in intracranial pressure.

   a. Cerebrospinal fluid (CSF)

   b. Brain tissue

   c. Blood tissue

2. Complete the following statements related to intracranial pressure.

   a. Normal intracranial pressure ranges from ________ to ________ mm Hg.

   b. Autoregulation to maintain constant blood flow to the brain becomes ineffective when the mean arterial pressure (MAP) is below _______ mm Hg and the brain becomes ____________. Autoregulation also becomes ineffective when MAP is greater than ________ mm Hg, because the vessels are maximally ______________.

   c. The cerebral perfusion pressure (CPP) is the blood pressure needed to ensure blood flow to the brain. Normal CPP is _______________ mm Hg. Calculate the cerebral perfusion pressure (CPP) of a patient whose blood pressure is 106/52 and ICP is 14 mm Hg: ____________ mm Hg.

   d. A patient with an ICP of 34 mm Hg and a systemic blood pressure of 108/64 has a CPP of _______________ mm Hg.

   e. Cerebral ischemia and neuronal death occurs when CPP is less than _________ mm Hg. Cellular ischemia and death result when CPP is less than ________ mm Hg.

3. The relationship of intracranial pressure to volume is affected by the brain's elastance and compliance in that

   a. as volume in the brain increases, there is decreased elastance.
   b. a decrease in compliance occurs as volume and pressure increase.
   c. with high elastance, an increase in volume does not increase intracranial pressure.
   d. with high compliance, a small increase in volume results in high changes in pressure.

4. Indicate whether the following factors increase (I) or decrease (D) cerebral blood flow.

_____ a. $PaCO_2$ of 30 mm Hg.

_____ b. PaO_2 of 45 mm Hg.

_____ c. decreased MAP

_____ d. increased ICP

_____ e. arterial blood pH of 7.3

5. Match the common causes of cerebral edema with their related types (answers may be used more than once).

_____ a. SIADH

_____ b. Increased permeability of blood-brain barrier

_____ c. Cerebral hypoxia

_____ d. Ingested toxins

_____ e. Hydrocephalus

1. Vasogenic
2. Cytotoxic
3. Interstitial

6. In the following events that occur in the progression of increased intracranial pressure (ICP), indicate whether the event is directly **caused by** (CB) increased ICP or is a **cause of** (CO) increased ICP (see Fig. 55-3).

_____ a. Tissue edema from initial insult

_____ b. Edema of necrotic tissue

_____ c. Compression of blood vessels

_____ d. Vasodilation

_____ e. Brainstem compression and herniation

7. The earliest signs of increased ICP the nurse should assess for include

a. Cushing triad.
b. unexpected vomiting.
c. decreasing level of consciousness.
d. dilated pupil with sluggish response to light.

8. The nurse recognizes the presence of Cushing triad in the patient with

a. increased pulse, irregular respiration, increased blood pressure.
b. increased pulse, decreased respiration, increased pulse pressure.
c. decreased pulse, irregular respiration, increased pulse pressure.
d. decreased pulse, increased respiration, decreased systolic blood pressure.

9. Increased intracranial pressure in the left cerebral cortex caused by intracranial bleeding causes displacement of brain tissue to the right hemisphere beneath the falx cerebri. The nurse knows that this is referred to as

   a. uncal herniation.
   b. tentorial herniation.
   c. cingulate herniation.
   d. temporal lobe herniation.

10. A patient has ICP monitoring with an intraventricular catheter. A priority nursing intervention for the patient is

   a. aseptic technique to prevent infection.
   b. constant monitoring of ICP waveforms.
   c. removal of CSF to maintain normal ICP.
   d. sampling CSF to determine abnormalities.

11. Identify whether the following statements are true or false. If a statement is false, correct the bold word(s) to make the statement true.

   _____ a. During intracranial pressure monitoring, the patient may be at risk for development of increased ICP when the height of the **P2 wave** is higher than the **P1 wave**.

   _____ b. P waves of ICP are normal and reflect changes in intracranial pressure with the **respiratory** cycle.

   _____ c. **A waves** in ICP waveforms indicate a sharp rise in ICP.

   _____ d. A complication of removal of CSF during intracranial pressure monitoring to control ICP is **ventricular collapse**.

12. Match the following treatments used to manage increased ICP with their effects.

_____	a. Oxygen administration	1. Decreased CSF production with decreased ICP
_____	b. Mild hyperventilation	2. Decreased cerebral metabolism with decreased ICP
_____	c. Osmotic diuretics	3. Prevention of hypoxia
_____	d. Loop diuretics	4. Decreased volume of brain water
_____	e. Dexamethasone (Decadron)	5. Cerbral arterial vasoconstriction
_____	f. Barbiturates	6. Decreased lesion edema

13. Metabolic and nutritional needs of the patient with increased intracranial pressure are best met with

   a. enteral feedings that are low in sodium.
   b. the simple glucose available in D_5W IV solutions.
   c. a fluid restriction that promotes a moderate dehydration.
   d. balanced, essential nutrition in a form that the patient can tolerate.

14. The three criteria for the definition of coma are that the patient is unable to

a.

b.

c.

15. A patient with an intracranial problem does not open his eyes to any stimulus, has no verbal response except muttering when stimulated, and flexes his arm in response to painful stimuli. The nurse records the patient's Glasgow Coma Scale score as

a. 6.
b. 8.
c. 9.
d. 11.

16. When assessing the body functions of a patient with increased intracranial pressure, the nurse should initially assess

a. corneal reflex testing.
b. extremity strength testing.
c. pupillary reaction to light.
d. circulatory and respiratory status.

17. Cranial nerve III originating in the midbrain is assessed by the nurse for an early indication of pressure on the brainstem by

a. assessing for nystagmus.
b. testing the corneal reflex.
c. testing pupillary reaction to light.
d. testing for oculocephalic (doll's eyes) reflex.

18. A patient has a nursing diagnosis of altered cerebral tissue perfusion related to cerebral edema. An appropriate nursing intervention for the patient is

a. avoiding positioning the patient with neck and hip flexion.
b. maintaining hyperventilation to a $PaCO_2$ of 15 to 20 mm Hg.
c. clustering nursing activities to provide periods of uninterrupted rest.
d. routine suctioning to prevent accumulation of respiratory secretions.

19. A patient with increased intracranial pressure is positioned in a lateral position with the head of the bed elevated 30 degrees. The nurse evaluates a need for lowering the head of the bed when the patient experiences

a. ptosis of the eyelid.
b. unexpected vomiting.
c. a decrease in motor functions.
d. decreasing level of consciousness.

20. An unconscious patient with increased intracranial pressure is on ventilatory support. The nurse notifies the physician when ABG results reveal a

a. pH of 7.43.
b. SaO_2 of 94%.
c. PaO_2 of 50 mm Hg.
d. $PaCO_2$ of 30 mm Hg.

21. While caring for a patient with increased intracranial pressure, the nurse monitors intake and output and urine specific gravity. A finding that indicates the presence of a posterior pituitary disturbance that may cause an increase in ICP is

a. increased urinary output and increased urine specific gravity.
b. decreased urinary output and increased urine specific gravity.
c. increased urinary output and decreased urine specific gravity.
d. decreased urinary output and decreased urine specific gravity.

22. While the nurse performs ROM on an unconscious patient with increased intracranial pressure, the patient experiences severe decerebrate posturing reflexes. The nurse should

a. use restraints to protect the patient from injury.
b. administer CNS depressants to lightly sedate the patient.
c. perform the exercises less frequently because posturing can increase ICP.
d. continue the exercises because they are necessary to maintain musculoskeletal function.

23. Match the following types of head injury with their descriptions.

_____ a. Linear skull fracture
_____ b. Depressed skull fracture
_____ c. Compound skull fracture
_____ d. Comminuted skull fracture
_____ e. Basilar skull fracture
_____ f. Posterior fossa fracture
_____ g. Frontal lobe skull fracture
_____ h. Orbital skull fracture
_____ i. Parietal skull fracture
_____ j. Temporal skull fracture
_____ k. Cerebral concussion
_____ l. Cerebral contusion

1. Depressed skull fracture and scalp lacerations with communication to intracranial cavity
2. Temporary, minor injury with transient reduction in neural activity and LOC
3. Possible pneumocranium, CSF rhinorrhea
4. Fractured skull without alteration in fragments
5. Bruising of brain, often associated with coup-contrecoup injury
6. May involve dural tear with CSF otorrhea, vertigo, and Battles' sign
7. Multiple linear fracture with fragmentation of bone
8. Causes periorbital ecchymosis
9. Inward indentation of skull with possible pressure on brain
10. Cortical blindness or visual field defects
11. Boggy temporal muscle because of extravasation of blood
12. May cause deafness, loss of taste, CSF otorrhea

24. A patient with a head injury has bloody drainage from the ear. To determine if CSF is present, in the drainage the nurse

    a. examines the tympanic membrane for a tear.
    b. tests the fluid with a glucose-identifying strip or stick.
    c. tests the fluid for a halo sign on a white 4 × 4 dressing.
    d. collects 5 ml of fluid in a test tube and sends it to the lab for analysis.

25. The nurse suspects the presence of an arterial epidural hematoma in the patient who experiences

    a. failure to regain consciousness following a head injury.
    b. a rapid deterioration of neurologic function within 24 to 48 hours following a head injury.
    c. nonspecific, nonlocalizing progression of alteration in LOC occurring over weeks or months.
    d. unconsciousness at the time of a head injury with a brief period of consciousness followed by a decrease in LOC.

26. Skull x-rays and a CT scan provide evidence of a depressed parietal fracture with a subdural hematoma in a patient admitted to the emergency department following an automobile accident. In planning care for the patient, the nurse anticipates that

    a. the patient will receive life-support measures until the condition stabilizes.
    b. immediate burr holes will be made to rapidly decompress the intracranial cavity.
    c. the patient will be treated conservatively with close monitoring for changes in neurologic status.
    d. the patient will be taken to surgery for a craniotomy for evacuation of blood and decompression of the cranium.

27. When a patient is admitted to the emergency department following a head injury, the nurse's first priority in management of the patient is

    a. maintaining cervical spine precautions.
    b. determining the presence of increased ICP.
    c. monitoring for changes in neurologic status.
    d. establishing IV access with a large-bore catheter.

28. A 54-year-old man is recovering from a skull fracture with a subacute subdural hematoma. He has return of motor control and orientation but appears apathetic and has reduced awareness of his environment. When planning discharge of the patient, the nurse explains to the patient and the family that

    a. continuous improvement in the patient's condition should occur until he has returned to pretrauma status.
    b. the patient's complete recovery may take years, and the family should plan for his long-term dependent care.
    c. the patient is likely to have long-term emotional and mental changes that may require continued professional help.
    d. role changes in family members will be necessary because the patient will be dependent on his family for care and support.

29. Identify whether the following statements are true or false. If a statement is false, correct the bold word(s) to make the statement true.

_____ a. Without treatment **only malignant** brain tumors will cause death as a result of increased growth leading to increased ICP and compression of vital brain centers.

_____ b. Symptoms of visual disturbances and seizures may indicate a tumor of the **temporal** lobe.

_____ c. The most common malignant brain tumor is **an astrocytoma**.

_____ d. Tumors that are considered inoperable are those located in the **upper brainstem** or **deep in the dominant hemisphere**.

_____ e. Radiation therapy for brain tumors may cause serious **increases in ICP**.

30. Assisting the family to understand what is happening to the patient is an especially important role of the nurse when the patient has a tumor of the

a. ventricles.
b. frontal lobe.
c. parietal lobe.
d. occipital lobe.

31. Match the following types of cranial surgery with their descriptions.

_____	a. Burr holes	1. Excision of cranial bone without replacement
_____	b. Craniotomy	2. Three-dimensional targeting of cranial tissue
_____	c. Craniectomy	3. Placement of tubes to redirect CSF from one area to another
_____	d. Cranioplasty	4. Opening into cranium with a drill to remove blood and fluid
_____	e. Sterotactic surgery	5. Replacement of part of the cranium with an artificial plate
_____	f. Shunt procedures	6. Opening into cranium with removal of bone flap to open dura

32. For the patient undergoing a craniotomy, the nurse provides information about the use of wigs and hairpieces or other methods to disguise hair loss

a. during preoperative teaching.
b. if the patient asks about their use.
c. in the immediate postoperative period.
d. when the patient expresses negative feelings about his or her appearance.

33. It is most important that the nurse position the patient who has had a craniectomy with an anterior fossae incision

a. on the unoperative side.
b. flat with the head slightly hyperextended.
c. with the head of the bed elevated 15 degrees.
d. on either side with the head elevated 30 degrees.

34. Successful achievement of patient outcomes for the patient with cranial surgery would best be indicated by

a. ability to return home in 6 days.
b. ability to meet all self-care needs.
c. acceptance of residual neurologic deficits.
d. absence of signs and symptoms of increased intracranial pressure.

35. Indicate whether the following descriptions are characteristic of meningitis (M) or encephalitis (E).

_____ a. Most frequently caused by bacteria

_____ b. Is an inflammation of the brain

_____ c. May be transmitted by insect vectors

_____ d. CSF production is increased

_____ e. Almost always has a viral cause

_____ f. Involves an inflammation of pia mater and arachnoid layer

_____ g. Has a rapid onset of symptoms

_____ h. Cerebral edema is a major problem

_____ i. Exudate may impair normal CSF flow and absorption

36. A patient is admitted to the hospital with possible bacterial meningitis. During the initial assessment, the nurse questions the patient about a recent history of

a. mosquito or tick bites.
b. chickenpox or measles.
c. cold sores or fever blisters.
d. an upper respiratory infection.

37. Classic symptoms of bacterial meningitis include

a. papilledema and psychomotor seizures.
b. high fever, nuchal rigidity, and severe headache.
c. behavioral changes with memory loss and lethargy.
d. positive Kernig's and Brudzinski's signs and hemiparesis.

38. Management of the patient with meningitis includes

a. administering antibiotics immediately following collection of specimens for culture.
b. waiting for results of a CSF culture to identify an organism before initiating treatment.
c. providing symptomatic and supportive treatment because drug therapy is not effective in treatment.
d. performing skull x-rays and CT scans to determine the extend of the disease before treatment is started.

39. Vigorous control of fever in the patient with meningitis is required to prevent complications. Identify four undesirable effects of fever in the patient with meningitis.

    a.

    b.

    c.

    d.

40. On physical examination of a patient with headache and fever, the nurse would suspect a brain abscess when the patient has

    a. seizures.
    b. nuchal rigidity.
    c. focal symptoms.
    d. signs of increased ICP.

CASE STUDY

NEUROLOGIC COMPLICATIONS

Patient Profile

Steven K., a 16-year-old unrestrained driver, suffered a compound fracture of the skull and facial fractures in a motor vehicle accident. On admission to the hospital he was immediately taken to surgery for evacuation of a right subdural hematoma in the temporal region and repair of facial fractures. On the fourth postoperative day, the nurse discovers the following findings during assessment of Steven.

Subjective Data

- Increasingly difficult to arouse

Objective Data

- Glasgow Coma Scale decreased from 10 to 5
- Signs of nuchal rigidity
- Temperature 102.2° F (39° C), BP 110/60, HR 114
- ICP ranges between 20 and 30 mm Hg despite CSF drainage and mannitol

Critical Thinking Questions

1. What is the probable cause of Steven's change in neurologic status?

2. What were the contributing factors that put Steven at risk for complications after a head injury and surgery?

3. Discuss the pathophysiologic basis for the symptoms exhibited by Steven.

4. On the basis of the nursing assessment, what are the priority interventions?

5. Discuss the possible areas for organisms to gain access to the meninges in the case of Steven.

6. Based on the assessment data presented, write one or more appropriate nursing diagnoses. Are there any collaborative problems?

CHAPTER 56 NURSING MANAGEMENT: STROKE

1. In promoting health maintenance for prevention of strokes, the nurse understands that the highest risk for the most common type of stroke is present in

   a. African-Americans.
   b. women who smoke.
   c. individuals with hypertension and diabetes.
   d. those who are obese with high dietary fat intake.

2. A thrombus that develops in a cerebral artery does not always cause a loss of neurologic function because

   a. the body can dissolve atherosclerotic plaques as they form.
   b. some tissues of the brain do not require constant blood supply to prevent damage.
   c. circulation through the circle of Willis may provide blood supply to the affected area of the brain.
   d. neurologic deficits occur only when major arteries are occluded by thrombus formation around an atherosclerotic plaque.

3. A patient comes to the emergency department immediately after experiencing numbness of the face and an inability to speak, but while the patient awaits examination, the symptoms disappear and the patient requests discharge. The nurse stresses that it is important for the patient to be evaluated, primarily because

   a. the patient has probably experienced an asymptomatic lacunar stroke.
   b. the symptoms are likely to return and progress to worsening neurologic deficit in the next 24 hours.
   c. neurologic deficits that are transient occur most often as a result of small hemorrhages that clot off.
   d. the patient has probably experienced a transient ischemic attack (TIA) that is a sign of progressive cerebral vascular disease.

4. Match the characteristics with their related type of stoke (answers may be used more than once).

	Characteristic	Type
_____	a. Onset unrelated to activity	1. Thrombotic
_____	b. Rupture of atherosclerotic vessels	2. Embolic
_____	c. Carries the poorest prognosis	3. Intracerebral hemorrhage
_____	d. Type most often signaled by TIAs	4. Subarachnoid hemorrhage
_____	e. Most common of sudden death	
_____	f. Creates mass that compresses brain	
_____	g. Symptoms of meningeal irritation	
_____	h. Commonly occur during or after sleep	
_____	i. Quick onset and resolution	
_____	j. Caused by rupture of intracranial aneurysm	
_____	k. Strong association with hypertension	
_____	l. Associated with sudden, severe headache	
_____	m. Associated with endocardial disorders	

5. A patient with right-sided paresthesias and hemiparesis is hospitalized and diagnosed with a thrombotic stroke. Over the next 72 hours the nurse plans care with the knowledge that the patient

   a. is ready for aggressive rehabilitation.
   b. will show gradual improvement of the initial neurologic deficits.
   c. may show signs of deteriorating neurologic function as cerebral edema increases.
   d. should not be turned or exercised to prevent extension of the thrombus and increased neurologic deficits.

6. The neurologic functions that are affected by a stroke are primarily related to

   a. the amount of tissue area involved.
   b. the rapidity of the onset of symptoms.
   c. the brain area perfused by the affected artery.
   d. the presence or absence of collateral circulation.

7. Indicate whether the following manifestations of a stroke are more likely to occur with right brain damage (R) or left brain damage (L).

   _____ a. Aphasia

   _____ b. Left homonymous hemianopia

   _____ c. Agnosia

   _____ d. Quick and impulsive behavior

   _____ e. Inability to remember words

   _____ f. Neglect of the left side of the body

8. Identify whether the following statements are true or false. If a statement is false, correct the bold word(s) to make the statement true.

   _____ a. **Receptive** aphasia is characterized by a lack of comprehension of both verbal and written language.

   _____ b. **Dysarthria** results from a disturbance in Broca's area and is an impairment in speaking and writing.

   _____ c. A lesion that affects both Wernicke's area and Broca's area is most likely to cause **global** aphasia.

   _____ d. A **nonfluent dysphagia** is characterized by the presence of speech that contains little meaningful communication.

   _____ e. The long-term effect of paralysis of an extremity resulting from a stroke is **flaccidity**.

9. A patient is admitted to the hospital with a left hemiplegia. To determine the size, location, and whether a stroke is ischemic or hemorrhagic the nurse anticipates that the physician will request a

   a. CT scan.
   b. lumbar puncture.
   c. cerebral arteriogram.
   d. positron emission tomography (PET).

10. A carotid endarterectomy is being considered as treatment for a patient who has had several TIAs. The nurse explains to the patient that this surgery

    a. is used to restore blood circulation to the brain following an obstruction of a cerebral artery.
    b. involves intracranial surgery to join a superficial extracranial artery to an intracranial artery.
    c. involves removing an atherosclerotic plaque in the carotid artery to prevent an impending stroke.
    d. is used to open a stenosis in a carotid artery with a balloon and stent to restore cerebral circulation.

11. The incidence of ischemic stroke in patients with TIAs and other risk factors is reduced with the administration of

    a. furosemide (Lasix).
    b. lovastatin (Mevacor).
    c. daily low-dose aspirin.
    d. nimodipine (Nimotop).

12. An essential intervention in the emergency management of the patient with a stroke is

    a. intravenous fluid replacement.
    b. administration of osmotic diuretics to reduce cerebral edema.
    c. initiation of hypothermia to decrease the oxygen needs of the brain.
    d. maintenance of respiratory function with a patent airway and oxygen administration.

13. A diagnosis of a ruptured cerebral aneurysm has been made in a patient with manifestations of a stroke. The nurse anticipates that treatment options that would be evaluated for the patient include

    a. hyperventilation therapy.
    b. surgical clipping of the aneurysm.
    c. administration of hyperosmotic agents.
    d. administration of thrombolytic therapy.

14. During the acute phase of a stroke, the nurse assesses the patient's vital signs and neurologic status q4h. A cardiovascular sign that the nurse would see as the body attempts to increase cerebral blood flow is

    a. hypertension.
    b. fluid overload.
    c. cardiac arrythmias.
    d. S_3 and S_4 heart sounds.

15. Identify four nursing diagnoses in which impaired neuromotor function can be an etiologic factor.

    a.

    b.

    c.

    d.

16. A nursing intervention that is indicated for the patient with hemiplegia is

    a. the use of a footboard to prevent plantar flexion.
    b. immobilization of the affected arm against the chest with a sling.
    c. positioning the patient in bed with each joint lower than the joint proximal to it.
    d. having the patient perform passive ROM of the affected limb with the unaffected limb.

17. A newly admitted patient who has suffered a right brain stroke has a nursing diagnosis of disturbed visual sensory perception related to homonymous hemianopsia. Early in the care of the patient, the nurse should

    a. place objects on the right side within the patient's field of vision.
    b. approach the patient from the left side to encourage the patient to turn the head.
    c. place objects on the patient's left side to assess the patient's ability to compensate.
    d. patch the affected eye to encourage the patient to turn the head to scan the environment.

18. Four days following a stroke, a patient is to start oral fluids and feedings. Before feeding the patient, the nurse should first

    a. check the patient's gag reflex.
    b. order a soft diet for the patient.
    c. raise the head of the bed to a sitting position.
    d. evaluate the patient's ability to swallow small sips of ice water.

19. An appropriate food for a patient with a stroke who has mild dysphagia is

    a. fruit juices.
    b. pureed meat.
    c. scrambled eggs.
    d. fortified milkshakes.

20. A patient who has suffered a stroke is experiencing urinary incontinence. Nursing management of the patient includes

    a. limiting fluid intake to 1000 ml/day.
    b. ambulating the patient to the bathroom q4hr.
    c. determining the pattern and cause of the incontinence.
    d. using incontinence briefs to reduce the effects of incontinence.

21. To promote communication during rehabilitation of the patient with aphasia, an appropriate nursing intervention is to

    a. use gestures, pictures, and music to stimulate patient responses.
    b. talk about activities of daily living that are familiar to the patient.
    c. structure statements so that the patient does not have to respond verbally.
    d. use flash cards with simple words and pictures to promote language recall.

22. A patient with a right hemisphere stroke has a nursing diagnosis of unilateral neglect related to sensory-perceptual deficits. During the patient's rehabilitation, it is important for the nurse to

    a. avoid positioning the patient on the affected side.
    b. place all objects for care on the patient's unaffected side.
    c. teach the patient to consciously care for the affected side.
    d. protect the affected side from injury with pillows and supports.

23. A patient with a stroke has a right-sided hemiplegia. The nurse prepares family members to help control behavior changes seen with this type of stroke by teaching them to

    a. ignore undesirable behaviors manifested by the patient.
    b. provide directions to the patient verbally in small steps.
    c. distract the patient from inappropriate emotional responses.
    d. supervise all activities before allowing the patient to pursue them independently.

24. The nurse can assist the patient and the family in coping with the long-term effects of a stroke by

    a. informing family members that the patient will need assistance with almost all ADLs.
    b. explaining that the patient's prestroke behavior will return as improvement progresses.
    c. encouraging the patient and family members to seek assistance from family therapy or stroke support groups.
    d. helping the patient and family understand the significance of residual stroke damage to promote problem solving and planning.

CASE STUDY

STROKE

Patient Profile

Mrs. C., a 38-year-old married woman, was admitted unconscious to the hospital after her family could not rouse her in the morning. She was accompanied by her husband and three daughters, ages 10, 13, and 15.

Subjective Data

- Has no history of hypertension or other health problems
- Had complained of a headache the day before she developed unconsciousness

Objective Data

- Diagnostic tests reveal a subarachnoid hemorrhage
- Vital signs: BP 150/82; RR 16; HR 56, T 101° F (38.3° C)
- Glasgow Coma Scale score: 5

Critical Thinking Questions

1. What diagnostic tests would be indicated to determine the cause of Mrs. C.'s unconsciousness?

2. What signs of increased intracranial pressure are present in Mrs. C.?

3. What should the family be told to expect in terms of Mrs. C.'s condition?

4. What nursing interventions have the highest priority for Mrs. C. at this stage of her illness?

5. What treatment modalities indicated for thrombotic strokes are contraindicated for Mrs. C.?

6. What therapeutic options are available for the patient with a hemorrhagic stroke resulting from a ruptured aneurysm?

7. Based on the assessment data presented, write one or more appropriate nursing diagnoses. Are there any collaborative problems?

CHAPTER 57 NURSING MANAGEMENT: CHRONIC NEUROLOGIC PROBLEMS

1. Match the following characteristics with their related type of headache (answers may be used more than once).

_____ a. Activation of trigeminal nerve causes facial vasomotor symptoms and pain

_____ b. Chronic, dull, persisting intermittently over months or years

_____ c. Strong family history

_____ d. Bilateral pressure or tightness sensation

_____ e. Commonly recur several times a day for several weeks

_____ f. May occur with or between migraine headaches

_____ g. Severe, steady, penetrating head pain

_____ h. Causes agitation, restlessness

_____ i. May be accompanied by systemic edema, nausea, and vomiting

_____ j. Abrupt onset lasting 30 to 90 minutes

_____ k. Unilateral or bilateral throbbing pain

_____ l. Prodrome phase followed by headache phase

1. Tension-type
2. Migraine
3. Cluster

2. The most important method of diagnosing functional headaches is

a. EMG.
b. CT scan.
c. cerebral blood flow studies.
d. a thorough history of the headache.

3. Drug therapy for acute migraine and cluster headaches that appears to alter the pathophysiologic process includes

a. serotonin antagonists such as methysergide (Sansert).
b. tricyclic antidepressants such as amitriptyline (Elavil).
c. beta-adrenergic blockers such as propranolol (Inderal).
d. vasoconstrictors such as ergotamine (Ergomar) and sumatriptan (Imitrex).

4. A nursing intervention that is appropriate for the patient with a nursing diagnosis of anxiety related to lack of knowledge of etiology and treatment of headache is to

a. help the patient examine lifestyle patterns and precipitating factors.
b. administer medications as ordered to relieve pain and promote relaxation.
c. provide a quiet, dimly lit environment to reduce stimuli that increase muscle tension and anxiety.
d. support the patient's use of counseling or psychotherapy to enhance conflict resolution and stress reduction.

5. During the nursing assessment of a patient with a headache, the nurse recognizes that the headache may be organic when the headache is associated with

   a. projectile vomiting.
   b. visual disturbances.
   c. weakness and paralysis.
   d. paresthesias and confusion.

6. Generalized seizures differ from partial seizures in that

   a. partial seizures are confined to one side of the brain and remain focal in nature.
   b. generalized seizures result in loss of consciousness while partial seizures do not.
   c. generalized seizures result in temporary residual deficits during the postictal phase.
   d. generalized seizures have no warning or aura because the entire brain is affected at the onset.

7. Match the following characteristics with their related types of seizures (answers may be used more than once).

	Characteristic	Type of seizure
_____	a. Also known as petit mal seizure	1. Generalized tonic-clonic
_____	b. Sudden, excessive jerk of body that may hurl the person to the ground	2. Typical absence
_____	c. Often involve behavioral, emotional, and cognitive functions with altered consciousness	3. Atypical absence
_____	d. Often accompanied by incontinence, tongue or cheek biting	4. Myoclonic
_____	e. Brief staring spell accompanied by peculiar behavior during seizure or postictal confusion	5. Atonic
_____	f. Focal motor, sensory, or autonomic symptoms without loss of consciousness	6. Simple partial
_____	g. Also known as grand mal seizure	7. Complex partial
_____	h. Falling spell from loss of muscle tone accompanied by brief unconsciousness	
_____	i. Staring spell lasting a few seconds	
_____	j. Psychomotor seizures with repetitive behaviors and lip smacking	
_____	k. Alterations in memory, sexual sensations, and distortions of visual or auditory sensations	
_____	l. Loss of consciousness, stiffening of the body with subsequent jerking of extremities	
_____	m. Known as temporal lobe seizures	
_____	n. Very brief and may occur in clusters	

8. Identify whether the following statements are true or false. If a statement is false, correct the bold word(s) to make the statement true.

_____ a. **Status epilepticus** is the effect that occurs when frequent seizures produce permanent changes in neuron excitability, increasing the likelihood of more seizures.

_____ b. Status epilepticus is most serious in **tonic-clonic seizures** because it can cause ventilatory insufficiency and hypoxemia.

_____ c. Permanent brain damage may occur from status epilepticus of **any type of** seizures.

_____ d. The most useful tool for diagnosing epilepsy is **the EEG**.

_____ e. Immediate medical care should be sought for **all** seizures.

_____ f. A tonic-clonic seizure with loss of consciousness that is preceded by an aura is a **partial** seizure that generalizes.

9. A patient admitted to the hospital following a generalized tonic-clonic seizure asks the nurse what caused the seizure. The best response by the nurse is

a. "So many factors can cause epilepsy that it is impossible to say what caused your seizure."
b. "Epilepsy is an inherited disorder. Does anyone else in your family have a seizure disorder?"
c. "In seizures, some type of trigger causes sudden, abnormal bursts of electrical brain activity."
d. "Scar tissue in the brain alters the chemical balance, creating uncontrolled electrical discharges."

10. A patient with a seizure disorder is being evaluated for surgical treatment of the seizures. The nurse recognizes that one of the requirements for surgical treatment is

a. identification of scar tissue that is able to be removed.
b. an adequate trial of drug therapy that had unsatisfactory results.
c. development of toxic syndromes from long-term use of antiseizure drugs.
d. the presence of symptoms of cerebral degeneration from repeated seizures.

11. The nurse teaches the patient taking antiseizure drugs that the method most commonly used to measure compliance and to monitor for toxicity is

a. monthly EEGs.
b. a daily seizure log.
c. urine testing for drug levels.
d. blood testing for drug levels.

12. When teaching a patient with a seizure disorder about the medication regimen, it is most important for the nurse to stress that

a. the patient should increase the dosage of the medication if stress is increased.
b. if gingival hypertrophy occurs the drug should be stopped and the physician notified.
c. stopping the medication abruptly may increase the intensity and frequency of seizures.
d. most over-the-counter and prescription drugs are safe to take with anticonvulsant drugs.

13. The nurse finds a patient in bed having a generalized tonic-clonic seizure. During the seizure activity, the nurse should

a. turn the patient to the side.
b. suction the patient and administer oxygen.
c. insert an oral airway into the patient's mouth.
d. restrain the patient's extremities to prevent soft tissue and bone injury.

14. Following a generalized tonic-clonic seizure, the patient is tired and sleepy. The nurse should

    a. suction the patient before allowing him to rest.
    b. allow the patient to sleep as long as he feels sleepy.
    c. stimulate the patient to increase his level of consciousness.
    d. check the patient's level of consciousness every 15 minutes for an hour.

15. During the diagnosis and long-term management of a seizure disorder, the nurse recognizes that one of the major needs of the patient is assistance to

    a. manage the complicated drug regimen of seizure control.
    b. cope with the effects of negative social attitudes toward epilepsy.
    c. adjust to the very restricted lifestyle required by a diagnosis of epilepsy.
    d. learn to minimize the effect of the condition in order to obtain employment.

16. Match the chronic neurologic disorders with their pathophysiologic descriptions.

	Disorder		Description
_____	a. Multiple sclerosis	1.	Degeneration of motor neurons in brainstem and spinal cord
_____	b. Parkinson's disease	2.	Deficiency of acetylcholine and GABA in basal ganglia and extrapyramidal system
_____	c. Myasthenia gravis	3.	Immune-mediated inflammatory destruction of myelin and replacement with glial scar tissue
_____	d. Huntington's disease	4.	Autoimmune antibody destruction of cholinergic receptors at the neuromuscular junction
_____	e. Amyotropic lateral sclerosis	5.	Degeneration of dopamine-producing neurons in substantia nigra of midbrain and basal ganglia

17. A 38-year-old woman has newly diagnosed multiple sclerosis (MS) and asks the nurse what is going to happen to her. The best response by the nurse is

    a. "You need to plan for a continuous loss of movement, sensory functions, and mental capabilities."
    b. "Most people with MS have periods of attacks and remissions, with progressively more nerve damage over time."
    c. "You will most likely have a steady course of chronic progressive nerve damage that will change your personality."
    d. "It is common for people with MS to have an acute attack of weakness and then not have any other symptoms for years."

18. During assessment of a patient admitted to the hospital with an acute exacerbation of MS, the nurse would expect to find

    a. tremors, dysphasia, and ptosis.
    b. bowel and bladder incontinence and loss of memory.
    c. motor impairment, visual disturbances, and paresthesias.
    d. excessive involuntary movements, hearing loss, and ataxia.

19. The nurse explains to a patient newly diagnosed with MS that the diagnosis is made primarily by

    a. MRI findings.
    b. T cell analysis of the blood.
    c. analysis of cerebrospinal fluid.
    d. history and clinical manifestations.

20. Mitoxantone (Novantrone) is being considered as treatment for a patient with progressive-relapsing MS. The nurse explains that a disadvantage of this drug compared with other drugs used for multiple sclerosis is that it

    a. must be given subcutaneously every day.
    b. has a lifetime dose limit due to cardiac toxicity.
    c. is an anticholinergic agent that causes urinary incontinence.
    d. is an immunosuppressant agent that increases the risk for infection.

21. A patient with MS has a nursing diagnosis of self-care deficit related to muscle spasticity and neuromuscular deficits. In providing care for the patient, it is most important for the nurse to

    a. teach the family members how to adequately care for the patient's needs.
    b. encourage the patient to maintain social interactions to prevent social isolation.
    c. promote the use of assistive devices so the patient can participate in self-care activities.
    d. perform all activities of daily living for the patient in order to conserve the patient's energy.

22. A patient with newly diagnosed MS has been hospitalized for evaluation and initial treatment of the disease. Following discharge teaching, the nurse evaluates that additional instruction is needed when the patient says

    a. "It is important for me to avoid exposure to those with upper respiratory infections."
    b. "When I begin to feel better, I should stop taking the prednisone to prevent side effects."
    c. "I plan to use vitamin supplements and a high-protein diet to help manage my condition."
    d. "I must plan with my family how we are going to manage my care if I become more incapacitated."

23. List the classic triad of signs associated with Parkinson's disease and identify one consequence in patient function for each of the signs.

    a.

    b.

    c.

24. A patient with a tremor is evaluated for Parkinson's disease. The nurse explains to the patient that Parkinson's disease can be confirmed by

    a. CT and MRI scans.
    b. relief of symptoms with administration of dopaminergic agents.
    c. the presence of tremors that increase during voluntary movement.
    d. a cerebral angiogram that reveals the presence of cerebral atherosclerosis.

25. An observation of the patient made by the nurse that is most indicative of Parkinson's disease is

    a. large and embellished handwriting.
    b. a weakness of one leg resulting in a limping walk.
    c. difficulty arising from a chair and beginning to walk.
    d. the onset of muscle spasms occurring with voluntary movement.

26. A patient with Parkinson's disease is started on levodopa. The nurse explains that this drug

    a. stimulates dopamine receptors in the basal ganglia.
    b. promotes the release of dopamine from brain neurons.
    c. is a precursor of dopamine that is converted into dopamine in the brain.
    d. prevents the excessive breakdown of dopamine in the peripheral tissues.

27. An appropriate nursing intervention to promote speech and swallowing in a patient with Parkinson's disease is

  a. massaging the facial and neck muscles.
  b. keeping the patient positioned in an upright position.
  c. encouraging deep breaths before speaking or attempting to swallow.
  d. suctioning the patient to remove pooled secretions and prevent aspiration.

28. To reduce the risk for falls in the patient with Parkinson's disease, the nurse teaches the patient to

  a. use an elevated toilet seat.
  b. use a walker or cane for support.
  c. consciously lift the toes when stepping.
  d. rock side to side to initiate leg movements.

29. A patient with myasthenia gravis is admitted to the hospital with respiratory insufficiency and severe weakness. A diagnosis of cholinergic crisis is made when

  a. the patient's respiration is impaired because of muscle weakness.
  b. administration of edrophonium (Tensilon) increases muscle weakness.
  c. the edrophonium (Tensilon) test results in improved muscle contractility.
  d. electromyography reveals decreased response to repeated stimulation of muscles.

30. During care of a patient in myasthenic crisis, the nurse's first priority for the patient is maintenance of

  a. mobility.
  b. nutrition.
  c. respiratory function.
  d. verbal communication.

31. A patient at the clinic for a routine health examination mentions that she is exhausted because her legs bother her so much at night that she can't sleep. The nurse questions the patient further about her leg symptoms with the knowledge that if she has "restless legs syndrome"

  a. the condition can be readily diagnosed with electromyography.
  b. other more serious nervous system dysfunctions may be present.
  c. dopaminergic agents are often effective in managing the symptoms.
  d. the symptoms can be controlled by vigorous exercise of the legs during the day.

32. When providing care for a patient with amyotrophic lateral sclerosis (ALS), the nurse recognizes that one of the most distressing problems experienced by the patient is

  a. painful spasticity of the face and extremities.
  b. retention of cognitive function with total degeneration of motor function.
  c. uncontrollable, writhing, twisting movements of the face, limbs, and body.
  d. the knowledge that there is a 50% chance the disease has been passed to any offspring.

33. In providing care for patients with chronic, progressive neurologic disease, the major goal of treatment that the nurse works toward is to

  a. meet the patient's personal care needs.
  b. return the patient to normal neurologic function.
  c. maximize neurologic functioning as long as possible.
  d. prevent the development of additional chronic diseases.

CASE STUDY

MULTIPLE SCLEROSIS

Patient Profile

Ms. S., a 32-year-old Caucasian woman, born and raised in Minneapolis, is diagnosed with multiple sclerosis after an episode of numbness and tingling on the left side of her body that started several months ago. Two years ago she had an episode of optic neuritis in the right eye.

Subjective Data

- Difficulty seeing out of the right eye
- Numbness and tingling on the left side that worsens in hot weather
- Tires easily
- Used all sick days at work; concerned about losing her job and her ability to care for her 3-year-old son

Objective Data

- Crying softly during the interview
- Appears tense and anxious
- Prolonged visual evoked response in right eye
- MRI scan of head shows several plaques in white matter

Critical Thinking Questions

1. What is the pathophysiology of multiple sclerosis?

2. What precipitating factors for multiple sclerosis are present in Ms. S.'s life?

3. Why did it take so long for a definitive diagnosis to be made for Ms. S.?

4. What teaching plan should be developed for Ms. S.?

5. What treatment would be appropriate for Ms. S.?

6. Based on the assessment data presented, write one or more appropriate nursing diagnoses for Ms. S. Are there any collaborative problems?

CHAPTER 58
NURSING MANAGEMENT: ALZHEIMER'S DISEASE AND DEMENTIA

1. The nurse assesses a postoperative patient who has Parkinson's disease for early signs of delirium based on the knowledge that

   a. anticholinergic medications used to treat Parkinson's disease can precipitate delirium in older adults.
   b. older patients are more likely to develop delirium and most patients with Parkinson's disease are older adults.
   c. decreased levels of dopamine in the CNS found in Parkinson's disease have also been shown to be related to the onset of delirium.
   d. the decreased production of acetylcholine in patients with Parkinson's disease may also be responsible for development of delrium.

2. A patient with metastatic cancer develops delirium. The nurse recognizes that a factor of the patient's disease that may be related to development of delirium is

   a. decreased production of WBC.
   b. decreased antibody production.
   c. decreased production of platelets.
   d. increased production of cytokines.

3. A 72-year-old woman is hospitalized in the intensive care unit (ICU) with pneumonia secondary to COPD. She has a fever, productive cough, and adventitious breath sounds throughout her lungs. In the past 24 hours her fluid intake was 1000 ml and her urine output was 700 ml. She was diagnosed with early stage Alzheimer's disease 6 months ago but has been able to maintain her ADLs with supervision. Identify at least six risk factors for the development of delirium in this patient.

   a.

   b.

   c.

   d.

   e.

   f.

4. A 68-year-old man is admitted to the emergency department with multiple blunt traumas following a one-vehicle car accident. He is restless; disoriented to person, place, and time; and agitated. He resists attempts at examination and calls out the name "Janice." The nurse suspects delirium rather than dementia in this patient based on

   a. the fact that he wouldn't have been allowed to drive if he had dementia.
   b. his hyperactive behavior, which differentiates his condition from the hypoactive behavior of dementia.
   c. the report of emergency personnel that he was noncommunicative when they arrived at the accident scene.
   d. the report of his family that although he has heart disease and is "very hard of hearing," this behavior is unlike him.

5. The management of a patient with delirium includes

   a. the use of restraints to protect the patient from injury.
   b. the use of short-acting benzodiazepines to sedate the patient.
   c. identification and treatment of underlying causes when possible.
   d. administration of high doses of an antipsychotic drug such as haloperidol (Haldol).

6. Identify the following manifestations of cognitive impairment as primarily characteristic of delirium (DL) or dementia (DM).

   _____ a. Delusions and hallucinations common

   _____ b. Impaired judgments

   _____ c. Sleep-wake cycle reversed

   _____ d. Distorted thinking and perception

   _____ e. Inability to perform purposeful acts

   _____ f. Lucid intervals

   _____ g. Insidious onset with prolonged course and duration

   _____ h. Struggles to perform well with mental status testing

   _____ i. Fluctuating impaired orientation

   _____ j. Generally normal alertness

7. Identify whether the following statements are true or false. If a statement is false, correct the bold word(s) to make the statement true.

   _____ a. The two major causes of dementia are **neurodegenerative conditions** and **multiinfarction**.

   _____ b. **Neurodegenerative** dementia can be diagnosed by brain lesions identified with neuroimaging techniques.

   _____ c. Dementia caused by hepatic or renal **encephalopathy** is potentially reversible.

   _____ d. Dementia resulting from **vascular** causes can be prevented.

   _____ e. A genetic mutation that has been found in some patients with Alzheimer's disease causes overproduction of **tau proteins**.

8. A patient with dementia has manifestations of depression. The nurse knows that treatment of the patient with antidepressants will most likely

   a. improve cognitive function.
   b. not alter the course of either condition.
   c. cause interactions with the drugs used to treat the dementia.
   d. be contraindicated because of the CNS depressant effect of antidepressants.

9. The wife of a patient who is manifesting deterioration in memory asks the nurse whether her husband has Alzheimer's disease. The nurse explains that a diagnosis of Alzheimer's disease is made when

   a. a CT scan of the brain indicates brain atrophy.
   b. a urine test indicates elevated levels of isoprostanes.
   c. all other possible causes of dementia have been eliminated.
   d. blood analysis reveals increased amounts of amyloid-beta protein.

10. The nurse uses the Mini-Mental State Examination to evaluate a patient with cognitive impairment primarily because this test

   a. is a good tool to evaluate mood and thought processes.
   b. indicates cognitive impairment if the score is more than 30 points.
   c. can help document the degree of cognitive impairment in delirium and dementia.
   d. is useful for initial evaluation of mental status, but additional tools are needed to evaluate cognition changes over time.

11. Collaborative care of patients with Alzheimer's disease focuses on

   a. replacement of deficient acetylcholine in the brain.
   b. drug therapy to enhance cognition and control undesirable behaviors.
   c. the use of memory-enhancing techniques to delay disease progression.
   d. prevention of other chronic diseases that hasten the progression of Alzheimer's disease.

12. Match each of the following medications used in the management of Alzheimer's disease with its classification and use.

		Medication	Classification
_____	_____	a. amitriptyline (Elavil)	1. Cholinesterase inhibitors
_____	_____	b. haloperidol (Haldol)	2. Selective serotonin reuptake inhibitors
_____	_____	c. donepezil (Aricept)	3. Tricyclic antidepressants
_____	_____	d. lorazepam (Ativan)	4. Conventional antipsychotics
_____	_____	e. risperidone (Risperdal)	5. Atypical antipsychotics
_____	_____	f. zolpidem (Ambien)	6. Benzodiazepines
_____	_____	g. doxepin (Sinequan)	7. Nonbenzodiazepine sedative-hypnotics
_____	_____	h. fluoxetine (Prozac)	**Use**
_____	_____	i. olanzapine (Zyprexa)	8. Improved cognition
_____	_____	j. rivastigmine (Exelon)	9. Behavior management
_____	_____	k. sertraline (Zoloft)	10. Treatment of depression
			11. Treatment of sleep disturbances

13. A patient with moderate Alzheimer's disease has a nursing diagnosis of disturbed thought processes related to effects of dementia. An appropriate nursing intervention for the patient is

    a. posting clocks and calendars in the patient's environment.
    b. monitoring the patient's activity to maintain a safe patient environment.
    c. establishing and consistently following a daily schedule with the patient.
    d. stimulating thought processes by asking the patient questions about recent activities.

14. The caregiver for a patient with Alzheimer's disease expresses an inability to make decisions, concentrate, or sleep. The nurse determines that the caregiver

    a. is also developing signs of Alzheimer's disease.
    b. is manifesting symptoms of caregiver role strain.
    c. needs a period of respite from the care of the patient.
    d. should ask other family members to participate in the patient's care.

15. The wife of a man with moderate Alzheimer's disease has a nursing diagnosis of social isolation related to diminishing social relationships and behavioral problems of the patient with Alzheimer's disease. A nursing intervention that would be appropriate to provide respite care and allow the wife to have satisfactory contact with significant others is to

    a. help the wife arrange for adult day care for the patient.
    b. encourage permanent placement of the patient in an Alzheimer's unit of a long-term care facility.
    c. refer the wife to a home health agency to arrange daily home nursing visits to assist with the patient's care.
    d. arrange for hospitalization of the patient for 3 or 4 days so that the wife can visit out-of-town friends and relatives.

CASE STUDY

ALZHEIMER'S DISEASE

Patient Profile

Mr. D. is a 79-year-old man whose wife noticed that he has become increasingly forgetful over the past 3 years. Recently he was diagnosed with Alzheimer's disease.

Subjective Data

- Wanders out of the house at night
- States that he "sees things that aren't there"
- Is able to dress, bathe, and feed himself
- Has trouble figuring out how to use his electric razor
- His wife is distressed about his cognitive decline
- His wife says she is depressed and can't watch him at night and get rest herself

Objective Data

- CT scan: moderate cerebral atrophy

Critical Thinking Questions

1. What pathophysiologic changes are associated with Alzheimer's disease?

2. How is a diagnosis of Alzheimer's disease made?

3. What progression of symptoms should Mr. D.'s wife be told to expect over the course of the disease?

4. What suggestions can the nurse make to relieve some of the stress on the wife?

5. What community resources might be available to Mr. D. and his wife?

6. Based on the assessment data presented, write one or more appropriate nursing diagnoses for Mr. D. Are there any collaborative problems?

7. Based on the assessment data presented, write one or more appropriate nursing diagnoses for Mr. D.'s wife. Are there any collaborative problems?

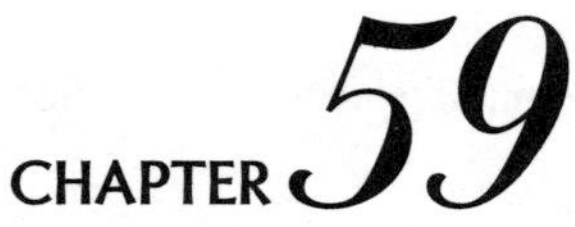

NURSING MANAGEMENT: PERIPHERAL NERVE AND SPINAL CORD PROBLEMS

1. Identify whether the following statements are true or false. If a statement is false, correct the bold word(s) to make the statement true.

_____ a. Trigeminal neuralgia affects the **sensory branches of the trigeminal nerve** while Bell's palsy affects the **motor branches of the facial nerve**.

_____ b. Herpes simplex virus infection is strongly associated as a precipitating factor in the development of **trigeminal neuralgia**.

_____ c. **Antiseizure drugs** are the drugs of choice for treatment of Bell's palsy.

_____ d. Gentle upward massage of the face may be indicated to maintain circulation in the patient with **trigeminal neuralgia**.

_____ e. A special need of patients with both trigeminal neuralgia and Bell's palsy is **oral hygiene**.

_____ f. Severe withdrawal behaviors and suicidal tendencies may be seen in patients with **trigeminal neuralgia**.

2. In planning care for the patient with trigeminal neuralgia, the nurse sets the highest priority on the patient outcome of

a. relief of pain.
b. protection of the cornea.
c. maintenance of nutrition.
d. maintenance of positive body image.

3. Surgical intervention is being considered for a patient with trigeminal neuralgia. The nurse recognizes that the procedure that has the least residual effects with a positive outcome is

a. glycerol rhizotomy.
b. suboccipital craniotomy.
c. microvascular decompression.
d. percutaneous radiofrequency rhizotomy.

4. In providing care for a patient with an acute attack of trigeminal neuralgia, the nurse should

a. carry out all hygiene and oral care for the patient.
b. use conversation to distract the patient from pain.
c. maintain a quiet, comfortable, draft-free environment.
d. have the patient examine the mouth after each meal for residual food.

5. A patient is admitted to the hospital with Guillain-Barré syndrome. She had a weakness in her feet and ankles that has progressed to weakness with numbness and tingling in both legs. During the acute phase of her illness, the nurse recognizes that

a. the most important aspect of care is to monitor the patient's vital capacity and ABGs.
b. early treatment with corticosteroids can suppress the immune response and prevent ascending nerve damage.
c. although voluntary motor neurons are damaged by the inflammatory response, the autonomic nervous system is unaffected by the disease.
d. the most serious complication of this condition is ascending demyelination of the peripheral nerves of the lower brainstem and cranial nerves.

6. A patient with Guillain-Barré syndrome asks if he is going to die as the paralysis spreads toward his chest. In responding to the patient, the nurse knows that

   a. patients who require ventilatory support almost always die.
   b. death occurs when nerve damage affects the brain and meninges.
   c. most patients with Guillain-Barré syndrome make a complete recovery.
   d. if death can be prevented, residual paralysis and sensory impairment are usually permanent.

7. Match the following characteristics with their related condition (answers may be used more than once).

_____	a. Results from dormant infection	1. Botulism
_____	b. Inhibits transmission of acetylcholine at myoneural junction	2. Tetanus
		3. Neurosyphilis
_____	c. Transmitted through wound contamination	
_____	d. Initially manifests with GI symptoms with subsequent absorption of neurotoxin	
_____	e. Primary prevention is immunization	
_____	f. May involve a meningoencephalitic infection	
_____	g. Blocks inhibitory transmitters in spinal cord and brain	
_____	h. Prevented by boiling food for 10 minutes	
_____	i. Severe, conscious, continuous tonic convulsions with apnea	
_____	j. Degenerative changes in spinal cord and brainstem	
_____	k. Motor and sensory loss	

8. In planning community education for prevention of spinal cord injuries, the nurse targets

   a. elderly men.
   b. teenage females.
   c. elementary school–age children.
   d. adolescent and young adult men.

9. A patient has a complete spinal cord transection at the C7 level. During the acute period, the nurse would expect the patient to have

   a. paraplegia with a flaccid paralysis.
   b. tetraplegia with total sensory loss.
   c. total hemiplegia with sensory and motor loss.
   d. flaccid tetraplegia with loss of pressure sensation.

10. Match the syndromes of incomplete spinal cord lesions with their descriptions.

_____ a. Central cord syndrome
_____ b. Anterior cord syndrome
_____ c. Brown-Sequard syndrome
_____ d. Posterior cord syndrome
_____ e. Caudio equina syndrome/ conus medullaris syndrome

1. Spinal cord damage resulting in ipsilateral motor paralysis and contralateral loss of pain and sensation below level of lesion
2. Damage to the most distal cord and nerve roots, resulting in flaccid paralysis of the lower limbs and areflexic bowel and bladder
3. Rare cord damage resulting in loss of proprioception below level of lesion with retention of motor control and temperature and pain sensation
4. Often caused by flexion injury with acute compression of cord resulting in complete motor paralysis and loss of pain and temperature sensation below the level of injury
5. Cord damage common in cervical region resulting in greater weakness in upper extremities than lower

11. An initial incomplete spinal cord injury often results in complete cord damage because of

a. edematous compression of the cord above the level of the injury.
b. continued trauma to the cord resulting from damage to stabilizing ligaments.
c. infarction and necrosis of the cord caused by edema, hemorrhage, and metabolites.
d. mechanical transection of the cord by sharp vertebral bone fragments after the initial injury.

12. A patient with a spinal cord injury has spinal shock. The nurse plans care for the patient based on the knowledge that

a. rehabilitation measures cannot be initiated until spinal shock has resolved.
b. the patient will need continuous monitoring for hypotension, tachycardia, and hypoxemia.
c. resolution of spinal shock is manifested by spasticity, hyperreflexia, and reflex emptying of the bladder.
d. the patient will have complete loss of motor and sensory functions below the level of the injury, but autonomic functions are not affected.

13. Two days following a spinal cord injury, a patient asks continuously about the extent of impairment that will result from the injury. The best response by the nurse is

a. "You will have more normal function when spinal shock resolves and the reflex arc returns."
b. "The extent of your injury cannot be determined until the secondary injury to the cord is resolved."
c. "When your condition is more stable, an MRI will be done that can reveal the extent of the cord damage."
d. "Because long-term rehabilitation can affect the return of function it will be years before we can tell what the complete effect will be."

14. Indicate the lowest level of acute spinal cord injury at which the following effects occur.

a. GI hypomotility with paralytic ileus and gastric distention

b. Loss of all respiratory muscle function

c. Respiratory diaphragmatic breathing

d. Hypofunction and distention of bladder and bowel

15. A patient is hospitalized following a spinal cord injury at the level of C8. A priority of nursing care for the patient is monitoring for

a. return of reflexes.
b. bradycardia with hypoxemia.
c. effects of sensory deprivation.
d. fluctuations in body temperature.

16. Match the following activities with the highest level of spinal cord injury that the activity can be expected (not all answers will be used).

_____ a. Ambulate with crutches and leg braces — 1. C1–C3

_____ b. Push wheelchair on flat surfaces — 2. C4

_____ c. Maintain bowel and bladder continence — 3. C5

_____ d. Have normal respiratory function — 4. C6

_____ e. Drive electric wheelchair with chin control — 5. C7–C8

_____ f. Be independent in self-care and wheelchair use — 6. T1–T6

7. T6–T12

8. L1–L2

9. L3–L4

17. One indication for surgical therapy of the patient with a spinal cord injury is when

a. there is incomplete cord lesion involvement.
b. the ligaments that support the spine are torn.
c. a high cervical injury causes loss of respiratory function.
d. evidence of continued compression of the cord is apparent.

18. A patient is admitted to the emergency department with a possible cervical spinal cord injury following an automobile accident. During the admission of the patient, the nurse places the highest priority on

a. maintaining a patent airway.
b. assessing the patient for head and other injuries.
c. maintaining immobilization of the cervical spine.
d. assessing the patient's motor and sensory function.

19. Immobilization and traction of the patient with a cervical spinal cord injury most frequently requires the use of

a. kinetic beds.
b. hard cervical collars.
c. skeletal traction with skull tongs.
d. sternal-occipital-mandibular immobilizer (SOMI) brace.

20. The current standard of care for spinal cord injury within the first 8 hours of injury is treatment with

    a. dopamine (Intropin).
    b. high-volume IV fluids.
    c. dexamethasone (Decadron).
    d. methylprednisolone (Medrol).

21. During the assessment of a patient with a spinal cord injury, the nurse determines that the patient has a poor cough with diaphragmatic breathing. Based on this finding, the nurse

    a. uses tracheal suctioning to remove secretions.
    b. assesses lung sounds and respiratory parameters q1-2hr.
    c. places the patient prone to promote drainage of respiratory secretions.
    d. explains to the patient that mechanical ventilation will be necessary to maintain respiratory function.

22. Following a T2 spinal cord injury, the patient develops paralytic ileus. While this condition is present, the nurse anticipates that the patient will need

    a. IV fluids.
    b. tube feedings.
    c. nasogastric suctioning.
    d. total parenteral nutrition.

23. Urinary function during the acute phase of spinal cord injury is maintained with

    a. an indwelling catheter.
    b. intermittent catheterization.
    c. insertion of a suprapubic catheter.
    d. use of incontinent pads to protect the skin.

24. A week following a spinal cord injury at T2, a patient experiences movement in his leg and tells the nurse he is recovering some function. The nurse's best response to the patient is

    a. "It is really still too soon to know if you will have a return of function."
    b. "That could be a really positive finding. Can you show me the movement?"
    c. "That's wonderful. We will start exercising your legs more frequently now."
    d. "I'm sorry, but the movement is only a reflex and does not indicate normal function."

25. A patient with a spinal cord lesion at C8 tells the nurse that he has a headache and feels flushed and warm. The first action by the nurse is to

    a. check the patient's temperature.
    b. take the patient's blood pressure.
    c. elevate the head of the patient's bed.
    d. assess the patient for a distended bladder or rectum.

26. Two weeks following a spinal cord injury, the patient has a neurogenic bladder. The nurse recognizes that a neurogenic bladder

    a. has no reflex detrusor contractions.
    b. has sensory function but no motor function.
    c. has hyperactive reflect detrusor contractions.
    d. requires diagnostic evaluation to determine the best management interventions.

27. The preferred method of long-term management of a neurogenic bladder in a paraplegic patient is

    a. surgical urinary diversion.
    b. indwelling catheterization.
    c. suprapubic catheterization.
    d. intermittent self-catheterization.

28. In counseling patients with spinal cord lesions regarding sexual function, the nurse advises a male patient with a complete lower motor neuron lesion that he

    a. is most likely to have reflexogenic erections, and may experience orgasm if ejaculation occurs.
    b. may have uncontrolled reflex erections, but that orgasm and ejaculation are usually not possible.
    c. has a lesion with the greatest possibility of successful psychogenic erection with ejaculation and orgasms.
    d. will probably be unable to have either psychogenic or reflexogenic erections, with no ejaculation or orgasm.

29. During the patient's process of grieving for the losses resulting from spinal cord injury, the nurse

    a. helps the patient understand that working through the grief will be a lifelong process.
    b. should assist the patient to move through all stages of the mourning process to acceptance.
    c. lets the patient know that anger directed at the staff or the family is not a positive coping mechanism.
    d. facilitates the grieving process so that it is completed by the time the patient is discharged from rehabilitation.

30. A patient with a metastatic tumor of the spinal cord is scheduled for removal of the tumor by a laminectomy. In planning postoperative care for the patient, the nurse recognizes that

    a. most cord tumors cause autodestruction of the cord as in traumatic injuries.
    b. metastatic tumors are commonly extradural lesions that can be removed completely.
    c. radiation therapy is routinely administered following surgery for all malignant spinal cord tumors.
    d. because complete removal of intramedullary tumors is not possible, the surgery is considered palliative.

CASE STUDY

SPINAL CORD INJURY

Patient Profile

Susan M. is a 16-year-old high school student who sustained a C7 spinal cord injury when she dove into a lake while swimming with her friends. Susan is admitted directly to the ICU.

Subjective Data

- Has patchy sensation in her upper extremities

Objective Data

- Very weak bicep and tricep strength bilaterally
- Moderate strength in both of her lower extremities
- Bowel and bladder control present
- X-rays show no fracture dislocation of the spine
- Placed on bed rest with a hard cervical collar
- Methylprednisolone administered per protocol

Critical Thinking Questions

1. What spinal cord syndrome is Susan experiencing?

2. What is the physiologic reason that Susan can move her lower extremities better than her upper extremities?

3. Why does Susan have a spinal cord injury without having sustained any spinal fracture?

4. What is the rationale for the use of the methylprednisolone?

5. What psychologic problems are anticipated?

6. What can be done to begin long-term plans for Susan?

7. Based on the assessment data presented, write one or more appropriate nursing diagnoses. Are there any collaborative problems?

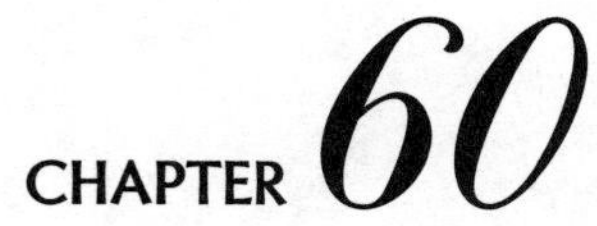

NURSING ASSESSMENT: MUSCULOSKELETAL SYSTEM

1. Using the list of terms below, identify the structures in the following illustration.

List of Terms

articular cartilage	epiphyseal growth plate
bone marrow	epiphysis
cancellous bone	medullary cavity
cortical bone	metaphysis
diaphysis	periosteum

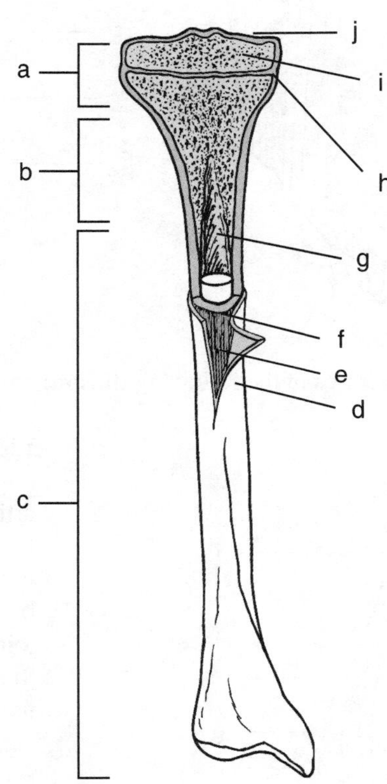

a. ______________________ f. ______________________

b. ______________________ g. ______________________

c. ______________________ h. ______________________

d. ______________________ i. ______________________

e. ______________________ j. ______________________

2. Using the terms below, identify the structures in the following illustration.

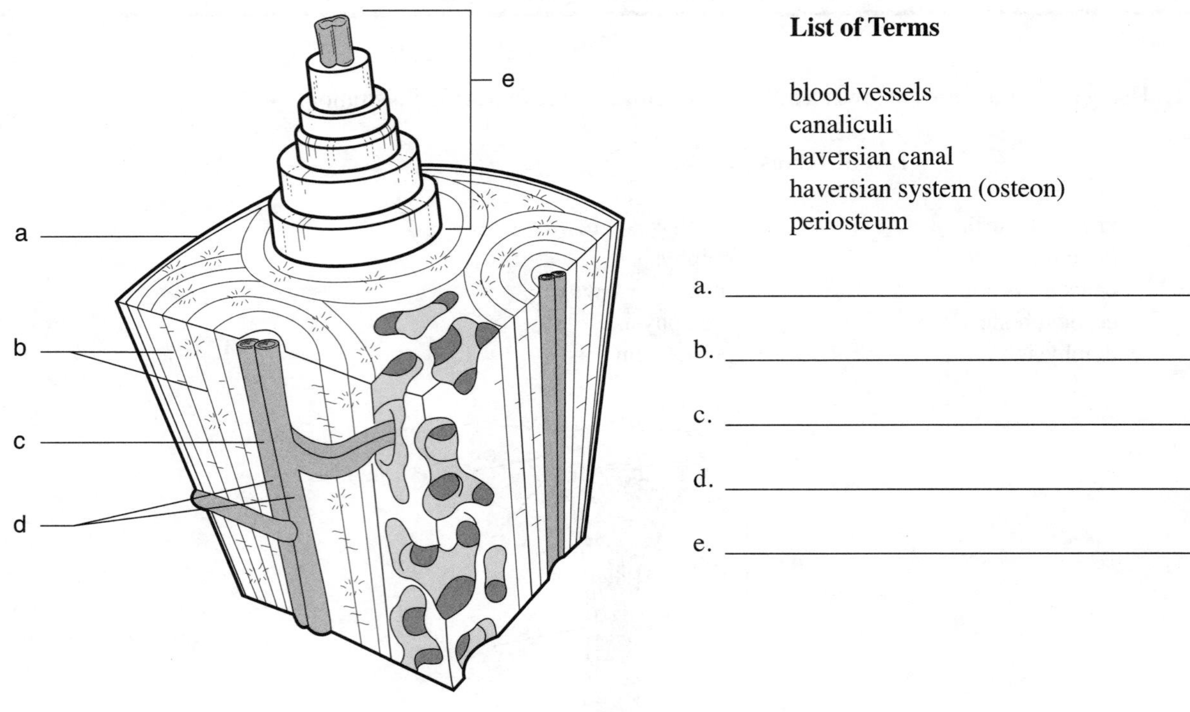

List of Terms

blood vessels
canaliculi
haversian canal
haversian system (osteon)
periosteum

a. ______________________

b. ______________________

c. ______________________

d. ______________________

e. ______________________

3. Using the terms below, identify the structures in the following illustration.

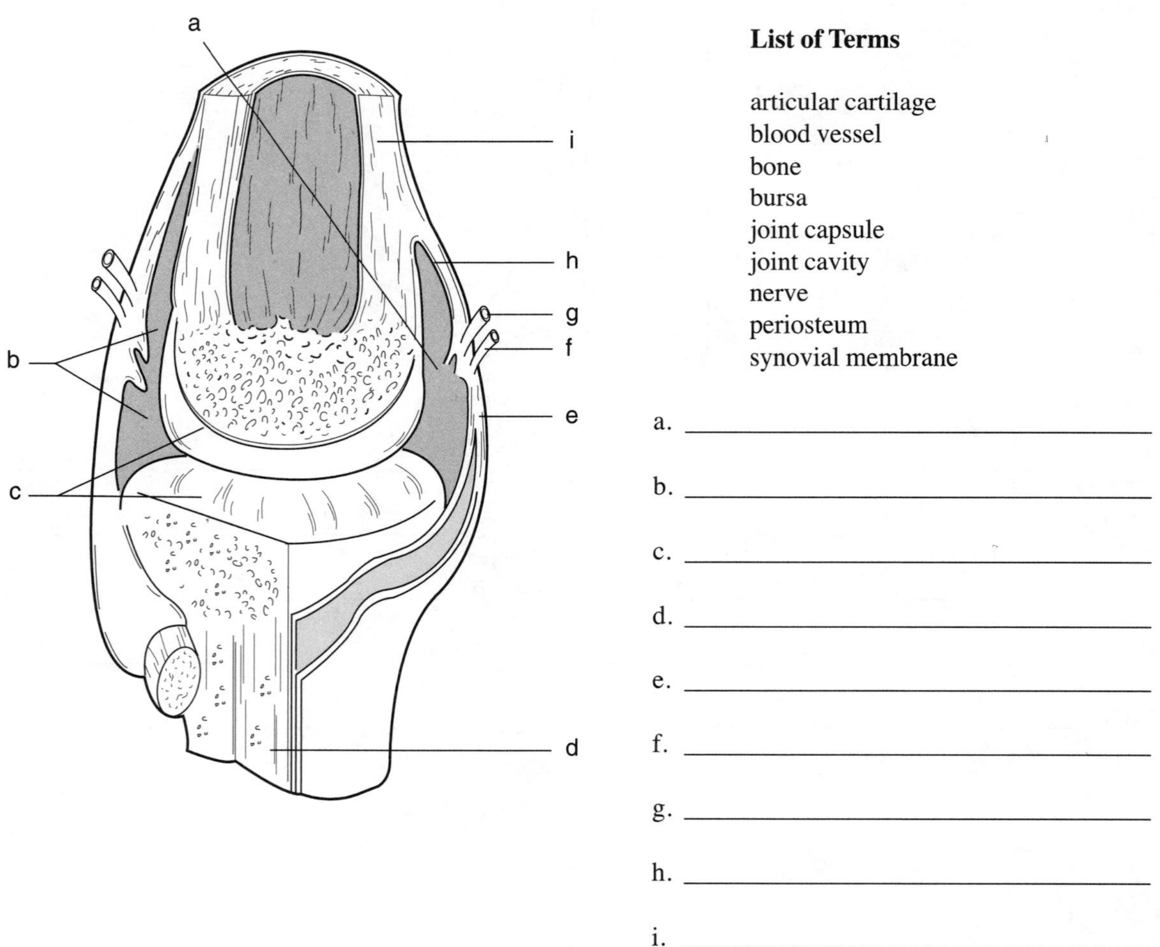

List of Terms

articular cartilage
blood vessel
bone
bursa
joint capsule
joint cavity
nerve
periosteum
synovial membrane

a. ______________________

b. ______________________

c. ______________________

d. ______________________

e. ______________________

f. ______________________

g. ______________________

h. ______________________

i. ______________________

4. Word Search: Find the words that are described by the clues given below. The words may be located horizontally, vertically, or diagonally, and may be reversed.

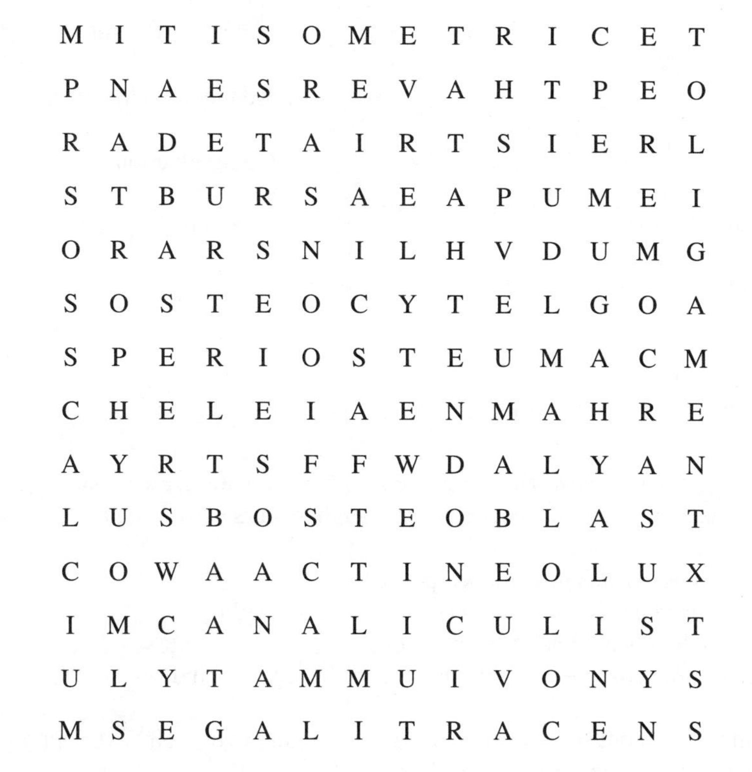

a. System of structural unit of compact bone
b. Contractile unit of myofibrils
c. Cancellous bone at end of long bones
d. Mature bone cell
e. Attaches muscles to bone
f. Connective tissue covering bone
g. Lining of joint capsule
h. Muscle contraction that produces hypertrophy
i. Mineral responsible for muscle contraction
j. Canals extending from lacunae to connect osteocytes
k. Bone cell responsible for resorption of bone
l. Decrease in size of muscle
m. Thin myofibril filaments
n. Small sacs of connective tissue lined with synovium and synovial fluid
o. Bone cell responsible for formation of bone
p. Lack of blood supply makes this tissue slow healing
q. Connects bone to bone at joint
r. Connective tissue surrounding muscle
s. Most common type of cartilage tissue
t. Characteristic of skeletal muscle

5. In performing ROM with a patient, the nurse puts each joint through its full movement. Match the type of movements that can be performed on the following joints (answers may be used more than once, and joints may have more than one movement).

_____	a. Knee	1. Flexion/extension
_____	b. Hip	2. Abduction/adduction
_____	c. Thumb	3. Circumduction
_____	d. Radioulnar joint	4. Rotation
_____	e. Shoulder	
_____	f. Elbow	
_____	g. Wrist	

6. While having his height measured during a routine health examination, a 79-year-old man asks the nurse why he is "shrinking." The nurse explains that decreased height occurs with aging because

   a. decreased muscle mass results in a stooped posture.
   b. loss of cartilage in the knees and hip joints cause a loss of height.
   c. long bones become less dense and shorten as bone tissue compacts.
   d. vertebrae become more compressed with thinning of intervertebral disks.

7. A 78-year-old woman has a physiologic change related to aging in her joints. An appropriate nursing diagnosis related to common changes of aging in the skeletal system is

   a. fatigue.
   b. risk for injury.
   c. impaired physical mobility.
   d. risk for impaired skin integrity.

8. When obtaining information about the patient's use of medications, the nurse recognizes that both bone and muscle function may be impaired when the patient reports taking

   a. corticosteroids.
   b. oral hypoglycemic agents.
   c. potassium-depleting diuretics.
   d. nonsteroidal antiinflammatory drugs (NSAIDs).

9. Identify one specific finding identified by the nurse during assessment of each of the patient's functional health patterns that indicates a risk factor for musculoskeletal problems or a patient response to an actual musculoskeletal problem.

   a. Health perception–health management

   b. Nutritional-metabolic

   c. Elimination

   d. Activity-exercise

   e. Sleep-rest

   f. Cognitive-perceptual

   g. Self-perception–self-concept

   h. Role-relationship

   i. Sexuality-reproductive

   j. Coping–stress tolerance

10. During muscle-strength testing, the patient has active movement against gravity and some resistance to pressure. The nurse scores this finding as

    a. 2.
    b. 3.
    c. 4.
    d. 5.

11. On observation of the patient, the nurse notes the presence of a gait disturbance. To further evaluate the patient, the nurse should

    a. palpate the hips for crepitation.
    b. measure the length of the limbs.
    c. evaluate the degree of leg movement.
    d. compare the muscle mass of one leg with the other.

12. A patient with severe joint immobility is receiving physical and exercise therapy. To evaluate the effect of the treatment the nurse may assess joint range of motion with a(n)

    a. myometer.
    b. ergometer.
    c. goniometer.
    d. arthrometer.

13. Match the following assessment abnormalities with their descriptions.

_____	a. Lordosis	1. Partial joint dislocation
_____	b. Varus	2. Shortening of muscle or ligament
_____	c. Ankylosis	3. Convex curve of the spine
_____	d. Subluxation	4. Grating sensation between bones
_____	e. Ganglion	5. Angulation of bone away from midline
_____	f. Scoliosis	6. Fluid-filled cyst
_____	g. Valgus	7. Angulation of bone toward the midline
_____	h. Crepitation	8. Lateral curvature of the spine
_____	i. Contracture	9. Fixed joint
_____	j. Kyphosis	10. Concave curve of the spine

14. Complete the following statements.

a. The most common diagnostic test used to assess musculoskeletal disorders is ______________________.

b. Insertion of a needle into a joint for aspiration and analysis of synovial fluid is known as a(n) ____________________.

c. A test that is specific for visualization of intervertebral disk abnormalities is a(n) ____________________.

d. A fast, precise measurement of the bone mass of the spine, forearm, and total body calcium to evaluate osteoporosis can be obtained with the use of ____.

e. The study in which needles are inserted into muscles to measure electrical activity of muscles is a(n) ____________________.

f. The enzyme that is most predominant in skeletal muscle is _________ ________________.

15. Identify three serologic tests that may be positive or elevated in rheumatic arthritis.

a.

b.

c.

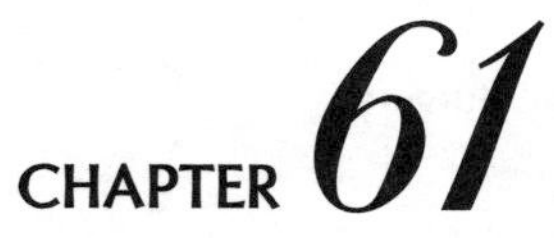

NURSING MANAGEMENT: MUSCULOSKELETAL TRAUMA AND ORTHOPEDIC SURGERY

1. A 72-year-old man tells the nurse that he cannot perform most of the physical activities he could do 5 years ago because of overall joint aches and pains. To prevent further deconditioning and the risk for developing musculoskeletal problems, the nurse can advise the patient to

   a. avoid the use of canes and walkers because they increase dependence on ambulation aids.
   b. limit weight-bearing exercise to prevent stress on fragile bones and possible hip fractures.
   c. increase his activity by more frequently climbing stairs in buildings and environments with steps.
   d. use aspirin or ibuprofen as prescribed by the physician to decrease inflammation and pain so that exercise can be maintained.

2. The nurse teaches individuals that one of the best ways to prevent musculoskeletal injuries during physical exercise is to

   a. increase muscle strength with daily isometric exercises.
   b. avoid exercising on concrete or hard pavement surfaces.
   c. perform stretching and warm-up exercises before exercise.
   d. wrap susceptible joints with elastic bandages or adhesive tape before exercise.

3. Match the following types of musculoskeletal soft-tissue injuries with their definitions.

   _____ a. Sprain
   _____ b. Strain
   _____ c. Dislocation
   _____ d. Subluxation
   _____ e. Repetitive strain injury
   _____ f. Bursitis
   _____ g. Carpal tunnel syndrome
   _____ h. Meniscus injury
   _____ i. Impingement syndrome
   _____ j. Rotator cuff injury

   1. Inflammation of synovial membrane sac at friction sites
   2. Incomplete separation of articular surfaces of joint due to ligament injury
   3. Compression of median nerve in wrist
   4. Entrapment of soft-tissue structures under coracoacromial arch of shoulder
   5. Tear within muscles or ligaments of shoulder
   6. Complete separation of articular surface of joint due to ligament injury
   7. Cartilage compression and tearing associated with rotational stress
   8. Tearing of a ligament
   9. Tendon and muscle strain with inflammation and decreased circulation
   10. Stretching of muscle and fascia sheath

4. Application of RICE (rest, ice, cold, compression, and elevation) is indicated for initial management of

   a. muscle spasms.
   b. sprains and strains.
   c. repetitive strain injury.
   d. dislocations and subluxations.

5. During the recovery phase of acute musculoskeletal soft-tissue injuries, management of the affected limb includes

   a. gradual, gentle exercise.
   b. immobilization and rest.
   c. alternating use of cold and heat.
   d. administration of antiinflammatory drugs.

6. Match the following types of fractures with their descriptions.

_____	a. Avulsion	1. Bone fragments driven into each other
_____	b. Comminuted	2. One side splintered and other side bent
_____	c. Open	3. Line of fracture twists along shaft of bone
_____	d. Oblique	4. Results from pulling effect of tendons or ligaments
_____	e. Impacted	5. Fracture with communication with external environment
_____	f. Pathologic	6. Slanted fracture line
_____	g. Greenstick	7. Fracture fragment overrides other bone fragment
_____	h. Displaced	8. Fracture with more than two fragments
_____	i. Transverse	9. Spontaneous fracture at site of bone disease
_____	j. Spiral	10. Line of fracture at right angle to longitudinal axis

7. Match the characteristics of the fracture healing process with their stages (answers may be used more than once).

_____	a. Invasion of osteoblasts and deposition of calcium	1. Hematoma
_____	b. Closure of space between bone fragments	2. Granulation
_____	c. Semisolid blood clot at ends of fragments	3. Callus formation
_____	d. Absorption of excess cells	4. Ossification
_____	e. Phagocytosis of necrotic byproducts	5. Consolidation
_____	f. Deposition and absorption of bone in response to stress	6. Remodeling
_____	g. Organization of hematoma into fibrous network	
_____	h. First stage to prevent movement at fracture site	
_____	i. Return to preinjury strength and shape	
_____	j. Formation of osteoid	
_____	k. Stage at which radiographic union first apparent	

8. A patient is brought to the emergency department following a fall while rock climbing that injured his left lower leg. The nurse identifies the presence of a fracture based on the cardinal sign of

   a. muscle spasms.
   b. obvious deformity.
   c. edema and swelling.
   d. pain and tenderness.

9. A patient with a fractured femur experiences the complication of malunion. The nurse recognizes that with this complication

   a. the fracture heals in an unsatisfactory position.
   b. the fracture fails to heal properly despite treatment.
   c. fracture healing progresses more slowly than expected.
   d. loss of bone substances occurs as a result of immobilization.

10. Identify whether the following statements are true or false. If a statement is false, correct the bold word(s) to make the statement true.

    _____ a. Realignment of bone fragments into anatomic position is known as **fixation**.

    _____ b. **Traction** may be used to both reduce a fracture and immobilize a fracture.

    _____ c. The disadvantage of open reduction and internal fixation of a fracture is that the patient has an increased risk for **complications related to immobility**.

    _____ d. Pressure causing circulatory, nerve, and skin impairment is most likely to occur with the use of **skeletal** traction.

    _____ e. Countertraction with Russell's traction may be achieved by elevating **the head of the bed**.

    _____ f. A cast or splint is a type of **external fixation**.

11. In planning care for the patient in traction, the nurse knows that elevation of the buttocks and back off the bed for linen changes, bedpan use, and skin care is possible for the patient with

    a. pelvic traction.
    b. Buck's traction.
    c. Russell's traction.
    d. balanced suspension traction.

12. When assessing the traction of a patient with a fracture femur, the nurse recognizes that a correction should be made if

    a. the weights are touching the floor.
    b. the ropes are in the center of the pulley.
    c. the patient exercises the unaffected limb.
    d. the patient is lying flat in the center of the bed.

13. A patient with a fractured femur has a hip spica cast applied. While the cast is drying, the nurse should

    a. elevate the legs above the level of the heart for 24 hours.
    b. turn the patient to both sides and prone to supine every 2 hours.
    c. cover the cast with a light blanket to avoid chilling from evaporation.
    d. assess the patient frequently for abdominal pain, nausea, and vomiting.

14. A patient is admitted with an open fracture of the tibia following a bicycle accident. During assessment of the patient, the nurse questions the patient specifically about

    a. any previous injuries to the leg.
    b. the status of tetanus immunization.
    c. the use of antibiotics in the last month.
    d. whether the injury was exposed to dirt or gravel.

15. A patient has fallen in the bathroom of the hospital room and complains of pain in the right upper arm and elbow. Before splinting the injury, the nurse knows that emergency management of a possible fracture should include

    a. elevation of the arm.
    b. application of ice to the site.
    c. notification of the physician.
    d. neurovascular checks below the site of the injury.

16. To assess for neurologic status in a patient with a fractured humerus, the nurse asks the patient to

    a. evert, invert, dorsiflex, and plantar flex the foot.
    b. abduct, adduct, and oppose the fingers, and pronate and supinate the hand.
    c. assess the location, quality, and intensity of pain below the site of the injury.
    d. assess the color, temperature, capillary refill, peripheral pulses, and presence of edema in the extremity.

17. A patient is discharged from the outpatient clinic following application of a synthetic fiberglass long arm cast for a fractured ulna. Before discharge, the nurse instructs the patient to

    a. never get the cast wet.
    b. move the shoulder and fingers frequently.
    c. place tape petals around the edges of the cast when it is dry.
    d. use a sling to support the arm at waist level for the first 48 hours.

18. A patient with a long leg cast is allowed to ambulate with crutches with no weight bearing on the affected leg. The nurse teaches the patient to use a

    a. swing-to gait.
    b. two-point gait.
    c. four-point gait.
    d. swing-through gait.

19. A patient with a fractured tibia accompanied by extensive soft-tissue damage initially has a splint applied and held in place with an elastic bandage. An early sign that would alert the nurse that the patient is developing compartment syndrome is

    a. paralysis of the toes.
    b. absence of peripheral pulses.
    c. progressive pain unrelieved by usual analgesics.
    d. the skin over the injury site is blanched when the bandage is removed.

20. Identify the problems that are indicated by each of the six Ps characteristic of an impending compartment syndrome.

a.

b.

c.

d.

e.

f.

21. Surgical treatment that is indicated for compartment syndrome is

a. fasciotomy.
b. amputation.
c. internal fixation.
d. release of tendons.

22. A fat embolism is most likely to occur

a. 24 to 48 hours following a fractured tibia.
b. 36 to 72 hours following a skull fracture.
c. 4 to 5 days following a fractured femur.
d. 5 to 6 days following a pelvic fracture.

23. The nurse suspects a fat embolism rather than a pulmonary embolism from a venous thrombosis in the patient with a fracture who develops

a. tachycardia and dyspnea.
b. a sudden onset of chest pain.
c. ECG changes and decreased PaO_2.
d. petechiae around the neck and upper chest.

24. Match the following characteristics with the related type of fracture (answers may be used more than once).

_____ a. Possible radial nerve and brachial artery damage

_____ b. Moving the patient may cause serious injury from bone fragments

_____ c. Often occurs when breaking a fall with an outstretched hand

_____ d. Airway patency is a major concern

_____ e. Balanced suspension traction and hip spica cast are treatment options

_____ f. Hanging arm cast may be used to reduce the fracture

_____ g. Most often a compression fracture

_____ h. High incidence of fat embolism and compartment syndrome

_____ i. Drastic change in appearance requires supportive care

_____ j. Fractured distal radius and possible styloid process of ulna

_____ k. Most serious complication is displacement of fracture

_____ l. May be accompanied by intraabdominal lacerations and ruptures

_____ m. Vulnerable site because of lack of anterior muscle covering

_____ n. Internal fixation with intermedullary rod or compression plates preferred

_____ o. Halo apparatus may be used for immobilization

1. Colles' fracture
2. Fractured humerus
3. Fractured pelvis
4. Femoral shaft fracture
5. Fractured tibia
6. Stable vertebral fracture
7. Facial fractures

25. Identify whether the following statements are true or false. If a statement is false, correct the bold word(s) to make the statement true.

_____ a. **Extracapsular** hip fractures often occur in individuals with osteoporosis and minor injury.

_____ b. An **intertrochanteric** fracture of the hip occurs between the greater and lesser trochanter.

_____ c. Avascular necrosis is a serious complication of displaced **subtrochanteric** fractures.

_____ d. The preferred treatment of extracapsular fractures is **pinning or nailing** while intracapsular frac tures are usually repaired with **hip prostheses**.

_____ e. **Intracapsular** hip fractures are also know as fractures of the neck of the femur.

26. An older adult woman is admitted to the emergency department after falling at home. The nurse suspects a fractured hip when assessment of the patient reveals

    a. inability to move the toes and ankle.
    b. edema of the thigh extending to the knee.
    c. internal rotation of the leg with groin pain.
    d. shortening and external rotation of the leg.

27. A patient with an extracapsular hip fracture is admitted to the orthopedic unit and placed in Russell's traction. The nurse explains to the patient that the purpose of the traction is to

    a. pull bone fragments back into alignment.
    b. immobilize the leg until healing is complete.
    c. reduce pain and muscle spasms before surgery.
    d. prevent damage to the blood vessels at the fracture site.

28. A patient with a fractured right hip has an open reduction and internal fixation of the fracture. Postoperatively, the nurse plans to

    a. get the patient up to the chair the first postoperative day.
    b. position the patient only on the back and unoperative side.
    c. keep leg abductor splints on the patient except when bathing.
    d. ambulate the patient with partial weight bearing by discharge.

29. Discharge instructions for the patient following a hip prosthesis include

    a. restrict walking for 2 to 3 months.
    b. take a bath rather than a shower to prevent falling.
    c. keep the leg internally rotated while sitting and standing.
    d. have a family member put on the patient's shoes and socks.

30. When preparing a patient for discharge following fixation of a mandibular fracture, the nurse determines that teaching has been successful when the patient says

    a. "I can keep my mouth moist by sucking on hard candy."
    b. "I should cut the wires with scissors if I begin to vomit."
    c. "I may use a bulk-forming laxative if my liquid diet causes constipation."
    d. "I should use a moist swab to clean my mouth every time I eat something."

31. A left above-the-knee amputation (AKA) is scheduled for a diabetic patient with ischemic gangrene of three toes. The patient asks why they cannot just amputate her toes. The best response by the nurse is

    a. "A prosthesis is easier to fit with this type of amputation."
    b. "The amputation must be high enough to have good circulation for healing."
    c. "There is infection in your lower leg that you cannot see that must be removed."
    d. "An amputation at this level will help prevent further circulatory problems in your leg."

32. A patient who suffered a traumatic below-the-elbow amputation in a boating accident is withdrawn, does not look at the arm, and asks to be left alone. An appropriate nursing diagnosis of the patient includes

    a. impaired adjustment.
    b. disturbed body image.
    c. impaired social interaction.
    d. ineffective individual coping.

33. A patient complains of pain in the foot of a leg that was recently amputated. The nurse recognizes that the pain

a. is caused by swelling at the incision.
b. should be treated with ordered analgesics.
c. will become worse with the use of a prosthesis.
d. can be managed with diversion since it is psychologic.

34. An immediate prosthetic fitting during surgery is used for a patient with a traumatic below-the-knee amputation (BKA). During the immediate postoperative period, it is most important for the nurse to

a. assess the site for hemorrhage.
b. monitor the patient's vital signs.
c. elevate the residual limb on pillows.
d. have the patient flex and extend the knee every hour.

35. The nurse positions a patient with an above-the-knee amputation with a delayed prosthetic fitting prone several times a day to

a. prevent flexion contractures.
b. assess the posterior skin flap.
c. reduce edema in the residual limb.
d. relieve pressure on the incision site.

36. A patient who had a below-the-knee amputation is to be fitted with a temporary prosthesis. It is most important for the nurse to teach the patient to

a. inspect the residual limb daily for irritation.
b. apply an elastic shrinker before applying the prosthesis.
c. perform ROM exercises to the affected leg four times a day.
d. apply alcohol to the residual limb every morning and evening to toughen the skin.

37. Match the following joint surgeries with their uses.

_____ a. Synovectomy

_____ b. Osteotomy

_____ c. Debridement

_____ d. Arthroplasty

_____ e. Arthrodesis

1. Reconstruction or replacement of a joint to relieve pain and correct deformity
2. Surgical fusion of a joint to relieve pain
3. Used in rheumatoid arthritis to remove the tissue involved in joint destruction
4. Correction of bone deformity by removal of a wedge or slice of bone
5. Arthroscopic removal of degenerative tissue in joints

38. A 65-year-old patient has undergone a right total hip arthroplasty with a cemented prosthesis for treatment of severe osteoarthritis of the hip. Patient activity that the nurse anticipates on the patient's first or second postoperative day includes

a. transfer from bed to chair bid only.
b. turning from back to unaffected side q2h only.
c. crutch walking with nonweight bearing on the operative leg.
d. ambulation and weight bearing on the right leg with a walker.

39. When positioning the patient with a total hip arthroplasty, it is important that the nurse maintains the affected extremity in

    a. adduction and flexion.
    b. extension and abduction.
    c. abduction and internal rotation.
    d. adduction and external rotation.

40. Following a knee arthroplasty, a patient has a continuous passive motion machine for the affected joint. The nurse explains to the patient that this device is used to

    a. relieve edema and pain at the incision site.
    b. promote early joint mobility and increase knee flexion.
    c. prevent venous stasis and the formation of a deep venous thrombosis.
    d. improve arterial circulation to the affected extremity to promote healing.

41. A patient with severe ulnar deviation of the hands undergoes an arthroplasty with reconstruction and replacement of finger joints. Postoperatively, it is most important for the nurse to

    a. position the fingers lower than the elbow.
    b. perform neurovascular assessments of the fingers q2-4h.
    c. encourage the patient to gently flex, extend, abduct, and adduct the fingers q4h.
    d. remind the patient that function of the hands is more important than their cosmetic appearance.

CASE STUDY

FRACTURE

Patient Profile

Mr. A., a 30-year-old telephone lineman, was seen in the emergency department after falling from a pole. His right lower extremity was splinted with a cardboard splint and a large bulky dressing.

Subjective Data

- Complains of severe pain in the right leg
- Expresses concern about notifying his wife about the accident and his whereabouts
- Asks how long he will be off work

Objective Data

- Avulsion of soft tissue on the anterolateral aspect of the tibia
- Obvious deformity, marked swelling, and ecchymosis in region of injury

Critical Thinking Questions

1. Was the immobilization of the fracture at the scene of the accident appropriate?

2. What is the appropriate nursing neurovascular assessment of the injured extremity?

3. What are the probable therapeutic and nursing interventions to prevent infection?

4. What specific nursing actions should the nurse implement to alleviate Mr. A.'s pain?

5. How would the nurse answer Mr. A.'s question about time off from work based on the stages of fracture healing?

6. How should the nurse notify Mrs. A. about her husband's accident?

7. Based on the assessment data presented, write one or more appropriate nursing diagnoses. Are there any collaborative problems?

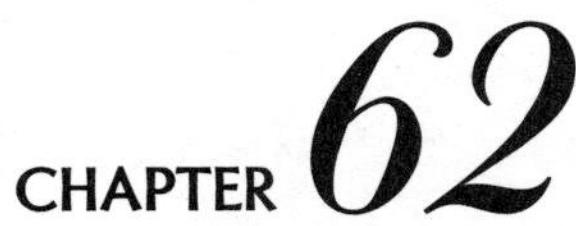

NURSING MANAGEMENT: MUSCULOSKELETAL PROBLEMS

1. A patient with chronic osteomyelitis has been hospitalized for surgical removal of the infection. The nurse explains to the patient that surgical treatment is necessary because

   a. the process of involucrum blocks the vascular supply to the bone.
   b. removal of the infection prevents the need for bone and skin grafting.
   c. formation of avascular scar tissue has led to a protected area of bacterial growth.
   d. antibiotics are not effective against microorganisms that cause chronic osteomyelitis.

2. A nursing intervention that is carried out to prevent the development of complications in the patient with osteomyelitis is

   a. providing ROM q4h to the involved extremity.
   b. gently handling the involved extremity during movement.
   c. using careful and appropriate disposal of soiled dressings.
   d. measuring the circumference of the affected extremity daily.

3. A patient who experienced an open fracture of the humerus 2 weeks ago is having increased pain at the fracture site. To determine the causative agent if the patient has developed an acute osteomyelitis at the site, the nurse would expect testing to include

   a. x-rays.
   b. a CT scan.
   c. a bone biopsy.
   d. WBC and erythrocyte sedimentation rate (ESR).

4. Following 2 weeks of IV antibiotic therapy, a patient with acute osteomyelitis of the tibia is prepared for discharge from the hospital. The nurse determines that additional instruction is needed when the patient says

   a. "I will need to continue antibiotic therapy for 4 to 8 weeks."
   b. "I should notify the physician if the pain in my leg becomes worse."
   c. "I shouldn't bear weight on my affected leg until healing is complete."
   d. "I can use a heating pad to my lower leg for comfort and to promote healing."

5. During a follow-up visit to a patient with acute osteomyelitis treated with IV antibiotics, the home care nurse is told by the patient's wife that she can hardly get the patient to eat because his mouth is so sore. In checking the patient's mouth, the nurse would expect to find

   a. a dry, cracked tongue with a central furrow.
   b. white, curdlike membranous lesions of the mucosa.
   c. ulcers of the mouth and lips surrounded by a reddened base.
   d. single or clustered vesicles on the tongue and buccal mucosa.

6. Match the following characteristics with their related types of bone cancer (answers may be used more than once).

_____	a. Involves medullary cavity of long bones	1. Multiple myeloma
_____	b. Involves bones with active marrow	2. Osteosarcoma
_____	c. Arises in cancellous ends of long bones	3. Osteoclastoma
_____	d. Often brought to attention by injury	4. Ewing's sarcoma
_____	e. Replacement of bone marrow by malignant plasma cells	
_____	f. Extremely malignant and metastasizes early	
_____	g. Locally destructive lesion without metastasis	

7. A 24-year-old patient with a 12-year history of Becker's muscular dystrophy is hospitalized with congestive heart failure. A nursing intervention that would be appropriate for this patient and any patient with muscular dystrophy is

   a. to feed and bathe the patient to avoid exhausting the muscles.
   b. frequent repositioning to avoid skin and respiratory complications.
   c. to provide hand weights for the patient to exercise the upper extremities.
   d. using orthopedic braces to promote ambulation to prevent muscle wasting.

8. Identify whether the following statements are true or false. If a statement is false, correct the bold word(s) to make the statement true.

   _____ a. **Chemotherapy** may be used in the management of all primary bone tumors.

   _____ b. The most common cause of low back pain is **herniation of an intervertebral disk**.

   _____ c. Use of **NSAIDs** for chronic low back pain is important in being able to maintain exercise and activity throughout the day.

   _____ d. The low back pain associated with a **lumbosacral instability** is usually accompanied by buttock and leg pain along the sciatic nerve.

   _____ e. **Degenerative disk disease** is a major factor in the development of herniated intervertebral disks.

9. The nurse teaches the patient with an acute episode of low back pain to

   a. perform daily exercise as a lifelong routine.
   b. sit in a chair with the hips higher than the knees.
   c. avoid occupations in which the use of the body is required.
   d. sleep on the abdomen or on the back with the legs extended.

10. To help prevent the patient with chronic low back pain from assuming sick-role behaviors, the nurse

   a. teaches the patient alternative methods of pain control.
   b. encourages activity and ambulation within the patient's limitations.
   c. discusses the nature of chronic pain and the need for lifestyle adjustments.
   d. monitors for decreased muscle strength that indicates the development of complications.

11. A patient with a herniated intravertebral disk and acute back pain is treated conservatively with rest and drug therapy. An important nursing intervention during this time is to

   a. monitor neurologic signs q4h.
   b. encourage foot and leg exercises q2-4h.
   c. assess the patient's use of body mechanics to identify teaching needs.
   d. maintain the patient in a supine position with the head slightly elevated and the knees flexed.

12. A laminectomy and spinal fusion is performed on a patient with a herniated lumbar intervertebral disk. During the postoperative period, the nurse notifies the physician when the patient experiences

   a. paralytic ileus.
   b. urinary incontinence.
   c. greater pain at the graft site than at the lumbar incision site.
   d. leg and arm movement and sensation unchanged from preoperative status.

13. Before repositioning the patient to the side after a lumbar laminectomy, the nurse

   a. raises the head of the bed 30 degrees.
   b. has the patient flex the knees and hips.
   c. places a pillow between the patient's legs.
   d. has the patient grasp the side rail on the opposite side of the bed.

14. Match the following foot problems with their characteristics (answers may be used more than once).

	Characteristic	Foot problem
_____	a. Breakdown of metatarsal arch	1. Hallux valgus (bunion)
_____	b. Papilloma growth on sole of foot	2. Hammer toe
_____	c. Local thickening of skin caused by pressure on bony prominences	3. Morton's neuroma
		4. Pes planus
_____	d. Deformity of second toe with callus on dorsum of proximal interphalangeal joint	5. Corn
_____	e. Tumor on nerve tissue between third and fourth metatarsal heads	6. Callus
		7. Plantar wart
_____	f. Lateral angulation of large toe toward second toe	
_____	g. Metatarsal joint support used in conservative treatment	
_____	h. May be trimmed with razor or scalpel after softening	
_____	i. Surgical treatment is removal of bursal sac and bony enlargement	
_____	j. Thickening of skin on weight-bearing part of foot	

15. In promoting healthy feet, the nurse recognizes the factor that is associated with most foot problems is

    a. poor foot hygiene.
    b. congenital deformities.
    c. improperly fitting shoes.
    d. peripheral vascular disease.

16. Match the following metabolic bone diseases with their characteristics (answers may be used more than once).

_____	a. Loss of total bone mass and substance	1. Osteomalacia
_____	b. Results from vitamin D deficiency	2. Paget's disease
_____	c. Replacement of normal marrow with vascular connective tissue	3. Osteoporosis
_____	d. Generalized bone decalcification with bone deformity	
_____	e. Most common in bones of spine, hips, and wrists	
_____	f. Abnormal remodeling and resorption of bone	
_____	g. Bowed legs and cranial enlargement	

17. The nurse determines that the woman with the highest risk for osteoporosis is a

    a. 60-year-old aerobic instructor.
    b. 65-year-old on estrogen therapy.
    c. 45-year-old obese African-American.
    d. 55-year-old Asian-American cigarette smoker.

18. Identify three methods of preventing osteoporosis in postmenopausal women.

    a.

    b.

    c.

CASE STUDY

HERNIATED INTRAVERTEBRAL DISK

Patient Profile

Howard Brown is a 38-year-old truck driver who slipped on a wet floor at work and landed on his buttocks.

Subjective Data

- Experienced immediate, severe lower back pain, with pain radiating into his right buttock
- Had worsening of pain in 3 days, with pain radiating down his entire leg into his foot
- Experienced tingling of his toes
- Rested at home for 2 weeks without relief
- Smokes 1 pack of cigarettes a day

Objective Data

- Is 5 ft 8 in tall; weighs 253 lbs
- Diagnostic studies: MRI revealed a large herniated disk at L 4-5 level.

Collaborative Care

- Underwent microdiskectomy at L 4-5
- Expected discharge 2 days after surgery

Critical Thinking Questions

1. What risk factors for low back pain does Mr. Brown have?

2. What preoperative teaching is indicated for Mr. Brown?

3. What postoperative activity restrictions will Mr. Brown need to follow?

4. What postoperative nursing assessments should be made?

5. What discharge teaching should be implemented with Mr. Brown?

6. Based on the assessment data presented, write one or more nursing diagnoses. Are there any collaborative problems?

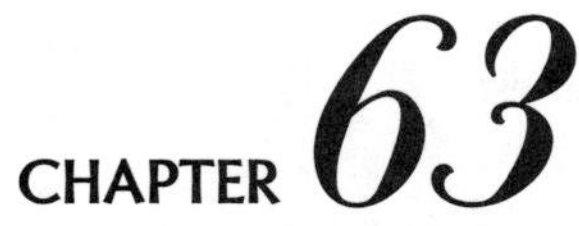

CHAPTER 63 NURSING MANAGEMENT: ARTHRITIS AND CONNECTIVE TISSUE DISEASES

1. A 60-year-old woman has pain on motion in her fingers and asks the nurse whether this is just a result of aging. The best response by the nurse includes the information that

   a. joint pain with functional limitation is a normal change that affects all people to some extent.
   b. joint pain that develops with age is usually related to previous trauma or infection of the joints.
   c. this is a symptom of a systemic arthritis that eventually affects all joints as the disease progresses.
   d. changes in the cartilage and bones of joints may cause symptoms of pain and loss of function in some people as they age.

2. Number in sequence from 1 to 6 the pathophysiologic processes that occur in osteoarthritis (OA).

   _____ a. Erosion of articular surfaces

   _____ b. Joint space narrows

   _____ c. Incongruity in joint surfaces leads to reduction in motion

   _____ d. Joint cartilage becomes yellow and rough

   _____ e. Osteophytes formed at joint margins

   _____ f. Cartilage becomes softer and less elastic

3. Identify whether the following statements are true or false. If a statement is false, correct the bold word(s) to make the statement true.

   _____ a. **Bouchard's nodes** are reddened, tender protuberances found at the distal interphalangeal joints in some patients with osteoarthritis.

   _____ b. The pain of latent osteoarthritis is most commonly caused by **swelling and stretching of soft tissue around the joint**.

   _____ c. Joint stiffness in OA can be caused by **crepitation**.

   _____ d. First-line drug therapy used in the management of osteoarthritis is **aspirin**.

   _____ e. Pain and immobility of osteoarthritis may be aggravated by **falling barometric pressure**.

4. To preserve function and the ability to perform activities of daily living, the nurse teaches the patient with osteoarthritis to

   a. avoid exercise that involves the affected joints.
   b. plan and organize less stressful ways to perform tasks.
   c. maintain normal activities during an acute episode to prevent loss of function.
   d. use mild analgesics to control symptoms when performing tasks that cause pain.

5. A patient with osteoarthritis uses NSAIDs to decrease pain and inflammation. The nurse teaches the patient that common side effects of these drugs include

   a. allergic reactions, fever, and oral lesions.
   b. fluid retention, hypertension, and bruising.
   c. skin rashes, gastric irritation, and headache.
   d. prolonged bleeding time, blood dyscrasias, and hepatic damage.

6. A patient with osteoarthritis asks the nurse whether he could try glucosamine and chondroitin for control of his symptoms. The best response by the nurse includes the information that

   a. although these substances may not help, there is no evidence that they can cause any untoward effects.
   b. glucosamine should not be used by patients with diabetes because it can decrease blood glucose levels.
   c. these supplements are a fad that has not been shown to reduce pain or increase joint mobility in patients with OA.
   d. only dosages of these supplements available by prescription are high enough to provide any benefit in treatment of OA.

7. A patient taking ibuprofen (Motrin) for treatment of OA has good pain relief but is experiencing increased dyspepsia and nausea with the drug's use. The nurse knows that an appropriate alternative with less GI effects than ibuprofen would be
   a. rofecoxib (Vioxx).
   b. naproxen (Naprosyn).
   c. diclofenac (Voltaren).
   d. indomethacin (Indocin).

8. The basic pathophysiologic process of rheumatoid arthritis is

   a. destruction of joint cartilage and bones by an autoimmune process.
   b. initiated by a viral infection that destroys the synovial membranes of joints.
   c. the presence of HLA-DR4 antigen that causes inflammatory responses throughout the body.
   d. an immune response that activates complement and produces inflammation of joints and other organ systems.

9. Indicate whether the following descriptions are most characteristic of osteoarthritis (O), rheumatoid arthritis (R), or both (B).

   _____ a. Most commonly occurs in women

   _____ b. Affects knees, hips, and spine

   _____ c. Asymmetric involvement of joints

   _____ d. Joint pain, stiffness, and limitation of motion

   _____ e. Inflammatory synovial fluid

   _____ f. Joint stiffness in morning and after periods of inactivity

   _____ g. Firm, subcutaneous, nontender nodules

   _____ h. Normal erythrocyte sedimentation rate (ESR)

   _____ i. Anemia and weight loss

   _____ j. Associated with normal life expectancy

   _____ k. Associated with autoantibodies to abnormal IgG

10. Number in sequence the pathophysiologic processes of rheumatoid arthritis.

_____ a. Invasion of joint capsule by granulation inflammatory tissue

_____ b. Calcification of fibrous tissue

_____ c. Joint inflammation

_____ d. Formation of pannus at juncture of synovium and cartilage

_____ e. Joint capsule occluded by tough fibrous connective tissue

_____ f. Bony ankylosis of joint with total immobilization

_____ g. Swelling of synovial membrane

11. During the physical assessment of the patient with moderate rheumatoid arthritis, the nurse would expect to find

a. hepatomegaly.
b. Heberden's nodes.
c. spindle-shaped fingers.
d. crepitus on joint movement.

12. Laboratory findings that the nurse would expect to be present in the patient with rheumatoid arthritis include

a. polycythemia.
b. increased IgG.
c. increased ESR.
d. decreased WBC.

13, Describe the three most common extraarticular manifestations of RA.

a.

b.

c.

14. Match the following drugs used in the management rheumatoid arthritis with their characteristics (answers may be used more than once).

_____ a. Requires monitoring for bone marrow depression

_____ b. Binds to TNF, blocking its effect in inflammation and immune responses

_____ c. Causes orange-yellow urine

_____ d. Antimalarial agent often used initially for mild RA

_____ e. Immunosuppresive agent that inhibits DNA and RNA synthesis

_____ f. Used intraarticularly for acute flare of one or two joints

_____ g. Blocks action of interleukin-1, decreasing inflammatory response

_____ h. Use requires periodic eye exam for retinal damage

_____ i. First drug of choice for patients with moderate-severe RA

_____ j. Systemic use limited to life-threatening exacerbations

_____ k. Sulfonamide with anti-inflammatory effects by blocking prostaglandin synthesis

_____ l. Antirheumatic agent that may take 3 to 6 months to have effect

_____ m. Often used with DMARDs for additional anti-inflammatory effect

_____ n. Systemic doses must be tapered to prevent exacerbation of symptoms

1. hydroxychloroquine (Plaquenil)
2. corticosteroids
3. anakinra (Kineret)
4. parenteral gold
5. sulfazalazine (Azulfidine)
6. etanercept (Enbrel)
7. methotrexate (Rheumatrex)
8. NSAIDs and aspirin
9. azathioprine (Imuran)

15. A 70-year-old patient is being evaluated for symptoms of rheumatoid arthritis. The nurse recognizes that a major problem in the management of rheumatoid arthritis in the older adult is that

a. rheumatoid arthritis is usually more severe in older adults.
b. older patients are not as likely to comply with treatment regimens.
c. drug interactions and toxicity are more likely to occur with multidrug therapy.
d. laboratory and other diagnostic tests are not effective in identifying rheumatoid arthritis in older adults.

16. After teaching a patient with rheumatoid arthritis about the prescribed therapeutic regimen, the nurse determines that further instruction is needed when the patient says

a. "It is important for me to perform my prescribed exercises every day."
b. "I should perform most of my daily chores in the morning when my energy level is highest."
c. "An ice pack to a joint for 10 minutes may help relieve pain and inflammation when I have an acute flare."
d. "I can use assistive devices such as padded utensils, electric can openers, and elevated toilet seats to protect my joints."

17. A patient recovering from an acute exacerbation of rheumatoid arthritis tells the nurse she is too tired to bathe. The nurse should

    a. give the patient a bed bath to conserve her energy.
    b. allow the patient a rest period before showering with the nurse's help.
    c. tell the patient that she can skip bathing if she will walk in the hall later.
    d. inform the patient that it is important for her to maintain self-care activities.

18. After teaching a patient with RA to use heat and cold therapy to relieve symptoms, the nurse determines that teaching has been effective when the patient says

    a. "Heat treatments should not be used if muscle spasms are present."
    b. "Cold applications can be aplied for 15-20 minutes to relieve joint stiffness."
    c. "I should use heat applications for 20 minutes to relieve the symptoms of an acute flare."
    d. "When my joints are painful I can use a bag of frozen corn for 10-15 minutes to relieve the pain."

19. The nurse teaches the patient with RA that one of the most effective methods of aerobic exercise is

    a. ballet dancing.
    b. casual walking.
    c. aquatic exercises.
    d. low-impact aerobic exercises.

20. Characteristics of spondyloarthritides associated with the HLA-B27 antigen include

    a. absence of extraarticular disease.
    b. symmetric polyarticular arthritis.
    c. presence of rheumatoid factor and autoantibodies.
    d. high involvement of sacroiliac joints and the spine.

21. An important nursing intervention for the patient with ankylosing spondylitis is to teach the patient to

    a. wear roomy shoes with good orthotic support.
    b. sleep on the side with the knees and hips flexed.
    c. keep the spine slightly flexed while sitting, standing, or walking.
    d. perform chest-cage stretching and deep chest breathing exercises.

22. Match the following characteristic with their related rheumatic disorders (answers may be used more than once).

_____ a. High association with stress and irritable bowel syndrome

_____ b. Characteristic symptom of erythema migrans

_____ c. Methotrexate is a treatment of choice

_____ d. Fever and extraarticular symptoms present in full attack

_____ e. Infection of a joint often caused by hematogenous route

_____ f. Inflammation and dysfunction of salivary and lacrimal glands

_____ g. Diagnosed by finding of hypersensitive tender points

_____ h. An inflammatory polyarthritis associated with psoriasis

_____ i. Increased risk in persons with decreased host resistance and prior joint disease

_____ j. Lymphatic infiltration of bone marrow and visceral organs may occur

_____ k. Systemic infection with migratory polyarthritis that may involve cardiac and neurologic function

_____ l. Self-limiting reactive arthritis following enteric or venereal infections

1. Psoriatic arthritis
2. Reiter's syndrome
3. Septic arthritis
4. Lyme disease
5. Sjögren's syndrome
6. Fibromyalgia

23. A patient is seen at the outpatient clinic for a sudden onset of inflammation and severe pain in the great toe. A diagnosis of gout is made on the basis of

a. a family history of gout.
b. elevated urine uric acid levels.
c. elevated serum uric acid levels.
d. the presence of sodium urate crystals in synovial fluid.

24. During treatment of the patient with an acute attack of gout, the nurse would expect to administer

a. aspirin.
b. colchicine.
c. allopurinol (Zyloprim).
d. probenecid (Benemid).

25. A patient with gout is treated with drug therapy to prevent future attacks. The nurse teaches the patient that it is most important to

a. avoid all foods high in purine, such as organ meats.
b. have periodic determination of serum uric acid levels.
c. perform active ROM of all joints that have been affected by gout.
d. increase the dosage of medication with the onset of an acute attack.

26. The pathophysiology of systemic lupus erythematosus (SLE) is characterized by

a. destruction of constituents of the cell nucleus by autoantibodies.
b. overproduction of collagen that disrupts the functioning of internal organs.
c. formation of abnormal IgG that attaches to cellular antigens, activating complement.
d. increased activity of T-suppressor cells with B cell hypoactivity, resulting in an immunodeficiency.

27. Identify the most common clinical manifestations of SLE that may occur in each of the following organ systems.

a. Skin

b. Musculoskeletal

c. Cardiac

d. Pulmonary

e. Renal

f. Central nervous

g. Hematologic

28. A patient with newly diagnosed SLE asks the nurse how the disease will affect her life. The best response by the nurse is

a. "You can plan to have a near-normal life as SLE rarely causes death."
b. "It is difficult to tell since the disease is so variable in its severity and progression."
c. "Life span is shortened somewhat in people with SLE, but the disease can be controlled with long-term use of corticosteroids."
d. "Most people with SLE have alternating periods of remissions and exacerbations with rapid progression to permanent organ damage."

29. During an acute exacerbation, a patient with SLE is treated with corticosteroids. The nurse would expect the steroids to begin to be tapered when serum laboratory results indicate

a. increased RBC.
b. decreased ESR.
c. decreased anti-DNA.
d. increased complement.

30. Teaching that the nurse plans for the patient with SLE includes

a. ways to avoid exposure to sunlight.
b. increasing dietary protein and carbohydrate intake.
c. the necessity of genetic counseling before planning a family.
d. the use of nonpharmacologic pain interventions instead of analgesics.

31. During an acute exacerbation of SLE, the patient has a nursing diagnosis of impaired skin integrity. An appropriate nursing intervention for the patient is to

    a. clean the skin with mild soap and water and keep it dry.
    b. apply moisturizing lotion to the skin several times a day.
    c. use a mild astringent on the face to stimulate circulation.
    d. teach the patient to use cosmetics to minimize the skin changes.

32. During assessment of the patient with systemic sclerosis, the nurse would expect to find

    a. cool, cyanotic fingers with thinning skin over the joints.
    b. swan-neck deformity or ulnar drift deformity of the hands.
    c. low back pain, stiffness, and limitation of spine movement.
    d. expressionless facial features with pursed lips and a small mouth.

33. When caring for the patient with CREST syndrome associated with systemic sclerosis, the nurse teaches the patient to

    a. avoid exposure to the sun or other UV light.
    b. maintain a fluid intake of at least 3000 ml/day.
    c. monitor and keep a log of daily blood pressure.
    d. protect the hands and feet from cold exposure and injury.

34. During the acute phase of dermatomyositis, an appropriate patient outcome is

    a. performs active ROM qid.
    b. relates improvement in pain.
    c. does not experience aspiration.
    d. maintains absolute rest of affected joints.

35. A 56-year-old man develops symptoms of dermatomyositis. The patient asks the nurse why his physician has ordered so many screening diagnostic exams. The best response by the nurse includes the information that

    a. the disease is often precipitated by a hidden, latent infection.
    b. dermatomyositis in older men is often associated with a malignancy.
    c. extensive diagnostic testing is required to determine the effects of the disease on internal organs.
    d. symptoms of dermatomyositis are so rare in older persons that diagnosis requires extensive testing.

36. During assessment of the patient diagnosed with fibromyalgia syndrome (FMS), the nurse would expect the patient to report

    a. generalized muscle twitching and spasms.
    b. nonrestorative sleep with resulting fatigue.
    c. profound and progressive muscle weakness that limits ADLs.
    d. widespread musculoskeletal pain that is accompanied by inflammation and fever.

37. One criteria for a diagnosis of FMS is

    a. fiber atrophy found on muscle biopsy.
    b. elimination of all other causes of musculoskeletal pain.
    c. the presence of the manifestations of chronic fatigue syndrome.
    d. the elicitation of pain upon palpation of at least 11 of 18 identified tender points.

38. One important nursing intervention for the patient with FMS is to teach the patient to

   a. rest the muscles as much as possible to avoid triggering pain.
   b. plan night-time sleep and naps to obtain 12-14 hours of sleep a day.
   c. use stress-management techniques such as biofeedback, guided imagery, or tai chi.
   d. try the use of food supplements such as glucosamine and chondroitin for relief of pain.

39. A patient with debilitating fatigue has been diagnosed with chronic fatigue syndrome. List the four major criteria that must be present for this diagnosis to be made.

   a.

   b.

   c.

   d.

CASE STUDY

RHEUMATOID ARTHRITIS

Patient Profile

Mrs. M. is a 36-year-old obese Caucasian woman who has rheumatoid arthritis. When her symptoms began to interfere with her daily activities, she sought medical help.

Subjective Data

- Has painful, stiff hands and feet
- Feels tired all of the time
- Reports an intermittent low grade fever
- Takes naproxen (Naprosyn) 500 mg twice daily
- Wears a copper bracelet on the advice of a neighbor

Objective Data

- Hands show mild ulnar drift and puffiness
- Temperature 100° F (37.8° C)
- Admitted to the hospital for examination and comprehensive treatment plan
- Methotrexate (Rheumatrex) therapy is to be initiated

Critical Thinking Questions

1. How might the nurse explain the pathophysiology of rheumatoid arthritis to Mrs. M.?

2. What manifestations does Mrs. M. have that suggest the diagnosis of rheumatoid arthritis?

3. What results may be expected from methotrexate therapy? What are the nursing responsibilities related to methotrexate therapy?

4. What are some suggestions that may be offered to Mrs. M. concerning home management and joint protection?

5. How can the nurse help Mrs. M. recognize ineffective, unproved methods of treatment?

6. What other sources of information regarding arthritis might the nurse suggest to Mrs. M.?

7. Based on the assessment data presented, write one or more appropriate nursing diagnoses. Are there any collaborative problems?

CHAPTER 64 NURSING MANAGEMENT: CRITICAL CARE

1. A primary difference in the skills of a certified critical care nurse compared with nurses certified in medical-surgical nursing is an ability to

   a. diagnose and treat life-threatening diseases.
   b. detect and manage early complications of health problems.
   c. provide intensive psychologic support to the patient and family.
   d. use advanced technology to assess and maintain physiologic function.

2. Identify which of the common three reasons patients are admitted to the ICU apply in the following situations.

   a. Patient with diabetic ketoacidosis

   b. Patient with nondisplaced skull fracture who is alert and oriented

   c. Postoperative patient with mitral valve replacement

   d. Comatose patient who had an anaphylactic reaction with cardiopulmonary arrest at home with reestablishment of cardiac function

3. A nursing intervention that is indicated for the patient in the ICU who has a nursing diagnosis of anxiety related to ICU environment and sensory overload is

   a. eliminating unnecessary alarms and overhead paging.
   b. providing flexible visiting schedules for family members.
   c. administering sedatives or psychotropic drugs to promote rest.
   d. allowing the patient to do as much self-care in daily activities as possible.

4. The critical care nurse includes family members of the patient in the ICU as part of the health care team primarily because

   a. the costs of critical care will affect the entire family.
   b. family members are responsible for making health care decisions for the patient.
   c. the extent of the family members' involvement affects the patient's clinical course.
   d. family members that are ignored are more likely to question the patient's quality of care.

5. Review the concepts of cardiac output (CO), preload, and afterload by indicating whether the following conditions cause an increase or a decrease in the parameters under normal conditions.

   a. If heart rate (HR) is decreased, CO is __________________.

   b. If stroke volume (SV) is increased, CO is ______________.

   c. A decrease in preload will _______________ SV.

   d. An increase in fluid administration will _______________ preload.

   e. A decrease in afterload causes _______________ CO.

   f. Increased systemic vascular resistance (SVR) ______________ afterload.

6. During hemodynamic monitoring, the nurse finds that the patient has a decreased CO with unchanged pulmonary artery wedge pressure (PAWP), HR, and SVR. The nurse identifies that the patient has a decrease in

   a. SV.
   b. preload.
   c. afterload.
   d. contractility.

7. Before taking hemodynamic measurements, the monitoring equipment must be referenced by

   a. confirming that when pressure in the system is zero, the equipment reads zero.
   b. positioning the stopcock nearest the transducer level with the phlebostatic axis.
   c. placing the transducer on the left side of the chest at the fourth intercostal space.
   d. placing the patient in a left lateral position with the transducer level with the top surface of the mattress.

8. Identify whether the following statements are true or false. If a statement is false, correct the bold word(s) to make the statement true.

   _____ a. When a patient has an arterial catheter placed for arterial blood gas (ABG) sampling, the low pressure alarm must be activated to detect **disconnection** of the line.

   _____ b. A pulmonary artery flow-directed catheter has a balloon at the distal tip that floats into the **left side of the heart**.

   _____ c. The pressure obtained when the balloon of the pulmonary artery catheter is inflated reflects the preload of the **right ventricle**.

   _____ d. In the absence of mitral value impairment, the left ventricular end-diastolic pressure is reflected by the **PAWP**.

   _____ e. A decrease in SVO_2 (mixed venous blood) when arterial oxygenation, hemoglobin, and tissue perfusion are unchanged indicates **increased oxygen consumption**.

9. In preparing the patient for insertion of a pulmonary artery catheter, the nurse

   a. obtains informed consent from the patient.
   b. places the patient in a high Fowler's position.
   c. ensures that the patient has continuous ECG monitoring.
   d. performs an Allen test to confirm adequate ulnar artery perfusion.

10. Describe the techniques the nurse uses to obtain the following data from the pulmonary artery catheter.

    a. PAWP

    b. Thermodilution CO (TDCO)

11. A patient in the ICU with hemodynamic monitoring has the following values:

BP 90/68 mm Hg
HR 124
PAWP 22 mm Hg
CO 3.2 L/min
RAP (CVP) 14 mm Hg
Pulmonary artery pressure 38/20 mm Hg

a. Calculate the additional values that can be determined from these findings.

MAP PAP

SV SVR

b. What interpretation can the nurse make about the patient's circulatory status and cardiac function from these values?

12. A patient has SVO_2 of 52%, CO of 4.8 L/min, SpO_2 of 95%, and unchanged hemoglobin level. The nurse should assess the patient for

a. arrhythmias.
b. pain or movement.
c. pulmonary edema.
d. signs of septic shock.

13. The nurse observes a pulmonary artery wedge pressure waveform on the monitor when the balloon of the patient's pulmonary artery catheter is deflated. The nurse recognizes that

a. the patient is at risk for embolism because of occlusion of the catheter with a thrombus.
b. the patient is developing pulmonary edema that has increased the pulmonary artery pressure.
c. the patient is at risk for an air embolus because the injected air cannot be withdrawn into the syringe.
d. the catheter must be immediately repositioned to prevent pulmonary infarction or pulmonary artery rupture.

14. The use of the intraaortic balloon pump (IABP) would be indicated for the patient with

a. an insufficient aortic valve.
b. a dissecting aortic aneurysm.
c. accelerating or crescendo angina.
d. generalized peripheral vascular disease.

15. Identify whether the following statements are true or false. If a statement is false, correct the bold word(s) to make the statement true.

_____ a. The rapid deflation of the intraaortic balloon causes a decreased **preload**.

_____ b. During intraaortic counterpulsation, the balloon is inflated during **diastole**.

_____ c. A primary effect of the intraaortic balloon pump is increased **systolic** pressure.

16. To prevent arterial trauma during the use of the IABP, the nurse should

    a. reposition the patient q2h.
    b. check the site for bleeding every hour.
    c. prevent hip flexion of the cannulated leg.
    d. cover the insertion site with an occlusive dressing.

17. A patient who is hemodynamically stable is weaned from the IABP. The nurse should

    a. decrease the augmentation pressure to zero.
    b. stop the machine when hemodynamic parameters are satisfactory.
    c. stop the infusion flow through the catheter when weaning is initiated.
    d. continue the pumping every third or fourth beat until the balloon is removed.

18. Ventricular assist devices are designed to

    a. provide permanent, total circulatory support when the left ventricle fails.
    b. temporarily partially or totally support circulation until a donor heart can be obtained.
    c. support circulation only when patients cannot be weaned from cardiopulmonary bypass.
    d. reverse the effects of circulatory failure in patients with acute myocardial infarction in cardiogenic shock.

19. A comatose patient with a possible cervical spine injury is intubated with a nasal endotracheal tube. The nurse recognizes that in comparison with an oral endotracheal tube, a nasal tube

    a. requires the placement of a bite block.
    b. is more likely to cause laryngeal trauma.
    c. requires greater respiratory effort in breathing.
    d. provides for easier suctioning and secretion removal.

20. In preparing an alert patient in the ICU for oral endotracheal intubation, the nurse

    a. tells the patient that the tongue should be extruded while the tube is inserted.
    b. explains that gagging and feelings of suffocation may be experienced during insertion of the tube.
    c. positions the patient supine with the head hanging over the edge of the bed to align the mouth and trachea.
    d. informs the patient that while it will not be possible to talk during insertion of the tube, speech will be possible after it is correctly placed.

21. A patient has an oral endotracheal tube inserted to relieve an upper airway obstruction and to facilitate secretion removal. The first responsibility of the nurse immediately following placement of the tube is to

    a. suction the tube to remove secretions.
    b. mark the tube where it exits the mouth.
    c. secure the tube to the face with adhesive tape.
    d. assess for bilateral breath sounds and symmetric chest movement.

22. The nurse uses the minimal occluding volume (MOV) to inflate the cuff on an endotracheal tube to minimize the incidence of

    a. infection.
    b. hypoxemia.
    c. tracheal necrosis.
    d. accidental extubation.

23. Complete the following statements related to the patient with an endotracheal tube.

a. After inflating an endotracheal tube cuff, the nurse monitors the cuff pressure every ________ hours with a manometer to verify that the cuff pressure is ________ mm Hg.

b. Equipment that should be at the bedside for all patients undergoing endotracheal intubation includes ________________ equipment and a ______________________________.

c. A catheter used to suction an endotracheal tube should be no larger than _____________ the diameter of the ET tube.

d. When suctioning an endotracheal tube, the nurse uses a suction pressure of ________ to ________ mm Hg.

e. During endotracheal tube suctioning, each suction pass should be no longer than ________ seconds.

f. To prevent hypoxemia during endotracheal suctioning, the nurse always ________________ the patient before and after suctioning.

24. The nurse suctions the patient's endotracheal tube when the patient

a. has peripheral crackles in all lobes.
b. has not been suctioned for 2 hours.
c. has coarse rhonchi over central airways.
d. needs stimulation to cough and deep breathe.

25. While suctioning the endotracheal tube of a spontaneously breathing patient, the nurse notes that the patient develops bradycardia with premature ventricular contractions. The nurse should

a. stop the suctioning and assess the patient for spontaneous respirations.
b. attempt to resuction the patient with reduced suction pressure and pass time.
c. stop suctioning and ventilate the patient with a BVM with 100% oxygen until the heart rate returns to baseline.
d. stop the suctioning and ventilate the patient with slow, small-volume breaths using the bag-valve-mask (BVM) device.

26. Identify two precautions the nurse should take during mouth care of the patient with an oral endotracheal tube to prevent and detect tube dislodgement.

a.

b.

27. A patient with an oral endotracheal tube has a nursing diagnosis of risk for aspiration related to presence of artificial airway. An appropriate nursing intervention for this patient is to

a. monitor the patient for an inability to speak.
b. inflate the cuff during tube feedings and mouth care.
c. keep the ventilator tubing cleared of condensed water.
d. use a small-bore, blunt ring-tipped catheter to suction the oropharynx.

28. When extubation of the patient is being performed, it is most important to

    a. observe the patient for respiratory distress after tube removal.
    b. have the patient cough to remove secretions before extubation.
    c. perform tracheal suctioning immediately following removal of the tube.
    d. obtain a blood specimen for ABGs immediately after the tube is removed.

29. Mechanical ventilation is indicated when a patient in respiratory distress has a

    a. $PaCO_2$ of 50 mm Hg.
    b. tidal volume of 8 ml/kg.
    c. resting minute ventilation of 5L/min.
    d. maximal inspiratory pressure of –15 cm H_2O.

30. Indicate whether the following are characteristic of negative pressure ventilators (N), positive pressure ventilators (P), or both (B).

_____ a. Reduce intrathoracic pressure causing air to be pulled into lungs

_____ b. Require an artificial airway

_____ c. Expiration is passive as machine cycles off

_____ d. Most similar to physiologic ventilation

_____ e. Applied to outside of the body

_____ f. Can provide control and assist-control ventilatory modes

_____ g. Most frequently used with acutely ill patients

_____ h. Frequently used in the home for neuromuscular or nervous system disorders

31. Match the following types of positive pressure ventilators with their descriptions (answers may be used more than once).

_____ a. Indicated for patients at risk for barotrauma

_____ b. Preset volume of gas delivered with pressure-limiting valve

_____ c. Inspiration terminated when preset airway pressure achieved

_____ d. Volume of gas delivery limited if obstructions or asynchronous breathing present

_____ e. Consistent volume and oxygen concentrations delivered despite lung resistance

1. Volume ventilator
2. Pressure ventilator

32. Identify the ventilatory settings and modes described below.

    a. Positive pressure applied throughout the entire respiratory cycle ____________ ____________

    b. Patient self-regulates the rate and depth of spontaneous respirations but may also receive preset volume and frequency breaths by ventilator____________ ____________

    c. Ventilator delivers gas independent of patient's ventilatory efforts ____________

    d. Positive pressure applied only during inspiration that supplies a rapid flow of gas

       ____

    e. Preset tidal volume delivered at set frequency but can be delivered more frequently if patient attempts to inhale ____________

    f. Positive pressure applied to airway during exhalation ____________ ____________

    g. Delivery of small tidal volumes at a rapid respiratory rate ____________ ____________

    h. Prolonged inspiration and shortened expiration set to promote alveolar expansion and prevent collapse ____________

33. A patient in acute respiratory failure is receiving assist-control mechanical ventilation with PEEP of 10 cm H_2O. A sign that alerts the nurse to undesirable effects of increased airway and thoracic pressure is

    a. decreased PaO_2.
    b. increased crackles.
    c. decreased blood pressure.
    d. decreased spontaneous respirations.

34. The nurse recognizes that a factor that is commonly responsible for sodium and fluid retention in the patient on mechanical ventilation is

    a. increased ADH release.
    b. increased release of atrial natriuretic factor.
    c. increased insensible water loss via the airway.
    d. decreased renal perfusion with release of renin.

35. A patient with chronic COPD who is on mechanical assist-control ventilation has $PaCO_2$ of 40 mm Hg, PaO_2 of 70 mm Hg, and pH of 7.45. The nurse determines that

    a. the patient is responding optimally to the ventilator settings.
    b. the ventilator setting for rate or volume should be decreased.
    c. PEEP is indicated to increase the PaO_2 and improve gas exchange.
    d. an inverse-ratio ventilation maneuver should be set on the ventilator.

36. A patient receiving mechanical ventilation is very anxious and agitated, and neuromuscular blocking agents are used to promote ventilation. The nurse recognizes that

   a. the patient will be too sedated to be aware of the details of care.
   b. visitors should be encouraged to provide stimulation and diversion.
   c. the patient should always be addressed and explanations of care given.
   d. communication will not be possible with the use of neuromuscular blocking agents.

37. Identify five problems associated with inadequate nutrition in the patient receiving prolonged mechanical ventilation.

   a.

   b.

   c.

   d.

   e.

38. The nurse determines that alveolar hypoventilation is occurring in a patient on a ventilator when

   a. the patient develops cardiac arrhythmias.
   b. auscultation reveals an air leak around the ET cuff.
   c. ABG results show a $PaCO_2$ of 32 mm Hg and a pH of 7.47.
   d. the patient tries to breathe faster than the ventilator setting.

39. When weaning a patient from a ventilator, the nurse plans

   a. to decrease the delivered FIO_2 concentration.
   b. intermittent trials of spontaneous ventilation follow by ventilatory support to provide rest.
   c. substitution of ventilator support with a manual resuscitation bag if the patient becomes hypoxemic.
   d. to implement weaning procedures around-the-clock until the patient does not experience ventilatory fatigue.

40. A patient is to be discharged to home with mechanical ventilation. Before discharge, it is most important for the nurse to

   a. teach the family members to care for the patient with a home ventilator.
   b. stress the advantages for the patient in being cared for in the home environment.
   c. help the family plan for the extent of time and financial resources required for home care.
   d. have the family arrange for around-the-clock home health nurses for the first several weeks.

CASE STUDY

CRITICALLY ILL PATIENT

Patient Profile

Mr. V., age 42, has a history of HIV infection with the development of manifestations of AIDS 2 years ago. He has been hospitalized and treated twice for *Pneumocystis carinii* pneumonia and is now admitted to ICU with a suspected cryptococcal meningitis. Intracranial pressure (ICP) monitoring is instituted, and an arterial line and flow-directed pulmonary artery catheter are inserted. Endotracheal intubation with assist-control mechanical ventilation at 12 breaths per minute, 15 cm H_2O PEEP, and FIO_2 of 50% is established. (Note: This patient is very critically ill and requires review of intracranial pressure, septic shock, multiple organ dysfunction syndrome, and respiratory failure.)

Subjective Data

- Friend relates that Mr. V. had two generalized tonic-clonic seizures in the 2 hours before admission.

Objective Data

- Glasgow Coma Scale score: 6
- ICP: 22 mm Hg
- Vital signs: T 102.2° F (39° C), HR 80, RR 26/min, BP 100/46 mm Hg
- Arterial blood gases: PaO_2 65 mm Hg, $PaCO_2$ 32 mm Hg, HCO_3 16 mEq/L, pH 7.26
- Other lab: glucose 228 mg/dl (12.6 mmol/L), lactate 3 mEq/L (3 mmol/L), WBC 18,500/μl
- Hemodynamic monitoring values: CO 6 L/min, PAP 8 mm Hg, PAWP 15 mm Hg, SVR 530 dyne sec/cm^5, SvO_2 90%, SaO_2 92%
- Skin warm and dry
- Foley catheter inserted with 30 ml urine return

Critical Thinking Questions

1. What are the best indicators to use in Mr. V.'s case to monitor his hemodynamic status?

2. What effect might the use of PEEP have on Mr. V.'s intracranial pressure?

3. What is Mr. V.'s MAP? What MAP would be necessary to promote tissue and cerebral perfusion and yet not increase ICP?

4. What drugs and fluids would be indicated for Mr. V.'s treatment?

5. How may Mr. V.'s condition be complicated by gastrointestinal ischemia?

6. Explain the processes that account for the abnormal assessment findings in Mr. V.

7. Based on the assessment data presented, write one or more appropriate nursing diagnoses. Are there any collaborative problems?

CHAPTER 65 NURSING MANAGEMENT: SHOCK AND MULTIPLE ORGAN DYSFUNCTION SYNDROME

1. The key factor in describing any type of shock is

   a. hypoxemia.
   b. hypotension.
   c. vascular collapse.
   d. inadequate tissue perfusion.

2. Match each type of shock with its major classification.

   _____ a. Anaphylactic shock
   _____ b. Cardiogenic shock
   _____ c. Hypovolemic shock
   _____ d. Neurogenic shock
   _____ e. Septic shock

   1. Low blood flow
   2. Maldistribution of blood

3. Match the following precipitating factors with their related types of shock (answers may be used more than once).

   _____ a Acute myocardial infarction
   _____ b. Insect bites
   _____ c. Burns
   _____ d. Severe pain
   _____ e. Ventricular arrhythmias
   _____ f. Spinal cord injury
   _____ g. Hemorrhage
   _____ h. Urinary tract infection
   _____ i. Vaccines
   _____ j. Ruptured spleen
   _____ k. Epidural block
   _____ l. Severe vomiting and diarrhea
   _____ m. Peritonitis
   _____ n. Pulmonary embolism

   1. Neurogenic
   2. Cardiogenic
   3. Anaphylactic
   4. Septic
   5. Hypovolemic

4. Identify whether the following statements are true or false. If a statement is false, correct the bold word(s) to make the statement true.

_____ a. **Cardiogenic shock** is characterized by increased systemic vascular resistance (SVR), decreased cardiac output (CO), and decreased pulmonary artery pressure (PAP).

_____ b. In septic shock bacterial endotoxins cause vascular changes that result in **decreased systemic vascular resistance** with **increased cardiac output**.

_____ c. Bradycardia with hypotension is characteristic of **neurogenic shock**.

_____ d. In anaphylactic shock, death may occur as a result of **respiratory** failure.

_____ e. Hypovolemic shock from **relative hypovolemia** may occur with diabetes insipidus.

_____ f. Hemodynamic monitoring in the patient with cardiogenic shock will reveal an **increased** PAWP and a **decreased** cardiac index.

5. Complete the following pathophysiologic mechanisms that occur in the compensated stage of hypovolemic shock, filling the blanks with the following words or phrases. (See Figure 65-6)

Aldosterone secretion
Alpha-adrenergic stimulation
Beta-adrenergic stimulation
Decreased capillary hydrostatic pressure
Increased blood pressure
Increased heart strength and rate
Increased serum osmolality
Increased venous return to heart
Release of ADH
Renal water reabsorption
Renin release

a. Decreased blood pressure → ______________________________ → Fluid movement into intravascular space.

b. Decreased blood pressure → Activation of sympathetic nervous system → ______________________________ → Decreased blood flow to lungs, skin, and GI tract.

c. Decreased blood pressure → Activation of sympathetic nervous system → ______________________________ → Coronary vasodilation and ______________________________.

d. Decreased kidney perfusion → ____________________ → Increased angiotensin I.

e. Increased angiotensin II → ______________________ → Increased renal sodium reabsorption.

f. Increased angiotensin II → Venous and arterial vasoconstriction → ______________________ and ______________________________.

g. Increased renal sodium reabsorption → ______________________ → ______________________

h. Increased ADH → ______________________________ → Increased blood volume.

6. From the data presented in question 5, identify six clinical manifestations that may be evident in a patient in the compensated stage of shock.

   a.

   b.

   c.

   d.

   e.

   f.

7. When caring for a patient with shock, the nurse knows that alterations in coagulation are more likely to manifest earlier and more severely in the patient with

   a. septic shock.
   b. neurogenic shock.
   c. hypovolemic shock.
   d. anaphylactic shock.

8. Progressive tissue hypoxia leading to anaerobic metabolism and metabolic acidosis is characteristic of the progressive stage of shock. Identify what changes occur in the following tissues to cause this increasing tissue hypoxia.

   a. Renal

   b. Lung

   c. Capillaries

   d. Cardiac

9. The major pathophysiologic characteristic of the irreversible or refractory stage of shock is

   a. cardiac failure.
   b. renal insufficiency.
   c. ischemia of the intestinal mucosa.
   d. failure of compensatory mechanisms.

10. An intervention that is appropriate in the emergency management of any type of shock is

   a. vasopressor therapy.
   b. high volume fluid resuscitation.
   c. administration of high flow oxygen (100%).
   d. endotracheal intubation and mechanical ventilation.

11. An abnormal finding that is common in early, compensated shock is

   a. metabolic acidosis.
   b. increased serum sodium.
   c. decreased blood glucose.
   d. increased serum potassium.

12. In late, irreversible shock in a patient with massive thermal burns the nurse would expect the patient's laboratory results to reveal

    a. respiratory alkalosis.
    b. increased liver enzymes.
    c. decreased urine specific gravity.
    d. decreased hemoglobin and hematocrit.

13. A patient with hypovolemic shock is receiving lactated Ringer's for fluid replacement therapy. During this therapy, it is most important for the nurse to monitor the patient's

    a. serum pH.
    b. serum sodium.
    c. serum potassium.
    d. hemoglobin and hematocrit.

14. A patient in shock weighs 198 pounds. Adequate fluid volume replacement in this patient would be indicated by minimum urine output of ________ ml/hr.

15. Large amounts of crystalloid fluids are administered to a patient in septic shock to maintain adequate blood volume. As a result of this therapy, the nurse would expect the patient to experience

    a. decreased CO.
    b. systemic edema.
    c. decreased PAWP.
    d. decreased urinary output.

16. When caring for a patient in cardiogenic shock, the nurse recognizes that the metabolic demands of turning and moving the patient exceed the oxygen supply when hemodynamic monitoring reveals a change in

    a. SvO_2 from 62% to 54%.
    b. SV from 52 to 68 ml/beat.
    c. CO from 4.2 L/min to 4.8 L/min.
    d. SVR from 1300 to 1120 dyne sec/cm^5.

17. During administration of intravenous norepinephrine (Levophed), the nurse should assess the patient for

    a. hypotension.
    b. marked diuresis.
    c. metabolic alkalosis.
    d. decreased tissue perfusion.

18. When administering any vasoactive drug during the treatment of shock, the nurse knows that the goal of the therapy is to

    a. increase urine output to 50 ml/hr.
    b. maintain a MAP of at least 60 mm Hg.
    c. dilate vessels to improve tissue perfusion.
    d. constrict vessels to maintain blood pressure.

19. Identify two medical therapies that are specific to each of the following types of shock.

    a. Cardiogenic

    b. Hypovolemic

    c. Septic

    d. Anaphylactic

20. Identify four drugs and their actions that are used in treatment of cardiogenic shock that are not generally used for other types of shock.

	Drug	**Actions**
a.		
b.		
c.		
d.		

21. The most important nursing responsibility in the prevention of shock is

    a. frequently monitoring all patients' vital signs.
    b. using aseptic technique for all invasive procedures.
    c. being aware of the potential for shock in all patients at risk.
    d. teaching patients health promotion activities to prevent shock.

22. Five indicators of tissue perfusion that should be monitored in critically ill patients are

    ______________________, ____________________, ________________, ________________________, and

    ______________________.

23. Match each assessment area with the frequency with which the nurse should monitor its status when caring for an unstable patient in the acute phases of shock (some answers may not be used).

_____	a. Renal function	1. Continuously
_____	b. HR, BP, CVP, and PAP	2. q15min
_____	c. Neurologic function	3. q1hr
_____	d. GI function	4. q2hr
_____	e. Respiratory rate and rhythm	5. q4hr
_____	f. Oxygen saturation	6. q8hr
_____	g. Breath sounds	
_____	h. Electrocardiogram	
_____	i. Response to medication and fluid administration	
_____	j. Normal body temperature	

24. A patient in the progressive stage of shock has rapid, deep respirations. The nurse determines that the patient's hyperventilation is compensating for a metabolic acidosis when the patient's arterial blood gas results include

a. pH 7.42, PaO_2 80 mm Hg.
b. pH 7.48, PaO_2 69 mm Hg.
c. pH 7.38, $PaCO_2$ 30 mm Hg.
d. pH 7.32, $PaCO_2$ 48 mm Hg.

25. A patient in shock has a nursing diagnosis of fear related to severity of condition and perceived threat of death as manifested by verbalization of anxiety about condition and fear of death. An appropriate nursing intervention for the patient is to

a. administer antianxiety agents.
b. call a member of the clergy to visit the patient.
c. allow family members to visit as much as possible.
d. inform the patient of the current plan of care and its rationale.

26. Identify whether the following statements are true or false. If a statement is false, correct the bold word(s) to make the statement true.

_____ a. Systemic inflammatory response syndrome (SIRS) is always present in a patient with **sepsis**.

_____ b. Multiple organ dysfunction syndrome (MODS) **may occur independently** from SIRS.

_____ c. All patients with septic shock develop **MODS**.

_____ d. A patient with direct multiple organ damage from massive trauma experiences **primary** MODS.

_____ e. A common initial mediator that causes endothelial damage leading to SIRS and MODS is **endotoxin**.

_____ f. Generally, the first organ system affected by mediator-induced injury in SIRS and MODS is the **central nervous system**.

27. Match the following clinical findings with their related primary pathophysiologic processes of SIRS and MODS (answers may be used more than once).

_____ a. Decreased preload

_____ b. Metabolic acidosis

_____ c. Warm skin

_____ d. Prolonged prothrombin time

_____ e. Cerebral edema and increased intracranial pressure

_____ f. Translocation of GI bacteria

_____ g. Decreased serum protein and albumin

_____ h. Stress ulcers

_____ i. Cardiac arrhythmias

_____ j. Decreased serum potassium

_____ k. Decreased serum calcium, phosphate, and magnesium

1. Increased capillary permeability
2. Impaired liver function
3. Gastrointestinal ischemia
4. Vasodilation
5. Release of aldosterone
6. Impaired kidney function

28. The nurse recognizes that SIRS is present in the patient who manifests

   a. a $PaCO_2$ of 48 mm Hg and a WBC of 13,000/μl.
   b. a heart rate of 88/min and a $PaCO_2$ of 30 mm Hg.
   c. a temperature of 101.2° F (38.4° C) and confusion.
   d. a respiratory rate of 24/min and a WBC of 3800/μl.

29. An intervention that may prevent GI bacterial and endotoxin translocation in a critically ill patient with SIRS is

   a. early enteral feedings.
   b. surgical removal of necrotic tissue.
   c. aggressive, multiple antibiotic therapy.
   d. strict aseptic technique in all procedures.

30. The development of MODS is confirmed in a patient who manifests

   a. a urine output of 30 ml/hr, a BUN of 65 mg/dl, and a WBC of 1120/μl.
   b. upper GI bleeding, Glasgow Coma Scale score of 7, and a hematocrit of 25%.
   c. a respiratory rate of 45/min, a $PaCO_2$ of 60, and a chest x-ray with bilateral diffuse patchy infiltrates.
   d. an elevated serum amylase and lipase, a serum creatinine of 3.8 mg/dl, and a platelet count of 15,000/μl.

CASE STUDY

SEPTIC SHOCK

Patient Profile

Mr. M. is an 81-year-old man who was brought to the emergency department via an ambulance from a local nursing home. He was found by the nurses on their 6 AM rounds to be very confused, restless, and hypotensive.

Past Health History

Mr. M. is a type 1 diabetic with a history of prostate cancer and congestive heart failure. He has been a resident of the nursing home for 3 years. He has had an indwelling urinary catheter in place for 5 days because of difficulty voiding. Until today, Mr. M. has been very oriented and cooperative. His current medications are digoxin, hydrochlorothiazide (HydroDiuril), isosorbide (Isordil), and insulin.

Subjective Data

- Denies any pain or discomfort

Objective Data

- Neurologic: lethargic, confused, easily aroused, does not follow commands; moves all extremities in response to stimuli
- Cardiovascular: B/P 80/60, HR 112 and regular, T 104° F (40° C) rectal; heart sounds normal without murmurs or S_3, S_4; peripheral pulses weak and thready
- Skin: warm, dry, flushed
- Respiratory: RR 34 and shallow; breath sounds audible in all lobes with crackles bilaterally in the bases
- GI/GU: abdomen soft with hypoactive bowel sounds; urinary catheter in place draining scant, purulent urine

In the emergency department, two 16-gauge IVs were inserted and 700 ml of normal saline was given over the first hour. The patient was placed on 40% oxygen via face mask. The urinary catheter was removed and cultured and blood cultures were drawn at three intervals. A new catheter was inserted. The patient was started on IV antibiotics and was transferred to the ICU with the diagnosis of septic shock due to gram-negative sepsis.

In the ICU, a pulmonary catheter was inserted in addition to an arterial line.

- ABG results were pH 7.25; PaO_2 60 mm Hg; $PaCO_2$ 28 mm Hg; HCO_3^- 12 mEq/L; and SaO_2 82%.
- Hemodynamic pressures taken were right atrial pressure (CVP), PAP, PAWP, cardiac output, and SVR.
- Lab results were WBC 21,000/µl, Na 133 mEq/L, K 4.5 mEq/L, Cl 96 mEq/L, glucose 230 mg/dl, creatinine 1.7 mg/dl, Hb 12 g/dl, Hct 36%.

Mr. M.'s blood pressure continued to drop despite several liters of crystalloids. Dopamine was started and titrated up as needed to try to maintain the patient's blood pressure, in addition to more fluid administration. Despite all efforts, including intubation and mechanical ventilation, Mr. M. died on the sixth hospital day. The cause was multiple organ dysfunction syndrome due to gram-negative sepsis.

Critical Thinking Questions

1. What risk factors for septic shock were present in Mr. M.?

2. What preventive measures could have been taken by the nursing home staff in regard to Mr. M.?

3. What are the major pathophysiologic changes associated with sepsis?

4. Discuss the mechanism for hypotension in the patient with septic shock.

5. Explain the physiologic reasons for the following assessment parameters found in this patient.

   Decreased LOC

   Warm, dry, and flushed skin

   Tachycardia

   Tachypnea

   Fever

Decreased SVR

Increased CO

Oliguria

Hyperglycemia

6. Why was a pulmonary artery catheter indicated for Mr. M.?

7. Analyze the results of the arterial blood gases.

8. Describe the changes in the hemodynamic pressure that would be expected in Mr. M.

9. Explain the rationale for fluid therapy and the use of dopamine.

10. Based on the assessment data provided, write one or more nursing diagnosis. What collaborative problems are present?

CHAPTER 66 NURSING MANAGMENT: RESPIRATORY FAILURE AND ACUTE RESPIRATORY DISTRESS SYNDROME

1. Respiratory failure can be defined as

   a. the absence of ventilation.
   b. any episode in which part of the airway is obstructed.
   c. inadequate gas exchange to meet the metabolic needs of the body.
   d. an episode of acute hypoxemia caused by a pulmonary dysfunction.

2. Indicate whether the following descriptions are characteristic of hypoxemic respiratory failure (HO) or hypercapnic respiratory failure (HC).

   _____ a. Primary problem is inadequate oxygen transfer

   _____ b. Most often caused by V/Q mismatch and shunt

   _____ c. Referred to as ventilatory failure

   _____ d. Exists when PaO_2 is 60 mm Hg or less, even when oxygen is administered at 60%

   _____ e. Risk of inadequate oxygen saturation of hemoglobin exists

   _____ f. The body is unable to compensate for acidemia of increased $PaCO_2$

   _____ g. Primary problem is insufficient carbon dioxide removal

   _____ h. Referred to as oxygenation failure

   _____ i. Results from an imbalance between ventilatory supply and ventilatory demand

3. Identify whether the following statements are true or false. If a statement is false, correct the bold word(s) to make the statement true.

   _____ a. A V/Q ratio of 1:1 (V/Q = 1) reflects an **alveolar ventilation** of 4 to 5 L that is matched by 4 to 5 L of **blood flow** to the lungs each minute.

   _____ b. The V/Q ratio is **1 or greater** when there is less ventilation to an area of the lung than perfusion.

   _____ c. An extreme V/Q imbalance resulting from blood leaving the heart without being exposed to ventilated areas of the lung is known as **a shunt**.

   _____ d. An intrapulmonary shunt occurs when an obstruction impairs the flow of **blood to ventilated areas of the lung**.

   _____ e. In differentiating between a V/Q mismatch and an intrapulmonary shunt, an increase in PaO_2 on oxygen administration occurs in the patient with **an intrapulmonary shunt**.

   _____ f. Gas transport is slowed in **shunt**, resulting in exertional hypoxemia that is not present at rest.

4. Match the following physiologic mechanisms of hypoxemia with their common causes.

_____	a. V/Q mismatch 1 or greater	1. Pulmonary fibrosis
_____	b. V/Q mismatch 1 or less	2. Ventricular septal defect
_____	c. Anatomic shunt	3. Pulmonary embolism
_____	d. Intrapulmonary shunt	4. Atelectasis
_____	e. Diffusion limitation	5. Pulmonary edema

5. Match the mechanisms of hypoxemic respiratory failure that may occur in the patient with pneumonia with the responsible factors.

_____	a. V/Q mismatch	1. Thickening of alveolar-capillary membrane from secretions and fluid accumulation
_____	b. Diffusion limitation	2. Consolidation of lung lobules with exudate and alveolar collapse
_____	c. Shunt	3. Decreased alveolar ventilation from obstruction of bronchioles and terminal respiratory units
_____	d. Alveolar hypoventilation	4. Pleuritic pain and inflammation

6. Hypercapnic respiratory failure is most likely to occur in the patient who has

a. rapid, deep respirations in response to pneumonia.
b. slow, shallow respirations as a result of sedative overdose.
c. large airway resistance as a result of severe bronchospasm.
d. poorly ventilated areas of the lung due to pulmonary edema.

7. Acute respiratory failure in a patient with chronic lung disease would most likely be indicated by arterial blood gas (ABG) results of

a. PaO_2 52 mm Hg, $PaCO_2$ 56 mm Hg, pH 7.4.
b. PaO_2 46 mm Hg, $PaCO_2$ 52 mm Hg, pH 7.36.
c. PaO_2 48 mm Hg, $PaCO_2$ 54 mm Hg, pH 7.38.
d. PaO_2 50 mm Hg, $PaCO_2$ 54 mm Hg, pH 7.28.

8. Indicate whether the following manifestations are primarily characteristic of hypoxemic (HO) or hypercapnic (HC) respiratory failure.

_____ a. Cyanosis

_____ b. Morning headache

_____ c. Rapid, shallow respirations

_____ d. Metabolic acidosis

_____ e. "Three-word" dyspnea

_____ f. Use of tripod position

_____ g. Respiratory acidosis

9. The nurse detects the early onset of hypoxemia in the patient who experiences

a. restlessness.
b. hypotension.
c. central cyanosis.
d. cardiac arrhythmias.

10. The nurse assesses that a patient in respiratory distress is developing respiratory fatigue and the risk of respiratory arrest when the patient

a. has an increased I/E ratio.
b. cannot breathe unless he is sitting upright.
c. uses the abdominal muscles during expiration.
d. has a change in respiratory rate from rapid to slow.

11. A patient has a PaO_2 of 50 mm Hg and a $PaCO_2$ of 42 mm Hg because of an intrapulmonary shunt. The patient is most likely to respond best to

a. positive pressure ventilation.
b. oxygen administration at a FIO_2 of 100%.
c. administration of oxygen per nasal cannula at 1 to 3L/min.
d. clearance of airway secretions with coughing and suctioning.

12. A patient with a massive hemothorax and pneumothorax has absent breath sounds in the right lung. To promote improved V/Q matching, the nurse positions the patient

a. on the left side.
b. on the right side.
c. in a reclining chair bed.
d. supine with the head of the bed elevated.

13. A patient in hypercapnic respiratory failure has a nursing diagnosis of ineffective airway clearance related to increasing exhaustion. An appropriate nursing intervention for the patient includes

a. inserting an oral airway.
b. performing augmented coughing.
c. teaching the patient "huff" coughing.
d. teaching the patient slow pursed-lip breathing.

14. Hemodynamic monitoring is instituted in severe respiratory failure primarily to

a. detect V/Q mismatches.
b. evaluate oxygenation and ventilation status.
c. evaluate cardiac status and blood flow to tissues.
d. continuously measure the arterial blood pressure.

15. Drug therapy that is indicated for the patient in acute respiratory failure includes

a. sedatives to reduce the work of breathing.
b. prophylactic antibiotics to prevent respiratory infection.
c. inhaled corticosteroids to relieve bronchospasm and inflammation.
d. agents that relieve symptoms and reverse the underlying disease process.

16. In caring for a patient in acute respiratory failure, the nurse recognizes that noninvasive positive pressure ventilation (NIPPV) may be indicated for a patient who

    a. is comatose and has high oxygen requirements.
    b. has copious secretions that require frequent suctioning.
    c. responds to hourly bronchodilator nebulization treatments.
    d. is alert and cooperative but has increasing respiratory exhaustion.

17. Although acute respiratory distress syndrome (ARDS) may result from direct lung injury or indirect lung injury as a result of systemic inflammatory response syndrome (SIRS), the nurse is aware that ARDS is most likely to occur in the patient with a host insult resulting from

    a. septic shock.
    b. oxygen toxicity.
    c. multiple trauma.
    d. prolonged hypotension.

18. Identify the three primary changes that occur in the injury or exudative phase of ARDS.

    a.

    b.

    c.

19. Patients with ARDS who survive the acute phase of lung injury and who progress to the fibrotic stage manifest

    a. chronic pulmonary edema and atelectasis.
    b. resolution of edema and healing of lung tissue.
    c. continued hypoxemia because of diffusion limitation.
    d. increased lung compliance due to breakdown of fibrotic tissue.

20. In caring for the patient with ARDS, the most characteristic sign the nurse would expect the patient to exhibit is

    a. refractory hypoxemia.
    b. bronchial breath sounds.
    c. progressive hypercapnia.
    d. increased pulmonary artery wedge pressure.

21. The nurse suspects the early stage of ARDS in any seriously ill patient who

    a. develops respiratory acidosis.
    b. has diffuse crackles and rhonchi.
    c. exhibits dyspnea and restlessness.
    d. has a decreased PaO_2 and an increased $PaCO_2$.

22. A patient with ARDS has a nursing diagnosis of risk for infection. To detect the presence of infections commonly associated with ARDS, the nurse monitors

    a. gastric aspirate for pH and blood.
    b. the quality, quantity, and consistency of sputum.
    c. for subcutaneous emphysema of the face, neck, and chest.
    d. the mucous membranes of the oral cavity for open lesions.

23. The best patient response to treatment of ARDS occurs when initial management includes

    a. treatment of the underlying condition.
    b. administration of prophylactic antibiotics.
    c. treatment with diuretics and mild fluid restriction.
    d. endotracheal intubation and mechanical ventilation.

24. When mechanical ventilation is used for the patient with ARDS, positive end-expiratory pressure (PEEP) is often applied to

    a. prevent alveolar collapse and open up collapsed alveoli.
    b. permit smaller tidal volumes with permissive hypercapnia.
    c. promote complete emptying of the lungs during exhalation.
    d. permit extracorporeal oxygenation and carbon dioxide removal outside the body.

25. The nurse suspects that a patient with PEEP is experiencing negative effects of this ventilatory maneuver upon finding a(n)

    a. increasing PaO_2.
    b. decreasing heart rate.
    c. decreasing blood pressure.
    d. increasing central venous pressure (CVP).

26. Prone positioning is considered for a patient with ARDS who has not responded to other measures to increase PaO_2. The nurse knows that this strategy

    a. increases the mobilization of pulmonary secretions.
    b. decreases the workload of the diaphragm and intercostals muscles.
    c. promotes opening of atelectic alveoli in the upper portion of the lung.
    d. promotes perfusion of nonatelectic alveoli in the anterior portion of the lung.

CASE STUDY

ACUTE RESPIRATORY FAILURE

Patient Profile

Mrs. C. is a 75-year-old married woman with severe oxygen- and corticosteroid-dependent COPD. She is admitted to the MICU with acute respiratory failure and pneumonia.

Subjective Data

- Complains of shortness of breath and difficulty breathing

Objective Data

- ABGs on 2 L oxygen/min: pH 7.3, $PaCO_2$ 55 mm Hg, PaO_2 60 mm Hg, SaO_2 84%
- Awake, alert, and oriented
- Sitting in tripod position and using pursed-lip breathing

Collaborative Care

- O_2 at 2 L/min per NIPPV
- Albuterol (Ventolin, Proventil) nebulization q1hr prn
- IV aminophylline
- IV antibiotics
- IV corticosteroids

Critical Thinking Questions

1. What type of respiratory failure is Mrs. C. primarily experiencing? Briefly describe how this situation illustrates the concept of acute on chronic respiratory failure.

2. What factors contributed to the development of respiratory failure in Mrs. C.?

3. What are the pathophysiologic effects and clinical manifestations of Mrs. C.'s respiratory failure?

4. How do the tripod position and pursed-lip breathing contribute to respiratory function?

5. What is NIPPV? When is it contraindicated?

6. Which of the treatments instituted for Mrs. C. is the most important in returning her to her usual level of respiratory function?

7. Based on the assessment data presented, write one or more appropriate nursing diagnoses. Are there any collaborative problems?

CHAPTER 67 NURSING MANAGEMENT: EMERGENCY CARE SITUATIONS

1. Triage the following patient situations that may be present in an emergency department as emergent (E), urgent (U), or nonurgent (N).

   _____ a. A 6-year-old child with a temperature of 103.2° F (39.6° C)

   _____ b. A 22-year-old woman with asthma in acute respiratory distress

   _____ c. An infant who has been vomiting for 2 days

   _____ d. A 50-year-old man with low back pain and spasms

   _____ e. A 32-year-old woman who is unconscious following an automobile accident

   _____ f. A 58-year-old man with midsternal chest pain

   _____ g. A teenager with an angulated forearm following a sports injury

2. The nurse performing a primary survey in the emergency department is assessing

   a. the acuity of the patient's condition to determine priority of care.
   b. the status of airway, breathing, circulation or presence of deformity.
   c. whether the patient is responsive enough to provide needed information.
   d. whether the resources of the emergency department are adequate to treat the patient.

3. Identify two life-threatening conditions that the nurse may identify during each step of the primary survey and one appropriate intervention for the conditions that may be performed during the assessment.

	Conditions	Interventions
A		
B		
C		
D		

4. During the secondary survey of a trauma patient in the emergency department, it is important that the nurse obtain details of the incident primarily because

   a. the mechanism of injury can indicate specific injuries.
   b. important facts may be forgotten when needed later for legal actions.
   c. alcohol use associated with many accidents can affect treatment of injuries.
   d. many types of accidents or trauma must be reported to government agencies.

5. Identify the five interventions that are performed during the "F" step of the secondary survey.

   a.

   b.

   c.

   d.

   e.

6. Placement of a nasogastric tube is contraindicated during emergency care when the patient has a possible

   a. inhalation injury.
   b. basilar skull fracture.
   c. cervical spine fracture.
   d. intraabdominal bleed.

7. In assessing the emergency patient's health history, what information is obtained with the use of the mnemonic AMPLE?

   a. A

   b. M

   c. P

   d. L

   e. E

8. A trauma patient has open wounds, and the nurse questions the patient regarding her tetanus immunization status. Tetanus immunoglobulin would be administered if the patient has

   a. had only 3 doses of tetanus toxoid.
   b. had less than 3 doses of tetanus toxoid.
   c. not had a dose of tetanus toxoid in the past 5 years.
   d. not had a dose of tetanus toxoid in the past 10 years.

9. Following the death in the emergency department of a 36-year-old man from a massive head injury, it would be appropriate for the nurse to

   a. ask the family members whether they have ever considered organ donation.
   b. notify an organ procurement agency that a death has occurred that could result in organ donation.
   c. explain to the family what a generous act it would be to donate the patient's organs to another who needs them.
   d. ask the family to check the patient's driver's license to determine whether he had designated approval of donation of his organs in case of death.

10. Match the heat-related emergencies with their characteristics (answers may be used more than once).

_____ a. Rectal temperature of 103.6° F (40° C)
_____ b. Treated with rapid cooling methods
_____ c. Related to salt deficiency following heavy work without adequate fluids
_____ d. High risk of mortality and morbidity
_____ e. Volume and electrolyte depletion
_____ f. Elevated core temperature without sweating
_____ g. Associated with prolonged standing and heat exposure
_____ h. Oxygen administration necessary
_____ i. Causes mild confusion, headache, and dilation of pupils
_____ j. Extremity swelling is only symptom

1. Heat edema
2. Heat cramps
3. Heat syncope
4. Heat exhaustion
5. Heat stroke

11. During rewarming of a patient's toes that have suffered deep frostbite, the nurse

a. applies sterile dressings to blisters.
b. places the feet in a cool water bath.
c. ensures that analgesics are administered.
d. massages the digits to increase circulation.

12. A patient is brought to the emergency department following a skiing accident in which he was not found for several hours. He is unconscious and has a slowed respiratory and heart rate. During the initial assessment of the patient, the nurse should

a. avoid moving the patient as much as possible.
b. initiate active core rewarming interventions.
c. monitor the core temperature via the axillary route.
d. expose the patient to check for areas of frostbite and other injuries.

13. A homeless man is brought to the emergency department in profound hypothermia with a temperature of 85° F (29.4° C). On initial assessment, the nurse would expect to find

a. shivering and lethargy.
b. fixed and dilated pupils.
c. respirations of 6 to 8 per minute.
d. blood pressure obtainable only by Doppler.

14. Indicate whether each of the following conditions occur with freshwater near-drowning (F), saltwater near-drowning (S), or both (B).

_____ a. Hypervolemia

_____ b. Pulmonary edema

_____ c. Hemoconcentration

_____ d. Destruction of surfactant

_____ e. Hypovolemia

_____ f. Metabolic acidosis

15. The priority of management of the near-drowning patient is

a. correction of hypoxia.
b. correction of acidosis.
c. maintenance of fluid balance.
d. prevention of cerebral edema.

16. A patient is admitted to the emergency department following a snakebite to the dorsal aspect of the hand. A nursing intervention that is appropriate for the patient is

a. application of ice.
b. elevation of the extremity.
c. application of a tourniquet.
d. removal of rings and watches.

17. The ascending paralysis caused by exposure to the dog tick may cause respiratory arrest unless

a. the tick is removed.
b. antibiotics are administered.
c. an antidote for the neurotoxin is administered.
d. hemodialysis is instituted to remove the neurotoxin.

18. Identify whether the following statements are true or false. If a statement is false, correct the bold word(s) to make the statement true.

_____ a. The type of bite that carries the highest risk of infection is **cat** bites.

_____ b. Rabies vaccination is always indicated when a bite is caused by a **carnivorous wild animal**.

_____ c. Emergency management of surface exposure to most toxins is **application of topical steroids**.

_____ d. Treatment of ingested toxic alkali substances includes administration of **activated charcoal**.

_____ e. A systemic response to a **brown recluse spider** bite may cause hemolysis leading to renal failure and death.

19. For the following ingested poisons, identify all those for which gastric lavage is indicated.

_____ a. Aspirin

_____ b. Cyanide

_____ c. Iron

_____ d. Bleach

_____ e. Acetaminophen

_____ f. Drain cleaner

20. Match the actions with the following agents used in the management of ingested toxins.

_____ a. Syrup of ipecac — 1. Neutralize and dilute strong acids or alkalis

_____ b. Milk — 2. Increase elimination of toxins from GI tract

_____ c. Activated charcoal — 3. Induce vomiting

_____ d. Cathartics — 4. Absorb poisons in GI tract preventing systemic absorption

21. A patient is admitted unconscious to the emergency department by his family, who brought an empty container of lithium found near the patient. A large oral-gastric tube is inserted and the nurse prepares to administer

a. cathartics.
b. syrup of ipecac.
c. a gastric lavage.
d. activated charcoal.

22. In the following diagram, check the columns that apply to each of the biologic agents of terrorism.

Agent	Bacterial	Viral	Person-to-Person Spread	Antibiotic Treatment	Active Vaccine	Passive Vaccine
Botulism						
Anthrax						
Plague						
Hemorrhagic Fever						
Tularemia						
Smallpox						

23. Match the following biologic agents of terrorism with their characteristics (answers may be used more than once).

_____	a. Ebola is a highly lethal type of this disease	1. Botulism
_____	b. The septicemic form is most lethal	2. Anthrax
_____	c. Toxins cause hemorrhage and destruction of lung tissue	3. Smallpox
		4. Plague
_____	d. Neurotoxins that cause paralysis respiratory failure	5. Tularemia
_____	e. Spread by flea bites	6. Hemorrhagic fever
_____	f. Hemorrhage of tissues with organ failure	
_____	g. Lesions are pustular vesicles	
_____	h. Skin lesions are most common form	
_____	i. Only agent without preventive or active treatment	
_____	j. Primarily an infection of rabbits	
_____	k. People under the age of 35 are the most vulnerable population	
_____	l. Death may occur within 24 hours of exposure	

24. A victim of a sublethal dose of whole body ionizing radiation exposure is admitted to the emergency department several hours after exposure. On assessment the nurse would expect the patient to report

a. hair loss.
b. nausea and vomiting.
c. bleeding from the gums and nose.
d. bruises on skin not covered by clothing.

CASE STUDY

HEAT STROKE

Patient Profile

Mr. M., age 72, was taking a short break from nailing new shingles on his roof during the summer when he lost consciousness and collapsed in his yard. He was brought by ambulance to the emergency department accompanied by his wife.

Subjective Data

- Wife states he has been working all week on the roof even though he has not felt well the last day or two

Objective Data

- Vital signs: T 106.6° F (41.4° C), HR 124 and weak and thready, RR 36 and shallow, BP 82/40
- Skin hot, dry, and pale

Critical Thinking Questions

1. What factors in Mr. M.'s history place him at risk for heat stroke?

2. What laboratory tests would the nurse anticipate to be ordered, and what alterations in these tests would be indications of heat stroke?

3. How would cooling for Mr. M. be carried out?

4. What supportive treatment is indicated for Mr. M.?

5. What should Mrs. M. be told about Mr. M.'s condition?

6. Based on the assessment data presented, write one or more appropriate nursing diagnoses. Are there any collaborative problems?

ANSWERS TO WORKSHEETS

CHAPTER 1

1. a, c, d, f
2. fear, anxiety, pain, impaired physical mobility of arm, disturbed body image, ineffective role performance, anticipatory grieving
3. b, d; the role and legal practice of advanced practice nurses are regulated by each state.
4. c. Rationale: Although evidence-based practice (EBP) uses results of research to improve quality and outcomes of health care, research utilization is not the only component of EBP. Research results are summarized into a single conclusion about the state of practice, and then it is translated into a clinical practice guideline for implementation based on the practitioner's expertise and the patient's unique circumstances.
5. c. Rationale: The classification of nursing interventions (NIC) and outcomes (NOC) provides a standardized language that describes outcomes that are responsive to nursing intervention and interventions that are appropriate for nursing diagnoses. The nurse individualizes care for a specific patient by selecting outcomes and interventions based on individual patient assessment and nursing diagnoses. Nursing diagnosis classified by NANDA is the language that is used to identify patient problems that are the specific domain of nursing practice.
6. a. North American Nursing Diagnosis Association (NANDA); b. Nursing Outcomes Classification (NOC); c. Nursing Intervention Classification (NIC)
7. a. 2; b. 3; c. 4; d. 1; e. 2; f. 5; g. 3; h. 2; i. 4; j. 5; k. 4
8. a. independent: assessment of physical and psychologic status, evaluation of response to medications, and dietary teaching
   b. collaborative: communication with physician regarding assessment findings and lab results and communication with dietician about dietary order and patient status
   c. dependent: administration of medication
9. a. I; A need is not a nursing diagnosis; b. I; Traction is not a treatable condition; c. I; Dyspnea is a symptom of activity intolerance, not the cause; d. C; e. I; Surgery is a medical pathologic situation that cannot be treated by nursing; f. C; g. I; Bowel obstruction is a medical pathologic situation; h. I; Cardiac monitoring is equipment, not a nursing diagnosis.
10. a. CP; b. ND; c. ND; d. CP; e. ND; f. ND; g. ND; h. CP; i. ND; j. CP
11. Activity intolerance related to prolonged bed rest as manifested by shortness of breath on exertion, weakness and fatigue, failure of pulse to return to preactivity level after 3 minutes.
12. a. Life-threatening problems; b. Maslow's hierarchy of needs; c. Patient's perception of importance; d. Identification of nursing diagnoses that may be managed simultaneously
13. For anorexia, nursing measures would include mouth care, odor control, presentation of foods, offering of favorite foods, etc. These measures are very different from those for difficulty swallowing, which would include checking gag reflex, positioning, offering small bites of formed foods, avoiding free liquids in the mouth, etc. The differences show how important it is to determine the correct etiology of a nursing diagnosis.
14. a. I; not measurable, behavioral, nor does it ensure he will take medications; b. C; c. I; not measurable, no criteria, no time designation; d. I; not measurable, not behavioral; e. C
15. There may be many correct answers. Examples include the following:
    a. Turn patient every 2 hours using the following schedule: L side → back → R side → L side → back; inspect and document all at-risk areas for blanching and erythema at each position change.
    b. Provide 8 ounces of fluids every 2 hours (even hours) while patient is awake (prefers cold liquids); assist patient to choose 5 fresh fruits or vegetables from menu each day.
16. a. The mistake was made during assessment when the nurse did not ask why the patient had not taken her medication regularly and the appropriate etiology for the nursing diagnosis was not validated.
    b. The nursing diagnosis should be changed in this case to reflect an etiology of lack of financial resources, and nursing interventions would not be teaching about the medications but rather perhaps consulting with the physician regarding the use of generic medications or a change in prescription and perhaps providing the patient with a list of discount drug sources. The patient outcome would remain the same.
17. a. More efficient (selection rather than writing); b. Increased availability to all appropriate health

care providers; c. Maintenance of patient anonymity and confidentiality; d. Contribute to evidence-based practice by easy tracking of the effectiveness of nursing interventions

CHAPTER 2

1. a. 5; b. 4; c. 7; d. 2; e. 9; f. 1; g. 6; h. 10; i. 3; j. 8
2. a. Learned through the processes of language acquisition and socialization; b. Shared by all members of the same cultural group; c. Adapted to specific conditions such as environmental factors; d. Dynamic and ever-changing
3. a. cultural knowledge; b. cultural awareness; c. cultural encounter; d. cultural skills
4. c. Rationale: Cultural competence is demonstrated by an awareness of traditional treatments that people of other cultures may use to treat illness. Southeast Asians and Hispanics may use cupping to treat a variety of disorders, and this procedure leaves bruising on the skin. The patient may be reluctant to disclose traditional treatments upon direct questioning, and the nurse should not presume abuse before considering cultural factors. Only in rare instances would a disease leave perfectly round cup-sized bruises on the skin.
5. Examples may include any instances of the following:
   a. Patients may be late for appointments, skip appointments entirely, or delay seeing a health care provider because social events are more important.
   b. Lack of health insurance, limited financial resources, or illegal immigrant status may deter patients from using the health care system.
   c. Ethnic foods may be high in sodium and fat or low in calcium and protein. If dietary changes required by health problems are not made within the context of the patient's normal diet, chances are high the patient will not make the changes.
   d. Personal space zones are a strong cultural trait. A patient may move closer to the nurse, causing a feeling of discomfort for the nurse, or if the nurse increases the personal space, the patient may be offended.
   e. Religious beliefs or practices, faith in folk medicine, or negative experiences with culturally insensitive health care may delay or prevent patients from seeking health care.
6. b. Rationale: Traditional Native American rituals may include healing ceremonies used in addition to conventional therapy to promote a balance of physical, spiritual, and emotional wholeness believed to be necessary for wellness. These rituals may or may not be part of formal religious beliefs and may positively alter the progression of physical illnesses.
7. b. Rationale: In some cultural groups, especially Asian, Hispanic, and Native American, there is an emphasis on interdependence rather than independence. The nurse should be aware that in other cultures decisions for the patient may be made by other family members or may be made collectively by the patient and his/her family. All of the other options reflect insensitive assumptions that the patient should make an autonomous decision.
8. b. Rationale: In the Arabic culture, male-female roles are strictly observed. A female should not be touched by a male other than her husband, nor should she be alone with another male. An Arabic woman would be very uncomfortable being cared for by a male nurse or would be put in the position of having to refuse the care.
9. cancer
10. a. beta-adrenergic blockers; b. atropine; c. antidepressants; d. antidysrhythmics; e. antiseizure drugs; f. mydriatrics; g. others: analgesics, antianxiety agents
11. b. Rationale: Susto is a culture-bound syndrome also known as "fright sickness" that is a traumatic anxiety-depressive state resulting from a frightening experience. Empacho causes abdominal pain and cramping from food balls forming in the intestinal tract; ghost sickness causes nightmares, weakness, and a sense of suffocation; and bilis brought on by strong anger causes headaches, stomach disturbances, and loss of consciousness.
12. a. Rationale: Knowledge of cultural beliefs and behaviors can be used to determine the degree to which the patient shares commonalities with a given culture, but the nurse must be careful not to stereotype the patient, assuming that all members of a specific culture are alike and share the same values and beliefs. Individual differences always exist within a culture, and just as the nurse is an individual within a culture, so are patients unique individuals.

13.	Native American Patient	Traditional Hispanic Patient
Communication	comfortable with silence; silence necessary for thinking; avoid direct eye contact and consider it disrespectful	expect eye contact from others but will not return direct gaze; comfortable with close personal space
Illness factors	family history of diabetes; less tolerance to alcohol; less pupillary dilation with mydriatrics; use of traditional healers	family history of diabetes; cancer of cervix, esophagus, gallbladder, stomach; less pupillary dilation with mydriatrics; intolerance to and side effects from antidepressants; use of traditional healers
Culture-bound syndromes	ghost sickness	empacho, susto, bilis or colera, nervios

CHAPTER 3

1. Yes. Although some of the information contained in the medical history may be useful to nursing, the medical history focuses on the diagnosis of patients' health problems, whereas the nursing history is used to gather data that will provide a health profile for comprehensive health care, including patients' potential and actual health problems and health promotion.
2. *Subjective:* short of breath; pain in chest upon breathing; coughing makes head hurt; aches all over. *Objective:* respiratory rate of 28; coughing yellow sputum; skin hot and most; temperature 102.2° F (39° C).
3. Examples: Many answers could be correct. It is helpful to preface the question with the reason it is being asked.
   a. "Many patients taking drugs for hypertension have problems with sexual function. Have you experienced any problems?"
   b. "Alcohol may interact dangerously with drugs you may receive or may cause withdrawal problems in the hospital. Can you describe what alcohol intake you have had recently?"
   c. "It is important to contact and treat others who may have the infection you do. Would you please tell me who you have been sexually intimate with in the last 6 weeks?"
   d. "Many people today use herbs or supplements for health reasons, but they may cause some interactions with medications. What types of herbs, vitamins, or supplements do you use?"
4. d. Rationale: Data are required regarding the immediate problem, but gathering additional information can be delayed. The patient should not receive pain medication before pertinent information related to allergies or the nature of the problem is obtained. Questions that require brief answers do not elicit adequate information for a health profile. A friend or family member may not be present or adequately informed, and the patient may not achieve a pain-free state.
5. c. Rationale: When a patient describes a feeling, the nurse should ask about the factors surrounding the situation to clarify the etiology of the problem. An incorrect nursing diagnosis may be made if the statement is taken literally and if the meaning is not explored with the patient. A sense of "tired and wrung-out" does not necessarily indicate a need for rest or sleep, and there is no way to know that treatment will relieve the problem.
6. There may be many correct answers. Examples include the following:
   a. "Can you tell me how you are feeling?"
   b. "Describe your relationship with your wife."
   c. "Can you describe your experience with this illness?"
   d. "What is your usual activity during the day?"
7. a. 1; b. 10; c. 10; d. 8; e. 4; f. 4, 6; g. 2, 3; h. 6; i. 6; j. 6; k. 7; l. 5; m. 3, 9; n. 2; o. 4; p. 12; q. 11; r. 2; s. 10; t. 13
8. d. Rationale: Abnormal lung sounds are usually associated with chronic bronchitis, and their absence is a negative finding. Chest pain is a positive finding, and radiation is not expected for all chest pain. Elevated blood pressure in hypertension is a positive finding, and pupils that are equal and react to light and accommodation is a normal finding.
9. a. Rationale: The screening physical examination is performed for health surveillance and health maintenance purposes. A regional examination addressing specific problems would be performed for the other conditions.
10. a. 2; b. 2; c. 3; d. 2; e. 1; f. 4

11. d. Rationale: The usual sequence of physical assessment techniques is inspection, palpation, percussion, and auscultation. However, because palpation and percussion can alter bowel sounds, in abdominal assessment the sequence should be inspection, auscultation, percussion, and palpation.
12. b. Rationale: A nurse should use the same efficient sequence each examination to avoid forgetting a procedure, a step in the sequence, or a body part, but a specific method is not required. Patient safety, comfort, and privacy are considerations but not the priorities. The nursing history data should be collected in an interview to avoid prolonging the examination.
13. *Across:* 1. Navajo; 7. sign in; 8. otitis; 9. atrium; 11. rash; 13. polyp; 15. uvula; 18. side; 20. ocular; 21. smooth; 22. inhale; 23. masses
    Down: 2. arthro; 3. artery; 4. ossas; 5. in situ; 6. anemia; 10. thud; 12. apsa; 13. ptosis; 14. laughs; 16. venous; 17. little; 19. irsem

CHAPTER 4

1. a. maintenance of health; b. management of illness; c. appropriate selection and use of treatment options; d. prevention of disease
2. a. adults approach learning as problem solving
   b. adults are independent learners; adults resist learning when conditions are incongruent with their self-concepts
   c. readiness to learn arises from life's changes; adults learn best when the topic is of immediate value
   d. adults approach learning as problem solving; adults see themselves as doers
   e. adults resist learning when conditions are incongruent with their self-concepts
   f. adults see themselves as doers
   g. past experiences are resources for learning
3. a. Rationale: During the action stage of behavior change, the patient may experience relapses, and the behavior has not become sustained over a period of time. Walking to manage osteoporosis is a recommended lifetime behavior, and the change is not in the maintenance stage until it is sustained without relapses. In the termination stage, the behavior is part of the person's lifestyle and no longer considered a change.
4. a. Example: a sudden episode (acute) where the heart muscle (myocardium) is damaged from a lack of blood supply (infarction)
   b. Example: the intravenous (IV) injection of a dye to visually record (gram) the kidneys (pyelo)
   c. Example: damage (pathy) to the retina (retino) of the eye as a complication of diabetes
5. a. Rationale: An empathetic approach to teaching requires that the nurse discover and understand the world of the patient and teach according to the patient's needs. The other options are important but not directly related to empathy.
6. a. Rationale: According to the Family Support Model, no part of the system is an independent agent because the well-being of the individual depends on support from the family, community resources, and the medical care system. The support provided by the family unit has been shown to affect a patient's health outcome, and thus teaching plans often include identified family members. Family members may not be responsible for continued care of the patient, and if patients and families have different educational needs, the nurse addresses this in planning teaching.
7. b. Rationale: To promote self-efficacy, it is important that the person is successful in new endeavors to strengthen the belief in his/her ability to manage a situation. To avoid early failure, the nurse should work with the patient to present simple concepts related to knowledge and skills the person already has. Motivation and relevancy are important factors in adult learning but are more often a result of self-efficacy, not a method of promoting it.
8. a. Use supplementary illustrations and written materials; provide audiotapes or audiovisual presentations with headphones that block environmental noise and promote auditory function.
   b. Support the patient during this time, and do not argue about the need for change in behavior; wait until the patient is ready to learn to begin teaching.
   c. Evaluate the medication schedule and change, if possible, to increase alertness; if sedation is the objective of the medication, consider teaching family members or other caregivers.
   d. Provide only brief explanations, and wait to present more detailed instruction until the pain has been controlled.
   e. Use anxiety-reducing interventions such as sitting with the patient or listening to patients talk about their feelings and fears to decrease anxiety before attempting to teach; present nonthreatening information first and allow time for gradual learning.
   f. Plan role-playing situations to allow patients to rehearse new behaviors; use peer groups to promote learning from those who have been in the same situation.

   g. Provide small amounts of information repeated very frequently; if impairment is marked, it will be necessary to teach a caregiver as well as the patient.
   h. Set goals for teaching that are most important, and refer the patient to a community agency for continued teaching and follow-up after discharge.
   i. Be sure that educational materials are written at an 8th grade level; use audiovisual materials with simple, lay language.
   j. Provide a variety of written educational materials; refer the patient to appropriate Internet resources for information.
9. b. Rationale: The nursing diagnosis should specify the exact nature of the knowledge deficit so that the objectives, strategies, implementation, and evaluation relate to the identified problem. The problem is deficient knowledge, and a nursing diagnosis that states that the knowledge deficit is related to a lack of interest is in error. The statement "potential for cardiac arrhythmias" is a collaborative problem rather than a nursing diagnosis.
10. Example: The patient (who) will select foods high in potassium (behavior) from a given list of common foods (condition) with 90% accuracy (criteria).
11. d. Rationale: The learning objectives should be jointly developed by the patient and the nurse, and once these have been identified, the nurse, the patient, and the patient's family should choose the strategies that are most beneficial to meet the objectives. This approach supports all interventions identified as successful to adult and patient education.
12. a. 5; b. 6; c. 1; d. 1; e. 3; f. 2; g. 4; h. 3; i. 7; j. 5; k. 7; l. 6; m. 8; n. 7
13. c. Rationale: If audiovisual and written materials do not help the patient meet the learning objectives, they are a waste of time and expense and the nurse should ensure that these materials are accurate and appropriate for each specific patient. Audio and visual materials are often supplementary either before or after other presentation of information and do not need to include all the information the patient needs to learn in order to be of value. Patients with auditory and visual limitations may find these materials useful because they can adjust volume and size of the images.
14. Example:
    Action: This medicine, atorvastatin, keeps the liver from making so much cholesterol.
    Uses: The medicine is used to lower cholesterol and fats in the blood. It helps prevent heart attacks and strokes.
    Side Effects: Overall, this medicine does not cause many side effects. Stomach upset or intestinal gas may occur. Other effects can include liver and pancreas problems, skin rashes and itching, hair loss, muscle pain, eye changes, and headache. Call your doctor if these problems occur or get worse.
    Precautions: Tell your doctor if you get any yellowing of your eyes or skin or have vomiting. Tell your doctor if you have any liver disease in the past, alcoholism, low blood pressure, bad infections, seizure disorders, diabetes or thyroid problems, physical injuries, or blood imbalances. Drink very little or no alcohol because this can damage your liver and cause more side effects. If you have other effects not listed above, call your doctor.
    Interactions: This medicine will interact with many other medicines to cause problems. Give your doctor a list of all medicines that you take. Do not start any new medicine while you are taking atorvastatin without checking with your doctor.
15. a. Direct observation
    b. Ask direct question or use a written measurement tool (ask patient to write the symptoms)
    c. Direct observation with observation of verbal and nonverbal cues
    d. Direct observation
16. b. Rationale: A statement that documents what the patient does as a result of teaching indicates whether the learning objective has been met and provides the best documentation of patient instruction. "Understand" is not a measurable behavior and does not validate that learning has occurred. The content and strategies of patient education are documented in the teaching plan and would not be repeated in charting related to the outcome of instruction.

CHAPTER 5

1. There are many correct responses. Examples include the following:
   a. Older people cannot learn new skills as well as younger people can ("can't teach an old dog new tricks").
   b. Most old people are ill.
   Also:
   - Old people are not (or should not be) sexually active.
   - Old people are terrible drivers.
   - Forgetfulness is a sign of senility.
2. a. Rationale: The sense of a life well lived and acceptance of death is characteristic of Erikson's ego-integrity, which is in contrast to the despair

that may occur when life review reveals missed opportunities and wrong directions taken. According to Havighurst, if earlier developmental tasks are met, the work of the older adult is adjusting to declining health and social role changes. Peck's developmental tasks for the older adult include transcending the body, and self-esteem is maintained through the use of wisdom and judgment. In Levinson's theory of development, late adulthood is characterized by periods of change and growth toward personal goals and periods of stability to maintain the life structures necessary to pursue the goals.

3. a. 2; b. 4; c. 3; d. 1; e. 2; f. 3; g. 1
4. b. Rationale: Four characteristics that are common to all adult developmental models include development occurring throughout the life span; self-identity and growth through developmental tasks; movement through hierarchic stages from simplicity, rigidity, and narrowness to complexity, flexibility, and comprehensiveness; ultimate goal of achieving autonomy, separateness, and independence.
5. a. 6; b. 4; c. 1; d. 7; e. 3; f. 8; g. 5; h. 2
6. There may be other correct responses, but examples include the following:
   a. decreased intestinal villae; decreased digestive enzyme production and secretion; decreased dentine and gingival retraction; increased taste threshold for salt and sugar
   b. decreased force of cardiac contraction; decreased cardiac muscle mass; increased fat and collagen
   c. decreased skeletal muscle mass; increased joint flexion; stiffening of tendons and ligament; decreased cortical and trabecular bone; changes in eye and ear that impair vision and hearing
   d. decreased bladder smooth muscle and elastic tissue; decreased sphincter control
   e. decreased ciliary action; decreased respiratory muscle strength; decreased elastic recoil
   f. decreased collagen and subcutaneous fat; decreased sebaceous gland activity; decreased sensory receptors; increased tissue fluid; increased capillary fragility; decreased pigment cells
   g. decreased vessel elastin and smooth muscle; increased arterial rigidity; thickened ventrical wall
   h. decreased blood flow to colon; decreased intestinal motility; decreased sensation to defecation
7. c. Rationale: Age-associated memory impairment is characterized by a memory lapse or benign forgetfulness that is not the same as a decline in cognitive functioning. Forgetting a name, date, or recent event is not serious, but the other examples indicate abnormal functioning.
8. a. S—sadness (mood); b. C—cholesterol (high); c. A—albumin (low); d. L—loss (or gain of weight); e. E—eating problems; f. S—shopping (and preparation problems)
9. c. Rationale: Older adults tend to underreport symptoms and treat symptoms of illness by altering their level of daily function to compensate for the symptoms. Delirium may cause a decline in functional health status, but other symptoms are more prominent. A decline in functional health is not typical with asymptomatic pathology, nor is it directly related to the development of illness.
10. a. Preventing and managing crisis; carrying out prescribed regimens
    b. Preventing social isolation; attempting to normalize interactions with others
    c. Carrying out prescribed regimens; controlling symptoms
    d. Preventing social isolation; attempting to normalize interactions with others
    e. Preventing and managing crisis; reordering time; adjusting to changes in the course of the disease; attempting to normalize interactions with others
    f. Controlling symptoms; reordering time; adjusting to changes in the course of the disease
    g. Reordering time; preventing and managing crisis
11. d. Rationale: Older adults with an ethnic identity often have disproportionately low incomes and may not be able to afford Medicare deductibles or medications to treat health problems. Although they often live in older urban neighborhoods with extended families, they are not isolated. Ethnic diets have adequate nutrition, but health could be impaired if money is not available for food.
12. b. Rationale: During an initial contact with an older adult, the nurse should perform a comprehensive nursing assessment that includes a history using a functional health pattern format, physical assessment, assessment of ADLs and IADLs, mental status evaluation, and a social-environmental assessment. If available, a comprehensive interdisciplinary geriatric assessment may then be done to maintain and enhance the functional abilities of the older adult. The older adult and the caregiver should be interviewed separately, and the older adult should identify his/her own needs.
13. a. Rationale: The results of mental status evaluation often determine whether the patient is able to manage independent living, a major issue in older adulthood. Other elements of comprehensive

assessment could determine eligibility for special problems, determination of frailty, and total service and placement needs.

14. b. Rationale: For the older adult, new learning must relate to the patient's actual experience to have meaning. Written instructions should supplement verbal explanations. Repetition is important, but it should not be excessive to the point of demeaning the patient. Long-term memory is resistant to aging, and relating information to the patient's experience is much more effective than reviewing basic concepts.
15. b. Rationale: An acute confusional state (delirium) is one of the most common consequences of unscheduled surgery because there is not enough time to physically stabilize or emotionally prepare the patient. The risk for other surgical complications is also high in the older adult but not necessarily because the surgery is unscheduled.
16. a. Rationale: Exercise for all older adults is important to prevent deconditioning and subsequent functional decline from many different causes. Walkers and canes may improve mobility but can also decrease mobility if they are too difficult for the patient to use. Nutrition is important for muscles, but muscle strength is primarily dependent on use. Risk appraisals are usually performed for specific health problems.
17. a. Rationale: When pain is a known complication of a particular condition, the nurse should offer pain medication at regular intervals in addition to assessing pain with verbal and visual pain scales. Older patients may not ask for pain medication because of cognitive impairment, age-related changes, or because they think pain should be endured. The use of a pain diary can be used for chronic pain that interferes with ADLs and functional ability.
18. a. Absorption of enalapril may be more complete because of delayed gastric emptying and slowed gastrointestinal motility. However, less of the drug may be metabolized to active enalaprilat because of decreased liver function. The drug is not highly plasma protein-bound, but decreases in serum albumin and total body water may make more active drug available. Decreased kidney function lengthens the half-life of the drug, prolonging its action. Overall, there is likely to be an increased effect of the drugs, with marked hypotension and development of side effects.
    b. When digoxin is added to the regimen for the patient, consideration must be made of not only the effect of digoxin but also its possible interaction with enalapril. Digoxin toxicity is much more likely to occur in the older patient because of increased absorption due to decreased GI motility and decreased kidney elimination. The half-life of digoxin may be much prolonged beyond the normally long 36 hours. Although digoxin is not highly plasma protein-bound, decreased serum albumin, decreased total body water, and competition between digoxin and enalapril for plasma proteins could increase the free (active) amount of both drugs.
    c. The nurse should monitor the patient's blood pressure and apical pulse for hypotension, bradycardia, or marked tachycardia before administration of the drugs, and because the digoxin has such a long half-life, vital signs should also be routinely monitored throughout the day. Periodic serum digoxin levels are also advised in the older adult because of the many physiologic changes that can affect the drug's pharmacokinetics.
19. a. Emphasize medications that are essential, attempting to reduce medication usage that is not essential for minor symptoms.
    b. Use a standard assessment tool to screen medication usage that includes OTC medications, eye and ear medications, and alcohol as well as prescription drugs.
    c. Monitor medication dosage strength; normally the strength should be 30%–50% less than that of a younger person.
    d. Encourage the use of one pharmacy, and work with physicians and pharmacists to establish routine drug profiles on all older adult patients.
20. a. Psychologic abuse and physical neglect; b. Caregiver role strain; c. Community caregiver support group; formal support system for respite care
21. a. Part A; b. Daily documentation of improvement in function; c. Only for a limited number of days and only if the patient improves in function; d. None; e. Adult day care programs
22. a. Rapid patient deterioration; b. Caregiver exhaustion; c. Alteration in or loss of family support system

CHAPTER 6

1. c. Rationale: The focus of community-based nursing is illness-oriented care of individuals and families in the community and home settings. Community-oriented nursing includes public health nursing, which focuses on the health care of the community, and community health nursing, which is concerned about the health care of individuals, families, and groups in a community. In community-based nursing, nurses provide direct patient care in addition to case management of the care.
2. a. Rationale: Government, employers, insurance companies, and regulating agencies have influenced the changes in health care delivery in an effort to control health care costs, primarily through changing coverage or reimbursement for health care services. Health care providers are free to price services at any level, but third-party payers limit payment to providers. The increase in the aging population strains the Medicare program, but the aging of America is not the primary factor in the shift to community-based care settings. Advances in technology provide for shorter hospital stays and outpatient treatment, but the technology has been pushed by a need for lower health care costs.
3. b. Rationale: A prospective payment system, such as Medicare reimbursement, pays for health care services at a predetermined flat rate. If a health care provider can provide quality care at a lesser amount, then the difference is profit to the provider; if not, the difference is a loss to the provider. Thus providers are instituting systems to provide quality care in a more cost-effective manner to maintain financial balance.
4. b. Rationale: A diagnosis-related group (DRG) was established by Medicare and is a form of prospective payment for health services of Medicare-qualified patients based on their diagnoses. An outlier is a patient whose treatment and care costs more than the flat rate Medicare pays for the patient's diagnosis and constitutes a loss to health care providers.
5. a. Socioeconomic conditions resulting in a demand for less expensive health care
   b. Increasing older population with complex medical and health care needs
   c. Increase in chronic illnesses that are better prevented and managed in the community
   d. Increased technology available in outpatient and home settings
   e. Consumer input into health care and patient preference for community-based care.
6. c. Rationale: The case manager is critical in managed care to coordinate and link health care services to the patient and family during an entire illness episode across all patient care settings. Most case management is performed when patients belong to managed health care organizations where all settings for health care services are provided. Case managers do not determine when hospitalization is required, nor do they set limits on health care expenses but rather coordinate patient needs with cost-effective health services.
7. a. special care unit; b. hospice care; c. subacute care unit; d. skilled nursing facility; e. ambulatory care center; f. residential care facility; g. acute rehabilitation; h. home health care; i. intermediate care facility; j. long-term acute care
8. Ambulatory care center
9. Home health care
10. Skilled nursing facility, intermediate care facility
11. Acute rehabilitation center, skilled nursing facility, home health care
12. b. Rationale: Medicare stipulates that registered nurses are the coordinators of patient care in the home and that they are accountable for the supervision of personal care services by home health aides and for case management services, including all aspects of care in the home. Care delivered in the home may be provided by any member of the home health care team, and the frequency is determined by the patient's and family's needs.
13. d. Rationale: Continuous quality management is a system of monitoring facets of clinical care such as infection rates and admissions to hospitals, evaluating care with respect to patient outcomes. It is a method of evaluating services related to the patient's progress toward realistic goals and reflects quality in services that promote positive outcomes for the patient.
14. Any of the following are appropriate:
   a. Caregiver role strain
   b. Interrupted family processes
   c. Decisional conflict
   d. Disabled family coping

CHAPTER 7

1. a. 5, 12; b. 3, 18; c. 4, 8; d. 1, 6; e. 2, 17; f. 1, 11; g. 2, 16; h. 1, 7; i. 4, 19; j. 4, 10; k. 3, 13; l. 2, 9; m. 2, 15; n. 1, 14
2. a. F; b. F; c. T; d. T
3. b. Rationale: Complementary and alternative therapies are harmonious with the values of nursing that include a view of humans as holistic beings, an emphasis on healing and partnership relationships with patients, and a focus on health promotion and illness prevention. CAM is not inexpensive, nor is it without adverse or even validated therapeutic effects.
4. a. Rationale: The basic concept of disease in Chinese medicine is that the opposing phenomena of yin and yang are out of balance, and this imbalance alters the movement of the vital energy of the body, known as Qi, that influences physiologic functions of the body. Acupoints are holes in the Qi meridians where the flow of Qi can be influenced but not released. Health phenomena are organized according to the five elements, but these are not directly a cause of illness.
5. b. Rationale: Acupuncture is used to regulate the flow of Qi with the insertion of needles at acupoints, areas where needles may be inserted to unblock obstruction of energy and reestablish the flow of Qi. Counterirritation and inflammation are not consistent with the theory of Qi, and although electrical stimulation may be applied to the needles in electroacupuncture, this procedure releases neuropeptides within the central nervous system.
6. b. Rationale: Complications from acupuncture are rare, but if they occur, they are most often related to infections from the use of contaminated, nonsterile needles. The other complications may occur but are not as frequent as infections or transmission of infection from one patient to another.
7. a. meditation; b. relaxation; c. imagery
8. c. Rationale: The ultimate goal of biofeedback is to teach patients to control normally involuntary physiologic responses. The process involves measurement of physiologic responses to provide information to persons about their neuromuscular and autonomic nervous system activity and demonstrate the effect of stress relaxation behaviors so that patients can control the physiologic functions.
9. b. Clinical studies have indicated that acupuncture is clearly effective in treating adult postoperative and chemotherapy-associated nausea and vomiting as well as postoperative dental pain. Rolfing is used to improve musculoskeletal movement and alignment, aromatherapy uses essential plant oils to promote and maintain overall health, and electromagnetic therapy is useful for relieving pain and promoting tissue healing.
10. a. Rationale: Patients sensitive to energy repatterning, such as premature infants, newborns, children, pregnant women, older people, and those in critical, unstable conditions, should avoid therapeutic touch. It has been reported to promote wound healing and sleep and enhance immune function.
11. d. Rationale: Chiropractic therapy holds that structural distortions of the vertebrae can lead to organ dysfunction and pain anywhere in the body, and as such, chiropractic manipulation is used to treat not only musculoskeletal abnormalities but also a variety of health problems, including dysmenorrhea. Generally, chiropractic practice does not include drug therapy.
12. a. Rationale: Because of a lack of governmental control for clinical testing of herbs or standardization of ingredient concentration or acceptable levels of contamination of pesticides, solvents, bacteria, and heavy metals, the safety and efficacy of herbal preparations is based on the manufacturer's standards. As such, the reputation and history of the manufacturer must be the major criteria for purchasing herbs. Herbs indeed can be toxic and are contraindicated or should be used with caution in certain persons.
13. b. Rationale: To serve as a resource for patients regarding complementary and alternative therapies, nurses must first develop their own knowledge base. To teach patients about their use, monitor for adverse effects and interactions with conventional therapies, and assist patients to use the therapies knowledgeably and safely, nurses themselves must be informed.
14. *Down:* 1. kava; 2. evening primrose; 4. comfrey; 5. valerian; 7. DHEA; 8. black cohosh; 11. saw palmetto; 13. aloe; 14. ginseng
    Across: 3. angelica; 6. chamomile; 9. ginseng; 10. bilberry; 12. feverfew; 13. angelica; 15. St. John's wort; 16. ginkgo biloba

CHAPTER 8

1. a. R—Selye; b. S—Holmes, Rahe, Masuda; c. T—Lazarus and Folkman; d. R—Selye; e. S—Holmes, Rahe, Masuda
2. stage of resistance
3. stage of exhaustion
4. Use Table 8-2 in the text to calculate your personal score and determine your illness risk.
5. b. Rationale: Daily hassles are experiences and conditions of daily living that have been

appraised as being harmful or threatening to a person's well-being. These are counteracted by uplifts, positive everyday experiences. Threat demands and challenge demands are concepts of the stress-as-transaction theory, and the concept of sense of coherence is a personality characteristic or coping style that is a powerful mediator of stress and illness.

6. c. Rationale: An individual with a sense of coherence is likely to perceive the illness experience as structured and predictable and as a challenge worthy of investment. Information regarding the nature of the illness would be a resource the patient would seek to meet the demand of the illness.

7. a. Stimulus: diabetes mellitus
   b. Primary appraisal outcome: stressful demand
   c. Type of demand: harm or loss
   d. Secondary appraisal outcome: using resources to learn about the disease and planning management of the disease

8.

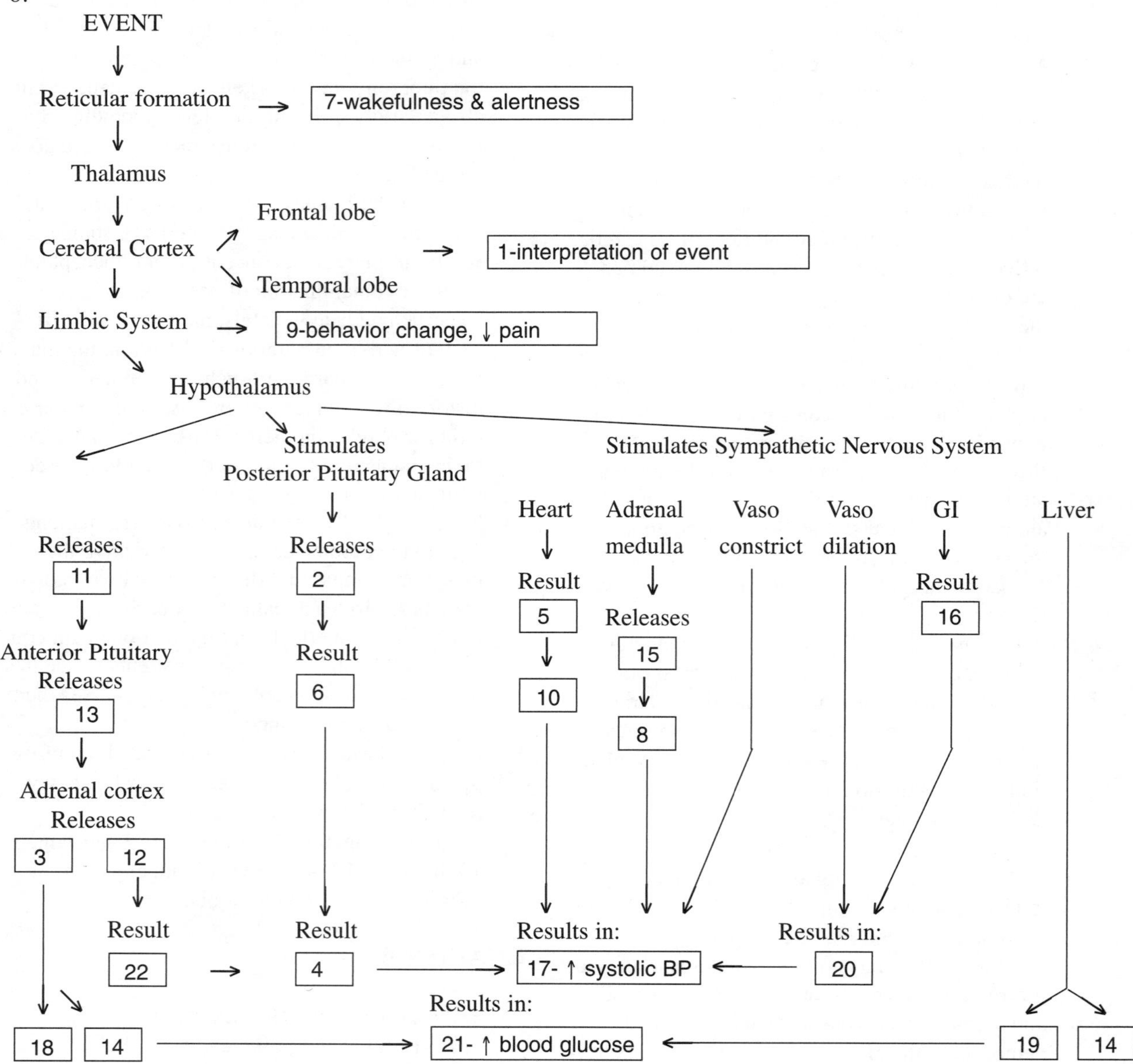

Word and Phrase List

1. interpretation of event, fear
2. ↑ ADH
3. cortisol
4. ↑ blood volume
5. ↑ HR and stroke volume
6. ↑ water retention
7. wakefulness and alertness reabsorption
8. ↑ sympathetic response
9. behavior change, ↑ pain perception
10. ↑ cardiac output
11. corticotropin-releasing hormone
12. aldosterone
13. ACTH
14. ↑ gluconeogenesis
15. ↑ epinephrine and norepinephrine
16. ↓ digestion
17. ↑ systolic blood pressure
18. ↓ inflammatory response
19. glycogenolysis
20. ↑ blood to vital organs and large muscles
21. ↑ blood glucose
22. ↑ Na and H_2O reabsorption

9.

Objective Manifestations:	**Subjective Findings:**
Increased heart rate	Anxiety, fear
Increased blood pressure	Decreased perception of pain
Cool, clammy skin	Verbalization of stress
Decreased bowel sounds	Wakefulness, restlessness
Hyperglycemia	
Decreased lymphocytes	
Decreased eosinophils	
Decreased urinary output	

10. a, c, e, f, g
11. c. Rationale: Allostasis refers to the mechanisms by which the body reestablishes homeostasis in the face of a challenge and includes many of the same physiologic responses that occur with any stress. If these allostatic (physiologic) responses do not terminate when they are no longer needed, or when stress occurs too frequently, the effects on the body create an allostatic load. Allostatic load is manifested by hypertension, salt and water retention, atherosclerosis, abdominal obesity, and other physical problems.
12. *Problem-focused:*
    - Attending cardiac rehabilitation program
    - Planning dietary changes
    - Starting an exercise program
    - Learning about medications

    Emotion-focused:
    - Sharing feelings with spouse or other family members
    - Using meditation
    - Setting aside private time
    - Doing favorite escape activities
13. a. Demands: Assessing the type, number, and duration of demands and prior experience with the demands; a specific assessment guide may be used for particular types of patients.
    b. Response to stress: Noting physiologic effects and the presence of diseases of adaptation; also observing behavioral and cognitive responses of the patient and significant others
    c. Coping: Assessing the patient's evaluation of coping resources and options and evaluating the use and effectiveness of problem-focused and emotion-focused coping efforts
14. c. Rationale: The coping behavior described is not adaptive, and the patient tells the nurse that she does not have the resources to cope with the demands of her illness. There is no evidence that emotional bonds with her family are disrupted, and her behavior does not match definitions of ineffective denial or impaired adjustment.
15. a. Sleeping regularly 7 to 8 hours per night
    b. Eating breakfast
    c. Eating regular meals with minimal or no snacking
    d. Eating moderately to maintain an ideal weight
    e. Exercising moderately
    f. Enjoying recreational and relaxing activities with friends
    g. Drinking alcohol in moderation or not at all
    h. Not smoking (best if have never smoked)
    i. Learning to successfully handle life's stressors and hassles

Case Study

1. Physiologic: fever, pain, anemia, the inflammatory disease itself
   Psychologic: no income, no insurance, the duration and chronicity of the disease, frequent hospital admissions, lack of social support systems
   Effects: Prolonged healing of illness, progression of the inflammatory disease
2. Her refusal to seek support from boyfriend
   Her depression, weakness
   Her experience with the illness and hospitalizations
   Her lack of financial resources
3. Increased weight, hemoglobin and hematocrit, strength
   Decreased body temperature, number of stools
4. One approach may be using a hospital stress rating scale to clarify the patient's perception of the situation. The nurse and the patient may not rate the stressors the same in intensity. Specific questions may include the following:

"What is the most stressful thing to you about being in the hospital?"
"Can you tell me what having this illness means to you?"

5. Reduce additional stressors, such as sleep deprivation, environmental stimuli
   Set short-term outcomes to achieve success
   Provide pain relief, measures for comfort, rest
   Provide stress-reducing interventions, such as relaxation and guided imagery
6. *Nursing diagnoses:*
   - Ineffective coping related to inadequate resources as manifested by crying, depression
   - Ineffective role performance related to lack of employment
   - Acute pain related to inflammatory process
   - Risk for impaired skin integrity related to frequent stools and emaciation
   - Imbalanced nutrition: less than body requirements related to nausea and frequent watery stools
   - Risk for deficient fluid volume related to frequent watery stools and low-grade fever

   Collaborative problems:
   Potential complications: fluid/electrolyte imbalances; intestinal obstruction; istula/fissure/abscess

CHAPTER 9

1. c. Rationale: Administering the smallest prescribed analgesic dose when given a choice is not consistent with current pain management guidelines and leads to inadequate pain control. This results in unnecessary suffering, impaired recovery from acute illness, and increased morbidity as a result of respiratory dysfunction, increased heart rate and cardiac workload, and other physical dysfunction.
2. c. Rationale: Because the patient's self-report is the most valid means of pain assessment, patients who have decreased cognitive function, such as those who are comatose, have dementia, or are mentally disabled, may not be able to report pain. In these cases, nonverbal information and behaviors are necessary to consider in pain assessment.
3. a. physiologic—the transmission of nociceptive stimuli to the brain
   b. sensory—how the pain is perceived
   c. affective—the emotions related to the pain
   d. behavioral—the behavioral responses to the pain
   e. cognitive—the beliefs, attitudes, and evaluations about the pain and pain control
4. a. 3; b. 2; c. 4; d. 4; e. 1; f. 3; g. 4
5. Information carried by large myelinated nerves, such as A-alpha and A-beta fibers, is communicated to the spinal cord faster than information carried by the smaller, slower primary afferent nociceptors (PANs) and may interfere with further transmission of PAN impulses.
6. b. Rationale: Although a peripheral nerve is one cell that carries an impulse directly from the periphery to the dorsal horn of the spinal cord with no synapses, the transmission of the impulse can be interrupted by drugs known as membrane stabilizers or sodium channel inhibitors, such as local anesthetics and some anticonvulsants. The nerve fiber produces neurotransmitters only at synapses, not during transmission of the action potential.
7. c. Rationale: Wide dynamic-range neurons in the dorsal horn of the spinal cord receive input from nociceptive fibers and A-beta fibers, and the message transmitted to the brain from these neurons causes pain to be perceived as originating from the body part innervated by the A-beta fiber rather than from the primary afferent nociceptors. Enlargement of the receptive field of a peripheral neuron with increased response to noxious stimuli is known as sensitization.
8. b. Rationale: It is known that the brain is necessary for pain perception, but because it is not clearly understood where in the brain pain is perceived, pain may be perceived even in a comatose patient who may not respond behaviorally to noxious stimuli. Any noxious stimulus should be treated as potentially painful.
9. c. Rationale: Modulation is primarily brought about by descending (efferent) fibers that release inhibitory neurotransmitters, such as serotonin, alpha-2 agonists, and opioids. Opioid receptors must be stimulated, not blocked, to change the transmission of nociceptive stimuli, and endorphins are not known to be released during the transduction step of pain.
10. d. Rationale: Limiting or adjusting daily physical activities to express or control pain is an example of the behavioral component of pain. The sensory component is recognition of the sensation as painful, the affective component refers to the emotional responses to pain, and the cognitive component refers to beliefs, attitudes, memories, and meaning attributed to the pain.
11. d. Rationale: Neuropathic pain is not well controlled by opioid analgesics alone and often includes the use of tricyclic antidepressants to help inhibit pain transmission. Neuropathic pain can be acute, intense, and either short-lived or lingering. Aching and throbbing are more characteristic of nociceptive pain.

12. a. P—pattern: daily pain pattern graph; b. A—area: body outline, pain map; c. I—intensity: pain intensity scale (simple descriptive or 0-10 numeric); d. N—nature: verbal description list, McGill Pain Questionnaire
13. a. Always believe the patient
    b. Every patient deserves adequate pain management
    c. Base treatment on the patient's goals
    d. Use a combination of drug and nondrug therapies
    e. Use a multidisciplinary approach
    f. Therapies must be evaluated
    g. Prevent and/or manage medication side effects
    h. Always include patient and family teaching
14. a. Rationale: Analgesics should be scheduled around the clock for patients with constant pain to prevent pain from escalating and becoming difficult to relieve. If pain control is not adequate, the analgesic dose may be increased or an adjunctive drug may be added to the treatment plan.
15. b. Rationale: When the patient's step 1 drugs are not effective, a step 2 drug should be added to the regimen and the step 1 drugs continued. Hydrocodone is a step 2 drug; morphine is a step 3 drug.
16. c. Rationale: Although tolerance to many of the side effects of opioids (nausea, sedation, respiratory depression, pruritis) develops within days, tolerance to opioid-induced constipation does not occur. A bowel regimen that includes a gentle stimulant laxative and a stool softener should be started at the beginning of opioid therapy and continue as long as the drug is taken.
17. PCA use is decreased at night when the patient sleeps, and without a continuous infusion of an analgesic, the patient is likely to awaken in pain that will require substantial time to bring under control.
18. a. 3; b. 2; c. 1; d. 2; e. 2; f. 4; g. 1; h. 3; i. 2; j. 4
19. The prototype is to reduce to an equivalent dose of morphine 30 mg PO/day. The following schedule would be used:
    Current use: 360 mg/day
    Day 1 and 2: 50% of 24-hour dose = 180 mg
    25% of 180 mg q6hr = 45 mg q6hr
    Day 3 and 4: Reduce dose by 25%
    75% of 180 mg = 36 mg q6hr (135 mg/day)
    Day 5 and 6: Reduce dose by 25%
    75% of 135 mg = 25 mg q6hr (101 mg/day)
    Day 7 and 8: Reduce dose by 25%
    75% of 101 mg = 19 mg q6hr (76 mg/day)
    Day 9 and 10: Reduce dose by 25%
    75% of 76 mg = 14 mg q6hr (57 mg/day)
    Day 11 and 12: Reduce dose by 25%
    75% of 57 mg = 10 mg q6hr (43 mg/day)
    Day 13 and 14: Reduce dose by 25%
    75% of 43 mg = 8 mg q6hr (32 mg/day)
    May stop drug completely after day 14.
20. "Nurses should not hesitate to use full and effective doses of pain medication for the proper management of pain in the dying patient. The increasing titration of medication to achieve adequate symptom control, even at the expense of life thus hastening death, is ethically justified."
21. b. Rationale: When a patient desires to be stoic about pain, it is important that he or she understand that pain itself can have harmful physiologic effects and that failure to report pain and participate in its control can result in severe unrelieved pain. No evidence is present in this situation that indicates fear of taking the medication.

Case Study

1. Assess the location, quality, and specifics of the pattern of the pain. Also assess his prior medication use, experience with narcotics, and any addictions.
2. Affective: worried about worsening of disease, afraid of narcotics
   Behavioral: posturing, slow gait, stays in bed with severe pain
   Cognitive: uses emptying mind to block pain
3. The symptoms he has in the mornings are related to withdrawal because of physical dependence and the long interval during the night that the narcotic is not used. An adjuvant drug should be added to his regimen, and it and the Percocet should be taken around the clock. If his pain is not controlled with this measure, a step 3 drug should be substituted for the Percocet around the clock.
4. Teach him to evaluate the dose required to control his pain, and see that he knows the range and frequency of his dose.
5. Explain that tolerance and physical dependence are expected with long-term opiate use and should not be confused with addiction. Addiction is a psychologic condition characterized by a drive to obtain and take substances for other than their prescribed therapeutic value. Less than 0.1% of patients receiving analgesics become addicted.
6. Dermal stimulation, such as massage and pressure; additional cognitive-behavioral therapies, such as relaxation and imagery. He has a potential for using cognitive-behavioral therapies successfully since he can already mentally block the pain somewhat.

7. *Nursing diagnoses:*
   - Chronic pain related to ineffective pain management
   - Anxiety related to effects of disease process and inadequate relief from pain-relief measures
   - Activity intolerance related to pain, fatigue

   Collaborative problems:
   Potential complications: drug-induced constipation; respiratory depression; negative nitrogen balance; narcotic toxicity

CHAPTER 10

1. a. Rationale: The goals of end-of-life care are to provide comfort and supportive care during the dying process, improve the quality of the remaining life, and help to ensure a dignified death. Grieving is a normal process and should be encouraged, but not all patients will progress through all stages of grieving in a systematic way.
2. a. 1) Cheyne-Stokes respiration
      2) death rattle (inability to cough and clear secretions)
      3) increased, then slowing respiratory rate
      Also: irregular breathing, terminal gasping
   b. 1) mottling on hands, feet, and legs that progresses to torso
      2) cold, clammy skin
      3) cyanosis on nose, nail beds, knees
      Also: waxlike skin when very near death
   c. 1) slowing of GI tract with accumulation of gas and abdominal distention
      2) loss of sphincter control with incontinence
      3) bowel movement prior to imminent death or at time of death
   d. 1) loss of muscle tone with sagging jaw
      2) difficulty speaking
      3) difficulty swallowing
      Also: loss of ability to move or maintain body position; loss of gag reflex
3. b. Rationale: Hearing is often the last sense to disappear with declining consciousness, and conversations can distress patients even when they appear unresponsive. Conversation around unresponsive patients should never be other than that which one would maintain if they were alert.
4. a. coma
   b. absent brainstem reflexes
   c. apnea
5. a. Rationale: Photos are a reflection of important people and events in an individual's life and can be an effective method of reviewing one's life experiences. Peacefulness usually comes with healthy grief resolution of an acceptance of the reality of death. Saying goodbyes involves talking with others and verbalizing their feelings of sadness, loss, and forgiveness, while anxiety about unfinished business requires completion of tasks important to the individual.
6. b. Rationale: Bargaining is demonstrated by "if-then" grief behavior that is described by Kubler-Ross and corresponds to Rando's confrontation. Avoidance is Rando's description of denial and shock that occur early in the grief process, and Martocchio's anguish, disorganization, and despair corresponds to Kubler-Ross's depression. Reorganization and restoration is Martocchio's acceptance and accommodation phase of grieving.
7. a. 3; b. 6; c. 4; d. 5; e. 1; f. 2
8. a. Rationale: Spiritual distress may surface when an individual is faced with a terminal illness, and it is characterized by verbalization about inner conflicts about beliefs and questioning the meaning of one's own existence. Individuals in spiritual distress may be able to resolve the problem and die peacefully with effective grief work, but referral to spiritual leaders should be of the patient's choice.
9. a. living will
   b. durable power of attorney for health care
   c. directive to physicians
   d. natural death acts
   e. Patient Self-Determination Act (Omnibus Reconciliation Act of 1990)
   f. advance directives
10. b. Rationale: Palliative care is aimed at symptom management rather than curative treatment for diseases that no longer respond to treatment and is focused on caring interventions rather than toward curative treatments. Palliative care and hospice are frequently used interchangeably.
11. b. Rationale: The hospice philosophy is to enhance the remaining time for the person who is terminally ill and to assist the patient and family with the task of preparing for death. Hospice care may be provided at home or in inpatient settings. Pain control and patient self-determination are important in hospice, but these may also be important care issues for terminally ill patients not admitted to a hospice program.
12. d. Rationale: In assisting patients with dying, end-of-life care promotes the grieving process, which involves saying goodbye. Physical care is very important for physical comfort, but assessments should be limited to essential data related to the patient's symptoms. Analgesics should be administered for pain, but patients who are sedated cannot participate in the grieving process.

Case Study

1. Additional assessment data should include Mr. and Mrs. J.'s reasons for not discussing her illness and impending death with their children, an assessment of their spiritual needs, what decisions, if any, they have made about where and how Mrs. J. prefers to die, and what resources they have used or could use to assist them through the dying process. In addition, assessment and evaluation of their coping skills is necessary. A functional assessment of Mrs. J.'s ADLs should also be made.
2. Maladaptive or dysfunctional grief is demonstrated in this family. Mrs. J. appears to have some degree of acceptance of her impending death but feels rejected by her children. The children may be experiencing fear, guilt, anger, powerlessness, and other emotions that they cope with by withdrawing from the family. Mr. J. is also feeling guilt at wishing the ordeal would be over. Healthy grieving is blocked in this family because communication has not occurred.
3. Pain patterns should be assessed and dosages and frequencies increased to provide pain relief that is acceptable to Mrs. J. without unnecessary sedation. Institute complementary therapies to enhance the effect of pain medication. As opioids are increased, constipation and abdominal distention could become a problem, and stool softeners may need to be used. Although she is underweight, patients tend to take in less food and fluid as death approaches, and maintaining food and fluid intake is not a high priority. Because she spends most of her time in bed and she is very thin, measures to prevent skin breakdown are essential. Oxygen therapy should be considered as a measure to relieve her shortness of breath.
4. Arrange for family meetings to discuss Mrs. J.'s condition and the feelings of the patient and the family. The hospice nurse or a grief counselor can help all members of the family express and acknowledge feelings of anger, fear, or guilt. The patient and family need to know that the grief reaction is normal, and they should be taught what to expect and how each individual's needs can be met as Mrs. J.'s death approaches.
5. A multidisciplinary team of nurses, physicians, pharmacists, dietitians, nursing assistants, social workers, clergy, and volunteers is available to this family to provide care and support to the patient and family through hospice care.
6. *Nursing diagnoses:*
   - Compromised family coping related to inadequate coping mechanisms
   - Dysfunctional grieving related to blocked communication and guilt
   - Chronic pain related to ineffective pain management
   - Risk for impaired skin integrity related to immobility and emaciation
   - Risk for constipation related to decreased oral intake and effects of drugs
   - Ineffective breathing pattern related to weakness
   - Impaired physical mobility related to pain

CHAPTER 11

1. a. 11; b. 6; c. 9; d. 1; e. 8; f. 2; g. 7; h. 10; i. 3; j. 4; k. 5
2. b. Rationale: Addictive drugs appear to increase the availability of dopamine in the mesolimbic system of the brain through several different methods. Opioids increase the firing rate of dopaminergic neurons, and cocaine decreases the reuptake of dopamine at synapses. Although other neurotransmitters are also increased, it appears that dopamine is responsible for the responses that lead to addiction.
3. a. Rationale: Tolerance results when the prolonged effect of an addictive drug reduces the responsiveness of dopamine receptors in the brain, and to even feel normal, the drug must be taken. To obtain the initial effects of the drug, larger and larger doses must be used.
4. c. Rationale: While all minority groups have a higher incidence of health problems associated with substance abuse, alcohol problems in Native Americans are more than four times that of the general population. Another major problem, although not as extensive, is drug-related AIDS in African-American women.
5. a. 1) chronic obstructive pulmonary disease (COPD)
      2) cancers: lung, mouth, esophagus, larynx, stomach, bladder, pancreas
      others: vascular disease: coronary and peripheral; peptic ulcer disease
   b. 1) cardiac arrhythmias, angina pectoris, myocardial infarction
      2) stroke
      others: pneumonia, nasal septum necrosis or perforation, sinusitis
   c. 1) cirrhosis of liver
      2) pancreatitis, gastritis
      others: cancers: esophagus, stomach, head and neck, lung

d. 1) bronchitis, chronic sinusitis
2) memory impairment
others: impaired immune function, reproductive dysfunction
6. a. 3; b. 1; c. 4; d. 1; e. 3; f. 2; g. 1; h. 2; i. 4; j. 2
7. a. stimulant; sedative-hypnotic
b. narcotic
c. hallucinogens
d. stimulant
e. sedative-hypnotics
f. narcotic; sedative-hypnotic
8. d. Rationale: Nicotine replacement contains the same nicotine as that in tobacco but with slower absorption. The nicotine will help prevent withdrawal symptoms as its use is gradually reduced. While the addiction is treated, the carcinogens and gases associated with tobacco smoke are eliminated.
9. a. 2; b. 3; c. 4; d. 1; e. 3; f. 4; g. 3
10. a. Rationale: Headache is a common symptom of caffeine withdrawal and often occurs in heavy caffeine users who are NPO for diagnostic tests and surgery. Nervousness, tremors, anxiety, and bronchial dilation are physiologic effects of caffeine.
11. b. Rationale: Of the two patterns of abuse and dependence recognized with sedative-hypnotic drugs, the one most likely in this patient is initial prescription use of the drug for treatment of anxiety or insomnia, with the patient increasing the dose and frequency of use without medical advice or indication. It is unlikely that this patient would have started a pattern with illegal sources.
12. a. gross tremors
b. seizures
c. hallucinations
d. delirium tremens (DTs)
13. c. Rationale: Open-ended questions that indicate that substance use is normal or at least understandable are helpful in eliciting information from patients who are reluctant to disclose substance use.
14. b. Rationale: This behavior is typical of ineffective denial—is unable to admit the impact of the disease/event on life patterns as manifested by minimizing symptoms or events and selectively integrating information and does not meet the definitions or defining characteristics of the other nursing diagnoses.
15. b. Rationale: Smoking is the single one most preventable cause of death, and most smokers start by the age of 16. If smoking in preadolescents and adolescents can be prevented, it is unlikely that they would start smoking at a later age. Health problems associated with smoking and future use of other addictive substances would be significantly reduced.
16. a. naloxone (Narcan) is given in case opioids are the cause of the CNS depression
b. flumazenil (Romazicon) is given in case benzodiazepines are the cause of the CNS depression
17. a. Rationale: The knowledge of when the patient last had alcohol intake will help the nurse anticipate the onset of withdrawal symptoms. In patients with alcohol tolerance, the amount of alcohol and the blood alcohol concentration do not reflect impairment as consistently as in the nondrinker. The type of alcohol ingested is not of importance because it is all alcohol in the body.
18. d. Rationale: An extreme autonomic nervous system response may be life-threatening and requires immediate intervention. A quiet room is recommended, but it should be well lighted to prevent misinterpretation of the environment and visual hallucinations. Cessation of alcohol intake causes low blood alcohol levels leading to withdrawal symptoms, and fluids should be carefully administered to prevent arrhythmias. Patients should not be restrained if at all possible because injury and exhaustion may occur as patients struggle against restraint.
19. a. Anesthesia requirements may be decreased as a result of cross-tolerance.
b. IV alcohol may be used to avoid acute withdrawal and delirium tremens triggered by surgery and the cessation of alcohol consumption.
c. Postoperative care will require close monitoring for signs of withdrawal and respiratory and cardiac problems.
d. Increased pain medications may be needed postoperatively if the patient is cross-tolerant to opiates.
20. a. Rationale: Because Wernicke's encephalopathy resulting from a thiamine deficiency is a possibility in chronic alcoholism, intravenous thiamine is often administered to intoxicated patients to prevent the development of Korsakoff's psychosis. Thiamine should be given before any glucose solutions because glucose may precipitate Wernicke's encephalopathy. Benzodiazepines may be used for sedation and to minimize withdrawal symptoms but would not be given before thiamine.
21. c. Rationale: This patient is demonstrating behavior characteristic of the precontemplation stage of behavior change. During this stage, the nurse should help the patient increase her awareness of the risks and problems related to alcohol use by asking the patient what she thinks could happen if

the behavior continues, providing evidence of the problem and offering factual information about the risks of the substance use.

22. d. Rationale: The elderly have the highest use of over-the-counter and prescription drugs, and simultaneous use of these drugs with alcohol is a major problem. Illegal drug use is minimal in the elderly except for long-term addicts.

Case Study

1. Because there is a tendency among substance abusers to take a variety of drugs simultaneously or in a sequence to obtain specific effects as shown by Mr. C.'s history, he should be assessed for his pattern of abuse. Regular alcohol use in addition to other drug use or the common use of cocaine in combination with heroin or phencyclidine hydrochloride could cause withdrawal symptoms and additional manifestations that would complicate his condition and direct his care. Information about all drugs he uses, including over-the-counter and prescription drugs, is necessary to avoid withdrawal syndromes, acute intoxication, overdose, or drug interactions that may be life-threatening.
2. The nurse should be aware that common behaviors that are likely to influence history taking from Mr. C. include manipulation, denial, avoidance, under-reporting or minimizing substance abuse, giving inaccurate information, and inaccurate self-reporting. To obtain reliable information about Mr. C.'s drug abuse patterns, the nurse should first explain that information about his drug use is very important in order to monitor for and prevent serious effects of the drugs while he already very ill. Providing a need for the information and explaining how the information will be used may facilitate more honest responses by Mr. C. The nurse should question him without judgment about his pattern of abuse with open-ended questions, such as "How much or how often do you use alcohol?" or "Can you describe how you use cocaine with other drugs?"
3. Physical effects of drug use that provide clues to drug abuse include collapsed and scarred veins used to inject drugs, nasal septum and mucosa damage, brown or black sputum production, and wound abscesses and cellulitis.
4. Continuous monitoring of Mr. C.'s vital signs, cardiac activity, level of consciousness, respiratory status, temperature, fluid and electrolyte balance, liver function, and renal function is necessary. Complications of cocaine toxicity that may occur and be detected by monitoring include myocardial ischemia or infarction, congestive heart failure, cardiopulmonary arrest, rhabdomyolysis with acute renal failure, stroke, respiratory distress or arrest, seizures, agitated delirium and hallucinations, electrolyte imbalances, and fever. In severe intoxication, the patient may progress rapidly through stages of stimulation and depression, which may result in death. Mr. C.'s use of cocaine with alcohol also increases his risk of liver injury and sudden death.
5. Assessment for neurologic, cardiovascular, and respiratory problems as described above is a critical nursing intervention in the patient with cocaine toxicity. In addition, the nurse should institute seizure precautions, provide airway management, keep open IV lines, administer medications aggressively as prescribed, and employ cardiac life support measures as indicated.
   Nursing interventions that are indicated for Mr. C.'s anxiety, nervousness, and irritability include explaining procedures, using short, simple, clear statements in a calm manner; providing a safe, secure environment; decreasing environmental stimuli; reinforcing reality orientation; and encouraging participation in relaxation exercises if possible.
6. Engaging an individual who is addicted to cocaine in treatment is difficult because of the intense craving for the drug and a strong denial that cocaine is addicting or that the individual cannot control it. Motivational interviewing is indicated in even this initial encounter with Mr. C. The nurse should help Mr. C. increase his awareness of risks and problems related to his current behavior and create doubt about the use of substances. Asking him what he thinks could happen if the behavior is continued, pointing out the physical symptoms he is experiencing, and offering factual information about the risks of substance abuse are indicated. Often the only motivation for a patient with a cocaine addiction to enter a treatment program is family threats, loss of job or professional license, legal action, or major health consequences, but a treatment program is indicated to provide him with new skills and an ability to deal with his addictive behavior.
7. *Nursing diagnoses:*
   - Ineffective health maintenance
   - Disturbed thought processes
   - Ineffective denial
   - Ineffective coping

   Collaborative problems:
   Potential complications: cardiopulmonary arrest, seizures, sudden death, cerebrovascular accident, acute renal failure

CHAPTER 12

1. a. 3; b. 1; c. 4; d. 5; e. 2; f. 6
2. mechanical trauma, heat, microbial, natural substances
3. a. Kupffer cells—fixed; b. alveolar macrophages—fixed; c. microglial cells—fixed; d. monocytes—free; e. histiocytes—free; f. osteoclasts—fixed; g. macrophages—free and fixed
4. Mediators/physiologic change:
   a. IL-1 released from mononuclear phagocytic cells and PGE2 synthesis/increases hypothalamic thermostatic set point
   b. histamine, kinins, prostaglandins/vasodilation and hyperemia
   c. histamine, kinins, prostaglandins/increased capillary permeability and fluid shift to tissues
   d. release of chemotactic factors at site of injury/increased release of neutrophils and monocytes from bone marrow
5. d. Rationale: *A shift to the left* is the term that is used to describe the presence of immature, banded nuclei neutrophils in the blood in response to an increased demand for neutrophils during tissue injury. Monocytes are increased in leukocytosis but are mature cells.
6. c. Rationale: Chemotaxis involves the release of chemicals at the site of tissue injury that attract neutrophils and monocytes to the site of injury. The attraction is chemotaxis, and when monocytes move from the blood into tissue, they are transformed into macrophages. The complement system is a pathway of chemical processes that results in cellular lysis, and vasodilation and increased capillary permeability cause the slowing of blood flow at the area.
7. c. Rationale: Eosinophils are white blood cells that are released in large quantities during allergic reactions and are involved in phagocytosis of allergen-antibody complexes. Neutrophils are the first white blood cells to increase in infection, followed by monocytes, which continue in high amounts in chronic infections. T lymphocytes are involved in immunity.
8. d. Rationale: The processes that are stimulated by the complement system include enhanced phagocytosis, increased vascular permeability, chemotaxis, and cellular lysis. Prostaglandins and leukotrienes are released by damaged cells, and body temperature is increased by action of prostaglandins and interleukins. All chemical mediators of inflammation increase the inflammatory response and, as a result, increase pain.
9. a. F, production of prostaglandins; b. T; c. F, cytokines; d. T; e. F, mononuclear phagocytic cells
10. b. Rationale: Labile cells of the skin, lymphoid organs, bone marrow, and mucous membranes divide constantly and regenerate rapidly following injury. Stable cells, such as those in bone, liver, pancreas, and kidney, regenerate only if injured, and permanent cells found in neurons and cardiac muscle do not regenerate when damaged.
11. a. 9; b. 5; c. 2; d. 8; e. 6; f. 1; g. 4; h. 10; i. 7; j. 3
12. c. Rationale: The process of healing by secondary intention is essentially the same as primary healing. With the greater defect and gaping wound edges of an open wound, healing and granulation take place from the edges inward and from the bottom of the wound up, resulting in more granulation tissue and a much larger scàr. Tertiary healing involves suturing two layers of granulation tissue together and may require debridement of necrotic tissue.
13. keloid formation, contracture, dehiscence, excess granulation tissue, and adhesions
14. methicillin-resistant *Staphylococcus aureus* (MRSA), vancomycin-resistant enterococci (VRE), penicillin-resistant *Streptococcus pneumoniae* (PRSP); hand washing.
15. c. Rationale: One of the most important factors in the development of antibiotic-resistant strains of organisms has been inappropriate use of antibiotics, and patients and their families should be taught to take full courses of prescribed antibiotics without skipping doses, not to request antibiotics for viral infections, not to take antibiotics prophylactically unless specifically prescribed, and not to take leftover antibiotics. Hand washing and avoiding others with infection are general measures to prevent transmission of infections.
16. b. Rationale: There is a 7% increase in metabolism for every degree Fahrenheit increase in temperature above 100 degrees or a 13% increase for every degree Centigrade increase. This patient has an increase of 1.2 degrees above 100, multiplied by 7% = a total increase of 8.4%. 8.4% of 1800 calories is 151, the amount calories should be increased for the patient during the fever.
17. a. 2; b. 4; c. 1; d. 3; e. 4; f. 1; g. 3; h. 2; i. 4
18. a. Rationale: Granulation tissue includes proliferating fibroblasts, capillary sprouts, white blood cells, exudate, and ground substance for laying collagen and epithelial tissues. Damage to granulation tissue prolongs healing. All open wounds heal with granulation tissue and must be protected with a sterile, moist environment. Topical antimicrobials may actually cause tissue damage,

and not all open wounds have excessive wound exudate that needs to be removed.

19. d. Rationale: Hand washing is the most important factor in preventing infection transmission and is recommended by the Centers for Disease Control for all types of isolation precautions in health care facilities.
20. d. Rationale: Although obesity, hyperglycemia, mental deterioration, malnutrition, old age, and incontinence contribute to development of pressure ulcers, the immobility of the comatose patient presents the greatest risk for tissue damage related to pressure.
21. c. Rationale: Relief of pressure on tissues is critical to prevention and treatment of pressure ulcers, and although pressure-reduction devices may relieve some pressure and lift sheets and trapeze bars prevent skin shear, they are no substitute for frequent repositioning of the patient.
22. a. 3; b. 4; c. 2; d. 1

Case Study

1. pain, redness of leg, edema of leg, fever
2. purulent; yellow wound
3. The WBC count is increased to 18,300/μl from a normal of 4000 to 11,000/μl, indicating a pronounced leukocytosis that would be seen in acute inflammation. Neutrophils are normally 50%–70% of the white cells, and hers are increased to 80%, indicating early response of neutrophils to tissue damage. She also has a "shift to the left" in that normally only 0%–8% of the neutrophils in the blood are immature, banded-nucleus cells, and she has 12% bands. All of these findings are consistent with an acute inflammatory process.
4. History of diabetes, with possible circulatory impairment to lower extremities and altered blood glucose levels; increased weight; inadequate nutrients for healing possible because confined to bed and has no one to help with meals; presence of infection in the wound
5. Aspirin interferes with the synthesis and release of PGs that are in part responsible for fever and also acts on the heat-regulating center in the hypothalamus, resulting in peripheral dilation and heat loss. Mild to moderate fevers (up to 103° F) are not usually harmful and may benefit defense mechanisms, and antipyretics are often only prescribed to control higher temperatures. To prevent acute swings in temperature and cycles of chilling/perspiring, antipyretics should be given regularly at 2- to 4-hour intervals.
6. The wound should be kept moist, with continuous cleansing to remove nonviable tissue and to absorb excessive drainage. Moist gauze or absorption dressings would be the best choice in the wound that is infected.
7. Hand washing—before application of clean gloves and immediately after gloves are removed
   Clean gloves—when in contact with infectious material, such as dressings or linens with exudate
   Biohazard disposal—of dressings, gloves;
   CDC Contact Precautions in addition to standard precautions if *Staphylococcus aureus* is methicillin resistant
8. *Nursing diagnoses:*
   - Pain related to inflammation of left leg
   - Hyperthermia related to inflammatory process
   - Risk for deficient fluid volume related to increased metabolic rate
   - Risk for imbalanced nutrition: less than body requirements related to decreased intake of essential nutrients

   Collaborative problems:
   Potential complication: septicemia

CHAPTER 13

1. a. 9; b. 3; c. 7; d. 5; e. 8; f. 10; g. 4; h. 1; i. 2; j. 11; k. 6
2. c. Rationale: Failure of the two chromosomes to separate during meiosis is known as *nondisjunction* and causes an abnormal number of chromosomes, such as in Down syndrome and Turner's syndrome. The result is two copies of the same chromosome, or sometimes a copy of a chromosome is missing. When genetic material is exchanged between the two chromosomes in a cell, *crossing over* occurs, creasing a greater amount of diversity in the genetic makeup of oocytes and sperm.
3.

		Mother H	Mother H
Father	H	HH unaffected	HH unaffected
Father	h	Hh affected	Hh affected

   a. 50%
   b. 0%
   c. 50%

4.

		Mother P	Mother p
Father	P	PP unaffected	Pp carrier
Father	P	PP unaffected	Pp carrier

a. 50%
b. 50%
c. 0%

5. c. Rationale: Gene therapy that involves using vectors, or gene carriers, can be done both in and outside the body. A common vector is a modified virus that can deliver genetic material into a cell. With ex vivo therapy, cells are removed from the body, transduced with a vector, and then reinfused back into the body. With in vivo therapy, the altered gene in the virus is directly installed into the body.
6. a. 3; b. 1; c. 4; d. 1; e. 2; f. 3; g. 2; h. 4
7. a. bone marrow and thymus gland; b. T lymphocytes, B lymphocytes, macrophages; c. spleen; d. bone marrow; thymus gland
8. a. Rationale: Both B and T lymphocytes must be sensitized by a processed antigen to activate the immune response. Processing involves the taking up of an antigen by macrophages and expression of the antigen on the macrophage cell membrane. Antigens need not be protein, and a few antigens may but may combine with larger molecules that are antigenic.
9. a. Rationale: T-cytotoxic cells directly attack antigens on the cell membrane of foreign pathogens and release cytolytic substances that destroy pathogens. CD4 cells (T-helper cells) and CD8 cells (T-suppressor cells) are involved in the regulation of humoral antibody response and cell-mediated immunity. Natural killer cells are involved in nonspecific killing of cells but are not considered T lymphocytes.
10. c. Rationale: Interferon produces an antiviral effect in cells by reacting with viruses and inducing the formation of an antiviral protein that prevents new viruses from becoming assembled. Most cytokines are immunomodulatory and do not directly affect antigens, and cytokines such as interleukins may stimulate activation of immune cells.
11. b. Rationale: Production of immunoglobulins by B lymphocytes is the essential component in humoral immunity. Tumor surveillance and production of cytokines are functions of T lymphocytes in cellular immunity, and B lymphocytes do not directly attack antigens.
12. a. Rationale: B lymphocytes activated by presentation of an antigen differentiate into many plasma cells that secrete immunoglobulins and only a few memory cells that retain recognition of the antigen as foreign. Helper cells are T lymphocytes, and natural killer cells are large granular lymphocytes that are neither B nor T lymphocytes.
13. a. 4; b. 5; c. 4; d. 3; e. 2; f. 1; g. 5; h. 1; i. 3
14. a. immunity against pathogens that survive inside cells; b. fungal infections; c. rejection of foreign tissue; d. contact hypersensitivity reactions; e. tumor surveillance
15. c. Rationale: Decline of T and B cell activity occurs with advancing age, but circulating autoantibodies increase. Increased autoantibodies are a factor in autoimmune diseases, which increase in persons over the age of 50. T-cell reduction is responsible for decreased tumor surveillance, resulting in an increase in cancer, and decreased hypersensitivity, resulting in anergy.
16. a. 2; b. 1; c. 4; d. 3
17. a. 2; b. 1; c. 1; d. 4; e. 3; f. 1; g. 4; h. 2; i. 1; j. 3; k. 1; l. 1; m. 4
18. a. 1) Edema and itching at injection site
    2) Rapid, weak pulse
    3) Hypotension
    4) Laryngeal spasm
    5) Dilated pupils
    b. 1) Maintain airway and provide oxygen
    2) Start IV for fluid and medication access
    3) Prepare to administer 5 ml of 1:10,000 epinephrine IV
    4) Position flat with legs elevated
    5) Have diphenhydramine (Benadryl) and aminophylline available
19. c. Rationale: Allergic individuals have elevated levels of IgE that react with allergens to produce symptoms of allergy. Immunotherapy involves injecting allergen extracts that will stimulate increased IgG that combines more readily with allergens without releasing histamine. The goal is to keep a "blocking" level of IgG high.
20. d. Rationale: Because there is always a possibility of an anaphylactic reaction when allergens are injected, a health care provider, emergency equipment, and essential drugs should always be available whenever injections are given. The allergen should always be administered in an extremity away from a joint so that a tourniquet can be applied for a severe reaction, and sites should be

rotated. The patient should be carefully observed for a reaction for 20 minutes after an injection.

21. d. Rationale: Two types of latex allergies can occur: a type IV allergic contact dermatitis that is caused by the chemicals used in the manufacturing process of latex gloves, and a type I allergic reaction that is a response to the natural rubber latex proteins, occurs within minutes of contact with the proteins, and may manifest with reactions ranging from skin redness to full-blown anaphylactic shock. Powder-free gloves and avoidance of oil-based hand creams when wearing gloves help prevent allergic reactions to latex.
22. genetic susceptibility and initiation of autoreactivity (a trigger)
23. c. Rationale: Plasmapheresis is the removal of plasma from the blood and in autoimmune disorders is used to remove pathogenic substances found in plasma, such as autoantibodies, complexes of antibodies and antigens, and inflammatory mediators. Circulating blood cells are not affected by plasmapheresis.
24. b. Rationale: The hereditary association that has been noted between HLA type and immune or autoimmune disorders may make it possible to identify members of a family at greatest risk for developing autoimmune disorders.
25. Histocompatibility refers to tissues that are genetically compatible with each other. Several genes determine what antigens are on the human leukocyte and all nucleated cells and platelets. These genes are grouped together on chromosome 6, are labeled as HLA-A, HLA-B, HLA-C, HLA-D, and HLA-DR, and have many possible alleles. If tissue is transplanted that has different antigens on cell surfaces, the recipient's body recognizes the tissue as foreign, and the immune system responds to destroy the tissue.
26. b. Rationale: At the current time, HLA typing is used to determine paternity and to match tissue for transplantation. As more knowledge is gained, there is a strong possibility that HLA associations with certain diseases can be specified and an individual's risk for disease identified.
27. drug-induced immunosuppression with antineoplastic agents and corticosteroids
28. graft-versus-host disease
29. c. Rationale: Standard immunotherapy involves the use of three different immunosuppressants that act in different ways: a calcineurin inhibitor (cyclosporin, tracolimus), a corticosteroid, and the antimetabolite, mycophenolate mofetil. Although cyclosporin is still used, tacrolimus is the most frequently prescribed calcineurin inhibitor.

Case Study

1. IgE is the immunoglobulin involved in most allergic reactions. Chemical mediators that would be active in the patient's allergic rhinitis include histamine, serotonin, slow-releasing substance of anaphylaxis (SRS-A), eosinophil chemotactic factor-anaphylaxis (ECF-A), and complement anaphylatoxins.
2. The procedure would involve either the scratch test or prick test technique. Intradermal allergy testing is not used unless these methods do not cause conclusive reactions. A positive result is manifested by a local wheal-and-flare response that occurs within minutes after insertion of the extract and may last for 8 to 12 hours.
3. Precautions to prevent or treat severe allergic reactions are important:
   Never leave the patient alone during the testing period.
   Always have the following available:
   Emergency equipment (oral airway, laryngoscope, endotracheal tubes, oxygen, tourniquet, IV therapy equipment, cardiac monitor with defibrillator)
   Essential drugs (epinephrine, antihistamines, corticosteroids, and vasopressors)
   Severe local reactions should be treated with removal of the extract and application of antiinflammatory topical cream to the site.
4. Antihistamines relieve allergic symptoms by competing with histamine for H1 receptor sites and thus block the effect of histamine. Action of most antihistamines is not very effective against histamine-induced bronchoconstriction. This patient should be taught to take antihistamines on a regular basis since he has perennial allergic rhinitis that is not limited to contact with seasonal allergens. He must also be cautioned about the common side effects of antihistamines: drowsiness and impaired coordination, dry mouth, GI upset, urinary retention, blurred vision, and dizziness.
5. Household dust is controlled with air conditioners and air filtration systems in the home, as well as daily damp dusting and frequent vacuuming with high-filtration vacuum bags.
6. Precautions:
   - Always have the following available:
     - Physician
     - Emergency equipment (oral airway, laryngoscope, endotracheal tubes, oxygen, tourniquet, IV therapy equipment, cardiac monitor with defibrillator)
     - Emergency drugs (epinephrine, antihistamines, corticosteroids, and vasopressors)

- Administer the extract in an extremity away from a joint so that a tourniquet can be applied for a severe reaction.
- Always aspirate for blood before injection of the allergen extract.
- Assess for systemic reactions manifested by pruritis, urticaria, sneezing, laryngeal edema, and hypotension.
- Observe patient for systemic reactions for 20 minutes following the injection.

7. *Nursing diagnoses:*
   - Ineffective health maintenance related to insufficient knowledge of medications, methods of decreasing exposure to allergens
   - Risk for injury related to effects of antihistamines

   Collaborative problems:
   Potential complication: anaphylaxis

CHAPTER 14

1. a. Rationale: Sexual contact is the most common method of HIV transmission. The other methods may transmit the virus but not as frequently.
2. a. women; b. vascular access; c. anal intercourse; d. whole blood; e. first 2 to 6 months of infection; f. mothers using no therapy; g. needle-stick exposure
3. a. 3; b. 5; c. 1; d. 6; e. 2; f. 7; g. 4
4. a. reverse transcriptase inhibitors: viral RNA is converted to single-strand viral DNA with assistance of the enzyme reverse transcriptase.
   b. protease inhibitors: long strands of viral RNA are cut in the presence of the enzyme protease.
5. c. Rationale: Activated CD4+ T cells are an ideal target for HIV because these cells are attracted to the site of concentrated HIV in the lymph nodes, where they become infected through viral contact with CD4 receptors. CD4+ T cells normally are a major component of the immune system, and their infection renders the immune system ineffective against HIV and other agents. The virus does not stimulate CD8+ T cells, and B lymphocytes are functional early in the disease, as evidenced by positive antibody titers against HIV. Monocytes do ingest infected cells and may become sites of HIV replication and spread the virus to other tissue, but this does not make the immune response ineffective.
6. a. Loss of cellular integrity from HIV budding; b. Syncytial formation may destroy cells that are not infected; c. Destruction of CD4+ T cells by circulating antibodies
7. a. 3; b. 1; c. 2; d. 1; e. 3; f. 2; g. 1; h. 3; i. 4; j. 3
8. d. Rationale: AIDS is diagnosed when an individual with HIV infection meets specific criteria, including development of an opportunistic disease such as *Pneumocystis carinii* pneumonia; a CD4+ T cell count of <200/ml; or candidiasis of the bronchi, trachea, lungs, or esophagus. Oral candidiasis may occur in intermediate chronic infection and is not a diagnostic criterion for AIDS. WBC count is not a criterion for AIDS diagnosis.
9. a. 3; b. 6; c. 8; d. 2; e. 5; f. 7; g. 1; h. 4
10. d. Rationale: Organisms that are nonvirulent or cause limited or localized diseases in an immunocompetent person can cause severe, debilitating, and life-threatening infections in persons with impaired immune function.
11. a. T; b. F, Western blot or immunofluorescence assay (IFA); c. F, CD4+ T cell counts or viral load tests; d. T; e. T
12. d. Rationale: All infants born to HIV-infected mothers will have a positive HIV antibody test because maternal antibodies cross the placental barrier. Within 4 weeks, detection of HIV in infants is possible with testing for the HIV antigen with the use of HIV DNA PCR, HIV RNA PCR, or viral culture. Only 25% of infants born to untreated HIV-infected women are infected with HIV.
13. b. Rationale: The use of potent combination antiretroviral therapy limits the potential for selection of antiretroviral-resistant HIV variants, the major factor limiting the ability of antiretroviral drugs to inhibit virus replication and delay disease progression. The drugs selected should be ones with which the patient has not been previously treated and that are not cross-resistant with antiretroviral agents previously used by the patient.
14. c. Rationale: Guidelines for initiating antiretroviral therapy (ART) are currently in a state of flux because of the development of alternative drugs and problems with long-term side effects and compliance with regimens. In the past, ART was always recommended at the time of HIV infection diagnosis, but today new guidelines suggest that treatment can be delayed until higher levels of immune suppression are observed. Whenever treatment is started, an important consideration is the patient's readiness to initiate ART because adherence to drug regimens is a critical component of the therapy.
15. b. Rationale: An undetectable viral load in the blood does not mean that the virus is gone—it is still present in lymph nodes and other organs. Transmission to others is still possible, and protective measures must be continued to be used.

16. c. Rationale: Pneumococcal, influenza, and hepatitis A and B vaccine should be given as early as possible in HIV infection while there is still immunological function. INH is used for 9-12 months only if a patient has reactive PPD greater than 5 mm, has had a high-risk exposure, or has prior untreated positive PPD. TMP-SMX is initiated when $CD4^+$ T cells are below 200/μl or when there is a history of PCP, and varicella-zoster immune globulin is indicated only after significant exposure to chickenpox or shingles in patients with no history of disease or a negative VZV antibody test.
17. d. Rationale: After a patient has positive HIV-antibody testing and is in early disease, the overriding goal is to keep the viral load as low as possible and to maintain a functioning immune system. The nurse should provide education regarding ways to enhance immune function to prevent the onset of opportunistic diseases in addition to teaching about the spectrum of the infection, options for care, signs and symptoms to watch for, and ways to adhere to treatment regimens.
18. Sexual intercourse:
    Abstain from sexual activity
    Noncontact sexual activities (outercourse)
    Use of barriers during sexual activity
    Drug use:
    Abstain from drug use
    Do not share equipment
    Use alterative routes to injecting
    Do not have sexual intercourse while under influence of drugs
19. d. Rationale: The nursing diagnosis of risk for impaired skin integrity addresses a nursing problem that occurs as a result of the diarrhea and wasting and is a problem that nursing can treat.
20. d. Rationale: All of the nursing interventions are appropriate for a patient with altered thought processes, but the priority is the safety of the patient when cognitive and behavioral problems impair the patient's ability to maintain a safe environment.

Case Study

1. Post-test counseling should include the following:
   Provide resources for medical and emotional support, with immediate assistance.
   Evaluate suicide risk.
   Determine need to test others who have had risky contact with patient.
   Discuss retesting to verify results.
   Encourage optimism: treatment is available, health habits can improve immune function, patient can visit HIV-infected people, and patient is infected with HIV but does not have AIDS.
2. Vague symptoms of fatigue, headaches, lymphadenopathy, and night sweats are characteristic of early chronic infection. $CD4^+$ T cell counts are usually >500/ml in early chronic infection. This patient experienced what could have been acute retroviral syndrome only 2 weeks ago, and it would be unlikely that he would be at a later stage than early chronic infection.
3. Additional testing at this visit should include the following:
   CBC
   Another $CD4^+$ T cell count
   Viral load assessment (bDNA or PCR)
   Hepatitis B serology
   PPD skin test by Mantoux method
4. pneumococcal, influenza, and hepatitis A & B vaccine
   INH if PPD is greater than 5 mm reactive or if he has had a high-risk exposure
   nutritional support and education
5. The drug therapy is not curative but has resulted in dramatic improvements in many HIV-infected patients by maintaining immune function and decreasing viral load. It is critical to take the drug combination specifically as prescribed to prevent development of resistance by the virus. If the drugs cannot be taken for any reason, the physician or nurse practitioner should be notified. There are many side effects of the drugs, some of which can be controlled and are not serious but some of which may prevent use of the drugs. It is important to report any changes in his condition or symptoms that develop. He will be closely monitored, and viral loads will be assessed 2 to 4 weeks after the therapy is started and periodically after that.
6. Genotype and phenotype testing can be done to test for resistance to antiretroviral drugs. The genotype assay detects drug-resistant viral mutations that are present in the reverse transcriptase and protease genes. The phenotype assay measures the growth of the virus in various concentrations of antiretroviral drugs (similar to bacteria-antibiotic sensitivity tests).
7. *Nursing diagnoses:*
   - Anxiety
   - Fear
   - Ineffective denial
   - Anticipatory grieving

   Collaborative problems:
   Potential complications: opportunistic infections; opportunistic malignancies; myelosuppression

CHAPTER 15

1. a. Rationale: Lung cancer is the leading cause of cancer deaths in the United States. Cancers of the reproductive organs are the second leading cause of cancer deaths.
2. d. Rationale: Malignant cells proliferate indiscriminately and continuously and also lose the characteristic of contact inhibition, growth on top of and in between other cells. Cancer cells do not usually proliferate at a faster rate than normal cells, nor can cell cycles be skipped in proliferation, but malignant proliferation is continuous, unlike normal cells.
3. a. Rationale: Cancer cells become more fetal and embryonic (undifferentiated) in appearance and function, and some produce new proteins, such as CEA and AFP, on cell membranes that reflect a return to more immature functioning.
4. c. Rationale: The major difference between benign and malignant cells is the ability of malignant tumor cells to invade and metastasize. Benign tumors are more often encapsulated and often grow at the same rate as malignant tumors. Benign tumors may cause death by expansion into normal tissues and organs.
5. a. 4; b. 1; c. 2; d. 6; e. 3; f. 5
6. a. T; b. T; c. F, reversible; d. T; e. F, initiation and promotion; f. T; g. F, metalloproteinase enzymes; h. T
7. a. rapid proliferation that causes mechanical pressure, leading to penetration of surrounding tissues
   b. decreased cell-to-cell adhesion, allowing cell movement to exterior of primary tumor and within other organ structures
   c. production of metalloproteinase enzymes capable of destroying the basement membrane of the tumor but also of lymph and blood vessels and other tissues
8. a. 5; b. 8; c. 1; d. 7; e. 4; f. 3; g. 6; h. 2
9. a. macrophages: stimulate T cells
   b. cytotoxic T cells: stimulate T cells, natural killer cells, B cells, and macrophages
   c. macrophages: augment natural killer cells
   d. cytotoxic T cells: stimulate macrophages
   e. macrophages: hemorrhagic necrosis of tumors
   f. macrophages: stimulate production and function of white blood cells
10. a. embryonal mesoderm—both
    b. meninges—both
    c. meningioma—benign; meningeal sarcoma—malignant
11. a. arose from epithelial tissue of the breast
    b. moderate differentiation as compared with slight differentiation or very abnormal
    c. small tumor size, with a small number of lymph nodes involved, with no evidence of distant metastases
12. a. men: annual digital rectal exam for prostate evaluation
    b. men: annual PSA blood test
    c. women: annual Pap test and pelvic exam
    d. women: annual professional breast exam
    e. women: annual mammogram
    f. annual fecal occult blood test, or flexible sigmoidoscopy q5yr, or annual fecal occult blood test and flexible sigmoidoscopy q5yr, or double-contrast barium enema every 5 to 10 years, or colonoscopy every 10 years
    g. cancer-related checkup every year
13. b. Rationale: Although other tests may be used in diagnosing cancer, biopsy is the only method by which cells can be determined to be malignant.
14. a. 3; b. 1; c. 4; d. 1; e. 2; f. 3; g. 1; h. 2
15. c. Rationale: Tissue that is actively proliferating, such as GI mucosa, esophageal and oropharyngeal mucosa, and bone marrow, exhibit early acute responses to radiation therapy. Cartilage, bone, kidney, and nervous tissue that proliferate slowly manifest subacute or late responses.
16. b. Rationale: Radiation ionization breaks chemical bonds in DNA, which renders cells incapable of surviving mitosis. This loss of proliferative capacity yields cellular death at the time of division for both normal cells and cancer cells, but cancer cells are more likely to be dividing because of the loss of control of cellular division. Cells are most radiosensitive in the M and G2 phases, but damage in cells that are not in the M phase will be expressed when division occurs. Normal tissues are usually able to recover from radiation damage but not always, and permanent damage may occur.
17. b. Rationale: Brachytherapy is the implantation or insertion of radioactive materials directly into the tumor or in proximity of the tumor and may be curative. The patient is a source of radiation, and in addition to implementing the principles of time, distance, and shielding, film badges should be worn by caregivers to monitor the amount of radiation exposure. Computerized dosimetry and simulation are used in external radiation therapy.
18. a. Rationale: Fatigue associated with radiation therapy may be severe and may be related to changes in cell cycle patterns, accumulation of metabolites from cell destruction, and other side effects of radiation therapy. Alopecia, bone marrow suppression, and skin reactions are local reactions when radiation is directed at specific areas of the body.

19. d. Rationale: Positive response of cancer cells to chemotherapy is most likely in tumors that arise from tissue that has a rapid rate of cellular proliferation, have a small number of cancer cells, are young tumors that have a greater percentage of proliferating cells, are not in a protected anatomic site, and have no resistant tumor cells. A state of optimum health and a positive attitude of the patient will also promote chemotherapy success.
20. a. 2; b. 1; c. 4; d. 3; e. 5
21. b. Rationale: One of the major concerns with the IV administration of chemotherapeutic agents is infiltration of drugs into tissue surrounding the infusion site. Many of these drugs are vesicants—drugs that, when infiltrated into the skin, cause severe local breakdown and necrosis. Specific measures to ensure adequate dilution, patency, and early detection of injury are important.
22. a. 4; b. 2; c. 5; d. 1; e. 3
23. a. Rationale: Right atrial catheters are vascular access devices inserted into central veins, which decrease the incidence of extravasation, provide for rapid dilution of chemotherapy, and reduce the need for venipunctures. Most right atrial catheters, except for a Groshong, need to be flushed with heparin to prevent clotting in the tubing. Regional chemotherapy administration delivers the drug directly to the tumor and is the only administration route that can decrease the systemic effects of the drugs.
24. b. Rationale: Patients should always be taught what to expect during a course of chemotherapy, including side effects and expected outcome. Side effects of chemotherapy are serious and may cause death, but it is important that patients are informed what measures can be taken to help them cope with the side effects of therapy. Hair loss related to chemotherapy is usually reversible, and short-term use of wigs, scarves, or turbans can be used during and following chemotherapy until the hair grows back.
25. d. Rationale: Alkylating chemotherapeutic agents and high-dose radiation are most likely to cause secondary resistant malignancies as a late effect of treatment. The other conditions are not known to be later effects of radiation or chemotherapy.
26. b. Rationale: Biologic therapies are normal components of the immune system, which have been identified and isolated and are used therapeutically to restore, augment, or modulate host immune system mechanisms to assist in immune activity against cancer cells.
27. a. Rationale: Virtually all biologic therapies may cause a flulike syndrome that includes headache, fever, chills, myalgias, fatigue, and anorexia. The other side effects may be caused by specific agents but not all biologic therapies.
28. a. Rationale: The most common cause of morbidity and death in cancer patients is infection. Decreased resistance to infection may be caused by bone marrow depression secondary to therapy or malignant infiltration of the bone marrow by cancer. Nursing measures include good handwashing techniques, monitoring WBC counts (especially neutrophils), noting even slight temperature elevations, and instituting protective isolation if the patient is severely immunosuppressed.
29. b. Rationale: An allogenic bone marrow transplant is one in which bone marrow from an HLA-matched donor is infused into a patient who has received high doses of chemotherapy, with or without radiation, to eradicate cancerous cells. In an autologous bone marrow transplant, the patient's own bone marrow is removed before therapy to destroy the bone marrow. The marrow is treated to remove cancer cells and may be infused right away or frozen and stored for later use. In either case, the new bone marrow will take several weeks to produce new blood cells, and protective isolation is necessary during this time.
30. c. Rationale: Tumor lysis syndrome may occur with chemotherapy and is the result of rapid destruction of large numbers of tumor cells. When the cells are destroyed, fatal biochemical changes can occur, especially hyperuricemia, hyperkalemia, hyperphosphatemia, and hypocalcemia.
31. a. Ability to cope with stressful events in the past
    b. Presence of effective support system
    c. Ability to express feelings and concerns
    d. Older age—usually have greater sense of mortality
    e. Feeling of control
    f. Possibility of cure or control

Case Study

1. Chemotherapy-induced bone marrow depression is probably the most relevant factor in his decreased WBC and neutrophil count. Inadequate protein intake would also contribute to impaired recovery of normal blood cells.
2. A temperature of 99. 4° F (37. 4° C) in an immunosuppressed patient is a significant finding for infection. He also has warm skin, with some degree of dehydration. His risk of infection is high with a WBC count of 3200/μl and neutrophils of 500/μl. The risk for infection increases when neutrophils are less than 1000/μl.

3. Assess for sore throat, chest pain, persistent cough, urinary symptoms, rectal pain, or confusion. Also note catheter site for chemotherapy as a possible source of infection.
4. His nausea, vomiting, and anorexia, as well as any other side effects of chemotherapy; negative attitude also promoted by lack of social support, an inability to cope with stress, and lack of information about expected results of treatment
5. Use antiemetic protocols to control treatment-related nausea and vomiting.
   Offer small, frequent feedings of bland, high-calorie, high-protein foods.
   Use relaxation techniques and distraction when the patient is nauseated.
   Offer any fluids or foods the patient can tolerate and that may be appealing to him.
   Avoid nagging or being judgmental about food intake.
6. Hand washing, for both staff and patient
   Careful sterile technique in caring for IV catheter site
   Avoid visitors with infection
7. *Nursing diagnoses:*
   - Hopelessness related to uncertainty about outcomes and insufficient knowledge about cancer and treatment
   - Imbalanced nutrition: less than body requirements related to decreased oral intake, increased metabolic demands of cancer
   - Deficient fluid volume related to decreased oral fluid intake
   - Risk for infection related to immunosuppression

   Collaborative problems:
   Potential complications: septicemia; negative nitrogen balance; myelosuppression

CHAPTER 16

1. a. F, 1000; b. F, 54 (90 kg x 60%); c. F, hyperkalemia; d. T; e. T; f. F, swell and burst, into; g. F, spaces that normally have little or no fluid; h. T
2. a. 4; b. 5; c. 6; d. 7; e. 2; f. 1; g. 3
3. 301 (2 x 147 + 126/18); increased
4. a. 1, 4; b. 2, 3; c. 1, 4; d. 2, 3
5. a. 1; oncotic pressure; b. 2; osmosis; c. 3; osmosis; d. 4; interstitial hydrostatic pressure; e. 1; plasma hydrostatic pressure; f. 1; tissue oncotic pressure; g. 4; interstitial hydrostatic pressure
6. a. serum osmolality increases as large amount of sodium absorbed
   b. stimulates ADH release from the posterior pituitary, which increases water reabsorption from the kidney, lowering the sodium concentration but increasing vascular volume and hydrostatic pressure, perhaps causing fluid shift into interstitial spaces
7. c. Rationale: Aldosterone is secreted by the adrenal cortex in response to a decrease in plasma volume (loss of water), serum sodium, or renal perfusion. It is also secreted in response to an increase in serum potassium.
8. b. Rationale: The action of aldosterone is to increase sodium reabsorption from the kidney, which retains water in the vasculature, and it also causes potassium excretion. ADH increases the permeability to water in the distal convoluted tubule and collecting duct, causing water retention but not sodium retention.
9. d. Rationale: A major cause of hypernatremia is a water deficit, which can occur in those with a decreased sensitivity to thirst, the major protection against hyperosmolality. All of the other conditions lead to hyponatremia.
10. d. Rationale: As water shifts into and out of cells in response to the osmolality of the blood, the cells that are most sensitive to shrinking or swelling are those of the brain, resulting in neurologic symptoms.
11. a. 8; b. 4; c. 6; d. 1; e. 7; f. 2; g. 9; h. 3; i. 10; j. 6; k. 1; l. 5
12. a. hypernatremia, hypokalemia, hypomagnesemia
    b. hyperkalemia, hypocalcemia, hyperphosphatemia, hypermagnesemia
    c. hypokalemia, hyponatremia, hypocalcemia
13. d. Rationale: Because of the osmotic pressure of sodium, water will be excreted with the sodium lost with the diuretic. A change in the relative concentration of sodium will not be seen, but an isotonic fluid loss will occur.
14. c. Rationale: Potassium maintains normal cardiac rhythm, transmission and conduction of nerve impulses, and contraction of muscles. Cardiac cells demonstrate the most clinically significant changes with potassium imbalances because of changes in cardiac conduction. Although paralysis may occur with severe potassium imbalances, cardiac changes are seen earlier and much more commonly.
15. b. Rationale: In a metabolic acidosis, hydrogen ions in the blood are taken into the cell in exchange for potassium ions as a means of buffering excess acids. This results in an increase in serum potassium until the kidneys have time to excrete the excess potassium.
16. d. Rationale: Chvostek's sign is a contraction of facial muscles in response to a tap over the facial nerve. This indicates the neuromuscular irritability of low calcium levels, and intravenous calcium is the treatment to prevent laryngeal spasms and respiratory arrest. Calcitonin is indicated for

treatment of high calcium levels, and loop diuretics may be used to decrease calcium levels. Oral vitamin D supplements are part of the treatment for hypocalcemia but not for impending tetany.

17. c. Rationale: Kidneys are the major route of phosphate excretion, a function that is impaired in renal failure. A reciprocal relationship exists between phosphorus and calcium, and high serum phosphate levels of kidney failure cause a low calcium concentration in the serum.
18. 7.35 to 7.45; 20 to 1
19. hydrogen ion concentration
20. a. 2; b. 4; c. 3; d. 2; e. 1; f. 4; g. 1; h. 2; i. 5; j. 1
21. c. Rationale: The amount of carbon dioxide in the blood directly relates to carbonic acid concentration and subsequently hydrogen ion concentration. The carbon dioxide combines with water in the blood to form carbonic acid, and in cases where carbon dioxide is retained in the blood, acidosis occurs.
22. a. Secretion of small amounts of hydrogen ions into renal tubule
    b. Combining hydrogen ions with ammonia (NH_3) to form ammonium (NH_4)
    c. Excreting weak acids
23. a. 4; b. 2; c. 1; d. 3
    Respiratory acid-base imbalances are associated with excesses or deficits of carbonic acid. Metabolic acid-base imbalances are associated with excesses or deficits of bicarbonate.
24. a. Kidney conservation of bicarbonate and excretion of hydrogen ions
    b. Deep, rapid respirations (Kussmaul's breathing) to increase CO_2 excretion
    c. Decreased respiratory rate and depth to retain carbon dioxide and kidney excretion of bicarbonate
25. a. 4; b. 3; c. 2; d. 1; e. 4; f. 3; g. 3; h. 2; i. 1
26. b. Rationale: Calculation of the anion gap by subtracting the serum chloride and bicarbonate levels from the serum sodium level should normally be 10-14 mmol/L. The anion gap is increased in metabolic acidosis associated with acid gain (e.g., diabetic acidosis) but remains normal in metabolic acidosis caused by bicarbonate loss (e.g., diarrhea).
27. a. 1. pH >7.45 indicates alkalosis
       2. $PaCO_2$ is low, indicating respiratory alkalosis
       3. HCO_3^- is normal
       4. Respiratory alkalosis matches the pH
       5. Although uncommon, if the HCO_3^- were decreased, compensation would be present.
       Interpretation: respiratory alkalosis
    b. 1. pH <7.35 indicates acidosis
       2. $PaCO_2$ is low, indicating a respiratory alkalosis
       3. HCO_3^- is low, indicating an metabolic acidosis
       4. Metabolic acidosis matches the pH
       5. The $PaCO_2$ does not match but is moving in the opposite direction, which indicates the lungs are attempting to compensate for the metabolic acidosis.
       Interpretation: metabolic acidosis; partially compensated
    c. 1. pH <7.35 indicates acidosis
       2. $PaCO_2$ is high, indicating a respiratory acidosis
       3. HCO_3^- is normal
       4. Respiratory acidosis matches the pH
       5. Normal HCO_3^- is found until the kidneys have time to retain bicarbonate.
       Interpretation: respiratory acidosis
    d. 1. pH >7.45 indicates alkalosis
       2. $PaCO_2$ is high, indicating a respiratory acidosis
       3. HCO_3^- is high, indicating a metabolic alkalosis
       4. Metabolic alkalosis matches the pH
       5. The $PaCO_2$ does not match but is moving in the opposite direction, indicating the lungs are attempting to compensate for the alkalosis.
       Interpretation: metabolic alkalosis, partially compensated
    e. 1. pH is within normal range but toward alkalosis
       2. $PaCO_2$ is high, indicating a respiratory acidosis
       3. HCO_3^- is high, indicating a metabolic alkalosis
       4. Because the body will not overcompensate, the metabolic alkalosis is a closer match with the pH.
       5. The high $PaCO_2$ indicates the ability of the lungs to compensate for the metabolic alkalosis.
       Interpretation: compensated or chronic metabolic alkalosis indicated by the high $PaCO_2$ and a pH within normal range
    f. 1. pH is within normal range but toward acidosis
       2. $PaCO_2$ is high, indicating a respiratory acidosis
       3. HCO_3^- is high, indicating a metabolic alkalosis
       4. Because the body will not overcompensate, the respiratory acidosis is a closer match with the pH.

5. The high HCO_3^- indicates the ability of the kidneys to compensate for the respiratory acidosis.
   Interpretation: compensated respiratory acidosis as reflected by high HCO_3^- and pH in normal range
28. b. Rationale: Fluids such as D_5W provide water that produces a movement of water from the extracellular fluid to the intracellular fluid. Although D_5W is physiologically isotonic, the dextrose is rapidly metabolized, leaving free water to shift into cells.
29. d. Rationale: An isotonic solution does not change the osmolality of the blood and does not cause fluid shifts between the extracellular fluid and intracellular fluid. In the case of extracellular fluid loss, an isotonic solution, such as lactated Ringer's solution, is ideal because it stays in the extracellular compartment. A hypertonic solution would pull fluid from the cells into the extracellular compartment, resulting in cellular fluid loss and possible vascular overload.

Case Study

1. Status: fluid volume deficit
   Physical assessment: decreased skin turgor; dry mucous membranes; weak pulses, low blood pressure; confusion
   Laboratory findings: elevated BUN; elevated hematocrit
   Status: hypokalemia
   Physical assessment: weakness, confusion; irregular heart rhythm, tachycardia
   Laboratory findings: potassium 2.5 mEq/L
   Etiology: diuretic therapy
2. ECG changes are associated with hypokalemia, metabolic alkalosis.
3. Metabolic alkalosis: pH 7.52
   base bicarbonate excess (43 mEq/L)
   Etiology: diuretic-induced hypokalemia is the primary factor.
   Compensation: compensation is not complete because the pH is out of normal range, but increased $PaCO_2$ and slow and shallow respirations indicate the attempt by the lungs to increase carbon dioxide to compensate for excess bicarbonate.
4. Less fluid reserve because older adults have less total body fluid; older adults also have decreased thirst sensation
5. Aldosterone would be secreted in response to a hyperkalemia, and in her case its release would be inhibited by the hypokalemia. However, her low blood pressure and extracellular fluid deficit would stimulate secretion of aldosterone to increase sodium and water retention but cause even more potassium loss.
6. General care: Encourage and assist with oral fluid intake
   Provide skin care with assessment, changes in position, no soap
   Assessments:
   Vital signs q4hr
   I&O; daily weights
   Cardiac monitoring until electrolytes and acid-base normal
   Type and rate of IV fluid and electrolyte replacement
   Lung sounds for signs of fluid overload in cardiac-compromised patient
   Daily serum electrolyte and blood gas levels
   Neurologic changes
7. *Nursing diagnoses:*
   - Deficient fluid volume related to excessive ECF loss or decreased fluid intake
   - Ineffective health maintenance related to lack of knowledge of drugs and preventive measures
   - Risk for injury related to confusion, muscle weakness
   - Risk for impaired skin integrity related to dehydration

   Collaborative problems:
   Potential complications: arrhythmias; hypovolemic shock; hypoxemia

CHAPTER 17

1. a. diagnosis; b. cosmetic; c. palliation; d. curative; e. curative
2. a. Rationale: Ambulatory surgery is usually less expensive and more convenient, generally involving fewer laboratory tests, fewer preoperative and postoperative medications, less psychologic stress, and less susceptibility to hospital-acquired infections. However, the nurse still is responsible for assessing, supporting, and teaching the patient undergoing surgery, regardless of where the surgery is performed.
3. a. Rationale: Excessive anxiety and stress can affect surgical recovery, and the nurse's role in psychologically preparing the patient for surgery is to assess for potential stressors that could negatively affect surgery. Specific fears should be identified and addressed by the nurse by listening and by explaining planned postoperative care. Falsely reassuring, ignoring her behavior, and telling her not to be anxious are not therapeutic.
4. a. Dong quai; b. feverfew; c. garlic; d. ginkgo biloba; e. ginseng; f. goldenseal
5. c. Rationale: Risk factors for latex allergies include a history of hay fever and allergies to

foods such as avocados, kiwi, bananas, potatoes, peaches, and apricots. When a patient identifies such allergies, the patient should be further questioned about exposure to latex and specific reactions to allergens.

6. a. Personal or family history of:
   Problems with anesthesia:
   - Possible malignant hyperthermia

   History of allergies:
   - Possible drug reactions

   Smoking:
   - Perioperative respiratory complications

   Medication/alcohol/drug use:
   - Interaction with anesthetics
   - Lab tests that should be evaluated
   - Impaired liver function

   b. Obesity
   - Predisposed to dehiscence, infection, herniation
   - Need for increased anesthesia

   Nutritional deficiencies:
   - Impaired healing

   c. Urinary retention:
   - Surgical drugs may increase retention postoperatively.

   Constipation:
   - Surgical drugs and analgesics may slow bowel motility.

   d. Respiratory disease:
   - URI may lead to cancellation of surgery.
   - Increased laryngeal-bronchospasm
   - Increased secretions

   Musculoskeletal problems:
   - Mobility restrictions affecting neck will alter intubation and airway management
   - Surgical positioning and postoperative ambulation may be altered.

   e. Use of sleeping medication:
   - Interaction with anesthetics
   - Need for preoperative sedation

   f. Pain tolerance:
   - Postoperative pain management plan

   Sensory devices:
   - Care of glasses, contacts, hearing aids

   g. Body image:
   - Alterations in self-perception and body image from surgery

   h. Fear and anxiety related to surgery; poor coping skills:
   - Stress management

7. d. Rationale: BUN, serum creatinine, and electrolytes are commonly abnormal in renal disease and should be evaluated before surgery. Other tests are often evaluated in the presence of diabetes, bleeding tendencies, and respiratory or heart disease.
8. a. Rationale: Obesity, as well as spinal, chest, and airway deformities, may compromise respiratory function during and after surgery. Dehydration may require preoperative fluid therapy, and an enlarged liver may indicate hepatic dysfunction that will increase perioperative risk related to glucose control, coagulation, and drug interactions. Weak peripheral pulses may reflect circulatory problems that could affect healing.
9. c. Rationale: All preoperative patients have the right to know what to expect and how to participate effectively in the surgical experience, including information related to preoperative preparation required before surgery. Specific measures such as teaching coughing and deep-breathing techniques and fluid and food restrictions are surgery-specific, and all patients may not receive actual descriptions of the surgical procedure, based on individual need for and response to information.
10. a. Rationale: The nurse may be responsible for obtaining and witnessing the patient's signature on the consent form, but the physician is ultimately responsible for obtaining informed consent. The nurse may be a patient advocate during the signature of the consent form, verifying that consent is voluntary and that the patient understands the implications of consent, but the primary legal action by the nurse is witnessing the patient's signature.
11. a. Notify the physician because the patient needs further explanation of the planned surgery.
    b. Sufficient comprehension
12. c. Rationale: Preoperative checklists are a tool to ensure that the many preparations and precautions performed before surgery have been completed and documented. Patient identification, instructions to the family, and administration of preoperative medications are often documented on the checklist that ensures that no details are omitted.
13. b. Rationale: Atropine, an anticholinergic medication, is frequently used preoperatively to decrease oral and respiratory secretions during surgery, and the addition of morphine will help relieve discomfort during the preoperative procedures. Antiemetics decrease nausea and vomiting during and after surgery, and scopolamine and some benzodiazepines induce amnesia. An actual sleep state is rarely induced by preoperative medications unless an anesthetic agent is administered before the patient is transported to the operating room.
14. c. Rationale: One of the major reasons that older adults need increased time preoperatively is the presence of impaired vision and hearing that slows understanding of preoperative instructions and

preparation for surgery. Thought processes and cognitive abilities may also be impaired in some older adults. The older adult's decreased adaptation to stress because of physiologic changes may increase surgical risks, and overwhelming surgery-related losses may result in ineffective coping that is not directly related to time needed for preoperative preparation. The involvement of family members in preoperative activities may be appropriate for patients of all ages.

Case Study

1. Family—children with cystic fibrosis that require extra care and expense and concern that wife will not be able to manage without him; fear of cancer and the unknown; anemia—contributes to fatigue and ability to cope
2. Three criteria:
   - Adequate disclosure of the diagnosis; nature and purpose of the proposed treatment; the risks and consequences of the proposed treatment; the probability of a successful outcome; the availability, benefits, and risks of alternative treatments; and the prognosis if treatment is not instituted
   - Sufficient comprehension of the information provided
   - Voluntary consent given without persuasion or coercion
3. General preoperative instruction: information related to preoperative routines and preparation, such as food and fluid restrictions, approximate length of surgery and postoperative recovery
   Outpatient instruction: when to arrive and the time of the surgery; how and where to register, what to wear and bring, and the need for a responsible adult for transportation home after the procedure
4. Smoking history increases the risk for postoperative respiratory complications—the longer the patient can stop smoking before surgery, the less the risk
   Mild obesity may contribute to problems with clearance of respiratory secretions and complete expansion of the lungs—should have preoperative instruction about deep-breathing and coughing techniques
   Fear of the diagnosis of cancer can alter adaptation and recovery—nurse can help minimize risk with specific information about the experience and with supportive listening
5. *Nursing diagnoses:*
   - Fear related to possible diagnosis of cancer
   - Interrupted family processes related to family roles shift
   - Ineffective health maintenance related to tobacco use

   Collaborative problems:
   Potential complications: hemorrhage; laryngospasm/bronchospasm; pneumonia

CHAPTER 18

1. b. Rationale: Although all the factors are important to the safety and well-being of the patient, the first consideration in the physical environment of the surgical suite is prevention of transmission of infection to the patient.
2. b. Rationale: Persons in street clothes or attire other than surgical scrub clothing can interact with personnel of the surgical suite in unrestricted areas, such as the holding area, nursing station, control desk, or locker rooms. Only authorized personnel wearing surgical attire and air covering are allowed in semirestricted areas, such as corridors, and masks must be worn in restricted areas, such as operating rooms, clean core, and scrub sink areas.
3. a. 2; b. 1; c. 4; d. 1; e. 2; f. 5; g. 1; h. 6; i. 3; j. 2; k. 5
4. a. Allergy to skin preparation agents, adhesive tapes, or latex; b. Musculoskeletal impairments requiring adaptations in positioning; c. Pain requiring adaptation in moving or procedures; d. Decreased level of consciousness requiring increased safety and protection techniques; e. Vision or hearing impairments requiring adaptations in communication
   Also: Skin conditions requiring special skin preparation and precautions against infection
5. a. Rationale: The most important procedure in admitting a patient to the operating room is a specific identification process that ensures that the correct patient is undergoing surgery. Verification of the patient's understanding of the risks of surgery and a thorough preoperative assessment with history and physical examination are completed preoperatively. Skin preparation is done as part of the surgical procedure.
6. a. Rationale: The protection of the patient from injury in the operating room environment is maintained by the circulating nurse by ensuring functioning equipment, preventing falls and injury during transport and transfer, and being with the patient during anesthesia induction.
7. a. Rationale: The mask covering the face is not considered sterile, and if in contact with sterile gloved hands, contaminates the gloves. The gown at chest level and to 2 inches above the elbows is considered sterile, as is the drape placed at the surgical area.

8. c. Rationale: Musculoskeletal deformities can be a risk factor for positioning injuries and require special padding and support on the operating table. Skin lesions and break in sterile technique are risk factors for infection, and electrical or mechanical equipment failure may lead to other types of injury.
9. c. Rationale: The Perioperative Nursing Data Set of outcome statements related to perioperative safety include the patient's freedom from any type of injury, including medications. Outcomes related to physiologic responses include those of physiologic function, such as respiratory function; behavioral responses include knowledge and actions of the patient and family, including the consistency of the patient's care with the perioperative plan and the patient's right to privacy.
10. thiopental sodium (Pentothal) and sodium methohexital (Brevital)
11. b. Rationale: The volatile liquid inhalation agents have very little residual analgesia, and patients experience early onset of pain when the agents are discontinued. They are associated with a low incidence of nausea and vomiting. Prolonged respiratory depression is not common because of their rapid elimination. Hypothermia is not related to use of these agents, but they may precipitate malignant hyperthermia in conjunction with neuromuscular blocking agents.
12. a. Rationale: Midazolam (Versed) is a rapid, short-acting, sedative-hypnotic benzodiazepine that is used to prevent recall of events under anesthesia because of its amnestic properties.
13. a. Maintenance anesthesia—monitor for laryngo/bronchospasm, respiratory depression, and early pain
    b. Dissociative anesthesia with analgesia and amnesia—monitor for agitation, hallucinations, nightmares
    c. Induction and maintenance of anesthesia; promote early analgesia—assess for nausea and vomiting, monitor respiratory status
    d. Produce deep muscle relaxation—monitor respiratory muscle movement, airway patency
14. a. 5; b. 4; c. 1; d. 3; e. 2
15. b. Rationale: During epidural and spinal anesthesia, a sympathetic nervous system blockade may occur that results in hypotension, bradycardia, and nausea and vomiting. A spinal headache may occur after, not during, spinal anesthesia, and unconsciousness and seizures are indicative of intravenous absorption overdose. Upward extension of the effect of the anesthesia results in inadequate respiratory excursion and apnea.
16. b. Rationale: Although malignant hyperthermia can result in cardiac arrest and death, if the patient is known or suspected to be at risk for the disorder, appropriate precautions taken by the ACP can provide for safe anesthesia for the patient. Because preventive measures are possible if the risk is known, it is critical that preoperative assessment include a careful family history of surgical events.

CHAPTER 19

1. d. Rationale: Technologic advances and shorter-acting anesthetic agents have made changes in anesthesia recovery. Ambulatory and outpatients often do not need as much time to recover, and different phases and recovery areas may be used to direct care. A collaborative PACU team should determine the standards for patient selection, anesthetics used, discharge criteria, and patient outcomes for fast tracking in a specific institution.
2. c. Rationale: Physiologic status of the patient is always prioritized with regard to airway, breathing, and circulation, and respiratory adequacy is the first assessment priority of the patient on admission to the PACU from the operating room. Following assessment of respiratory function, cardiovascular, neurologic, and renal function should be assessed, as well as the surgical site.
3. c. Rationale: The admission of the patient to the PACU is a joint effort between the ACP, who is responsible for supervising the postanesthesia recovery of the patient, and the PACU nurse, who provides care during anesthesia recovery. It involves a verbal report by the ACP of the details of the surgical and anesthetic course, preoperative conditions influencing the surgical and anesthetic outcome, and PACU treatment plans to ensure patient safety and continuity of care.
4. b. Rationale: Even before patients awaken from anesthesia, their sense of hearing returns, and all activities should be explained by the nurse from the time of admission to the PACU to assist in orientation and decrease confusion.
5. a. Rationale: ECG monitoring is performed on patients to assess initial cardiovascular problems during anesthesia recovery. Fluid and electrolyte status is an indication of renal function, and determination of ABGs and direct arterial blood pressure monitoring are used only in special cardiovascular or respiratory problems.
6. a. 3; b. 1; c. 3; d. 1; e. 2; f. 2; g. 1; h. 3
7. d. Rationale: An unconscious or semiconscious patient should be placed in a lateral position to protect the airway from obstruction by the tongue. Deep breathing and elevation of the head of the bed are implemented to facilitate gas

exchange when the patient is responsive. Oxygen administration is often used, but the patient must first have a patent airway.

8. c. Rationale: Hypotension with normal pulse and skin assessment is typical of residual vasodilating effects of anesthesia and requires continued observation. An oxygen saturation of 88% indicates hypoxemia, while a narrowing pulse pressure accompanies hypoperfusion. A urinary output >30 ml/hr is desirable and indicates normal renal function.
9. c. Rationale: A distended bladder may cause both hypertension and emergence delirium. Although hypoxemia is a common cause of emergence delirium, it is associated with hypotension. Delayed awakening may result from neurologic injury, and cardiac arrhythmias most often result from specific respiratory, electrolyte, or cardiac problems.
10. a. Rationale: During hypothermia, oxygen demand is increased, and metabolic processes slow down. Oxygen therapy is used to treat the increased demand for oxygen. Antiarrhythmics and vasodilating drugs would be used only if the hypothermia caused symptomatic cardiac arrhythmias and vasoconstriction. Sedatives and analgesics are not indicated for hypothermia.
11. a. patient awake; b. vital signs stable; c. no excess bleeding or drainage; d. no respiratory depression; e. oxygen saturation greater than 90%
12. *Nursing diagnoses:*
    - Ineffective airway clearance related to decreased respiratory excursion
    - Impaired physical mobility related to decreased muscle strength
    - Constipation related to decreased physical activity and impaired GI motility
    - Risk for infection related to surgical incision, immobility, and decreased circulation

    Collaborative problems:
    Potential complications:
    thromboembolism; paralytic ileus; urinary retention; pneumonia
13. c. Rationale: Incisional pain is often the greatest deterrent to patient participation in effective ventilation and ambulation, and adequate and regular analgesic medications should be provided to encourage these activities. Controlled breathing may help the patient manage pain but does not promote coughing and deep breathing. Explanations of rationale and use of an incentive spirometer help gain patient participation but are more effective if pain is controlled.
14. c. Rationale: Secretion and release of aldosterone and cortisol from the adrenal gland and ADH from the posterior pituitary as a result of the stress response cause fluid retention during the first 2 to 5 days postoperatively, and fluid overload is possible during this time. Aldosterone causes renal potassium loss with possible hypokalemia, and blood coagulation is enhanced by cortisol.
15. a. 1) leg exercises 10 to 12 times every 1 to 2 hours
       2) no pillows under knees, no knee gatch on bed
    b. 1) slow progression to ambulation—elevate head of bed 1 to 2 min; dangle legs, stand by bed
       2) sit if becomes faint; if fainting occurs, lower to floor
    c. 1) promote normal position for voiding or use bedside commode or ambulate to bathroom
       2) run water from faucet; pour warm water over perineum
    d. 1) encourage to expel flatus
       2) reposition in bed frequently; position on right side
    e. 1) use sterile technique for wound care; use proper drain management
       2) frequent assessment of wound
16. a. 2; b. 4; c. 1; d. 1; e. 3; f. 4
17. c. Rationale: Dressings over surgical sites are initially removed by the surgeon unless otherwise specified and should not be changed. Some drainage is expected for most surgical wounds, and the drainage should be evaluated and recorded to establish a baseline for continuing assessment.
18. d. Rationale: During the first 24 to 48 postoperative hours, temperature elevations to 100.4° F (38° C) are a result of the inflammatory response to surgical stress. Dehydration and lung congestion or atelectasis in the first 2 days will cause a temperature elevation above 100.4° F (38° C). Wound infections usually do not become evident until 3 to 5 days postoperatively and manifest with temperatures above 100° F (37.8° C).
19. d. Rationale: Before administering all analgesic medications, the nurse should first assess the nature and intensity of the patient's pain to determine if the pain is expected, if prior doses of the medication have been effective, and if any undesirable side effects are occurring. The administration of prn analgesic medication is based on the nursing assessment. If possible, pain medication should be in effect during painful activities, but activities may be scheduled around medication administration.
20. c. Rationale: All postoperative patients need discharge instruction regarding what to expect and what self-care can be assumed during recovery.

Diet, activities, follow-up care, symptoms to be reported, and instructions about medications are individualized to the patient.

Case Study

1. Orienting as patient recovers from the sedating medication; promoting voiding; providing oral fluids and intake
2. Syncope is possible because of the effects of the drug and instrumentation of the bladder. The patient should be slowly progressed to ambulation by elevating the head of the bed, then dangling the legs, then standing at the side of the bed before attempting ambulation.
3. Inability to void is the most likely problem. The patient could also have respiratory depression or unstable vital signs because of the effects of the drugs or have complications such as bladder bleeding.
4. By standard discharge criteria for PACUs: stable vital signs, oxygen saturation greater than 90%, awake and oriented, no excessive bleeding or drainage, and no respiratory depression, in addition to the specific criteria ordered for this patient
5. An outpatient also needs to be mobile and alert with the ability to provide self-care near the level of preoperative functioning. Postoperative pain, nausea, and vomiting must be controlled, and the patient must be accompanied by an adult to drive her home.
6. *Nursing diagnoses:*
   - Impaired urinary elimination related to bladder irritation
   - Risk for infection related to incomplete bladder emptying
   - Risk for injury related to sedation
   - Acute pain related to bladder irritation

   Collaborative problems:
   Potential complications: hemorrhage; infection

CHAPTER 20

1. a. anterior compartment; b. posterior chamber; c. anterior chamber; d. iris; e. cornea; f. pupil; g. lens; h. suspensory ligaments; i. ciliary body; j. sclera; k. choroids; l. retina; m. optic nerve; n. posterior compartment
2. a. zonules; b. aqueous humor; c. vitreous humor; d. cornea; e. ciliary body; f. rods; g. lens; h. cones; i. sclera; j. limbus; k. conjunctiva; l. puncta; m. optic disc; n. choroids; o. canal of Schlemm; p. iris; q. pupil

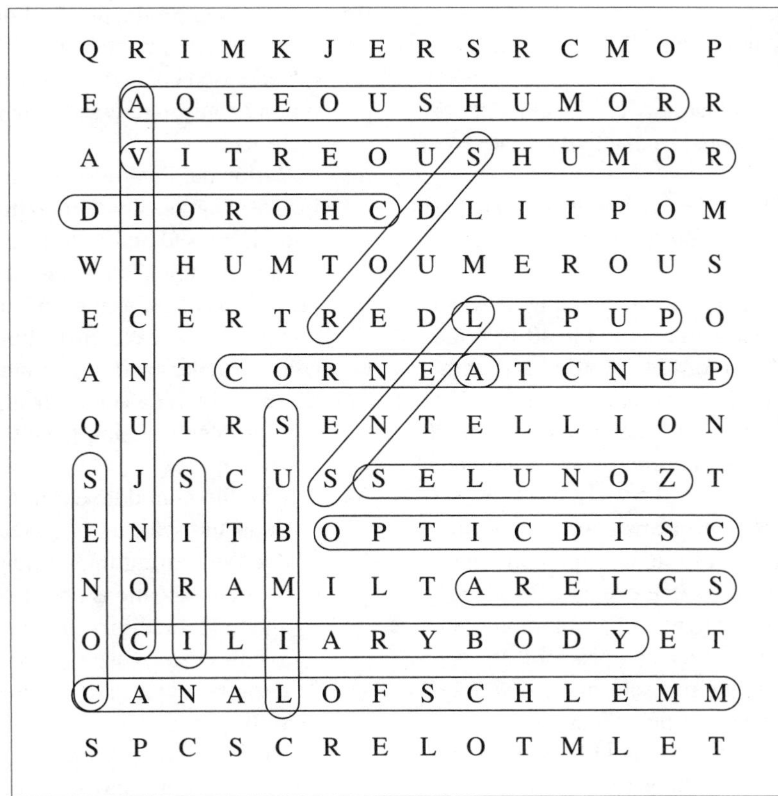

3. a. F, myopia; b. T; c. F, nearsightedness/myopia; d. T; e. F, tears
4. a. 2; b. 5; c. 2; d. 3; e. 2; f. 3; g. 6; h. 4; i. 2; j. 4; k. 1
5. a. Loss of orbital fat; b. Chronic exposure to UV light or other environmental irritants; c. Cholesterol deposits in the peripheral cornea; d. Liquifaction and detachment of vitreous; e. Decreased cones; f. Increased rigidity of iris; g. Deposition of lipids; h. Decreased tear secretion
6. a. Rationale: The use of corticosteroids has been associated with the development of cataracts and glaucoma. Use of oral hypoglycemic agents alerts the nurse to the presence of diabetes and risk for diabetic retinopathy. Antihistamine and decongestant drugs may cause eye dryness, while beta-adrenergic blocking agents may cause additive effects in patients with glaucoma for whom these medications may be prescribed.
7. a. UV light exposure; age-related eye problems, improper contact lens care, family history of ocular problems or diseases affecting the eye
   b. Deficiencies of zinc, vitamins C and E
   c. Constipation and straining to defecate increases intraocular pressure
   d. Work and leisure activities that increase eye strain, lack of protective eyewear during sports
   e. Lack of sleep
   f. Presence of eye pain
   g. Decreased self-concept and self-image, loss of independence
   h. Loss of roles and responsibilities, occupational eye injuries
   i. Eye medications that may cause fetal abnormalities; change in sexual activity related to self-image
   j. Grief related to loss of vision, emotional stress
   k. Values and beliefs that limit treatment decisions
8. With the right eye, the patient standing at 20 feet from a Snellen chart can read to the 40-foot line on the chart with two or fewer errors, and with the left eye, the patient can read only to the 50-foot line on the chart. This patient can read at 20 feet what a person with normal vision can read at 40 and 50 feet.
9. d. Rationale: PERRLA means pupils equal (in size), round, and react to light (pupil constricts when light shines into same eye and also constricts in the opposite eye) and accommodation (pupils constrict with focus on near object). Nystagmus on far lateral gaze is normal but is not part of the assessment of pupil function.
10. a. Confrontation test; b. Cardinal field of gaze; c. Jaeger chart; d. Snellen chart; e. Tono-pen tonometry
11. b. Rationale: A normal yellowish hue to the normally white sclera is found in dark-pigmented persons and the older adult. Infants and some older adults may exhibit a normal blue cast to the sclera because of thin sclera. Iris color does not affect the color of the sclera, and inflammatory conditions of the eye may cause dilation of small blood vessels in the normally clear bulbar conjunctiva, reddening the sclera and conjunctiva.
12. b. Rationale: Fluorescein is a dye that is used topically to identify corneal irregularities; irregularities stain a bright green on application of the dye. A tonometer is used to measure intraocular pressure. Corneal reflex testing establishes the function of the trigeminal nerve (CN V) and should not be done in the patient who may have a corneal abrasion. Corneal light reflex testing is performed to evaluate eye position.
13. a. 3; b. 7; c. 6; d. 5; e. 1; f. 8; g. 4; h. 2
14. c. Rationale: Although fluorescein dye can be used topically to identify corneal lesions, in angiography the dye is injected intravenously and outlines the vasculature of the retina, locating areas of retinopathy. A mirrored lens is used in gonioscopy to examine the anterior chamber angle, and electroretinography is the measurement of the electrical response of the retina to a flash of light.
15. a. 5; b. 1; c. 4; d. 7; e. 9; f. 6; g. 3; h. 8; i. 2
16. a. increased production and dryness of cerumen, increased hair; b. atrophy of the eardrum; c. decreased cochlear efficiency due to decreased blood supply, decreased hair cells, and decreased neurons
17. d. Rationale: Presbycusis is a sensorineural hearing loss that occurs with aging and is associated with decreased ability to hear high-pitched sounds. Tinnitus is present in some, but not all, presbycusis. A sensation of fullness in the ears is related to a blocked eustachian tube, and difficulty in understanding the meaning of words is associated with a central hearing loss occurring with problems arising from the cochlea to the cerebral cortex.
18. a. Childhood middle ear infections with perforations and scarring of the eardrum lead to conductive hearing impairments in adulthood.
    b. Many medications are ototoxic, causing damage to the auditory nerve. Over-the-counter agents such as aspirin and nonsteroidal antiinflammatory agents are potentially ototoxic, as well as prescription diuretics, antibiotics, and chemotherapeutic drugs.
    c. A head injury may damage areas of the brain to which auditory and vestibular stimuli are

transmitted, with a resultant loss of hearing or balance.
d. Some congenital hearing disorders are hereditary, and the age of onset of presbycusis also follows a familial pattern.
e. It is well documented that exposure to loud noises causes damage to the auditory organs and hearing loss. Noise exposure earlier in life also can result in increased hearing loss with age.
f. Persons with hearing loss may withdraw from social relationships because of difficulty with communication. A hearing loss often leaves the patient feeling isolated and cut off from valued relationships.

19. a. T; b. F, upward and backward; c. F, the umbo instead of the cone of light; d. T; e. F, left; f. T; g. F, acute otitis media
20. a. SHL; b. CHL; c. CHL; d. SHL; e. CHL; f. SHL
21. a. Rationale: Hearing is most sensitive between 500 and 4000 Hz, and a 40 to 45 dB loss in the frequency between 4000 and 8000 Hz will cause difficulty in distinguishing high-pitched consonants. A 10 dB loss is not significant at 8000 Hz. A hearing aid is rarely recommended for a hearing loss of less than 26 dB, and problems in everyday communication situations occur only when the thresholds are 25 dB or higher.
22. b. Rationale: Irrigation of the external ear with water causes a disturbance in the endolymph that normally results in nystagmus directed opposite the side of instillation. The absence of nystagmus indicates that peripheral or central vestibular functions are impaired. An improvement in hearing would occur only if there was an obstruction of the ear canal, which would not be an indication for caloric testing. Severe pain upon irrigation would not be related to vestibular function.

CHAPTER 21

1. a. 4; b. 5; c. 2; d. 2; e. 1; f. 1; g. 1; h. 4; i. 3; j. 2; k. 2; l. 1
2. b. Rationale: A soft lens should be moved off the cornea and then gently pinched to release it from the eye. A small suction cup may be used for hard lenses, but cotton balls should not be placed on the lenses. Blinking will not remove soft lenses, and an unconscious patient may not have a blink reflex.
3. d. Rationale: The most common correction for absence of the crystalline lens today is surgical replacement with an intraocular lens. In the past, aphakic spectacles or contact lenses were used, but they are heavy and cause marked magnification. Photorefractive keratectomy involves the use of a laser to reshape the cornea to correct refractive errors.
4. d. Rationale: A person who is legally blind has some usable vision that will benefit from vision enhancement techniques. A person with total blindness has no light perception and no usable vision, and one with functional blindness has the loss of usable vision but some light perception. Dependency on others from visual impairment is individual and cannot be assumed.
5. a. Address patient, not others with the patient, in normal conversational tones
   b. Face patient and make eye contact
   c. Introduce self when approaching the patient and let patient know when leaving
   d. Orient to sounds, activities, and physical surroundings
   e. Use sighted-guide technique to ambulate and orient patient
   f. Do not move objects positioned by patient without knowledge and consent of patient
   g. Ask patient what help is needed and how to provide it
6. c. Rationale: Emergency management of foreign bodies in the eye includes covering and shielding the eye, with no attempt to treat the injury, until an ophthalmologist can evaluate the injury. Irrigations are performed as emergency management in chemical exposure. Pressure should never be applied because it may further injure the eye.
7. a. 4; b. 5; c. 7; d. 6; e. 1; f. 3; g. 2
8. d. Rationale: All infections of the conjunctiva or cornea are transmittable, and frequent, thorough hand washing is essential to prevent spread from one eye to the other or to other persons. Artificial tears are not normally used in external eye infection. Photophobia is not experienced by all patients with eye infections, and cold compresses are indicated for some infections.
9. d. Rationale: Although cataracts do become worse with time, surgical extraction is considered an elective procedure and is usually performed when the patient decides that he wants or needs to see better for his lifestyle. There are no known measures to prevent cataract development or progression. Surgical extraction is safe, but the patient will still need glasses for near vision and for any residual refractive error of the implanted lens.
10. c. Rationale: The lens opacity of cataracts causes a decrease in vision, abnormal color perception, and glare. Blurred vision, halos around lights, and eye pain are characteristic of glaucoma; light flashes, floaters, and "cobwebs" or "hairnets" in the field of vision followed by a painless, sudden

loss of vision are characteristic of detached retina.

11. a. Rationale: Assessment of the visual acuity in the patient's unoperated eye enables the nurse to determine how visually compromised the patient may be while the operative eye is patched and healing and to plan for assistance until vision improves. The patch on the operative eye is usually removed within 24 hours, and although vision in the eye may be good, it is not unusual if visual acuity is reduced immediately after surgery. Activities that are thought to increase intraocular pressure, such as bending, coughing, and Valsalva's maneuver, are restricted postoperatively.
12. a. vitreous shrinking during aging, pulling and tearing the retina; b. rhegmatogenous; c. laser photocoagulation, cryopexy; d. scleral buckling
13. a. Rationale: Postoperatively the patient must position the head so that the bubble is in contact with the retinal break and may have to maintain this position for up to 16 hours a day for 5 days. The patient may go home within a few hours of surgery or may remain in the hospital for several days. No matter the type of repair, reattachment is successful in 90% of retinal detachments. Postoperative pain is expected and is treated with analgesics.
14. b. Rationale: The patient with ARDM can benefit from low-vision aids in spite of increasing loss of vision, and it is important to promote a positive outlook by not giving patients the impression that "nothing can be done" for them. Laser treatment may help a few patients with choroidal neovascularization, and photodynamic therapy is indicated for a small percent of patients with wet ARDM, but there is no treatment for the increasing deposit of extracellular debris in the retina.
15. c. Rationale: Verteporfin, the dye used with photodynamic therapy to destroy abnormal blood vessels, is a photosensitizing drug that can be activated by exposure to sunlight or other high-intensity light. Patients must cover all their skin to avoid thermal burns when exposed to sunlight. Blind spots occur with laser photocoagulation used for dry ARMD. Head movements and position are not of concern following this procedure.
16. a. Rationale: In glaucoma, increased intraocular pressure ultimately damages the optic nerve and retina. Deposition of drusen and degeneration of the macula are characteristic of age-related macular degeneration, and aqueous humor clouding and ciliary body paralysis are not specifically related to eye disorders.
17. c. Rationale: Because glaucoma develops slowly and without symptoms, it is important that intraocular pressure be evaluated every 2 to 4 years in persons between the ages of 40 and 64 and every 1 to 2 years in those over 65 years old. More frequent measurement of intraocular pressure should be done in a patient with a family history of glaucoma, the African-American patient, and the patient with diabetes or cardiovascular disease. The disease is chronic, but vision impairment is preventable in most cases with treatment.
18. a. POAG; b. PACG; c. PACG; d. PACG; e. POAG; f. PACG; g. POAG; h. POAG; i. POAG; j. PACG
19. a. beta-adrenergic blocking agent that decreases aqueous humor production
    b. adrenergic agonist that decreases production of aqueous humor
    c. cholinergic agent that stimulates iris sphincter contraction leading to miosis and opening of the trabecular network, increasing aqueous outflow
    d. carbonic anhydrase inhibitor that decreases aqueous humor production
20. To remove the prosthesis, pull the lower lid down and toward the cheekbone. To insert the prosthesis, open the upper lid with pressure on the upper bony orbit, place the top of the prosthesis under the upper lid, and pull the lower lid down, slipping the lower edge of the prosthesis under the lower lid with a little pressure on the prosthesis.
21. a. Rationale: Patients receiving ototoxic drugs should be monitored for tinnitus, hearing loss, and vertigo to prevent further damage caused by the drugs. Ears should not be cleaned with anything but a washcloth and finger, and ear protection should be used in any environment with noise levels above 90 dB. Exposure to the rubella virus during the first 16 weeks of pregnancy may cause fetal deafness, and the vaccine should never be given during pregnancy.
22. a. 6; b. 2; c. 3; d. 1; e. 5; f. 4
23. Advanced age; use of three potentially ototoxic drugs (aspirin, quinidine, and furosemide)
24. d. Rationale: Antibiotic eardrops for external otitis should be applied without touching the auricle to avoid contaminating the dropper and the solution, and the patient should hold the ear upward for several minutes to allow the drops to run down the canal. An ear wick may be placed in the canal to help deliver the drops, but it remains in the ear throughout the course of treatment. The use of lubricating eardrops followed by irrigation is performed for impacted cerumen. "Swimmer's ear" is best prevented by avoiding swimming in contaminated waters; prophylactic antibiotics are not used.

25. a. F, antibiotics; b. F, cholesteatoma; c. T; d. T; e. F, chronic; f. T; g. F, with the head of bed elevated 30 degrees
26. a. Rationale: Valsalva's maneuver can be used in serous otitis media to open the eustachian tube and equalize the negative pressure that develops in the middle ear. Measures that prevent an increase in middle ear pressure, such as nose blowing, coughing, or positioning, are not indicated.
27. a. Rationale: Otosclerosis is an autosomal dominant hereditary disease that causes fixation of the footplate of the stapes, leading to conductive hearing loss. Tuning fork testing in conductive hearing loss would result in a negative Rinne test and lateralization to the poor ear or ear with the greater hearing loss upon Weber testing. During a stapedectomy, the patient often reports an immediate improvement in hearing, but the hearing level decreases temporarily postoperatively.
28. b. Rationale: Stimulation of the labyrinth intraoperatively may cause postoperative dizziness, increasing the risk for falls. Nystagmus on lateral gaze may result from perilymph disturbances but does not constitute a risk for injury. A tympanic graft is not performed in a stapedectomy, nor is postoperative tinnitus common.
29. a. vertigo; b. sensorineural hearing loss; c. tinnitus
30. b. Rationale: Nursing care should minimize vertigo by keeping the patient in a quiet, dark environment. Movement aggravates the whirling and roaring sensations, and the patient should be moved only for essential care. Fluorescent lights or television flickering may also increase vertigo and should be avoided. Side rails should be raised when the patient is in bed, but there is no indication for padding.
31. d. Rationale: The benign acoustic neuroma can compress the facial nerve and arteries in the internal auditory canal and may expand into the cranium, but if removed when small, hearing and vestibular function can be preserved. During surgery for a tumor that has expanded into the cranium, preservation of hearing and the facial nerve is reduced.
32. a. C; b. C; c. C; d. C; e. S; f. C; g. S; h. S; i. S; j. C
33. c. Rationale: Initial adjustment to a hearing aid should include voices and household sounds and experimenting with volume in a quiet environment. The next recommended exposure is small parties, the outdoors and, finally, uncontrolled areas, such as shopping areas.

Case Study

1. Her race, her family history of glaucoma, and her increasing age place her at a high risk for glaucoma. Glaucoma is the leading cause of blindness among African Americans, and in older persons, 1 in 10 African Americans has glaucoma. African-Americans in every age category should have examinations more often than persons without risk factors because of the increased incidence and more aggressive course of glaucoma in these individuals.
2. To prevent systemic absorption of the drug; Mrs. G. already uses one beta-adrenergic blocker (metoprolol) for her hypertension, and systemic absorption of the betaxolol could cause additive effects.
3. The antihistamine comes into question because of its anticholinergic effects. It is allowed because Mrs. G. has open-angle glaucoma with no abnormal angle on gonioscopy. In angle-closure glaucoma the drug is contraindicated because anticholinergic effects of the antihistamine would dilate the pupil, obstructing an already narrowed angle.
4. No, because glaucoma is a chronic disease with no cure. It can be controlled with medication and some surgical interventions but not cured.
5. Alternatives to topical therapy for POAG include a trabeculoplasty that opens outflow channels in the trabecular meshwork, a trabeculectomy in which part of the iris and trabecular meshwork are removed, or cyclocryotherapy in which parts of the ciliary body are destroyed, decreasing production of aqueous humor.
6. Optic disc cupping with the disc becoming wider, deeper, and paler occurs with progression of glaucoma. Visual complaints with increasing damage include increasing peripheral visual field loss with eventual tunnel vision and loss of sight.
7. *Nursing diagnoses:*
   - Anxiety related to potential permanent visual impairment
   - Ineffective health maintenance related to lack of routine assessments for glaucoma
   - Risk for ineffective therapeutic regimen management related to lack of knowledge about disease, treatment, administration of eyedrops, follow-up recommendations

   Collaborative problems:

   Potential complications: increased intraocular pressure, blindness

CHAPTER 22

1. a. hair shaft; b. stratum corneum; c. stratum germinativum; d. melanocyte; e. sebaceous gland; f. eccrine sweat gland; g. apocrine sweat gland; h. blood vessels; i. nerves; j. adipose tissue; k. hair follicle; l. arrector pili muscle; m. connective tissue; n. subcutaneous tissue; o. dermis; p. epidermis
2. a. 5; b. 3; c. 1; d. 6; e. 2; f. 8; g. 1; h. 4; i. 4; j. 7; k. 2
3. a. Decreased subcutaneous fat, decreased elasticity, collagen stiffening, UV exposure, gravity; b. Decreased extracellular fluid, decreased sweat and sebaceous gland activity; c. Increased capillary fragility and permeability; d. Decreased blood supply, increased keratin
4. d. Rationale: A careful medication history is important because many medications cause dermatologic side effects and patients also use many over-the-counter preparations to treat skin problems. Freckles are common in childhood and are not related to skin disease. Communicable childhood illnesses are not directly related to skin problems, although varicella viruses may affect the skin in adulthood. Patterns of weight gain and loss are not significant, but the presence of obesity may cause skin problems in overlapping skin areas.
5. a. Poor skin hygiene, excessive or unprotected sun exposure, family history of alopecia, ichthyosis, psoriases, history of skin cancer
   b. Decreased intake of vitamins A, D, E, or C, malnutrition, food allergies, obesity
   c. Incontinence, fluid imbalances
   d. Exposure to carcinogens or chemical irritants
   e. Itching that interferes with sleep
   f. Pain, decreased perception of heat, cold, and touch
   g. Feelings of rejection, prejudice, loss of self-esteem, and decreased body image
   h. Exposure to irritants and allergens, altered relationships with others
   i. Changes in sexual intimacy because of appearance, pain
   j. Skin problems exacerbated by stress
   k. High social value placed on appearance and skin condition with tanning, use of cosmetics
6. d. Rationale: It is necessary for the patient to be completely undressed for an examination of the skin. Gowns should be provided and exposure minimized as the skin is inspected generally first, followed by a lesion-specific examination. Skin temperature is best assessed with the back of the hand, and turgor is best assessed with the skin over the sternum.
7. b. Rationale: Discolored lesions that are caused by intradermal or subcutaneous bleeding do not blanch with pressure, while those caused by inflammation and dilated blood vessels will blanch and refill after palpation. Varicosities are engorged, dilated veins that may empty with pressure applied along the vein.
8. a. Vesicles; b. Discrete, localized to chest and abdomen; c. Color, size, and configuration
9. a. 9; b. 5; c. 4; d. 7; e. 10; f. 8; g. 1; h. 11; i. 2; j. 6; k. 3
10. d. Rationale: An excoriation is a focal loss of epidermis, does not involve the dermis and, as such, does not scar with healing. Ulcers do penetrate into and through the dermis, and scarring does occur with these deeper lesions. Epidermal and dermal thinning is atrophy of the skin but does not involve a break in skin integrity. Both excoriations and ulcers have a break in skin integrity and may develop crusts or scabs over the lesions.
11. d. Rationale: During assessment of the skin in dark-skinned persons, inspection of skin color should be done where the epidermis is thin or in areas of least pigmentation. The nailbeds can be used or the mucosa of the eyes or mouth. In African-American individuals, the sclera is normally yellow tinged and is not a good site for evaluating color changes. The palms of the hands and soles of the feet are secondary choices to mucosa.
12. d. Rationale: A shave biopsy is done for superficial lesions that can be scraped with a razor blade, removing the full thickness of stratum corneum. Excisional biopsy is done when the entire removal of a lesion is desired. Punch biopsies are done with larger nodules to examine for pathology, as are incisional biopsies.
13. a. Rationale: A culture can be done to distinguish among fungal, bacterial, and viral infections. A Tzanck test is specific for herpesvirus infections, potassium hydroxide slides are specific for fungal infections, and immunofluorescent studies are specific for infections that cause abnormal antibody proteins.
14. a. 9; b. 5; c. 7; d. 8; e. 1; f. 4; g. 3; h. 10; i. 2; j. 6

CHAPTER 23

1. a. F, ultraviolet B (UVB); b. F, thiazide; c. T; d. T; e. F, B-complex vitamins
2. a. Rationale: Exposure to the sun is the one most important factor in the development of skin cancer and premature aging from loss of elasticity and thinning, wrinkling, and drying of the skin. Radiation exposure and alkaline soaps are less common causes of 2 skin problems, as is indiscriminate self-treatment with over-the-counter skin medications.
3. a. 5; b. 3; c. 5; d. 1; e. 4; f. 1; g. 4; h. 5; i. 2; j. 3
4. A: Asymmetry—one half unlike the other half; B: Border—irregular and poorly circumscribed; C: Color—varied within lesion; D: Diameter—larger than 6 mm
5. c. Rationale: Because of the high potential for metastasis, wide surgical excision with a margin of normal skin is the initial treatment for malignant melanoma. Mohs' surgery is used for cutaneous malignancies, such as basal or squamous cell carcinomas, where there is concern for preservation of normal tissue. Radiation may be used after excision for malignant melanoma, depending on staging of the disease. Topical nitrogen mustard may be used for treatment of cutaneous T cell lymphoma.
6. a. Chronic disease; b. Obesity; c. Recent antibiotic therapy; d. Recent corticosteroid therapy
7. a. 7; b. 10; c. 6; d. 11; e. 8; f. 14; g. 4; h. 12; i. 1; j. 15; k. 3; l. 9; m. 2; n. 5; o. 13
8. Kaposi's sarcoma, candidiasis, herpes zoster
9. b. Rationale: Urticaria is inflammation and edema in the upper dermis, most commonly caused by histamine released during an antibody-allergen reaction. The best treatment for all types of allergic dermatitis is avoidance of the allergen. Sunlight and warmth would increase the edema and inflammation. Antihistamines may be used for an acute outbreak but not to prevent the dermatitis. Topical γ-benzene hexachloride is used to treat pediculosis.
10. a. Rationale: Pediculosis (head lice and body lice) causes very small, red, noninflammatory lesions that progress to papular wheal-like lesions and causes severe itching. Lice live on the body as nits (tiny white eggs) that are firmly attached to the hair shaft in head and body lice. Burrows, especially in interdigital webs, are found with scabies.
11. a. Rationale: A lotion is a suspension of insoluble powders in water, which has cooling and drying properties, useful when itching is present. Creams and ointments have an oil and water base that lubricates and protects skin, while a paste is a mixture of powder and ointment.
12. d. Rationale: Psoralen is absorbed by the lens of the eye, and eyewear that blocks 100% of UV light must be used for 24 hours after taking the medication. Since UVA penetrates glass, the eyewear must also be worn indoors when near a bright window. Psoralen does not affect the accommodative ability of the eye.
13. a. Clean skin; no occlusive dressings
    b. Diagnosis of lesion first; thin layers; massaged in at prescribed frequency
    c. Advise of side effects and risks associated with driving or operating heavy machinery
    d. Avoid sunlight; causes photosensitivity; warn patient it will cause painful, eroded dermatitis before healing
14. a. 4; b. 1, 2, 3, 5; c. 1, 3; d. 2, 3, 6; e. 2, 6
15. a. Rationale: Dressings used to treat pruritic lesions should be cool to cause vasoconstriction and to have an antiinflammatory effect. Water is most commonly used, and it does not need to be sterile. Acetic acid solutions are bacteriocidal and are used to treat skin infections.
16. b. Rationale: Tepid or warm solutions should be used when the purpose is debridement, and saline is a common debridement solution. Baths are appropriate for debridement, but sodium bicarbonate and oatmeal are used for pruritus.
17. a. Vasoconstriction; b. Decrease inflammation and blood flow; c. Decrease vasodilation and stop itch sensation; d. Vasoconstriction and stop itch sensation
18. b. Rationale: Defining characteristics for body image problems include verbalization of self-disgust and reluctance to look at lesions as evidenced in this patient. Social isolation is indicated only if there is evidence of decreased social activities and of anxiety by verbalization of anxiety or frustration. Impaired therapeutic regimen management is indicated by evidence of a lack of self-care or understanding of the disease process.
19. a. Rationale: Lichenification is thickening of the skin, caused by chronic scratching or rubbing, and can be prevented by controlling itching. It is not an infection, nor is it contagious, as the other options indicate.
20. b. Rationale: Nursing interventions for nursing diagnoses should address the etiology of the problem. In this case, if appearance causes the anxiety, the nurse should help the patient improve appearance. A male patient especially may need to be taught skillful use of cosmetics and cover-up techniques to enhance appearance.

21. a. Rationale: Improvement of body image is the most common reason for undergoing cosmetic surgery, with appearance being an important part of confidence and self-assurance. Acne scars, pigmentation problems, and wrinkling can also be treated with cosmetic surgery, but the surgery does not prevent the skin changes associated with aging.
22. a. Face lift; b. Liposuction; c. Dermabrasion; d. Chemical face lift/peel; e. Topical tretinoin
23. a. Rationale: Skin flaps as grafts include moving skin and subcutaneous tissue to another part of the body and are used to cover wounds with poor vascular beds, add padding, and cover wounds over cartilage and bone. Both types of free grafts include just skin, and soft tissue extension involves placement of an expander under the skin, which stretches the skin over time to provide extra skin for covering the desired area.

Case Study

1. Mr. J. B. should have cleansed the wound with soap and water and sought medical care for cleaning and suturing. A sterile dressing should have been applied and the arm elevated to reduce edema.
2. *Staphylococcus aureus* and streptococcus
3. That systemic antibiotics will be necessary and that warm, moist packs or dressings should be used to help localize the infection; hospitalization will be necessary if it becomes severe.
4. Gangrene of the extremity; possible septicemia
5. *Nursing diagnoses:*
   - Impaired skin integrity related to trauma
   - Acute pain related to inflammatory process
   - Hyperthermia related to inflammatory process

   Collaborative problems:
   Potential complications: gangrene; septicemia

CHAPTER 24

1. a. 4; b. 1; c. 2; d. 4; e. 1; f. 3; g. 3
2. a. T; b. F, alkaline substances; c. F, chemical; d. T; e. F, electrical burn
3. a. major; b. major; c. moderate uncomplicated; d. major; e. minor (or superficial partial-thickness may not be classified)
4. a. Rationale: Dry, waxy white, leathery, or hard skin is characteristic of full-thickness burns in the emergent phase, and they may turn brown and dry in the acute phase. Deep partial-thickness burns in the emergent phase are red, shiny, and have blisters. Edema may not be as extensive in full-thickness burns because of thrombosed vessels.
5. a. $3\frac{1}{2} + 1 + 7\frac{1}{2} + 2 + 3\frac{1}{2} = 17\frac{1}{2}$
   b. $4\frac{1}{2} + 9 + 4\frac{1}{2} = 18$
   c. No, because edema and inflammation obscure the demarcation of zones of injury
   d. Major
6. d. Rationale: The first intervention is to remove the source and stop the burning process. Airway maintenance would be second, then establishing IV access, followed by assessing for other injuries.
7. a. Fluid loss and formation of edema—usually 24 to 48 hours but may be up to 5 days; b. Mobilization of fluid and diuresis—weeks to months; c. Burned area covered and wounds healed—weeks to months
8. a. Rationale: With increased capillary permeability, water, sodium, and plasma proteins leave the plasma and move into the interstitial spaces, decreasing serum sodium and albumin. Less sodium is excreted from the kidney because serum levels are low. Serum potassium is elevated because injured cells and hemolyzed RBCs release potassium from cells. An elevated hematocrit is caused by water loss into the interstitium, creating a hemoconcentration. Urine specific gravity increases because of water preservation by the kidneys during hypovolemia.
9. a. Rationale: Although all the selections add to the hypovolemia that occurs in the emergent burn phase, the initial and most pronounced effect is caused by fluid shifts out of the blood vessels as a result of increased capillary permeability.
10. a. Rationale: Burn injury causes widespread impairment of the immune system, with depression of neutrophil activity, decreased T-helper cells, and decreased levels of interleukins.
11. c. Rationale: Because of the hypovolemia and relative fluid loss, intense thirst is a common finding in the initially burned patient. Severe pain is not common in full-thickness burns, nor is unconsciousness unless there are other factors present. Fever is a sign of infection in later burn phases.
12. d. Rationale: In circumferential burns, circulation to the extremities can be severely impaired, and pulses should be monitored closely for signs of obstruction by edema. Swelling of the arms would be expected, but it becomes dangerous when it occludes vessels. Pain and eschar are also expected.
13. b. Rationale: Patients with major injuries involving burns to the face and neck require intubation within 1 to 2 hours after burn injury to prevent the necessity for emergency tracheostomy, which is done if symptoms of upper respiratory obstruction occur. Carbon monoxide poisoning is treated with 100% oxygen, and eschar constriction of the chest is treated with an escharotomy.

14. d. Rationale: Acute tubular necrosis occurs when kidney tubules are mechanically blocked by myoglobin (from muscle cell breakdown) and hemoglobin (from RBC breakdown). Fluid intake at a rate to maintain urinary output at 75 to 100 ml/hr, osmotic diuretics such as mannitol, and sodium bicarbonate to alkalinize the urine help flush the myoglobin and hemoglobin from the circulatory system through the kidneys.
15. To calculate fluid replacement, the patient's weight in pounds must be converted to kilograms: 132 lb = 60 kg.
    a. lactated Ringer's; 9600 ml (4 ml x 60 x 40)
    b. 4800, 1015 to 1730; 2400, 1730 to 0130; 2400, 0130 to 0930
    c. serum sodium levels
    d. urine output (30 to 50 ml/hr); VS (BP ≥90 mm Hg, P ≤100, R 16 to 20); alert, oriented to time, place, and person
16. d. Rationale: When the patient's wounds are exposed with open method, the staff must wear hats, masks, gowns, and gloves. Sterile water is not necessary in the debridement tank, and topical antiinfective agents should be applied with sterile gloves. Open method of treatment does not use dressings.
17. a. Rationale: Morphine is the drug of choice for pain control, and during the emergent phase, it should be administered IV because GI function is impaired and IM injections will not be absorbed adequately.
18. b. Rationale: The patient with large burns often develops paralytic ileus within a few hours, and a nasogastric tube is inserted and connected to low, intermittent suction. After GI function returns, feeding tubes may be used for nutritional supplementation and H_2 blockers may be used to prevent Curling's ulcers. Free water is not given to drink because of the potential for water intoxication.
19. c. Rationale: Patients with ear burns are not allowed to use pillows, because of the danger of the burned ear sticking to the pillowcase, and patients with neck burns are not allowed to use pillows, because contractures of the neck can occur.
20. a. hypermetabolic state resulting from increased plasma catacholamines and substrate mobilization
    b. massive catabolism resulting from protein breakdown and increased gluconeogenesis
    c. calories and protein for tissue repair
21. c. Rationale: At the end of the emergent phase, fluid mobilization moves potassium back into the cells and sodium returns to the vascular space, causing a hypokalemia and a hypernatremia. As diuresis in the acute phase continues, sodium will be lost in the urine and potassium will continue to be low unless replaced. Excessive fluid replacement with 5% dextrose in water without potassium supplementation can cause a hyponatremia with a hypokalemia. Prolonged hydrotherapy and free oral water intake can cause a decrease in both sodium and potassium.
22. c. Rationale: The limited range of motion in this situation is related to the patient's inability or reluctance to exercise the joints because of pain, and the appropriate intervention is to help control the pain so that exercises can be performed. The patient is probably never without some pain, and although exercises and enlisting the help of the physical therapist are important, neither of these interventions addresses the cause.
23. a. Rationale: Early signs of sepsis include an elevated temperature and increased pulse and respiratory rate accompanied by decreased BP and, later, decreased urine output and perhaps paralytic ileus. A burn wound may become locally infected without causing sepsis.
24. a. Dementia; b. Curling's ulcer; c. Stress diabetes
25. a. Cultured epithelial autograft; b. Eschar (or necrotic tissue), split-thickness grafts; c. Aspirating the fluid with a TB syringe or rolling the fluid with a sterile swab to an opening in the peripheral margin of the graft
26. a. Rationale: Midazolam is useful when patients' anticipation of the pain experience increases their pain because it causes a short-term memory loss, and if given before a dressing change, the patient will not recall the event. A dosage range of morphine is useful, as is patient-controlled analgesia, but seldom will these doses effectively relieve the discomfort of dressing changes. Buprenorphine has an analgesic action but is a narcotic antagonist and so cannot be used with other narcotics.
27. a. Rationale: Pressure garments help keep scars flat and prevent elevation and enlargement above the original burn injury area. Lotions and splinting are used to prevent contractures. Avoidance of sun is necessary for 1 year to prevent hyperpigmentation and sunburn injury to healed burn areas.

Case Study

1. Discharge planning should be initiated at the time of admission, when the patient is stabilized. Resuming a functional role in society and accomplishing functional and cosmetic reconstruction are the end goals toward which all care is directed. The nurse should coordinate the discharge process with the whole health care team involved with Kim's care—the physician, physi-

cal and occupational therapists, dietician, home care nurses, and counselors.

2. Kim will continue to need a high-calorie, high-protein diet but not to the extent as during the acute phase. She should be taught about her diet and also to monitor for unwanted weight gain and reduce calories as indicated. She may also have a functional disability in feeding herself and may need padded utensils or special assistive devices.
3. Kim will need to continue the splinting and exercise routines diligently until healing is complete—probably for at least a year.
4. Stress that exercise and performance of activities of daily living will decrease the tightness and limitation of movement. Set achievable short-term goals with her that can be measured, or have her identify a few activities she wants most to do that are realistic and work toward success with those. She is receiving a secondary gain from her husband in her dependence and regression, and the nurse should help her husband see the importance of her reestablishing independence and enlist his help in coaching the patient with exercises.
5. Provide information and expected outcomes related to the healing of her injuries to both patient and husband. Encourage both the patient and her husband to participate in the patient's care, and have them identify how care can be managed at home. Let them know that it is possible to maintain contact with hospital personnel after discharge to answer questions and give them support.
6. Kim and her family may experience a wide range of emotional responses—fear, anxiety, anger, guilt, or depression—and Kim may be very concerned about her children's reactions to the appearance of her injuries. The nurse should encourage the patient's expression of negative feelings and fears while still hospitalized. Arranging for short visits from her children while she is still hospitalized and while the visits can be controlled would be helpful. Preparation of the family can also be enhanced by helping all family members become aware of routines and activities that will need to be continued during rehabilitation.
7. The procedures for dressing changes and graft care should be formally demonstrated to the patient and her husband with time for them to practice and return the demonstrations. It is most likely the husband must be involved because she will be unable to manage dressings to her hands. Referral to home care nurses is essential for follow-up and evaluation when the patient is discharged to ensure that rehabilitation is continuing.
8. *Nursing diagnoses:*
   - Anticipatory grieving related to impact of injury on appearance, relationships, and lifestyle
   - Anxiety related to appearance
   - Self-care deficit related to inability or unwillingness to participate in self-care
   - Impaired therapeutic regimen management related to insufficient knowledge of wound care, follow-up care
   - Situational low self-esteem related to effects of burn on appearance, increased dependence on others, and disruption of lifestyle and role responsibilities
   - Risk for disuse syndrome related to effects of immobility

   Collaborative problems:
   Potential complications: graft rejection/infection; contractures

CHAPTER 25

1. a. nasal cavity; b. right main-stem bronchi; c. segmental bronchi; d. terminal bronchiole; e. alveolar duct; f. alveoli; g. septa; h. pores of Kohn; i. respiratory bronchiole; j. cilia; k. goblet cell; l. mucus; m. dust particle; n. left main-stem bronchi; o. carina; p. trachea; q. larynx; r. epiglottis; s. pharynx
2. a. right midclavicular line; b. right anterior axillary line; c. right upper lobe; d. right middle lobe; e. right lower lobe; f. left lower lobe; g. left upper lobe; h. angle of Louis; i. first rib; j. suprasternal notch; k. trachea; l. larynx; m. thyroid cartilage; n. midsternal line; o. vertebral line; p. spinal processes; q. left upper lobe; r. left lower lobe; s. right lower lobe; t. right upper lobe; u. scapular line

3. a. thoracic cage; b. epiglottis; c. trachea; d. carina; e. dead space; f. surfactant; g. alveolar sacs; h. compliance; i. larynx; j. turbinates; k. angle of Louis; l. parietal pleura; m. phrenic nerve; n. cilia; o. visceral; p. empyema

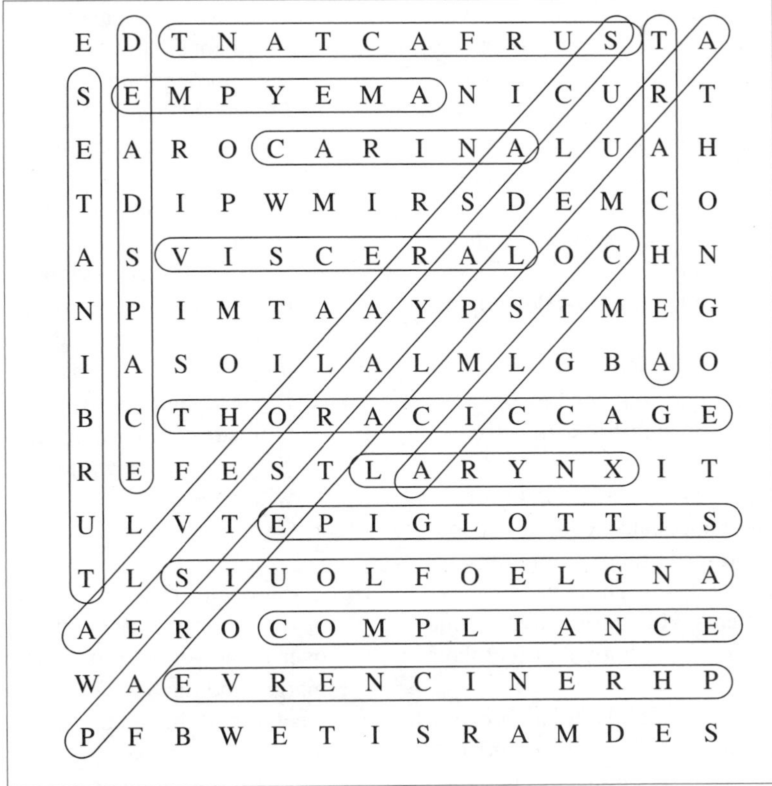

4. a. F, arterial oxygen saturation, as a percent; b. F, arterial oxygen tension, in mm Hg; c. T; d. T; e. F, 65 mm Hg
5. a. Rationale: When the oxygen-hemoglobin curve shifts to the right, blood picks up less oxygen from the lungs but delivers oxygen more readily to the tissues, thus low concentrations of oxygen may be given to prevent oxygen toxicity. Shifts to the right occur with acidosis, hyperthermia, and increased $PaCO_2$. Alkalosis, hypothermia, and decreases in $PaCO_2$ cause a leftward shift of the oxygen-hemoglobin curve, which may be treated with higher concentrations of oxygen to compensate for decreased oxygen unloading in the tissues.
6. c. Rationale: Normally, an SaO_2 of 85% correlates with a PaO_2 of about 60 mm Hg. In a leftward shift of the oxygen-hemoglobin curve, oxygen is less readily delivered to the tissues and a lower PaO_2 is present. In a rightward shift of the curve, an SaO_2 of 85% would reflect a higher PaO_2 than normal, about 65 mm Hg. Leftward shifts are commonly caused by alkalosis, hypothermia, and decreases in $PaCO_2$.
7. b. Rationale: Normal findings in arterial blood gases in the older adult include a decreased PaO_2 and SaO_2 but normal pH and $PaCO_2$. A normal PaO_2 for a 75-year-old patient would be determined by the following equation:
   PaO_2 (mm Hg) = 103.5 – (.42 x age [yr]) or
   103.5 – 31.5 = 72 mm Hg
   Normal PaO_2 levels are expected in patients of 60 years of age or less.
8. c. Rationale: Normal venous blood gas values reflect the normal uptake of oxygen from arterial blood and release of carbon dioxide from cells into the blood, with a decrease in pH due to higher $PvCO_2$ and also much lower PvO_2 and SvO_2. Mixed venous blood gases are used when patients are hemodynamically unstable to evaluate the amount of oxygen delivered to the tissue and the amount of oxygen consumed by the tissues.
9. c. Rationale: Pulse oximetry is inaccurate if the probe is loose, if there is low perfusion, or if there is dark skin color, and before other measures are taken, the nurse should check the probe site. If the probe is intact at the site and perfusion

is adequate, an ABG analysis should be done to verify accuracy, and oxygen may be administered depending on the patient's condition and assessment of respiratory and cardiac status.

10. c. Rationale: Poor peripheral perfusion that occurs with hypovolemia or other types of conditions that cause peripheral vasoconstriction will cause inaccurate pulse oximetry, and ABGs may need to be used to monitor oxygenation status and ventilation status in these patients. It would not be affected by fever or anesthesia and is a method of monitoring arterial oxygen saturation in patients receiving oxygen therapy.
11. a. How the patient's SpO_2 compares with the expected normal values
    b. Determining the trend and rate of development of the hypoxemia
    c. Assessing for the presence of other signs and symptoms of inadequate oxygenation
    d. What the oxygenation status is with activity or exercise
12. c. Rationale: An SpO_2 of 88% and a PaO_2 of 55 mm Hg indicate inadequate oxygenation and are the criteria for prescription of continuous oxygen therapy (Table 25-3). These values may be adequate for patients with chronic hypoxemia if no cardiac problems occur but will affect their activity tolerance.
13. c. Rationale: Lowering of the pH of cerebrospinal fluid by the combination of excess CO_2 and water to form carbonic acid stimulates chemoreceptors in the medulla to increase respiratory rate and volume to provide elimination of the excess CO_2. Peripheral chemoreceptors in the carotid and aortic bodies also respond to increases in $PaCO_2$ to stimulate the respiratory center. Excess CO_2 does not increase the amount of hydrogen ions available in the body but does combine with the hydrogen of water to form an acid.
14. c. Rationale: Ciliary action impaired by smoking and increased mucus production may be caused by the irritants in tobacco smoke, leading to impairment of the mucociliary clearance system. Smoking does not directly affect filtration, the cough reflex, or reflex bronchoconstriction, but it does impair the respiratory defense mechanism provided by alveolar macrophages.
15. a. Decreased functional alveoli, small airway closure earlier in expiration
    b. Decreased elastic recoil and decreased chest wall compliance
    c. Decreased functional cilia, decreased force of cough
    d. Decreased alveolar macrophage activity, decreased IgA
16. a. Smoking history; gradual change in health status; family history of lung disease
    b. Decreased fluid intake; anorexia and weight loss
    c. Constipation; incontinence
    d. Decreased exercise tolerance; dyspnea on rest or exertion; sedentary habits
    e. Sleep apnea; awakening with dyspnea, wheezing, or cough; night sweats
    f. Decreased cognitive function with restlessness, irritability; chest pain or pain with breathing
    g. Inability to maintain lifestyle; altered self-esteem
    h. Loss of roles at work or home; exposure to respiratory toxins at work
    i. Sexual activity altered by respiratory symptoms
    j. Dyspnea-anxiety-dyspnea cycle; poor coping with stress of chronic respiratory problems
    k. Noncompliance with treatment plan; conflict with values
17. a. 1; b. 2; c. 3; d. 2; e. 1; f. 2; g. 4; h. 4; i. 1; j. 1
18. a. Rationale: To assess the extent and symmetry of chest movement, the nurse places the hands over the lower anterior chest wall along the costal margin and moves them inward until the thumbs meet at midline, then asks the patient to breathe deeply and observes the movement of the thumbs away from each other. To determine tracheal position, the nurse places the index fingers on either side of the trachea just above the suprasternal notch and gently presses backward. The palms are placed against the chest wall to assess tactile fremitus.
19. b. Rationale: An increased anteroposterior diameter is characteristic of a barrel chest, in which the anteroposterior diameter is about equal to the side-to-side diameter. Normally the anteroposterior diameter should be one-third to one-half the side-to-side diameter. A prominent protrusion of the sternum is pectus carinatum, and diminished movement of the two sides of the chest indicates decreased chest excursion. Lack of lung expansion due to kyphosis of the spine results in shallow breathing with decreased chest expansion.
20. d. Rationale: Bronchovesicular breath sounds are normal breath sounds when they are heard anteriorly over the main-stem bronchi on either side of the sternum and posteriorly between the scapula. However, if they are heard in the peripheral lung fields, they are considered abnormal breath sounds. Adventitious lungs sounds are crackles, rhonchi, wheezes, and pleural friction rubs.

21. a. 7; b. 6; c. 5; d. 8; e. 1; f. 2; g. 4; h. 3
22. d. Rationale: Because antibody production in response to infection with the TB bacillus may not be sufficient to produce a reaction to TB skin testing immediately after infection, two-step testing is recommended for individuals likely to be tested often, such as health care providers. An initial negative skin test should be repeated in 1 to 3 weeks, and if the second test is negative, the individual can be considered uninfected. All of the other answers indicate a negative response to skin testing but, as single testing, do not allow for delay in antibody production.
23. c. Rationale: Samples for arterial blood gas must be iced to keep the gases dissolved in the blood, unless the specimen is to be analyzed in less than 1 minute and taken directly to the lab. The syringe used to obtain the specimen is rinsed with heparin before taking the specimen, and pressure is applied to the arterial puncture site for 5 minutes after obtaining the specimen. Changes in oxygen therapy or interventions should be avoided for 20 minutes before the specimen is drawn because these changes may alter blood gas values.
24. a. Rationale: A pulmonary angiogram involves the injection of an iodine-based radiopaque dye into the pulmonary artery or the right side of the heart, and iodine or shellfish allergies should be assessed before injection. A bronchoscopy requires NPO status for 6 to 12 hours before the test, and invasive tests, such as bronchoscopy, mediastinoscopy, or biopsies, require informed consent. Nuclear scans use radioactive materials for diagnosis, but the amounts are very small, and no radiation precautions are indicated for the patient.
25. c. Rationale: To prevent damage to the lung tissue and to facilitate entry into the pleural cavity, the patient having a thoracentesis is seated upright, with the elbows or arms on an overbed table.
26. c. Rationale: The greatest chance for a pneumothorax occurs with a bronchoscopic lung biopsy because of the possibility of lung tissue injury during this procedure. Air could enter the pleural space during a thoracentesis, but this is rare. A ventilation-perfusion scan and positron emission tomography involve injections, but no manipulation of the respiratory tract is involved.
27. d. Rationale: A pulmonary arteriogram outlines the pulmonary vasculature and is useful to diagnose obstructions or pathologic conditions of the pulmonary vessels, such as a pulmonary embolus. The tissue changes of TB and cancer of the lung may be diagnosed by chest x-ray, CT, MRI, or PET. Airway obstruction is most often diagnosed with pulmonary function testing.
28. a. 3; b. 7; c. 2; d. 4; e. 5; f. 6; g. 1

CHAPTER 26

1. a. F, nasal septoplasty; b. T; c. T; d. F, seasonal; e. T
2. a. Rationale: Direct pressure on the entire soft lower portion of the nose for 10 to 15 minutes is indicated for epistaxis, in addition to sitting the patient upright, leaning forward, to prevent swallowing of blood. Ice compresses to the nose may be used in addition to having the patient suck ice to constrict the nasal vessels.
3. a. Rationale: After packing of the posterior nasopharynx, some patients experience a decrease in PaO_2 and an increase in $PaCO_2$ because of impaired respiration, and the nurse should monitor respiratory rate and rhythm and SpO_2. The nares are cleaned and petroleum jelly is applied after the packing is removed. A low-grade fever may be an indication of infection and is not expected, and nonsteroidal antiinflammatory drugs should not be used because their antiplatelet effects may prolong bleeding.
4. b. Rationale: The most important factor in managing allergic rhinitis is identification and avoidance of triggers of the allergic reactions. Immunotherapy may be indicated if specific allergens are identified and cannot be avoided. Drug therapy is an alternative to avoidance of the allergens, but long-term use of decongestants may cause rebound nasal congestion.
5. d. Rationale: Dyspnea and purulent sputum in a patient who has a viral URI indicate lower respiratory involvement and a possible secondary bacterial infection. Bacterial infections are indications for antibiotic therapy, but unless symptoms of complications are present, injudicious administration of antibiotics may produce resistant organisms. Elevated temperature, purulent nasal drainage, cough, sore throat, and myalgia are common symptoms of viral rhinitis and influenza.
6. d. Rationale: The influenza vaccine is recommended for individuals at increased risk for influenza-related complications, such as those age 50 and older, residents of long-term care facilities, adults with chronic diseases, health care workers, and providers of care to at-risk persons. It is also recommended for any person wishing to reduce chances of acquiring influenza. Antiviral agents will help reduce the duration and severity of influenza in those at high risk, but immunization is the best control.

7. c. Rationale: Echinacea, goldenseal, and zinc have been shown to be effective stimulants of the immune system, and all three may help reduce symptoms and duration of the common cold. Echinacea and goldenseal should be taken for limited periods, usually only for the duration of the problem. Antibiotics should not be used for a common cold.
8. c. Rationale: Classic antihistamines available without a prescription increase mucus viscosity and promote continued symptoms of sinusitis and should be avoided. Antibiotics should be taken for at least 1 week after symptoms are relieved, and aspirin products may be used to relieve sinus pain or fever. Nasal irrigations with a saline solution may also be used.
9. c. Rationale: Although inadequately treated β-hemolytic streptococcal infections may lead to rheumatic heart disease or glomerulonephritis, antibiotic treatment is not recommended until strep infections are definitely diagnosed with culture or antigen tests. The manifestations of viral and bacterial infections are similar, and appearance is not diagnostic except when candidiasis is present.
10. c. Rationale: During apneic periods of sleep, severe hypoxemia and hypercapnia stimulate ventilation and awaken the patient, perhaps as many as 200 to 400 times a night, resulting in frequent awakening, insomnia, and excessive daytime sleepiness. Morning headaches also may occur. The degree of mattress firmness and a history of upper respiratory infections are not relevant factors.
11. d. Rationale: Compliance is poor with the use of the nasal BiPAP device, but it is highly effective, and the patient should be supported in its use. Emphasizing that it can eliminate the problems of snoring, personality changes, and cardiovascular complications associated with sleep apnea, encourage its use. The device should be used every night, and nighttime sedatives are contraindicated to prevent relaxation of pharyngeal muscles that contributes to airway closure. Head-of-bed elevation is not indicated.
12. a. Stridor; b. Use of accessory muscles; c. Suprasternal and intercostal retractions; d. Wheezing
    Others: restlessness, tachycardia, cyanosis
13. b. Rationale: With a tracheostomy rather than an endotracheal tube, patient comfort is increased because there is no tube in the mouth, and because the tube is more secure, mobility is improved. It is preferable to perform a tracheotomy in the operating room because it requires careful dissection, but it can be performed with local anesthetic in ICU or in an emergency. With a cuff, tracheal pressure necrosis is as much a risk with a tracheostomy tube as with an endotracheal tube, and infection is also as likely to occur since the defenses of the upper airway are bypassed.
14. a. 2; b. 1; c. 4; d. 2; e. 3; f. 4; g. 3; h. 1; i. 4
15. c. Rationale: An inner cannula is a second tubing that fits inside of the outer tracheostomy tube and can be removed and cleaned of mucus that has accumulated on the inside of the tube. Many tracheostomy tubes today do not have inner cannulas because if humidification is adequate, accumulation of mucus should not occur.
16. a. Keep a replacement tube of equal or smaller size at the bedside for emergency reinsertion.
    b. Tracheostomy tapes should not be changed the first 24 hours after insertion.
    c. The first tube change is performed by the physician no sooner than 7 days after tracheostomy.
17. b. Rationale: Cuff pressure should be monitored every 8 hours to ensure that an air leak around the cuff does not occur and that the pressure is not too high to allow adequate tracheal capillary perfusion (Table 26-5). Tracheostomy tubes are not usually changed sooner than 7 days after a tracheotomy. Mouth care should be performed a minimum of every 8 hours and more often as needed to remove dried secretions. ABGs are not routinely assessed with tracheostomy tube placement unless symptoms of respiratory distress continue.
18. b. Rationale: If a tracheostomy tube is dislodged, the nurse should immediately attempt to replace the tube by grasping the retention sutures (if available) and spreading the opening. The obturator is inserted in the replacement tube, water-soluble lubricant is applied to the tip, and the tube is inserted in the stoma at a 45-degree angle to the neck. The obturator is immediately removed to provide an airway. If the tube cannot be reinserted, the physician should be notified, and the patient should be assessed for the level of respiratory distress, positioned in semi-Fowler's position, and ventilated with an MRB only if necessary until assistance arrives.
19. d. Rationale: If colored secretions are coughed or suctioned from the trachea after the patient has attempted to swallow colored water, it indicates that swallowing is not functional and aspiration has occurred. Uncolored water is not discernable as aspirate, and aspiration of small amounts may not cause any respiratory symptoms. The presence of a gag reflex does not ensure that a patient can adequately swallow with a tracheostomy tube

in place, and no fluids except clear liquids should be used to assess aspiration risk.

20. b. Rationale: The primary risk factors associated with head and neck cancers are heavy tobacco and alcohol use and family history. Chronic infections are not known to be risk factors, and while oral cancer may cause a change in the fit of dentures, denture use is not a risk factor for oral cancer.
21. a. Rationale: If laryngeal tumors are small, radiation is the treatment of choice because it can be curative and can preserve voice quality. Surgical procedures are used if radiation treatment is not successful or if larger or advanced lesions are present.
22. a. Rationale: With removal of the larynx, the patient will not be able to communicate verbally, and it is important to arrange with the patient a method of communication before surgery so that postoperative communication can take place. Dry mouth and stomatitis results from radiation therapy. Vigorous coughing is not encouraged immediately postoperatively, and information related to community resources is usually introduced during the postoperative period.
23. a. Rationale: Following a radical neck dissection, drainage tubes are often used to prevent fluid accumulation in the wound, as well as possible pressure on the trachea. A tracheostomy tube is in place, but mechanical ventilation is usually not indicated. The patient has placement of a nasogastric tube to suction immediately after surgery, which will later be used to administer tube feedings until swallowing can be accomplished.
24. c. Rationale: A supraglottic laryngectomy involves the removal of the epiglottis and false vocal cords, and the removal of the epiglottis allows food to enter the trachea. Supraglottic swallowing requires performance of Valsalva's maneuver before placing food in the mouth and swallowing. The patient then coughs to remove food from the top of the vocal cords, swallows again, and then breathes after the food has been removed from the vocal cords.
25. b. Rationale: Suctioning of the tracheostomy with the use of a mirror is a self-care activity that the patient is taught before discharge. Voice rehabilitation is usually managed by a speech therapist or speech pathologist, but the nurse should discuss the various types and the advantages and disadvantages of the different options. The laryngectomy stoma should be covered with a shield during showering and covered with light scarves or fabric when aspiration of foreign materials is likely.
26. a. Rationale: The voice prosthesis provides the most normal voice reproduction but requires surgical insertion of the device into a fistula made between the esophagus and the trachea. Esophageal speech involves trapping air in the esophagus and releasing it to form sound, but only 10% of patients can develop fluent speech with this method. The electrolarynx, whether mouth placed or held to the neck, allows for speech with a metallic or robotic sound.

Case Study

1. Assessment of respiratory status—rate, depth, and rhythm; observation of surgical site for hemorrhage and edema
2. Elevate the head of the bed to semi-Fowler's position to decrease edema; minimize facial movement; apply 4 x 4 dressings dipped in ice water over the incision for the first 24 hours; administer analgesics (nonaspirin) and teach the patient schedule; may have PO fluids when awake, and cold fluids will help decrease swelling
3. His face will become more normal as the swelling decreases; most of the swelling will be relieved in 1 month, but it may be 8 months before it entirely subsides.
4. How to clean his nose and nares with cotton swabs and water or hydrogen peroxide and to apply water-soluble jelly to the nares; to report any continued drainage of serosanguinous fluid from nose after 24 hours or any fresh bleeding; not to use aspirin or aspirin-containing products for pain relief
5. *Nursing diagnoses:*
   - Disturbed body image related to postoperative edema and changed facial appearance
   - Acute pain related to incisional edema
   - Risk for ineffective breathing pattern related to presence of packing and nasal edema

   Collaborative problems:

   Potential complication: nasal hemorrhage

CHAPTER 27

1. c. Rationale: Acute bronchitis is the greatest threat to those who have chronic bronchitis, and they often are provided with antibiotics to take at the first symptoms, which include fever, increased productive cough, and exertional dyspnea. Diffuse rhonchi and wheezing may be heard on auscultation but would not usually be noted by the patient. Pleuritic pain may also occur, but the cough is productive.

2. a. Aspiration from the nasopharynx or oropharynx; b. Inhalation of microbes in the air; c. ematogenous spread from infections elsewhere in the body
3. c. Rationale: Pneumonia that onsets in the community is usually caused by different microorganisms than pneumonia that develops during hospitalization, and treatment can be empirical—based on observations and experience without knowing the exact cause. In at least half the cases of pneumonia, a causative organism cannot be identified from cultures, and treatment is based on experience.
4. a. 3; b. 2; c. 2; d. 1; e. 2; f. 1; g. 2; h. 2; i. 1; j. 3; k. 1
5. a. Red hepatization; b. Resolution; c. Congestion; d. Gray hepatization
6. d. Rationale: Community-acquired pneumonia usually has an acute onset with fever, chills, productive cough with purulent or bloody sputum, and pleuritic chest pain. A recent loss of consciousness or altered consciousness is common in those pneumonias associated with aspiration, such as anaerobic bacterial pneumonias.
7. d. Rationale: Prompt treatment of pneumonia with appropriate antibiotics is important in treating bacterial and mycoplasma pneumonia, and antibiotics are often administered on the basis of the history, physical exam, and a chest x-ray showing a typical pattern characteristic of a particular organism, without further testing. Sputum and blood cultures take 24 to 72 hours for results, and microorganisms often cannot be identified with either Gram stains or cultures. Whether the pneumonia is community-acquired or hospital-acquired is more significant than severity of symptoms.
8. c. Rationale: Pneumococcal meningitis is a metastatic complication of pneumococcal pneumonia, as well as infectious pericarditis, arthritis, or endocarditis. Pleurisy, empyema, and pleural effusion may also result from pneumococcal pneumonia, but these conditions are caused by local spread rather than a hematogenous route.
9. a. advanced generation macrolides; b. trimethoprim/sulfamethoxazole (Bactrim); c. aminoglycoside; d. vancomycin; e. cephalosporin
10. a. Patient with altered consciousness: position to side, protect airway
    b. Patient with feeding tube: check placement of tube before feeding, residual feeding, keep head of bed up after feedings or continuously with continuous feedings
    c. Patient with CNS-depressant drugs: monitor respiration, alertness; avoid oversedation
    d. Patient with local anesthetic to throat: check gag reflex before feeding or offering fluids
    e. Patient with difficulty swallowing: cut food in small bites, encourage thorough chewing, provide soft foods that are easier to swallow than liquids
11. a. Rationale: Secretions are liquefied and more easily removed by coughing when fluid intake is at least 3 L/day. Positioning and oxygen administration may help ineffective breathing patterns and impaired oxygen exchange but are not indicated for retained secretions. Deep breaths are necessary to move mucus from distal airways.
12. b. Rationale: The patient with pneumococcal pneumonia is acutely ill with fever and the systemic manifestations of fever, such as chills, thirst, headache, and malaise. Interventions that monitor temperature and aid in lowering body temperature are appropriate. Diarrhea is not associated, nor is disorientation and confusion unless the patient is very hypoxemic. Pleuritic pain is a local manifestation of pneumococcal pneumonia, not a systemic manifestation.
13. b. Rationale: The pneumococcal vaccine is good for a lifetime except for immunosuppressed patients, who should receive the vaccine every 5 to 6 years. The influenza virus undergoes minor changes each year, and the vaccine should be taken by those at risk for influenza and lower respiratory infections annually in the fall before exposure to the flu virus occurs. Antibiotic therapy is not appropriate for all upper respiratory infections unless secondary bacterial infections develop.
14. b. Rationale: Drug-resistant strains of TB have developed because TB patients' compliance to drug therapy has been poor and there has been general decreased vigilance in monitoring and follow-up of TB treatment. Antituberculous drugs are almost exclusively used for TB infections. TB can be effectively diagnosed with sputum cultures. The incidence of TB is at epidemic proportions in patients with HIV, but this does not account for drug-resistant strains of TB.
15. d. Rationale: The tubercular bacilli create a cellular immune response with development of an epithelioid granuloma that is surrounded by lymphocytes. The central portion of the granuloma undergoes necrosis characterized by a cheesy appearance and is named caseous necrosis and eventually heals with fibrosis and calcification.
16. b. Rationale: A patient with class 3 TB has clinically active disease, and respiratory isolation is required for active disease until the patient has been on drug therapy for at least 2 weeks or until smears are negative on 3 consecutive days. A TB

infection without clinical evidence of TB is class 2, class 4 includes patients with a history of TB but without current disease, and class 5 includes those suspected of having TB pending definite diagnosis.

17. b. Rationale: TB usually develops insidiously with fatigue, malaise, low-grade fevers, and night sweats. Chest pain and a productive cough may also occur, but hemoptysis is a late symptom.
18. a. infected with; b. latent; c. 9, 6; d. INH; e. 6; f. positive smear and culture
19. A four-drug regimen consisting of isoniazid, rifampin, pyrazinamide, and either ethambutol or streptomycin
20. d. Rationale: The nurse should notify the public health department if drug compliance is questionable so that follow-up of patients can be made by directly observed treatment (DOT) by a public health nurse or a responsible family member. A patient who cannot remember to take the medication usually will not remember to come to the clinic daily or will find it too inconvenient. Additional teaching, or support from others, is not usually effective for this type of patient.
21. c. Rationale: Amphotericin B is a toxic drug with many side effects, including hypersensitivity reactions, fever, chills, malaise, nausea and vomiting, and abnormal renal function, but it does not commonly cause immunosuppression. The side effect that would most commonly intensify when a patient also receives chemotherapeutic agents would be the nausea and vomiting.
22. d. Rationale: Almost all forms of bronchiectasis are associated with bacterial infections that damage the bronchial walls. The incidence of bronchiectasis has decreased with use of measles and pertussis vaccines and better treatment of lower respiratory tract infections.
23. d. Rationale: Mucus production is increased in bronchiectasis and collects in the dilated, pouched bronchi. A major goal of treatment is to promote drainage and removal of the mucus, primarily through deep breathing, coughing, and postural drainage.
24. b. Rationale: The most common cause of lung abscesses is aspiration of oropharyngeal materials into the lung, especially when oral and dental hygiene are poor. Positioning to protect the airway and prevent aspiration in patients with altered consciousness is an important measure.
25. b. Rationale: Although all of the precautions identified in this question are appropriate in decreasing the risk of occupational lung diseases, using masks and effective ventilation systems to reduce exposure is the most efficient and affects the greatest number of employees.
26. a. Rationale: Smoking is responsible for approximately 80%-90% of cases of lung cancer, and enough cannot be said about its contribution to lung cancer as well as many other diseases. To prevent lung cancer, avoid exposure to cigarette smoke. Chest x-rays and evaluation of cough are diagnostic means once cancer has already developed.
27. b. Rationale: SIADH is one manifestation of a paraneoplastic endocrine disturbance associated with small cell lung cancer. Small cell lung cancer is associated with cigarette smoking and has the poorest prognosis because of high malignancy and early spread. Surgical resection of squamous cell lung cancer and adenocarcinoma is possible if localized, and large cell tumors are somewhat radiosensitive. Adenocarcinoma is associated with lung scarring and chronic interstitial fibrosis.
28. d. Rationale: Although chest x-rays, lung tomograms, CT scans, MRI, and PET can identify tumors and masses, exact diagnosis of a lung malignancy requires identification of malignant cells either in sputum specimens or biopsies. It is important to note that a negative sputum cytology does not rule out the possibility of cancer, but positive findings can confirm it.
29. a. 3; b. 6; c. 8; d. 7; e. 1; f. 5; g. 2; h. 4
30. d. Rationale: The most successful programs for smoking cessation combine behavioral approaches to alter habits with pharmacologic intervention to decrease the physical addiction to nicotine. Other methods may work for some individuals and include hypnosis, education, environmental control, and social support.
31. b. Rationale: Before making any judgments about the patient's statement, it is important to explore what meaning he finds in the pain. It may be that he feels it is deserved punishment for smoking, but further information needs to be obtained from the patient. Immediate referral to a counselor negates the nurse's responsibility in helping the patient, and there is no indication that he is not dealing effectively with his feelings.
32. a. Open pneumothorax; b. flail chest; c. hemothorax; d. closed pneumothorax; e. tension pneumothorax; f. chylothorax; g. chest tube, water-seal drainage
33. b. Rationale: A tension pneumothorax causes many of the same symptoms as a pneumothorax, but severe respiratory distress from collapse of the entire lung with movement of the mediastinal structures and trachea to the unaffected side are present in a tension pneumothorax. Percussion dullness on the injured site indicates the presence of blood or fluid, and decreased movement and diminished breath sounds are characteristic of a

pneumothorax. Muffled and distant heart sounds indicate a cardiac tamponade.

34. a. Collection of air and fluid from chest cavity with air vented to second chamber
    b. Water-seal chamber allowing escape of air but preventing its reentry to collection chamber
    c. Suction-control chamber to which water is added to control the amount of suction
35. b. Rationale: The water-seal chamber should bubble intermittently as air leaves the lung with exhalation in a spontaneously breathing patient, and continuous bubbling indicates a leak. The water in the suction-control chamber will bubble continuously, and the fluid in the tubing in the water-seal chamber fluctuates with the patient's breathing. Water in the suction-control chamber, and perhaps in the water-seal chamber, evaporates and may need to be replaced periodically.
36. d. Rationale: Although stripping or milking chest tubes to promote drainage is somewhat controversial, there is no indication to milk the tubes when there is no bloody drainage, as in a pneumothorax. Tubing should be looped on the bed without any dependent loops to promote drainage, and patients should cough and deep breathe at least every 2 hours to aid in lung reexpansion. Clamping of chest tubes may cause a tension pneumothorax, but tubes may be clamped momentarily to check for leaks in the system.
37. a. 3; b. 5; c. 1; d. 6; e. 4; f. 2
38. d. Rationale: A thoracotomy incision is large and involves cutting into bone, muscle, and cartilage, resulting in significant postoperative pain. The patient has difficulty deep breathing and coughing because of the pain, and analgesics should be provided before attempting these activities. Water intake is important to liquefy secretions, but it is not indicated in this case, nor should a patient with chest trauma or surgery be placed in Trendelenburg's position because it increases intrathoracic pressure.
39. a. 2; b. 6; c. 5; d. 7; e. 9; f. 8; g. 1; h. 3; i. 4
40. a. 3; b. 1; c. 2; d. 4
41. b. Rationale: High pressure in the pulmonary arteries increases the workload of the right ventricle and eventually causes right ventricular hypertrophy and dilation, known as cor pulmonale. Eventually decreased left ventricular output may occur because of decreased return to the left atrium, but it is not the primary effect of pulmonary hypertension. Alveolar interstitial edema is pulmonary edema associated with left ventricular failure. Pulmonary hypertension does not cause systemic hypertension.
42. d. Rationale: If possible, the primary management of cor pulmonale is treatment of the underlying pulmonary problem that caused the heart problem. Low-flow oxygen therapy will help prevent hypoxemia and hypercapnia that causes pulmonary vasoconstriction.
43. c. Rationale: Acute rejection may occur as early as 5-7 days after surgery and is manifested by low-grade fever, fatigue, and oxygen desaturation with exertion. Complete remission of symptoms can be accomplished with bolus corticosteroids. CMV and other infections can be fatal but usually occur weeks after surgery and manifest with symptoms of pneumonia. Obliterative bronchiolitis is a late complication of lung transplantation, reflecting chronic rejection.

Case Study

1. Low-flow oxygen; calcium channel blocking agents (nifedipine [Adalat], diltiazem [Cardizem]); prostacyclins (epoprostenol [Flolan], bosentan [Tracleer]); diuretics
2. Yes, since she is a medical treatment failure and can be potentially treated with either a lung or heart-lung transplant. She meets additional criteria of being less than 60 years old and a nonsmoker.
3. A heart-lung transplant is indicated for the patient because she has heart damage from the pulmonary hypertension, although there is evidence that even a single-lung transplant can markedly correct pulmonary hypertension and the resultant cor pulmonale.
4. Ability to cope with the postoperative regimen that includes the following:
    - Strict adherence to immunosuppressive drugs
    - Continuous monitoring and reporting of manifestations of infection
    - Financial resources for the procedure, drugs, and follow-up care
    - Social/emotional support system since she is a single mother
5. *Nursing diagnoses:*
    - Activity intolerance related to fatigue secondary to hypoxemia
    - Excess fluid volume related to pump failure
    - Impaired gas exchange related to mechanical failure
    - Ineffective role performance related to inability to perform role responsibilities
    - Anxiety related to breathlessness
    - Risk for impaired skin integrity related to edema

    Collaborative problems:

    Potential complications: arrhythmias; hypoxemia

CHAPTER 28

1. c. Rationale: Obstructive pulmonary diseases are those in which there is increased resistance to airflow as a result of airway obstruction by accumulated secretions, edema, swelling of the inner lumen, bronchospasm, or destruction of lung tissue. In emphysema and chronic bronchitis, the obstruction is relatively constant, but with asthma the obstruction varies. Air trapping and hyperinflation of the lungs are characteristic.
2. a. 3; b. 5; c. 1; d. 4; e. 6; f. 7; g. 2
3. d. Rationale: Respiratory infections are one of the most common precipitating factors of an acute asthma attack. Sensitivity to food and drugs may also precipitate attacks, and exercise-induced asthma probably occurs to some extent in all patients with asthma. Psychologic factors can interact with the asthmatic response to worsen the disease, but it is not a psychosomatic disease.
4. a. Rationale: Diminished or absent breath sounds may indicate a significant decrease in air movement resulting from exhaustion and an inability to generate enough muscle force to ventilate and is an ominous sign. The other symptoms are expected in an asthma attack.
5. d. Rationale: Early in an asthma attack an increased respiratory rate and hyperventilation create a respiratory alkalosis with increased pH and decreased $PaCO_2$, accompanied by a hypoxemia. As the attack progresses, pH shifts to normal, then decreases, with ABGs that reflect respiratory acidosis with hypoxemia.
6. c. Rationale: There are no absolute criteria by which a decision is made to intubate and mechanically ventilate a patient with status asthmaticus, but as the patient becomes more fatigued, more carbon dioxide is retained, and exhaustion of respiratory effort is a major consideration in instituting mechanical ventilation.
7. c. Rationale: Peak expiratory flow rates (PEFRs) normally are up to 600 L/min and in status asthmaticus may be as low as 100 to 150 L/min. An SaO_2 of 85% and FEV1 of 85% of predicted are typical of mild to moderate asthma, and a flattened diaphragm may be present in the patient with long-standing asthma but does not reflect current bronchoconstriction.
8. a. 2, 3; b. 1, 6; c. 1, 6; d. 2, 8; e. 1, 7; f. 1, 4; g. 1, 6; h. 2, 7; i. 1, 3; j. 1, 5; k. 2, 3; l. 1, 6; m. 1, 4; n. 1, 3
9. Correct instructions are: a, b, d, f, g, i, j, k
10. b. Rationale: The patient who is in an acute asthma attack is very anxious and fearful. It is important to stay with the patient and interact in a calm, unhurried manner. Helping the patient breathe with pursed lips will facilitate expiration of trapped air and help the patient gain control of breathing.
11. b. Rationale: Initial drug therapy for acute respiratory distress involves the use of aerosolized albuterol or other beta-adrenergic agonists by nebulization every 20 minutes to 4 hours as necessary. The other medications may be added if the patient does not respond to inhaled beta-adrenergic agonists.
12. b. Rationale: A yellow zone indicated on the peak flow meter indicates that the patient's asthma is getting worse, and quick-relief medications should be used. The meter is routinely used only each morning before taking medications and does not have to be on hand at all times. The meter measures the ability to empty the lungs and involves blowing through the meter.
13. b. Rationale: Nonprescription drugs should not be used by patients with asthma because of dangers associated with rebound bronchospasm, interactions with prescribed drugs, and undesirable side effects. All of the other responses are appropriate for the patient with asthma.
14. a. 3; b. 3; c. 3; d. 3; e. 1; f. 4; g. 2; h. 3; i. 2; j. 1
15. a. AAT; b. smoking, inhaled irritants, infection; c. collagen, elastin; d. ATT; e. smoking, hereditary ATT deficiency; f. smoking
16. b. Rationale: The destruction of the alveolar walls and loss of lung elasticity in emphysema lead to the characteristic air trapping in the alveoli. There is increased lung compliance in emphysema because the lungs can be easily inflated but can deflate only partially.
17. c. Rationale: Chronic bronchitis is characterized by chronic inflammation of the bronchial lining, with edema and increased mucus production. Collapse of small bronchioles on expiration is common in emphysema, and abnormal dilation of the bronchi because of destruction of the elastic and muscular structures is characteristic of bronchiectasis.
18. a. B; b. CB; c. B; d. CB; e. E; f. CB; g. E; h. CB; i. B; j. CB; k. E; l. CB
19. b. Rationale: Constriction of the pulmonary vessels, leading to pulmonary hypertension, is caused by alveolar hypoxia and the acidosis that results from hypercapnia. Polycythemia is a contributing factor in cor pulmonale but because it increases the viscosity of blood and the pressure needed to circulate the blood. Long-term low-flow oxygen therapy dilates pulmonary vessels and is used to treat cor pulmonale, and high oxygen administration is not related to cor pulmonale.

20. a. Because of air trapping in the lungs, bronchial collapse on exhalation, and bronchial narrowing, the amount of air that can be exhaled in the first second is decreased.
    b. VC is the maximum volume of air that can be exhaled after maximum inspiration, and the same factors that decrease FEV1 decrease VC.
    c. The residual volume of air left in the lungs after forced expiration is increased because of the air trapping.
    d. Air trapping also increases the total lung capacity, as the lungs become overdistended with air that cannot be exhaled, and also leads to the barrel chest and flattened diaphragm seen in COPD.
21. a. Rationale: Respiratory acidosis with hypercapnia and hypoxemia are characteristic of COPD. Bicarbonate levels are increased in an attempt to buffer the acid load of the increased carbon dioxide. In early stages of COPD, ABGs may be normal or show only slightly decreased PaO_2 and a normal $PaCO_2$.
22. d. Rationale: Smoking cessation is the one most important factor in preventing further damage to the lungs in COPD, but prevention of infections that further increase lung damage is also important. The patient is very susceptible to infections, and infections make the disease worse, creating a vicious cycle. Bronchodilators, inhaled steroids, and lung volume reduction surgery help control symptoms, but these are symptomatic measures.
23. a. 4; b. 6; c. 5; d. 1; e. 3; f. 7; g. 2
24. a. F, carbon dioxide narcosis; b. T; c. F, nitrogen; d. T; e. T; f. F, ≤55 mm Hg, ≤88%
25. a. Rationale: Liquid oxygen reservoirs will last approximately 7 to 10 days when used at 2L/min, and the portable units will hold about 6 to 8 hours of oxygen. Compressed oxygen comes in various tank sizes, but generally it will require weekly deliveries of four to five large tanks to meet a 7- to 10-day supply. Oxygen concentrators or extractors are more expensive; they continuously supply oxygen, but they must be kept out of the bedroom because they are noisy and interfere with sleep.
26. c. Rationale: Pursed-lip breathing prolongs exhalation and prevents bronchiolar collapse and air trapping, while diaphragmatic breathing emphasizes the use of the diaphragm to increase maximum inhalation and to slow the respiratory rate. Thoracic breathing is not as effective as diaphragmatic breathing and is the method most naturally used by patients with COPD. Huff coughing is a technique used to increase coughing patterns to remove secretions.
27. c. Rationale: Many postural drainage positions require placement in Trendelenburg's position, but patients with heart disease, hemoptysis, chest trauma, or severe dyspnea should not be placed in these positions. Postural drainage should be done 1 hour before and 3 hours after meals if possible. Coughing, percussion, and vibration are all performed after the patient has been positioned.
28. b. Rationale: Eating is an effort for patients with COPD, and frequently they do not eat because of fatigue, dyspnea, and difficulty holding their breath while swallowing. Foods that require much chewing cause more exhaustion and should be avoided. A low-carbohydrate diet is indicated if the patient has hypercapnia because carbohydrates are metabolized into carbon dioxide. Fluids should be avoided at meals to prevent a full stomach, and cold foods seem to give less of a sense of fullness than hot foods.
29. d. Rationale: The tripod position with an elevated backrest and supported upper extremities to fix the shoulder girdle maximizes respiratory excursion and an effective breathing pattern. Staying with the patient and encouraging pursed-lip breathing also helps. Bronchodilators may help but can also increase nervousness and anxiety. Postural drainage is not tolerated by a patient in acute respiratory distress, and oxygen is titrated to an effective rate based on ABGs because of the possibility of carbon dioxide narcosis.
30. c. Rationale: Specific guidelines for sexual activity help preserve energy and prevent dyspnea, and maintenance of sexual activity is important to the healthy psychologic well-being of the patient. Open communication between partners is needed so that the modifications can be made with consideration of both partners.
31. c. Rationale: Shortness of breath usually increases during exercise, but the activity is not being overdone if breathing returns to baseline within 5 minutes after stopping. Bronchodilators can be administered 10 minutes before exercise but should not be administered for at least 5 minutes after activity to allow recovery. Patients are encouraged to walk 15 to 20 minutes a day with gradual increases, but actual patterns will depend on patient tolerance. Dyspnea most frequently limits exercise and is a better indication of exercise tolerance than is heart rate in the patient with COPD.
32. c. Rationale: Cystic fibrosis is an autosomal recessive, multisystem disease involving altered function of the exocrine glands of the lungs, pancreas, and sweat glands. Abnormally thick, abundant secretions from mucous glands lead to a chronic, diffuse, obstructive pulmonary disorder in almost all patients, while exocrine pancreatic insufficiency occurs in about 85%-90% of patients with CF.

33. d. Rationale: The major objective of therapy in CF is to promote removal of the secretions, and performance of postural drainage, vibration, and percussion has been the mainstay of treatment. Aerobic exercise also seems to be effective in clearing the airways and is an important part of treatment. Antibiotics are used for early signs of infection, and long courses are necessary, but they are not used prophylactically. Bronchodilators have no long-term benefit. Although CF has become a leading indication for heart-lung transplant, such remedy is not available for most patients.
34. a. Rationale: The presence of a chronic disease that is present at birth and significantly lowers life span affects all relationships and development of those patients who live to young adulthood. Children of a parent with CF will either be carriers of CF or have the disease; many men with CF are sterile, and women have difficulty becoming pregnant. Educational and vocational goals may be met in those who maintain treatment programs and health.

Case Study

1. Change in the amount and color of sputum; LLL percussion dullness indicates the consolidation found with pneumonia; the other sounds are typical of COPD; elevated temperature
2. Improve ventilation and promote secretion removal; promote patient comfort
3. Decreased macrophage activity in the lungs of patients with chronic bronchitis increases the risk of infection; increased inhaled irritants from dust or agricultural chemicals; infection will almost always cause an exacerbation of COPD
4. Respiratory acidosis: low pH; low PaO_2, elevated $PaCO_2$
5. Pulmonary rehabilitation involving bronchial hygiene, exercise conditioning, breathing retraining, and energy conservation; home oxygen therapy; nutrition to increase protein and calories; PEFR monitoring; evaluation of medication administration and instruction if needed
6. *Nursing diagnoses:*
   - Ineffective airway clearance related to expiratory airflow obstruction
   - Ineffective breathing pattern related to increased work of breathing
   - Impaired gas exchange: hypoxemia and hypercapnia related to alveolar hypoventilation
   - Imbalanced nutrition: less than body requirements related to lowered energy level and shortness of breath
   - Hyperthermia related to infectious process

   Collaborative problems:

   Potential complications: respiratory acidosis; respiratory failure; cor pulmonale

CHAPTER 29

1. a. 7; b. 8; c. 6; d. 7; e. 1; f. 4; g. 3; h. 5; i. 3; j. 6; k. 4; l. 8; m. 3; n. 2; o. 5; p. 3
2. a. neutrophils, basophils, eosinophils; b. erythropoietin; c. iron, vitamin B_{12}, folic acid; d. lymphedema; e. liver, spleen, lymph nodes
3. a. 3; b. 2; c. 1; d. 2; e. 1; f. 3; g. 1; h. 3; i. 2
4. b. Rationale: Plasmin causes clot dissolution by attacking fibrinogen or fibrin, the primary component of a clot. Heparin antagonizes thrombin and is an anticoagulant, not a fibrinolytic. As coagulants, fibrinogen is a precursor of fibrin, and prothrombin is a precursor of thrombin.
5. c. Rationale: During fibrinolysis by plasmin, the fibrin clot is split into smaller molecules known as fibrin split products (FSPs) or fibrin degradation products (FDPs). These molecules contribute to anticoagulation by impairing platelet aggregation, reducing prothrombin, and preventing clot stabilization. Tissue thromboplastin, which is released from injured tissues to activate the extrinsic coagulation pathway, is not affected by these products.
6. c. Rationale: Hemoglobin levels decrease in both women and men after middle age and continue to decline with age, although the actual number of RBCs are not significantly reduced. And although leukocyte reserve may be diminished in old age, normally the total WBC count is not affected, and platelets are unaffected by aging.
7. c. Rationale: A pancytopenia is a reduction in all of the blood cells produced by the bone marrow and indicates bone marrow suppression. The liver, spleen, and lymph nodes may filter excessive blood cells but do not cause pancytopenia.
8. b. Rationale: The parietal cells of the stomach secrete intrinsic factor, a substance necessary for the absorption of cobalamin (vitamin B_{12}), and if all or part of the stomach is removed, the lack of intrinsic factor can lead to impaired red cell production and pernicious anemia. Recurring infections indicate decreased WBCs and immune response, and corticosteroid therapy may cause a neutrophilia and lymphopenia. Oral contraceptive use is strongly associated with changes in blood coagulation.

9. a. family history of hematologic disorders; alcohol and cigarette use
   b. deficiencies of iron, vitamin B_{12}, and folic acid; GI bleeding
   petechiae or bruising of the skin
   fever, lymph node swelling
   c. frankly bloody or dark, tarry stools, dark or bloody urine
   d. fatigue and weakness, change in ability to perform normal ADLs
   e. fatigue unrelieved by sleep
   f. pain, especially in joints, bones
   paresthesias, numbness, tingling
   changes in hearing, vision, taste, mental status
   g. altered self-perception because of lymph node enlargement, skin changes
   h. home or work exposure to radiation or chemicals; military history
   i. menstrual history and characteristics of bleeding
   intrapartum or postpartum bleeding problems
   impotence
   j. lack of support to meet daily needs; methods of coping with stress
   k. value conflicts with treatment, especially blood products or bone marrow transplants
10. a. Rationale: Superficial lymph nodes are evaluated by light palpation, but they are not normally palpable. It may be normal to find small (<1.0 cm), mobile, firm, nontender nodes. Deep lymph nodes are detected with x-ray.
11. b. Rationale: Petechiae are small, flat, red or reddish-brown pinpoint microhemorrhages that occur on the skin when platelet levels are low, and when they are numerous, they group, causing reddish bruises known as purpura. Jaundice occurs when anemias are of a hemolytic origin, resulting in accumulation of bile pigments from red blood cells. Enlarged, tender lymph nodes are associated with infection, and sternal tenderness is associated with leukemias.
12. d. Rationale: A smooth, shiny, reddened tongue is an indication of iron-deficiency anemia or pernicious anemia that would be reflected by a decreased hemoglobin level. The increased WBC could be indicative of an infection; the decreased neutrophils, of a neutropenia; and the increased RBC, of polycythemia.
13. d. Rationale: A platelet count of 80,000/μl is a thrombocytopenia and could place the patient at risk for bleeding, necessitating consideration in nursing care. Chemotherapy may cause bone marrow suppression and a depletion of all blood cells. The other factors are all within normal range.
14. a. iron-deficiency anemia; b. inflammatory conditions of any kind; c. infection; d. heparin therapy; e. hemolysis of red blood cells; f. multiple myeloma
15. c. Rationale: A patient with O Rh^+ blood has no A or B antigens on the red cell but does have anti-A and anti-B antibodies in the blood and has an Rh antigen. AB Rh^- blood has both A and B antigens on the red cell but no Rh antigen and no anti-A or anti-B antibodies. If the AB Rh^- blood is given to the patient with O Rh^+ blood, the antibodies in the patient's blood will react with the antigens in the donor blood, causing hemolysis of the donor cells. There will be no Rh reaction because the donor blood has no Rh antigen.
16. a. Rationale: A contrast CT involves the use of an iodine-based dye that could cause a reaction if the patient is sensitive to iodine. Metal implants or internal appliances and claustrophobia should be determined before magnetic resonance imaging (MRI). Prior blood transfusions are not a factor in this diagnostic test.
17. d. Rationale: The preferred, and the most easily aspirated, sites for bone marrow examination are the anterior and posterior iliac crests. Alternative sites in adults are the sternum and the scapulae because they contain red marrow, but the tibia has only yellow marrow in adults.
18. c. Rationale: The aspiration of bone marrow contents is done with local anesthesia at the site of the puncture, but the aspiration causes a suction pain that is quite painful, but very brief. There generally is no residual pain following the test.
19. d. Rationale: Lymph node biopsy is usually done to determine if malignant cells are present in lymph nodes and can be used to diagnose lymphomas as well as metastatic spread from any malignant tumor in the body. Leukemias may infiltrate lymph nodes, but biopsy of the nodes is more commonly used to detect any type of neoplastic cells.

CHAPTER 30

1. a. 2, 4; b. 3, 4; c. 2, 4; d. 1, 4; e. 1, 4; f. 3, 4; g. 1, 6; h. 1, 6; i. 1, 5; j. 3, 4; k. 1, 4; l. 3, 4
2. b. Rationale: The patient's hemoglobin (Hb) level indicates a moderate anemia, and at this severity, additional findings usually include dyspnea and fatigue. Pallor, smooth tongue, and sensitivity to cold usually manifest in severe anemia when the Hb level is below 6 gm/dl (60 gm/L).
3. a. Rationale: Nutritional deficiencies account for the majority of anemia seen in older adults, and

the drugs that many older adults use for chronic illness may contribute to anemia. Anemias that are familial usually manifest before older adulthood, and exposure to chemical toxins as a source of anemia is not as common as nutritional deficiencies. Although postmenopausal bleeding can contribute to anemia in a susceptible older woman, it is rarely significant.

4. c. Rationale: Tachycardia occurs in severe anemia as the body compensates for hypoxemia and the low viscosity of the blood contributes to the development of systolic murmurs and bruits. Depression of the CNS is common with fatigue, lethargy, and malaise. Poor skin turgor may be present, but fever is not associated with anemia. The skin and mucous membranes are pale, with a bluish tinge to the sclera.
5. d. Rationale: Patients with any type of anemia have decreased hemoglobin and symptoms of hypoxemia, leading to activity intolerance. Impaired skin integrity and body image disturbance may be appropriate for patients with jaundice from hemolytic anemias, and altered nutrition is indicated when iron, folic acid, or vitamin B intake is deficient.
6. a. 2; b. 7; c. 5; d. 1; e. 8; f. 4; g. 3; h. 1; i. 3; j. 2; k. 3; l. 7; m. 6; n. 5; o. 1; p. 2; q. 4
7. a. The hypoxia resulting from loss of RBCs in chronic blood loss stimulates the kidney to release erythropoietin, stimulating production of RBCs and reticulocytes, but in pernicious anemia, normal reticulocytes are not produced because of the lack of cobalamin.
   b. Sickle cell anemia is a hemolytic anemia involving an accelerated RBC breakdown leading to increased serum bilirubin levels, while acute blood loss results in loss of the RBC and the bile pigments from the body.
   c. The mean corpuscular volume (MCV) is a determination of the relative size of an RBC, and macrocytic anemias, such as folic acid deficiency and cobalamin deficiency, are characterized by the production of large, immature RBCs that would reflect an increased MCV. In iron-deficiency anemia, the MCV is low because of the lack of hemoglobin in the cells.
8. b. Rationale: Constipation is a common side effect of oral iron supplementation, and increased fluids and fiber should be consumed to prevent this effect. Because iron can be bound in the GI tract by food, it should be taken before meals unless gastric side effects of the supplements necessitate its ingestion with food. Black stools are an expected result of oral iron preparations. Taking iron with ascorbic acid or orange juice enhances absorption of the iron, but enteric-coated iron often is ineffective because of unpredictable release of the iron in areas of the GI tract where it can be absorbed.
9. c. Rationale: Parenteral iron is very irritating and can stain the skin, so needles are changed between withdrawing and administering the medication; 0.5 ml of air is left in the syringe to completely clear the solution from the syringe during administration; it is administered Z-track in the large upper outer quadrant of the buttocks; and the site is not massaged after administration.
10. d. Rationale: To replace the body's iron stores, iron supplements should be continued for 2 to 3 months after the hemoglobin (Hb) level returns to normal, but if the cause of the iron deficiency is corrected, the supplements do not need to be taken for a lifetime. Milk and milk products are poor sources of dietary iron. Activity should be gradually increased as Hb levels return to normal since aerobic capacity can only be increased when adequate Hb is available.
11. b. Rationale: Pernicious anemia is a type of cobalamin (vitamin B_{12}) deficiency that results when parietal cells in the stomach fail to secrete enough intrinsic factor to absorb ingested cobalamin. Extrinsic factor IS cobalamin and may be a factor in some cobalamin deficiencies but not in pernicious anemia.
12. a. Rationale: Neurologic manifestations of weakness, paresthesias of the feet and hands, and impaired thought processes are characteristic of pernicious anemia. Cardiovascular effects are most common with acute blood loss, and aplastic anemias include a leukopenia that leads to decreased immunologic responses.
13. a. Rationale: Without cobalamin replacement, individuals with pernicious anemia will die in 1 to 3 years, but the disease can be controlled with cobalamin supplements for life. Hematologic manifestations can be completely reversed with therapy, but long-standing neuromuscular complications may not be reversed. Since pernicious anemia results from an inability to absorb cobalamin, dietary intake of the vitamin is not a treatment option, nor is a bone marrow transplant.
14. b. Rationale: A common cause of folic acid deficiency is chronic alcohol abuse. Lab results in folic acid deficiency include decreased serum folate levels and increased mean corpuscular hemoglobin concentration (MCHC) due to the large cell size. Achlorhydria and macrocytic RBCs are characteristic of pernicious anemia, and increased indirect bilirubin and increased reticulocytes are characteristic of thalassemia and sickle cell anemia.

15. d. Rationale: Because red meats are the primary dietary source of cobalamin, a strict vegetarian is most at risk for cobalamin-deficiency anemia. Meats are also an important source of iron and folic acid, but whole grains, legumes, and green leafy vegetables also supply these nutrients. Thalassemia is not related to dietary deficiencies.
16. d. Rationale: The anemia of aplastic anemia may cause an inflamed, painful tongue; the thrombocytopenia may contribute to blood-filled bullae in the mouth and gingival bleeding; and the leukopenia may lead to stomatitis and oral ulcers and infections.
17. b. Rationale: Hemorrhage from thrombocytopenia and infection from neutropenia are the greatest risks for the patient with aplastic anemia. The patient will experience fatigue from anemia, but bleeding and infection are the major causes of death in aplastic anemia.
18. a. F, clinical symptoms; b. T; c. F, blood transfusions or iron supplements; d. T; e. F, kidney; f. T
19. b. Rationale: Because red cells are abnormal in sickle cell anemia, the mean RBC survival time is 10 to 15 days (rather than the normal 120 days) because of accelerated RBC breakdown by the liver and spleen. Antibody reactions with RBCs may be seen in other types of hemolytic anemias but are not present in sickle cell anemia.
20. b. Rationale: During a sickle cell crisis, the sickling cells clog small capillaries, and the resulting hemostasis promotes a self-perpetuating cycle of local hypoxia, deoxygenation of more erythrocytes, and more sickling. Administration of oxygen may help control further sickling, but additional oxygen does not reach areas of local hypoxia caused by occluded vessels.
21. d. Rationale: Because pain usually accompanies a sickle cell crisis and may last for 4 to 6 days, pain control is an important part of treatment. Rest is indicated to reduce metabolic needs, and fluids and electrolytes are administered to reduce blood viscosity and maintain renal function. Although thrombosis does occur in capillaries, elastic stockings that primarily affect venous circulation are not indicated.
22. d. Rationale: The patient with sickle cell disease is particularly prone to infection, and infection can precipitate a sickle cell crisis. Patients should seek medical attention quickly to counteract upper respiratory infections because pneumonia is the most common infection of the patient with sickle cell disease. Fluids should be increased to decrease blood viscosity, which may precipitate a crisis, and moderate activity is permitted.
23. a. T; b. T; c. F, bleeding; d. F, increased agglutination function of platelets; e. F, petechiae; f. T; g. T; h. F, increased
24. b. Rationale: Thrombus and embolization are the major complications of polycythemia vera because of increased hypervolemia and hyperviscosity. Active or passive leg exercises and ambulation should be implemented to prevent thrombus formation. Hydration therapy is important to decrease blood viscosity, but because the patient already has hypervolemia, a careful balance of intake and output must be maintained and fluids are not injudiciously increased.
25. b. Rationale: Corticosteroids are used in initial treatment of ITP because they suppress the phagocytic response of splenic macrophages, decreasing platelet destruction. They also depress autoimmune antibody formation and reduce capillary fragility and bleeding time. All of the other therapies may be used but only in patients who are unresponsive to corticosteroid therapy.
26. c. Rationale: The major complication of thrombocytopenia is hemorrhage, and it may occur in any area of the body. Cerebral hemorrhage may be fatal, and evaluation of mental status for CNS alterations to identify CNS bleeding is very important. Fever is not a common finding in thrombocytopenia. Protection from injury to prevent bleeding is an important nursing intervention, but strict bed rest is not indicated. Oral care is performed very gently with minimum friction and soft swabs.
27. d. Rationale: A prolonged partial thromboplastin time occurs when there is a deficiency of clotting factors, such as factor VIII associated with hemophilia A. Factor IX is deficient in hemophilia B, and prolonged bleeding time and decreased platelet counts are associated with platelet deficiencies.
28. c. Rationale: Although whole blood and fresh frozen plasma contain the clotting factors that are deficient in hemophilia, specific factor concentrates have been developed that are more pure and safer in preventing infection transmission. Thromboplastin is factor III and is not deficient in patients with hemophilia.
29. b. Rationale: During an acute bleeding episode in a joint, it is important to totally rest the involved joint and slow bleeding with application of ice. Drugs that decrease platelet aggregation, such as aspirin or NSAIDs, should not be used for pain. As soon as bleeding stops, mobilization of the affected area is encouraged with ROM exercises and physical therapy.
30. a. 5; b. 8; c. 3; d. 6; e. 2; f. 7; g. 1; h. 4

31. d. Rationale: Both recognition of patients who are at risk for DIC and early detection of bleeding, both occult and overt, are primary nursing goals in the care of patients who could develop DIC. Management of the primary problem is important, but it does not necessarily assist in early recognition of acute DIC, and susceptible patients are not treated unless symptoms develop. Although DIC causes microvascular thrombosis, detection is usually made with signs of bleeding.
32. a. Yes—WBC below 5000/μl; b. 920/μl (2300 x 40%); c. Yes—neutrophils less than 1000 to 1500/μl; d. Moderate—neutropenia of 500 to 1000/μl
33. a. Rationale: An elevated temperature is of most significance in recognizing the presence of an infection in the neutropenic patient because there is no leukocytic response, and when the WBC count is depressed, the normal phagocytic mechanisms of infection are impaired, and the classic signs of inflammation may not occur. Cultures are indicated if temperature is elevated but are not used to monitor for infection.
34. d. Rationale: Despite its seeming simplicity, hand washing before, during, and after care of the patient with neutropenia is the major method to prevent transmission of harmful pathogens to the patient. HEPA filtration and LAF rooms may reduce the number of aerosolized pathogens, but they are expensive, and LAF use is controversial. Antibiotics are administered when febrile episodes occur but are not used prophylactically to prevent development of resistance.
35. a. Rationale: Although myelodysplastic syndromes, like leukemia, are a group of disorders in which hematopoietic stem cells of the bone marrow undergo clonal change and may cause eventual bone marrow failure, the primary difference from leukemias is that myelodysplastic cells have some degree of maturation and the disease progression is slower than in acute leukemias.
36. a. 4; b. 4; c. 1; d. 2; e. 3; f. 2; g. 3; h. 1; i. 3; j. 2; k. 4
37. b. Rationale: Induction therapy is aggressive treatment with chemotherapeutic agents, which often causes the patient to become devastatingly ill and predisposed to complications because the bone marrow is even further suppressed by the drugs. Induction therapy is usually administered for 10 days and may be followed by intensification therapy that involves high-dose therapy for several months.
38. c. Rationale: Almost all leukemias cause some degree of hepatosplenomegaly because of infiltration of these organs as well as the bone marrow, lymph nodes, bones, and CNS by excessive white blood cells in the blood.
39. d. Rationale: Whether the donor bone marrow is from a matched donor or taken from the patient during a remission for later use, bone marrow transplant always involves the use of combinations of chemotherapy and total body radiation to totally eliminate leukemic cells and the patient's bone marrow stem cells before IV infusion of the donor cells. There is a severe pancytopenic period following the transplant, during which the patient must be in protective isolation and during which RBC and platelet transfusions may be given.
40. b. Rationale: A patient newly diagnosed with leukemia is most likely to respond with anxiety about the effects and outcome of the disease, and the risk of infection from altered WBCs is always present, even if other blood cells are not yet affected by the disease.
41. a. NHL; b. HD; c. B; d. NHL; e. HD; f. NHL; g. HD; h. B; i. HD; j. HD
42. a. Rationale: GM-CSF is a type of colony-stimulating factor that is a naturally produced protein which stimulates proliferation and differentiation of granulocytes and monocytes. It is used to hasten recovery from bone marrow depression after chemotherapy or decrease bone marrow suppression associated with chemotherapy administration. Monoclonal antibodies, such as rituximab and ibritumomab tiuxetan, as well as interferons may be used to destroy malignant cells of NHL.
43. a. F, determine treatment; b. T; c. F, B cells, bone; d. T
44. d. Rationale: The laboratory results typical in multiple myeloma reflect the excessive production of plasma cells that produce abnormal and excessive amounts of immunoglobulin, known as myeloma protein, and the results of bone destruction by these cells and substances. Bone destruction results in increased serum levels of calcium and uric acid, and excretion of excessive uric acid and myeloma protein can result in kidney damage. Bone marrow damage results in neutropenia, anemia, and thrombocytopenia. A neutrophilic leukocytosis and anemia are seen in Hodgkin's disease.
45. c. Rationale: Splenectomy may be indicated for treatment for ITP, and when the spleen is removed, platelet counts increase significantly in most patients. In any of the disorders in which the spleen removes excessive blood cells, splenectomy will most often increase peripheral RBC, WBC, and platelet counts.

46. a. Rationale: Chills and fever are symptoms of an acute hemolytic or febrile transfusion reaction, and if these develop, the transfusion should be stopped, saline infused through the IV line, the physician and blood bank notified immediately, the ID tags rechecked, and vital signs and urine output monitored. Addition of a leukocyte reduction filter may prevent a febrile reaction but is not helpful once the reaction has occurred. Mild and transient allergic reactions indicated by itching and hives might permit restarting of the transfusion after treatment with antihistamines.
47. b. Rationale: Because platelets adhere to the plastic bags, the bag should be gently agitated throughout the transfusion. Platelets do not have A, B, or Rh antibodies, and ABO compatibility is not a consideration. Baseline vital signs should be taken before the transfusion is started, and the nurse should stay with the patient during the first 15 minutes. Platelets are stored at room temperature and should not be refrigerated.
48. a. 3; b. 2; c. 1; d. 1; e. 5; f. 2; g. 1; h. 5; i. 3; j. 4

Case Study

1. Traumatized placental and uterine tissues that release tissue factor into circulation, initiating the coagulation cascade
2. Venipuncture site bleeding, oozing of blood from other sites; respiratory problems, such as tachypnea, hemoptysis, and orthopnea; hematuria; hematemesis
3. Elevated FSPs; reduced factors V, VII, VIII, X; elevated D-dimers (cross-linked fibrin fragments); prolonged prothrombin and partial thromboplastin times; prolonged thrombin time; reduced fibrinogen, platelets
4. In the bleeding patient, therapy is administered on the basis of specific component deficiencies. Platelets are given to correct thrombocytopenia, cryoprecipitate replaces factor VIII and fibrinogen, and fresh frozen plasma replaces all clotting factors except platelets and provides a source of antithrombin. This patient is not manifesting symptoms of thrombosis, so anticoagulation is probably not indicated at this time.
   Treatment of the underlying condition may include a D&C or even a hysterectomy, if necessary, to remove the stimulus of DIC.
5. *Nursing diagnoses:*
   - Ineffective tissue perfusion: cardiopulmonary, cerebral, peripheral, and renal related to blood loss and thrombosis
   - Decreased cardiac output related to fluid volume deficit
   - Risk for impaired tissue integrity related to altered coagulation
   - Anxiety/fear related to disease process and therapy

   Collaborative problems:
   Potential complication: hemorrhage; thrombosis; hypovolemia/shock; renal failure

CHAPTER 31

1. a. mitral valve; b. tricuspid valve; c. ventricular septum; d. cusp; e. chordae tendineae; f. papillary muscle
2. a. aorta; b. superior vena cava; c. aortic semilunar valve; d. right atrium; e. right coronary artery; f. right marginal artery; g. posterior interventricular artery; h. right ventricle; i. left ventricle; j. anterior interventricular artery; k. left marginal artery; l. circumflex artery; m. left atrium; n. left coronary artery; o. pulmonary trunk; p. aorta; q. superior vena cava; r. right atrium; s. small cardiac vein; t. middle cardiac vein; u. right ventricle; v. left ventricle; w. great cardiac vein; x. coronary sinus; y. posterior vein; z. left atrium; aa. pulmonary trunk
3. a. right coronary artery, left anterior descending artery, left circumflex artery; b. right coronary artery; c. diastolic
4. a. 4; b. 7; c. 2; d. 5; e. 8; f. 1; g. 3; h. 6
5. a. 2; b. 4; c. 2; d. 1; e. 4; f. 5; g. 3; h. 3; i. 1
6. a. preload (decreased); CO decreased
   b. preload (decreased); CO decreased
   c. afterload (increased); CO decreased
   d. contractility (increased); CO increased
   e. preload (decreased); CO decreased
   f. preload (decreased); CO decreased
7. a. 2; b. 3; c. 1; d. 2; e. 2; f. 3
8. a. increased heart rate, increased force of contraction, vasoconstriction; b. decreased heart rate; c. stimulation of baroreceptors (in aortic arch and carotid sinus); d. 60, 96 mm Hg
9. a. loss of vascular distensibility and elastic recoil during systole; b. increased collagen and decreased elastin; c. decrease in SA node cells and bundle of His fibers; d. decreased number and function of receptors; e. valvular lipid accumulation and calcification
10. d. Rationale: Recreational or abused drugs, especially stimulants, such as cocaine and methamphetamine, are a growing cause of cardiac arrhythmias and problems associated with tachycardia, and IV injection of abused drugs is a risk factor for inflammatory and infectious conditions of the heart. Streptococcal, but not viral, pharyngitis is a risk factor for rheumatic heart disease.

Although calcium is involved in contraction of muscles, calcium supplementation is not a significant factor in heart disease, nor is metastatic cancer.

11. a. hyperlipidemia, hypertension, smoking, obesity, sedentary or stressful lifestyle, history of hereditary or familial cardiovascular disease, diabetes mellitus
    b. obesity, high intake of sodium, fat, cholesterol, and triglycerides
    c. dependent edema, incontinence or constipation; use of diuretics with increased urinary output
    d. lack of aerobic exercise; decreased activity tolerance; symptoms during exercise
    e. attacks of shortness of breath interrupting sleep; use of several pillows to sleep
    f. chest pain; pain in legs with walking; vertigo, cognitive changes
    g. loss of self-esteem resulting from fatigue and decreased activity
    h. stress or conflict in roles
    i. change in sexual activity caused by shortness of breath or fatigue; impotence
    j. high stress, anxiety, denial/anger/hostility as coping mechanisms
    k. treatment conflict with value system
12. d. Rationale: Normal reduction in blood pressure in a standing position is up to 15 mm Hg in the systolic pressure and from 3 to 5 mm Hg in the diastolic pressure. Reductions greater than these are abnormal and may be caused by drugs, fluid loss, or pathologic conditions.
13. d. Rationale: A palpable vibration of a blood vessel is called a thrill and usually indicates turbulent blood flow through the vessel. A weak, thready pulse has very little pressure and is difficult to palpate. A bruit is an abnormal buzzing or humming sound that may be auscultated over pathologic vessels, and a bounding pulse is an extra full, hard pulse that may occur with atherosclerosis or hypervolemia.
14. a. 1; b. 6; c. 4; d. 5; e. 7; f. 2; g. 3; h. 6; i. 6; j. 3
15. a. S_2; b. S_1; c. S_2; d. S_1; e. S_1; f. S_1; g. S_2; h. S_2; i. S_1
16. a. 7; b. 4; c. 9; d. 10; e. 8; f. 2; g. 1; h. 3; i. 6; j. 5
17. c. Rationale: In a Cardiolite scan, technetium-99 Sestimibi is injected at the maximum heart rate on a bicycle or treadmill and used to evaluate blood flow in different parts of the heart. It is taken up in an area of cardiac damage from myocardial infarction, producing hot spots. Simply monitoring electrocardiographic activity during exercise is an exercise stress test, and an echocardiogram uses transducers to bounce sound waves off the heart. Insertion of electrodes into the heart chambers via the venous system to record intracardiac electrical activity is an electrophysiology study.
18. b. Rationale: Holter monitoring involves placing electrodes on the chest, attached to a recorder that will record ECG rhythm for 24 to 48 hours while the patient engages in normal daily activities. The recording is later analyzed for cardiac arrhythmias. Frequent, but not continuous, ECGs are serial ECGs. An electrophysiology study is an invasive test that records intracardiac electrical activity in different cardiac structures, and positron emission tomography uses radioisotopes to evaluate myocardial perfusion and metabolic function.
19. c. Rationale: Because there is a significant risk for clotting around the catheter insertion site, causing obstruction of arterial blood flow, it is very important to access circulation to the extremity distal to the site frequently following a cardiac catheterization. Some swelling and pain at the site are expected, but the site is also monitored for bleeding, and a pressure dressing and perhaps a sandbag may be applied. Frequent vital signs and cardiac assessment are also necessary. Identification of iodine sensitivity should be done before the test.
20. a. Rationale: Troponin is a myocardial muscle protein that is released into circulation after injury and is specific to myocardial tissue. Apoproteins are water-soluble proteins that combine with lipids to form lipoproteins and may be associated with cardiac risk but do not indicate cardiac damage. LDH and AST are tissue enzymes that may indicate cardiac damage, but these tests have been replaced by CK-MB and troponin testing.
21. d. Rationale: A risk assessment for coronary artery disease is determined by comparing the total cholesterol to HDL, and a ratio can be calculated by dividing the total cholesterol level by the high-density lipoprotein level. The ratio provides more information than either value alone, and an increased ratio indicates an increased risk. The female patient has a ratio of 3.56 compared with the male patient's ratio of 6.56.

CHAPTER 32

1. a. B; increased rate and contractility of the heart (stroke volume) increases CO stimulation of renin production, causing increased SVR and increased CO
   b. B; peripheral arteriole vasoconstriction and increased contractility of the heart
   c. SVR; constriction of selected vascular beds
   d. SVR; vasoconstriction
   e. SVR; arteriole vasoconstriction
   f. CO; increased vascular volume
   g. CO; increased vascular volume
2. The vasoconstriction caused by the α_1-adrenergic agent raises the blood pressure, stimulating the baroreceptors. The baroreceptors send impulses to the sympathetic vasomotor center in the brainstem, which inhibit the sympathetic nervous system, resulting in a decreased heart rate, decreased force of contraction, and vasodilation.
3. Lower blood pressure because of decreased stroke volume and decreased heart rate, both of which decrease cardiac output
4. c. Rationale: Hypertension is diagnosed when the average of two or more resting BP measurements on at least three different occasions reveals an SBP of 140 mm Hg or greater or a DBP of 90 mm Hg or greater. Elevations of either SPB or DBP meet the criteria.
5. b. Rationale: Stage 2 hypertension is moderate hypertension, with BP ranges of 160 to 179/100 to 109. An average BP of 155/88 is stage 1, and the average BPs of 160/110 and 182/106 are stage 3.
6. a. Age—hypertension progresses with increasing age; b. Gender—hypertension is more prevalent in men to age 55, then more in women; c. Race—African Americans have twice the incidence of hypertension than do Caucasians; d. Family history—hypertension is strongly familial.
7. c. Rationale: Secondary hypertension has an underlying cause that can often be treated, in contrast to primary or essential hypertension, which has no single known cause. Isolated systolic hypertension occurs when the systolic BP is consistently elevated over 160 mm Hg, but the diastolic BP remains less than 90 mm Hg, which is more prevalent in the older adult. The only type of hypertension that does not cause target organ damage is pseudohypertension.
8. a. Rationale: Hypertension is often asymptomatic, especially if mild or moderate, and has been called the "silent killer." The absence of symptoms often leads to noncompliance with medical treatment and a lack of concern about the disease in patients. With severe hypertension, symptoms usually occur and may include a morning occipital headache, fatigability, dizziness, palpitations, angina, and dyspnea.
9. b. Rationale: Elevated blood pressure causes the entire inner lining of arterioles to become thickened from hyperplasia of connective tissues in the intima and affects coronary circulation, cerebral circulation, peripheral vessels, and renal and retinal blood vessels. The narrowed vessels lead to ischemia, and ultimately damage, of these organs.
10. b. Rationale: The increased systemic vascular resistance of hypertension directly increases the workload of the heart, and congestive heart failure occurs when the heart can no longer pump effectively against the increased resistance. The heart may be indirectly damaged by atherosclerotic changes in the blood vessels, as are the brain, retina, and kidney.
11. a. Elevated BUN and creatinine may indicate destruction of glomeruli and tubules of the kidney resulting from hypertension.
    b. Serum potassium levels are decreased when hypertension is associated with hyperaldosteronism.
    c. Fasting glucose levels are elevated when hypertension is associated with glucose intolerance and insulin resistance.
    d. An increased uric acid level may be caused by diuretics used to treat hypertension.
    e. An elevated LDL indicates an increased risk for atherosclerotic changes in the patient with hypertension.
12. a. Dietary modifications to restrict sodium; maintain intake of potassium, calcium, and magnesium; and promote weight reduction if overweight
    b. Moderation or cessation of alcohol intake
    c. Daily moderate-intensity physical activity for at least 30 minutes
    d. Cessation of smoking if a smoker
13. a. Rationale: The recommendation for initial pharmacologic management of hypertension is monotherapy with either a diuretic or a beta blocker. Other drugs used for initial monotherapy include calcium channel blockers, ACE inhibitors, alpha-adrenergic blockers, and the combined alpha-beta–adrenergic blockers. If the BP is not controlled in a few months with monotherapy, the dose of the first-line drug can be increased, a second drug from a different class can be substituted, or a second drug from a different class can be added.
14. a. 4; b. 5; c. 8; d. 6; e. 2; f. 7; g. 1; h. 3
15. d. Rationale: Hydrochlorothiazide is a thiazide diuretic that causes sodium and potassium loss through the kidney. High-potassium foods should

be included in the diet, or potassium supplements used, to prevent hypokalemia. Enalapril and spironolactone may cause hyperkalemia by inhibiting the action of aldosterone, and potassium supplements should not be used by patients taking these drugs. As a combined alpha-beta blocker, labetalol does not affect potassium levels.

16. b. Rationale: Prazosin is an alpha-adrenergic blocker that causes dilation of arterioles and veins and causes orthostatic hypotension. The patient may feel dizzy, weak, and faint when assuming an upright position after sitting or lying down and should be taught to change positions slowly, avoid standing for long periods of time, do leg exercises to increase venous return, and lie or sit down when dizziness occurs. Direct-acting vasodilators often cause fluid retention, dry mouth occurs with diuretic use and centrally acting alpha blockers, and beta blockers may cause bradycardia.
17. c. Rationale: Sexual dysfunction that may occur with many of the antihypertensive drugs, including thiazide and potassium-sparing diuretics and beta blockers, can be a major reason that a male patient does not adhere to his treatment regimen. It is helpful for the nurse to raise the subject because sexual problems may be easier for the patient to discuss and handle once it has been explained that the drug may be the source of the problem.
18. a. Rationale: Centrally acting alpha blockers may cause severe rebound hypertension if the drugs are abruptly discontinued, and patients should be taught about this effect because many are not consistently compliant with drug therapy. Diuretics should be taken early in the day to prevent nocturia, and the profound orthostatic hypotension that occurs with first-dose alpha-adrenergic blockers can be prevented by taking the initial dose at bedtime. Aspirin use may decrease the effectiveness of ACE inhibitors.
19. d. Rationale: Correct technique in measuring blood pressure includes taking and averaging two or more readings taken at least 2 minutes apart. If the first two readings differ by more than 5 mm Hg, additional readings should be obtained. Initially BP measurements should be taken in both arms to detect any differences, and if there is a difference, the arm with the higher reading should be used for all subsequent BP readings. The cuff should be inflated 10 to 20 mm Hg above the point that no brachial pulse is felt in the arm being used, and the pressure is released at 2 mm Hg per second to provide an accurate reading.
20. c. Rationale: A major problem in the long-term management of the patient with hypertension is poor compliance with the prescribed treatment regimen. Before adding or substituting medications because of a poor response to drug therapy, it is important to ensure that patients have been taking their medication as prescribed. Although drug-related causes and progressive renal damage may be responsible for lack of responsiveness to drug therapy, nonadherence to therapy for a variety of reasons is the most common factor.
21. b. Rationale: Hypertensive emergency, a type of hypertensive crisis, is a situation that develops over hours or days in which a patient's BP is severely elevated with evidence of acute target organ damage, especially to the central nervous system. The neurologic manifestations are often similar to the presentation of a CVA, but it does not show the focal or lateralizing symptoms of CVA. Hypertensive crises are defined by the degree of organ damage and how rapidly the BP must be lowered, not specific BP measurements. A hypertensive urgency is a less severe crisis in which a patient's BP becomes severely elevated over days or weeks, but there is no evidence of target organ damage.
22. c. Rationale: Hypertensive crises are treated with IV administration of antihypertensive drugs, including the vasodilators sodium nitroprusside, nitroglycerin, diazoxide, and hydralazine; adrenergic blockers such as phentolamine, labetalol, and methyldopa; and the ACE inhibitor IV enalaprilat. Sodium nitroprusside is the most effective parenteral drug for hypertensive emergencies. Drugs that are used specifically for hypertensive emergencies include sodium nitroprusside, nitroglycerin, and diazoxide.
23. c. Rationale: Initially the treatment goal in hypertensive emergencies is to reduce the MAP by 10%-20% in the first 1 to 2 hours, with further gradual reduction over the next 24 hours. Lowering the BP too far or too fast may cause hypotension in a person whose body has adjusted to hypertension and could cause a stroke, MI, or visual changes. Only when the patient has an aortic dissection, angina, or signs of MI does the systolic BP need to be lowered to 100 to 120 mm Hg as quickly as possible.
24. d. Rationale: Hypertensive urgencies are often treated with oral drugs on an outpatient basis, but it is important for the patient to be seen by a health professional within 24 hours to evaluate the effectiveness of the treatment. Hourly urine measurements, ECG monitoring, and titration of IV drugs are indicated for hypertensive emergencies.

Case Study

1. Increasing age, which leads to loss of elasticity in large arteries from atherosclerosis; more prevalent in women (and African Americans)
2. High sodium intake from canned foods; sedentary lifestyle; weight gain
3. Sodium restriction to 2 g/day; decrease fat to no more than 30% of diet; cholesterol intake of less than 200 mg/day; increase high-potassium foods
4. Regular daily aerobic exercise; need for stress management indicated by weight gain in response to husband's death; teaching about pathology, complications, and management of hypertension
5. Because of her low potassium, a potassium-saving diuretic, such as spironolactone, amiloride, or triamterine, could be used. If a stronger diuretic was needed, potassium supplementation would be indicated.
6. *Nursing diagnoses:*
   - Ineffective health maintenance related to increased caloric intake and deficiency of potassium sources
   - Ineffective coping related to use of food as coping mechanism

   Collaborative problems:
   Potential complications: cerebrovascular accident; myocardial infarction, renal failure

CHAPTER 33

1. a. fatty streak, age 15; b. raised fibrous plaque, age 30; c. complicated lesion, over age 30
2. a. F, endothelial injury; b. T; c. T; d. T; e. F, complicated lesion; f. F, older with chronic ischemia
3. a. elevated serum lipids, modifiable; b. hypertension, modifiable; c. cigarette smoking, modifiable
4. d. Rationale: The Caucasian woman has one unmodifiable risk factor (age) and two major modifiable risk factors (hypertension and physical inactivity). Her gender risk is as high as a man's because of her age. The Caucasian man has one unmodifiable risk factor (gender), one major modifiable risk factor (smoking), and one minor modifiable risk factor (stressful lifestyle). The African-American man has a an unmodifiable risk factor related to age, one major modifiable risk factor (hypertension), and one minor modifiable risk factor (obesity), but African-American men are at less risk for CAD than are Caucasians of the same age. The Asian woman has only one major modifiable risk factor (hyperlipidemia), and Asians in the United States have fewer MIs than do Caucasians.
5. a. 3; b. 5; c. 2; d. 1; e. 1; f. 3; g. 1; h. 6; i. 2; j. 4; k. 2
6. a. <200 mg/dl (5.2 mmol/L)
   b. <190 mg/dl (2.15 mmol/L)
   c. <130 mg/dl (3.4 mmol/L)
   d. >37 mg/dl (.97 mmol/L) men
   e. >40 mg/dl (1.05 mmol/L) women
7. a. Rationale: Increased exercise without an increase in caloric intake will result in weight loss, reducing the risk associated with obesity, and exercise increases lipid metabolism and increases HDL2, reducing CAD risk. Exercise may also indirectly reduce the risk of CAD by controlling hypertension, promoting glucose metabolism in diabetes, and reducing stress. Although research is needed to determine whether a decline in homocysteine can reduce the risk of heart disease, it appears that dietary modifications will be indicated for risk reduction.
8. d. Rationale: Stress related to a type A behavior pattern is associated with increased sympathetic nervous system stimulation, increasing heart rate and contractility and thus the workload of the heart. Hypertension also increases the workload of the heart by requiring more force to pump blood through the diseased arterial vasculature. Smoking also increases the workload by causing catecholamine release. Elevated serum lipids and diabetes are associated with causing vascular changes that decrease oxygen supply. It is not known how physical inactivity directly affects CAD, but exercise is known to increase HDL levels and reduce clot formation.
9. a. Rationale: Step 1 dietary changes include decreased intake of saturated fat and cholesterol and the substitution of skim or 1% milk for whole milk. A step 2 diet is used if the patient does not show a trend toward lower blood cholesterol within 6 months of using a step 1 diet. A step 2 diet includes only the very leanest cuts of meats (but red meat can be used) and only one egg yolk per week. Restriction of alcohol and simple sugars is indicated for control of elevated serum triglyceride levels.
10. a. Rationale: Diet therapy is indicated for a patient without CAD who has two or more risk factors and an LDL level equal to or greater than 130 mg/dl. When the patient's LDL levels are equal to or greater than 160 mg/dl, drug therapy would be added to diet therapy. Exercise is indicated to reduce risk factors throughout treatment.
11. c. Rationale: This patient has elevated cholesterol, LDLs, and triglyceride levels, and nicotinic acid is highly effective in lowering both cholesterol and triglyceride levels by interfering with their synthesis. Gemfibrozil primarily affects

VLDL and triglyceride levels, lovastatin primarily decreases liver synthesis of LDL and thus cholesterol, and cholestyramine primarily lowers LDL cholesterol and increases HDL levels.

12. a. stable angina
    b. unstable angina, non-ST-segment-elevation myocardial infarction
    c. ST-segment-elevation myocardial infarction
    d. infarct
13. a. increased oxygen demand, decreased oxygen supply; b. increased oxygen demand; c. decreased oxygen supply; d. decreased oxygen supply; e. decreased oxygen supply; f. increased oxygen demand; g. increased oxygen demand; h. increased oxygen demand
14. c. Rationale: When the coronary arteries are occluded, contractility ceases after several minutes, depriving the myocardial cells of glucose and oxygen for aerobic metabolism. Anaerobic metabolism begins and lactic acid accumulates, irritating myocardial nerve fibers that then transmit a pain message to the cardiac nerves and upper thoracic posterior roots. The other factors may occur during vessel occlusion but are not the source of pain.
15. d. Rationale: An increased heart rate decreases the time the heart spends in diastole, which is the time of greatest coronary blood flow. Unlike other arteries, coronary arteries are perfused when the myocardium relaxes and blood backflows from the aorta into the sinuses of Valsalva, which have openings to the right and left coronary arteries. Thus the heart has a decreased oxygen supply at a time when there is an increased oxygen demand.
16. c. Rationale: Location and areas of MIs correlate with the coronary arteries and the areas of the heart they normally perfuse. Anterior wall infarctions are usually caused by lesions in the left anterior descending artery; lateral wall infarctions by occlusion of the left circumflex or descending artery; inferior wall infarctions by occlusion of the right coronary artery or left circumflex artery; and posterior wall infarctions by lesions in the left circumflex artery.
17. c. Rationale: At 10 to 14 days after MI, the myocardium is considered to be especially vulnerable to increased stress because of the unstable state of healing at this point, and this is the time that the patient is also increasing physical activity. At 2 to 3 days, removal of necrotic tissue is taking place by phagocytic cells, and by 4 to 10 days, the tissue has been cleared and a collagen matrix for scar tissue has been deposited. Healing with scar tissue replacement of the necrotic area is usually complete by 6 weeks.
18. a. 6; b. 3; c. 5; d. 1; e. 5; f. 3; g. 1; h. 2; i. 4; j. 2
19. c. Rationale: Unstable angina is associated with deterioration of a once stable atherosclerotic plaque that ruptures, exposing the intima to blood and stimulating platelet aggregation and local vasoconstriction with thrombus formation. Patients with unstable angina require immediate hospitalization and monitoring because the lesion is at increased risk of complete thrombosis of the lumen with progression to MI. Any type of angina may be associated with severe pain, ECG changes, and arrhythmias, and Prinzmetal's, or variant, angina is characterized by coronary artery spasm.
20. a. Rationale: One of the primary differences between the pain of angina and the pain of an MI is that angina pain is usually relieved by rest or nitroglycerin, which reduces the oxygen demand of the heart, while MI pain is not. Both angina and MI pain can cause a pressure or squeezing sensation; may radiate to the neck, back, arms, fingers, and jaw; and may be precipitated by exertion.
21. b. Rationale: An exercise stress test will reveal ECG changes that indicate impaired coronary circulation when the oxygen demand of the heart is increased. A single ECG is not conclusive for CAD, and negative findings do not rule out CAD. Echocardiograms of various types may identify abnormalities of myocardial wall motion under stress but are indirect measures of CAD. Coronary angiography can detect narrowing of coronary arteries but is an invasive procedure.
22. d. Rationale: The pain of an MI is usually severe, is usually unrelieved by nitroglycerin, rest, or position change, and usually lasts more than the 15 or 20 minutes typical of angina pain. All of the other symptoms may occur with angina as well as an MI.
23. c. Rationale: The most common complication of MI is cardiac arrhythmias, especially ventricular arrhythmias that may be life-threatening. Continuous cardiac monitoring allows for identification and treatment of arrhythmias that may cause further deterioration of the cardiovascular status. Measurement of hourly urine output and vital signs is indicated to detect symptoms of the complication of cardiogenic shock, and crackles, dyspnea, and tachycardia may indicate the onset of congestive heart failure.
24. a. 4; b. 5; c. 2; d. 1; e. 3
25. c. Rationale: Creatine kinase, MB band, is a tissue enzyme that is specific to cardiac muscle and is released into the blood when myocardial cells die. CK-MB levels begin to rise about 6 hours

after an acute MI, peak in about 24 hours, and return to normal within 2 or 3 days, and this increase can demonstrate the presence of cardiac damage and the approximate extent of the damage. Troponin, a myocardial muscle protein released with myocardial damage, rises as quickly as CK and remains elevated for 2 weeks. ECG changes often are not apparent immediately after infarct and may be normal when the patient seeks medical attention. An enlarged heart determined by x-ray indicates cardiac stress but is not diagnostic of acute MI.

26. c. Rationale: A differentiation is made between myocardial infarcts that have ST-segment elevations on ECG and those that do not. Chest pain that is accompanied by ST-segment elevations is associated with prolonged and complete coronary thrombosis and is treated with reperfusion therapy.
27. a. nitrates; b. nitrates, calcium channel blocking agents; c. antiplatelet aggregation agents, including aspirin; d. beta-adrenergic blocking agents; e. nitrates, calcium channel blocking agents, beta-adrenergic blocking agents; f. beta-adrenergic blocking agents, calcium channel blocking agents
28. b. Rationale: A common complication of nitrates is dizziness caused by orthostatic hypotension, so the patient should sit or lie down and place the tablet under the tongue. The tablet should be allowed to dissolve under the tongue, and to prevent the tablet from being swallowed, water should not be taken with it. If the pain is not relieved, 2 more tablets may be taken at 5-minute intervals, but if the pain is present after 15 minutes and 3 tablets, the patient should seek medical attention. Headache is also a common complication of nitrates, which usually resolves with continued use of nitrates, and may be controlled with mild analgesics.
29. a. Rationale: The body has a tendency to develop tolerance not only to the side effects of nitrates but also to the antianginal effect. Providing a nitrate-free period of at least 8 hours within each 24-hour period for any route of administration is usually effective in preventing development of tolerance. Night is the best time to remove the patch unless the patient has nocturnal angina. Patches are designed for continuous nitrate therapy and should not be used on a prn basis. The sites should be changed daily to prevent skin irritation and alterations in absorption, but this does not affect tolerance.
30. a. 4; b. 5; c. 2; d. 1; e. 2; f. 3; g. 6; h. 5; i. 3; j. 1
31. d. Rationale: The most common method of coronary artery bypass involves using segments of a resected saphenous vein to carry blood from the aorta to the coronary artery distal to the site of an obstruction. Synthetic grafts are not used as coronary bypass grafts, although they may be used for other vessels. The internal mammary artery may be diverted from its delivery to the chest wall and attached to a coronary artery distal to an obstruction, but it is left attached to its origin from the subclavian artery.
32. b. Rationale: Although the inferior epigastric artery and the gastroepiploic artery are excellent conduits for bypassing obstructed coronary arteries, their use creates the need for a laparotomy, increasing the length of the surgery and chances of wound complications at the harvest site. Cardiopulmonary bypass during the surgery is used for all coronary bypass surgeries except the minimally invasive direct coronary artery bypass graft (MIDCABG).
33. a. Rationale: Because an NSTEMI is an acute coronary syndrome that indicates a transient thrombosis or incomplete coronary artery occlusion, treatment involves intensive drug therapy with antithromboics and heparin to prevent clot extension, in addition to nitroglycerine IV. Reperfusion therapy using fibrinolytics, CABG, or PCI are used for treatment of STEMI.
34. d. Rationale: Fibrinolytic therapy causes dissolution of the clot and, if given early in the infarct process, can reperfuse the myocardium before cellular death occurs. Treatment with antiarrhythmic drugs helps prevent development of lethal arrhythmias, and anticoagulant therapy, such as heparin, may be used to prevent formation of new clots following thrombolytic therapy or to prevent extension of established clots. In cases of severe left ventricular dysfunction and cardiogenic shock, an intraaortic balloon pump may be used to assist ventricular ejection and promote coronary artery perfusion.
35. a. Rationale: Indications that the coronary artery that was occluded is patent and blood flow to the myocardium is reestablished following thrombolytic therapy include relief of chest pain, return of ST segment to baseline on the ECG, the presence of reperfusion arrhythmias, and marked, rapid rise of the CK enzyme within 3 hours of therapy. If chest pain is unchanged, it is an indication that reperfusion was not successful.
36. a. 4; b. 5; c. 6; d. 2; e. 1; f. 3
37. a. agent of choice in CAD to prevent platelet aggregation around atheroma; administration at the time of unstable angina may prevent progression to MI
    b. IV infusion to prevent abrupt closure of intracoronary stents during placement; may be used

in combination with aspirin in patients with unstable angina

c. used as anticoagulants in patients with unstable angina undergoing PCI

d. alternative antiplatelet agents for those who cannot use aspirin

38. a. Rationale: This patient is indicating positive coping with a realization that recovery takes time and that lifestyle changes can be made as needed. The patient who is just going to get on with his life is probably in denial about the seriousness of the condition and the changes that need to be made. Nervous questions about the expected duration and effect of the condition indicate the presence of anxiety, as does the statement regarding the health care professionals' role in treatment.

39. a. Administer oxygen; b. Take vital signs; c. Arrange for ECG; d. Administer nitroglycerin or narcotic analgesic; e. Perform a physical assessment of the chest; f. Position the patient for comfort

40. a. dependence; b. anxiety/fear; c. depression; d. anger; e. denial

41. a. Rationale: Golfing is a moderate-energy activity that expends about 5.0 METs and is within the 3 to 5 METs activity level desired of a patient by the time of discharge from the hospital following MI. Walking at 5 mph and mowing the lawn by hand are high-energy activities, and cycling at 13 mph is an extremely high-energy activity.

42. c. Rationale: Phase III of rehabilitation is the time at which an exercise program, commonly walking, begins. Phase I occurs while the patient is in the hospital and includes rest, Phase II includes self-care activities, and Phase IV includes involvement with the community program for continuing physical training and fitness.

43. b. Rationale: Any activity or exercise that causes dyspnea and chest pain should be stopped in the patient with CAD. The training target for a healthy 58-year-old is 80% of maximum heart rate, or 132 beats/min, but in a patient with cardiac disease undergoing cardiac conditioning, the heart rate should not exceed 20 beats/min over the resting pulse rate. Heart rate, rather than respiratory rate, determines the parameters for exercise.

44. b. Rationale: Resumption of sexual activity is often difficult for patients to approach, and it is reported that most cardiac patients do not resume sexual activity after MI. The nurse can give the patient permission to discuss concerns about sexual activity by introducing it as a physical activity when other physical activities are discussed. Physicians may have preferences regarding the timing of resumption of sexual activity, and the nurse should discuss this with the physician and the patient, but addressing the patient's concerns is a nursing responsibility. Patients should be informed that impotence after MI is common but that it usually disappears after several attempts.

45. d. Rationale: It is not uncommon for a patient who experiences chest pain on exertion to have some angina during sexual stimulation or intercourse, and the patient should be instructed to use nitroglycerin prophylactically. Orogenital sex places no undue strain on the heart, and it and positions during intercourse are a matter of individual choice. Foreplay is desirable because it allows a gradual increase in heart rate.

46. c. Rationale: The majority of persons who experience sudden cardiac death as a result of CAD do not have an acute MI but have arrhythmias that cause death, probably as a result of electrical instability of the myocardium. Primary LV outflow obstruction is a less common cause of sudden cardiac death. Accidental or traumatic causes of cardiac arrest are not considered sudden cardiac death.

47. d. Rationale: An older adult often has altered responses to CAD and MI, resulting in atypical symptoms, and sudden dyspnea and profound weakness should be investigated. Heart rate does not rise as quickly because of decreased responsiveness to catacholamines, and diaphoresis is often not present. Pain perception is also blunted in older adults, and pain may not be a presenting symptom.

48. a. Rationale: Orthostatic hypotension may cause dizziness and falls in older adults taking antianginal agents that decrease preload, and they should be cautioned about changing positions slowly. Exercise programs are indicated for the older adult and may increase performance, endurance, and ability to tolerate stress. A change in lifestyle behaviors may increase quality of life and reduce the risks of CAD even in the older adult. Aspirin is commonly used in these patients and is not contraindicated.

49. d. Rationale: CAD is the number-one killer of American women, and they have a much higher mortality rate within 1 year following MI than do men. Recent research indicates that estrogen replacement does not reduce the risk for CAD even though estrogen lowers LDL and raises HDL cholesterol. Smoking carries specific problems for women because smoking has been linked to a decrease in estrogen levels and to early menopause and has been identified as the most powerful contributor to CAD in women under the age of 50. Men have a higher incidence of sudden cardiac death.

Case Study

1. Diabetes mellitus; smoking history; obesity; physical inactivity; stress response
2. Mrs. C. appears little motivated to assume responsibility for her health, and in the absence of symptoms, has not had a desire to make lifestyle changes. First, assist Mrs. C. to clarify her personal values. Then by explaining the risk factors and having her identify her personal vulnerability to various risks, you may help her recognize her susceptibility to CAD. Help her set realistic goals, and allow her to choose which risk factor to change first.
3. Anxiousness with fist clutching; radiation of the burning from epigastric area into the sternum; prior episodes of chest pain with activity, relieved by rest
4. ST segment changes, elevations
5. Procardia is a calcium channel blocker that decreases cardiac oxygen demand by reducing systemic vascular resistance and decreasing myocardial contractility and heart rate. It also increases oxygen supply by dilating coronary arteries.
6. Inform her that she will have continuous cardiac monitoring while she walks on a treadmill with increasing speed and elevation to evaluate the effects of exercise on the blood supply to her heart. Her pulse, respiration, and blood pressure will be measured while she walks and after the test until they return to normal, and the cardiac monitor will be used after the test until any changes return to normal.
7. *Nursing diagnoses:*
   - Acute pain related to ischemic myocardium
   - Anxiety related to possible diagnosis and uncertain future
   - Ineffective denial related to reluctance to receive medical care or change lifestyle
   - Ineffective coping related to lack of effective coping skills
   - Imbalanced nutrition: more than body requirements related to intake of calories in excess of calorie expenditure

   Collaborative problems:
   Potential complications: myocardial infarction; cardiac arrhythmias

CHAPTER 34

1. a. F, diastolic failure; b. T; c. T; d. F, arrhythmias; e. F, reduced
2. a. ↑ CO: increased force of contraction by stretching of cardiac muscle
   Detrimental effect: overstrain the muscle fibers; mitral valve incompetence
   b. ↑ CO: increased contractile force of muscle;
   Detrimental effect: increased myocardial oxygen need
   c. ↑ CO: increased heart rate and force of contraction; increased preload
   Detrimental effect: increased myocardial oxygen need; overwhelming preload; increased afterload
   d. 1) ↑ CO: increased fluid retention and vasoconstriction to maintain blood pressure;
   Detrimental effect: increased preload and afterload
   2) ↑ CO: increased water retention
   Detrimental effect: increased blood volume when already overloaded
   3) ↑ CO: decreased afterload and preload by vasodilation
   Detrimental effect: depletion occurs with prolonged atrial distention
3. a. 4; b. 10; c. 12; d. 5; e. 24; f. 7, 8; g. 10; h. 3
4. 2, 14, 16, 22
5. b. Rationale: In left-sided heart failure, blood backs up into the pulmonary veins and capillaries. This increased hydrostatic pressure in the vessels causes fluid to move out of the vessels and into the pulmonary interstitial space. When increased lymphatic flow cannot remove enough fluid from the interstitial space, fluid moves into the alveoli. This results in pulmonary edema and impaired alveolar oxygen and carbon dioxide exchange. Initially the right side of the heart is not involved.
6. a. Rationale: Clinical manifestations of acute left-sided heart failure are those of pulmonary edema, with bubbling crackles; frothy, blood-tinged sputum; severe dyspnea; tachypnea; and orthopnea. Severe tachycardia and cool, clammy skin are present as a result of stimulation of the sympathetic nervous system from hypoxemia. Systemic edema reflected by jugular vein distention, peripheral edema, and hepatosplenomegaly are characteristic of right-sided heart failure.
7. d. Rationale: Paroxysmal nocturnal dyspnea (PND) is awakening from sleep with a feeling of suffocation and a need to sit up to be able to breathe, and patients learn that sleeping with the upper body elevated on several pillows helps prevent PND. Orthopnea is an inability to breathe

effectively when lying down, and nocturia occurs with heart failure as fluid moves back into the vascular system during recumbency, increasing renal blood flow.

8. d. Rationale: Liver damage and failure indicated by increased liver enzyme levels may occur from severe hepatic venous congestion and edema and is considered a major complication of congestive heart failure. Increased weight gain and ascites are symptoms of right-sided failure, and restlessness and confusion are symptoms of the hypoxemia that occurs with heart failure.
9. b. Rationale: Thrombus formation occurs in the heart when the chambers do not contract normally and empty completely. Both atrial fibrillation and very low left ventricular output (LV ejection fraction of <20%) lead to thrombus formation that is treated with anticoagulants to prevent emboli release into the circulation.
10. a. Rationale: Because congestion of the pulmonary vessels, pulmonary edema, and pulmonary effusions, as well as the degree of cardiac enlargement, can be seen on chest x-ray, it is an important tool to diagnose and monitor the progress of the patient in heart failure. Exercise stress testing and cardiac catheterization are more important tests to diagnose coronary artery disease, and although the BUN may be elevated in congestive heart failure, it is a reflection of decreased renal perfusion. .
11. a. 20; b. 12, 23; c. 1, 8, 12; d. 4, 24; e. 1, 18, 19, 7, 10, 14; f. 5; g. 1, 5
12. a. 11; b. 4; c. 10; d. 8; e. 6; f. 7; g. 9; h. 1; i. 2; j. 5; k. 3
13. c. Rationale: Hypokalemia is one of the most common causes of digitalis toxicity because low serum potassium levels enhance ectopic pacemaker activity. When a patient is receiving potassium-losing diuretics, such as hydrochlorothiazide and furosemide, it is essential to monitor the patient's serum potassium levels to prevent digitalis toxicity.
14. a. Rationale: Spironolactone is a potassium-sparing diuretic, and when it is the only diuretic used in the treatment of congestive heart failure, moderate to low levels of potassium should be maintained to prevent development of hyperkalemia. Sodium intake is usually reduced to at least 2,400 mg/day in patients with CHF, but salt substitutes cannot be freely used because most contain high concentrations of potassium.
15. d. Rationale: Although all of these drugs may cause hypotension, nitroprusside is a potent dilator of both arteries and veins and may cause such marked hypotension that dobutamine administration may be necessary to maintain the blood pressure during its administration. Milrinone has a positive inotropic effect, in addition to direct arterial dilation, and nitroglycerine primarily dilates veins. Furosemide may cause hypotension because of diuretic-induced intravascular fluid volume depletion.
16. c. Rationale: All foods that are high in sodium should be eliminated in a 2,400-mg sodium diet, in addition to the elimination of salt during cooking. Examples include obviously salted snack foods as well as pickles, processed prepared foods, and many sauces and condiments.
17. a. Hypertension: use of medications, diet, and exercise to control
    b. Valvular defects: surgical replacement before CHF occurs; prophylactic antibiotics
    c. Ischemic heart disease: fibrinolytic treatment or PTCA for occlusions
    d. Arrhythmias: antiarrhythmic agents or pacemakers to control
18. c. Rationale: Successful treatment of congestive heart failure is indicated by absence of symptoms of pulmonary edema and hypoxemia, such as clear lung sounds and a normal heart rate. Weight loss and diuresis, and warm skin, less fatigue, and improved level of consciousness may occur without resolution of pulmonary symptoms. Chest pain is not a common finding in congestive heart failure unless coronary artery perfusion is impaired.
19. d. Rationale: A high Fowler's position increases the thoracic capacity, improving ventilation, and sitting with the legs dependent helps pool blood in the extremities and decrease venous return, or preload. Coughing and deep breathing will not clear the lungs of pulmonary edema. I&O and daily weights should be done to monitor the effects of treatment but do not directly address impaired gas exchange. During periods of acute dyspnea, rest is necessary to decrease oxygen demand.
20. d. Rationale: Further teaching is needed if the patient believes that a weight gain of 2 to 3 pounds in 2 days is an indication for dieting. In a patient with congestive heart failure, this type of weight gain reflects fluid retention and is a sign of CHF that should be reported to the health care provider.
21. a. H; b. D; c. R; d. D; e. H; f. D; g. D; h. H; i. D; j. H; k. R; l. H
22. b. Rationale: Patients will all types of cardiomyopathy should avoid strenuous activities that increase the workload of the heart and impair ventricular filling. Alcohol is prohibited in alcohol-induced dilated cardiomyopathy, and the patient with hypertrophic cardiomyopathy should increase fluids to prevent dehydration. Intermit-

tent dobutamine infusions may be prescribed for the patient with dilated cardiomyopathy.

23. d. Rationale: The 52-year-old woman does not have any contraindications for cardiac transplantation even though she lacks the indication of adequate financial resources. The postoperative transplant regimen is complex and rigorous, and patients who have not been compliant with other treatments or may not have the means to understand the care would not be good candidates. A history of drug or alcohol abuse is usually a contraindication to heart transplantation.
24. b. Rationale: Because of the need for long-term immunosuppressant therapy to prevent rejection, the patient with a transplant is at high risk for infection, the leading cause of death in transplant patients. Acute rejection episodes may occur in patients with transplants, but many can be successfully treated with augmented immunosuppressive therapy.

Case Study

1. Right-sided failure: jugular vein distention, peripheral edema, hepatomegaly
   Left-sided failure: dyspnea, ↓ SpO_2, PMI displacement, pulmonary crackles, ↓ BP, S_3, S_4 heart sounds
   Present with both: fatigue, ↑ HR, arrhythmias
2. In dilated CMP the atria and ventricles are enlarged (cardiomegaly) because of dilation rather than hypertrophy, as occurs in congestive heart failure. Decreased contractile function occurs because of degeneration of myocardial fibers rather than of ventricular remodeling.
3. Chest x-ray: cardiomegaly, pulmonary venous hypertension, pleural effusion
   ECG: tachycardia and arrythmias of conduction disturbances
   Echocardiogram: reveals thin, dilated ventricular walls; low LV ejection fraction
   Cardiac catheterization and coronary angiography: normal coronary arteries, thin-walled ventricles
   Endomyocardial biopsy: degenerative myocardium
4. Calm, reassuring approach because of his anxiety and critical condition
   Explanations of rationales for all diagnostic tests and medications
   Administration of oxygen, sit upright with legs out straight or dependent
   Provide emotional and physical rest
   Constant monitoring of cardiovascular and respiratory function
   Start I&O measurements
5. a. atrial fibrillation, increase myocardial strength
   b. diuresis to decrease circulating blood volume and preload
   c. inotropic effect and dilate vascular smooth muscle to decrease preload and afterload
   d. by blocking renin-angiotensin-aldosterone system reduce afterload by vasodilation and preventing sodium and water retention
   e. block sympathetic response to failure and decrease heart rate
6. Although some patients with dilated CMP respond to drug and nutritional therapy, many do not, and heart transplantation is the primary alternative for a good prognosis for survival. However, donor hearts are in short supply, and many patients with dilated CMP die while awaiting heart transplantation. Experimental artificial hearts are the only other alternative for patients who do not respond to conventional therapy.
7. *Nursing diagnoses:*
   - Death anxiety related to feeling of dying
   - Impaired gas exchange related to increased circulating blood volume
   - Ineffective tissue perfusion related to pump failure
   - Decreased cardiac output related to altered cardiac rate and rhythm
   - Activity intolerance related to imbalance between oxygen supply and demand
   - Risk for impaired skin integrity related to edema

   Collaborative problems:
   Potential complications: cardiogenic shock; ventricular arrhythmias; emboli; liver/renal failure, cardiac arrest

CHAPTER 35

1. a. F, depolarization; b. F, QRS complex; c. F, 80 beats/min; d. T; e. F, negative, positive; f. T; g. F, 40 to 60; h. T; i. F, ectopic foci
2. a. 4; b. 6; c. 5; d. 1; e. 2; f. 3
3. d. Rationale: The normal PR interval is 0.12 to 0.20 seconds and reflects the time taken for the impulse to spread through the atria, AV node and bundle of His, the bundle branches, and Purkinje fibers. A PR interval of six small boxes is 0.24 seconds and indicates that the conduction of the impulse from the atria to the Purkinje fibers is delayed.
4. c. Rationale: Electrophysiologic testing involves electrical stimulation to various areas of the atrium and ventricle to determine the inducibility of arrhythmias and frequently induces ventricular tachycardia or ventricular fibrillation. The patient may have "near-death" experiences and requires emotional support if this occurs.
5. a. 8; b. 7; c. 13; d. 1; e. 3; f. 11; g. 10; h. 6; i. 12; j. 2; k. 4; l. 5; m. 9
6. a. third-degree (total) heart block, pacemaker; b. sinus tachycardia; c. paroxysmal supraventricular tachycardia; d. type I, second-degree heart block; e. ventricular tachycardia, ventricular fibrillation
7. d. Rationale: In the presence of heart disease, a slow SA impulse may allow for escape arrhythmias and premature beats that can lead to further arrhythmias and decreased cardiac output. Asystole refers to total absence of ventricular activity, and SA activity may be present for a short time. Heart block occurs when the impulse from the SA node is not conducted normally to the ventricles, and sinus arrest is a rare complication of sinus bradycardia.
8. d. Rationale: Although many factors may cause a sinus tachycardia, in the patient who has had an acute MI, a tachycardia increases myocardial oxygen need in a heart that already has impaired circulation and may lead to increasing angina and further ischemia and necrosis.
9. a. Rationale: A distorted P wave with normal conduction of the impulse through the ventricles is characteristic of a premature atrial contraction. This arrhythmia is frequently associated in a normal heart with emotional stress or the use of caffeine, tobacco, or alcohol. Aerobic conditioning and holding the breath during exertion (Valsalva's maneuver) often cause bradycardia. Sedatives rarely may slow heart rate.
10. b. Rationale: When a P wave is absent, there is no SA node impulse, and the impulse is arising elsewhere in the heart. The most common site for impulse formation after the SA node is the AV node, creating a junctional rhythm. Normally junctional rhythm is 40 to 60 beats/min, but in this case it is accelerated, and an accelerated junctional rhythm is most often associated with acute inferior MI, digitalis toxicity, and acute rheumatic fever.
11. a. Rationale: A rhythm pattern that is normal except for a prolonged PR interval is characteristic of a first-degree heart block. First-degree heart blocks are not treated but are observed for progression to higher degrees of heart block. Defibrillation is used only for ventricular fibrillation, atropine is administered for bradycardias, and pacemakers are used for higher-degree heart blocks.
12. b. Rationale: Symptoms of decreased cardiac output related to cardiac arrhythmias include a sudden drop in blood pressure and symptoms of hypoxemia, such as decreased mentation, chest pain, and dyspnea. Peripheral pulses are weak, and heart rate may be increased or decreased, depending on the type of arrhythmia present.
13. c. Rationale: Premature ventricular contractions in a patient with an MI indicate significant ventricular irritability that may lead to ventricular tachycardia or ventricular fibrillation. Antiarrhythmics, such as α-adrenergic blockers, procainamide, aminodarone, or lidocaine, may be used to control the arrythmias. Valsalva's maneuver may be used to treat paroxysmal supraventricular tachycardia.
14. a. Rationale: The PVC is an ectopic beat that causes a wide, distorted QRS complex, greater than 0.12 second, because the impulse is not conducted normally through the ventricles. Because it is premature, it precedes the P wave and the P wave may be hidden in the QRS complex, or the ventricular impulse may be conducted retrograde and the P wave may be seen following the PVC. Continuous wide QRS complexes with a rate between 110 and 250 are seen in ventricular tachycardia, while sawtoothed P waves are characteristic of atrial flutter.
15. d. Rationale: The most common arrhythmias to occur when the myocardium is reperfused following thrombolytic therapy or angioplasty are PVCs and ventricular tachycardia, and their presence may be an indicator of the success of the therapy.
16. b. Rationale: In a monitored care area where the arrhythmia is identified and a defibrillator is readily available, it should be used immediately, with the initiation of CPR if the initial shock is not successful. IV drugs are rarely successful without defibrillation and CPR because there is no circulation or cardiac output during ventricular fibrillation.

17. c. Rationale: The intent of defibrillation is to apply an electrical current to the heart that will depolarize the cells of the myocardium so that subsequent repolarization of the cells will allow the SA node to resume the role of pacemaker. An artificial pacemaker provides an electrical impulse that stimulates normal myocardial contractions. Cardioversion involves delivery of a shock that is programmed to occur during the QRS complex of the ECG, but this cannot be done during ventricular fibrillation because there is no normal ventricular contraction or QRS complex.
18. a. Rationale: During asystole or pulseless electrical activity, CPR must be initiated immediately to maintain minimal cardiac output and oxygenation, followed by intubation and administration of epinephrine and atropine. Defibrillation is not effective because the myocardial cells are in a state of depolarization.
19. a. Rationale: In preparation for defibrillation, the nurse should apply conductive materials, such as saline pads, electrode gel, or defibrillator gel pads, to the patient's chest to decrease electrical impedance and prevent burns. For defibrillation the initial shock is 200 joules, and the synchronizer switch that is used for cardioversion must be turned off. Sedatives may be used before cardioversion if the patient is conscious, but the patient in ventricular fibrillation is unconscious.
20. a. Rationale: If the cardioverter-defibrillator delivers a shock, the patient has experienced a lethal arrhythmia and needs to lie down to allow recovery from the arrythymia. If the patient loses consciousness or if there is repetitive firing, 991 should be called.
21. b. Rationale: High-output electrical generators or large magnets, such as those used in MRI, can reprogram pacemakers and should be avoided. Microwave ovens pose no problems to pacemaker function, but the arm should not be raised above the shoulder for 1 week following placement of the pacemaker. The pacing current of an implanted pacemaker is not felt by the patient, but an external pacemaker may cause uncomfortable chest muscle contractions.
22. c. Rationale: This patient is manifesting behaviors that are characteristic of a nursing diagnosis of fear related to perceived vulnerability and reliance on a pacemaker, as evidenced by refusal to move or participate in care. It is important for the nurse to teach the patient what activity restrictions are necessary to prevent damage to the pacemaker (avoid direct blows to the generator site) and to affirm that the pacemaker can enhance physiologic function and the quality of the patient's life.
23. c. Rationale: Catheter ablation therapy uses radiofrequency energy to ablate or "burn" accessory pathways or ectopic sites in the atria, AV node, or ventricles that cause tachyarrhythmias.
24. c. Rationale: One of the most common causes of syncope is neurocardiogenic syncope or "vasovagal" syncope. In this type of syncope, there is accentuated adrenergic activity in the upright position, with intense activation of cardiopulmonary receptors resulting in marked bradycardia and hypotension. Normally testing with the upright tilt table causes activation of the renin-angiotensin system and compensation to increase cardiac output and maintain blood pressure when blood pools in the extremities. However, patients with neurocardiogenic syncope experience a marked decrease in blood pressure and heart rate.
25. d. Rationale: Because brain cells start to die within 6 minutes of anoxia, it is critical that CPR be initiated within 4 to 6 minutes of cardiac or pulmonary arrest. Rapid intervention is the most important factor in preventing biologic death or the death of brain cells.
26. a. 2; b. 5; c. 8; d. 4; e. 1; f. 3; g. 7; h. 6
27. b. Rationale: Chest compressions are stopped for no more than 10 seconds at the end of the first minute of CPR to determine if the victim has resumed spontaneous breathing and circulation. Four cycles of compressions and ventilations should take 1 minute.
28. b. Rationale: The most important factor in the successful resuscitation of a person in cardiopulmonary arrest is rapid intervention to prevent death or brain cell death. It is also critical to use correct CPR technique because the best technique provides only about 30% of the normal cardiac output. Absence of underlying cardiac disease is a factor in successful resuscitation but only if resuscitation is rapidly instituted.
29. b. Rationale: Management of a foreign body airway obstruction in a conscious adult who cannot speak requires the administration of abdominal thrusts until the foreign body is expelled or the patient loses consciousness. For a patient who is sitting in a chair, the abdominal thrusts should be performed with the patient in the chair. If the patient loses consciousness, she or he should be positioned on the floor with the nurse astride the patient to deliver the abdominal thrusts.
30. d. Rationale: It is important to know what cardiac activity is present or absent before administering drugs in a cardiac emergency. Arrhythmia identification with monitoring is essential to determine the guidelines that should be used for definitive treatment of specific cardiac emergencies. Endotracheal intubation does not have to be performed

before drug administration, nor would defibrillation be performed in the absence of ventricular fibrillation.

31. a. third-degree block; b. atrial flutter; c. premature ventricular contraction; bigeminal; d. sinus bradycardia; e. second-degree block; Type I; f. premature atrial contraction; g. second-degree block, Type II; h. sinus tachycardia; i. first-degree block; j. ventricular fibrillation; k. premature ventricular contraction; trigeminal; l. atrial fibrillation; m. premature atrial contraction; n. normal sinus rhythm; o. ventricular tachycardia

Case Study

1. The immediate goal of drug therapy is to decrease the rapid ventricular response to the atrial fibrillation because it leads to decreased cardiac output.
2. Cardioversion may be used to convert the fibrillation to a normal sinus rhythm. Cardioversion is administered with an initial dose of 50 joules synchronized with the QRS complex of the ECG, and the patient may be sedated before the procedure.
3. Digoxin is used to treat atrial fibrillation because it decreases the ventricular response by increasing the refractory period of the AV node and it also decreases atrial automaticity.
   Diltiazem is indicated for treatment of atrial fibrillation because it inhibits the influx of calcium ions during depolarization of cardiac cells and slows the AV nodal conduction time, decreasing the ventricular response.
   Coumadin is used to prevent thrombus formation, or extension, in the atria where blood pools because of ineffective atrial contraction. If thrombi form in the left atria, arterial embolization may occur.
4. During atrial fibrillation there is total disorganization of atrial electrical activity and no effective atrial contraction. Fibrillatory waves or undulations occur at a rate of 300 to 600 per minute in the atria, and although not all electrical activity is conducted to the ventricles, the ventricular rate is usually 100 to 160 beats/min and irregular.
5. Atrial rhythm is chaotic, and although no definite P wave can be observed, fibrillatory waves can be seen as a jagged, irregular baseline between QRS complexes. The PR interval cannot be measured. The ventricular rhythm is usually irregular, but QRS complexes are usually of normal contour.
6. *Nursing diagnoses:*
   - Decreased cardiac output related to arrhythmia
   - Activity intolerance related to inadequate cardiac output
   - Impaired gas exchange related to increased preload
   - Anxiety related to vulnerability and cardiac disease

   Collaborative problems:
   Potential complications: embolism; congestive heart failure; cardiogenic shock

CHAPTER 36

1. a. Rationale: The primary cause of right-sided infective endocarditis is intravenous drug use, because venous contamination is first carried to the right side of the heart. Left-sided endocarditis is more common in patients with other bacterial infections and underlying heart disease.
2. a. Rationale: Although a CBC will reveal a mild leukocytosis and ESR rates will be elevated in patients with infective endocarditis, these are nonspecific findings, and blood cultures are the primary diagnostic tool for infective endocarditis. Transesophageal echocardiograms can identify vegetations on valves but are used when blood cultures are negative, and cardiac catheterizations are used when surgical intervention is being considered.
3. a. 3; b. 5; c. 2; d. 1; e. 4
4. b. Rationale: Drug therapy for patients who develop endocarditis of prosthetic valves is often not successful in eliminating the infection and preventing embolization, and early valve replacement followed by prolonged drug therapy is recommended for these patients.
5. d. Rationale: The dyspnea, crackles, and restlessness the patient is manifesting are symptoms of congestive heart failure and decreased cardiac output that occurs in up to 80% of patients with aortic valve endocarditis as a result of aortic valve incompetence. Vegetative embolization from the aortic valve occurs throughout the arterial system and may affect any body organ. Pulmonary emboli occur in right-sided endocarditis.
6. d. Rationale: The patient with outpatient antibiotic therapy requires vigilant home nursing care, and it is most important to determine the adequacy of the home environment for successful management of the patient. The patient is at risk for life-threatening complications, such as embolization and pulmonary edema, and must be able to access a hospital if needed. Bed rest will not be necessary for the patient without heart damage. Avoiding infections and planning diversional activities are indicated for the patient but are not most important while he is on outpatient antibiotic therapy.

7. c. Rationale: Prophylactic antibiotic therapy should be initiated before invasive dental, medical, or surgical procedures to prevent recurrence of endocarditis. Continuous antibiotic therapy is indicated only in patients with implanted devices or ongoing invasive procedures. Symptoms of infection should be treated promptly, but antibiotics are not used for exposure to infection.
8. c. Rationale: The stethoscope diaphragm at the left sternal border is the best method to use to hear the high-pitched, grating sound of a pericardial friction rub. The sound does not radiate widely and occurs with the heartbeat.
9. b. Rationale: The patient is experiencing a cardiac tamponade that consists of excess fluid in the pericardial sac, which compresses the heart and the adjoining structures, preventing normal filling and cardiac output. Fibrin accumulation, a scarred and thickened pericardium, and adherent pericardial membranes occur in chronic constrictive pericarditis.
10. a. F, expiration; heard throughout the respiratory cycle; b. T; c. F, drop in the patient's blood pressure of 30 mm Hg or more from baseline; d. T; e. T
11. d. Rationale: Relief from pericardial pain is often obtained by sitting up and leaning forward. Pain is increased by lying flat. The pain has a sharp, pleuritic quality that changes with respiration, and patients take shallow breaths. Antiinflammatory medications may also be used to help control pain, but narcotics are not usually indicated.
12. b. Rationale: Viruses are the most common cause of myocarditis in the United States, and early manifestations of myocarditis are often those of systemic viral infections. Myocarditis may also be associated with systemic inflammatory and metabolic disorders as well as with other microorganisms, drugs, or toxins. The heart has increased sensitivity to digoxin in myocarditis, and it is used very cautiously, if at all, in treatment of the condition.
13. d. Rationale: A patient who has had rheumatic fever is more susceptible to recurrent attacks after another streptococcal infection, and the most common cause of recurrent infection is failure to take continued prophylactic antibiotics following the first episode of rheumatic fever.
14. d. Rationale: Initial attacks of rheumatic fever and the development of rheumatic heart disease can be prevented by adequate treatment of Group A β-hemolytic streptococcal pharyngitis. Because streptococcal infection accounts for only about 20% of acute pharyntitis, cultures should be done to identify the organism and direct antibiotic therapy. Viral infections should not be treated with antibiotics. Prophylactic therapy is indicated in those who have valvular heart disease or have had rheumatic heart disease.
15. a. Rationale: Although it is unproven, the manifestations of ARF appear to be related to an abnormal immunologic response to an upper respiratory infection with group A β-hemolytic streptococci, and antibodies produced in response to the streptococcal antigens cross-react with normal body tissues. It is known that streptococci are not demonstrable in lesions of rheumatic fever, and active streptococcal infection is not apparent when rheumatic fever occurs.
16. c. Rationale: Major criteria for the diagnosis of rheumatic fever include evidence of carditis, polyarthritis, chorea (often very late), erythema marginatum, and subcutaneous nodules. Minor criteria include all laboratory findings as well as fever, arthralgia, and a history of previous rheumatic fever.
17. d. Rationale: The mitral valve is most often involved in chronic rheumatic carditis, and the valve becomes thickened and fibrosed, and leaflets may fuse, leading to stenosis or regurgitation. The aortic valve and tricuspid valve are involved less often and rarely is the pulmonary valve.
18. a. To eliminate any residual group A β-hemolytic streptococci, prevent spread of infection, prevent recurrent infection
    b. Antiinflammatory effect to control fever, arthritic and joint manifestations
    c. Antiinflammatory effect to control fever, inflammation of severe carditis
19. d. Rationale: When carditis is present in the patient with rheumatic fever, ambulation is postponed until any symptoms of heart failure are controlled with treatment, and full activity cannot be resumed until antiinflammatory therapy has been discontinued. In the patient without cardiac involvement, ambulation may be permitted as soon as acute symptoms have subsided, and normal activity can be resumed when antiinflammatory therapy is discontinued.
20. b. Rationale: The dosage of maintenance prophylactic antibiotics is not adequate for protection when the patient with rheumatic heart disease undergoes invasive procedures, and additional doses are necessary at this time. Prophylactic therapy following rheumatic fever should continue for life for those who had rheumatic heart disease, for at least 5 years for those without carditis after the age of 18, or indefinitely for patients with frequent exposure to group A streptococcus.
21. a. F, decreased, hypertrophy; b. F, valvular stenosis; c. F, mitral; d. F, mitral valve prolapse
22. a. 5; b. 6; c. 2; d. 4; e. 8; f. 1; g. 7; h. 3

23. a. 6; b. 8; c. 2; d. 1; e. 3; f. 4; g. 5; h. 7; i. 5; j. 1; k. 8; l. 2; m. 3
24. b. Rationale: Because normal blood flow through the heart chambers is impaired in all valvular disorders, prophylactic anticoagulation therapy is used to prevent systemic or pulmonary embolization. Nitrates are contraindicated for the patient with aortic stenosis because an adequate preload is necessary to open the stiffened aortic valve. Antiarrhythmics are used only if arrhythmias occur, and α-adrenergic or β-adrenergic blocking agents may be used to control heart rate as needed.
25. b. Rationale: Arrhythmias frequently cause palpitations, light-headedness, and dizziness, and the patient should be carefully attended to prevent falls. Hypervolemia and paroxysmal nocturnal dyspnea (PND) would be apparent in the patient with congestive heart failure.
26. d. Rationale: Although the long-term results of percutaneous transluminal balloon valvuloplasty are not known, the procedure poses fewer complications and postprocedural care than does open valve repair or replacement and is used for those patients, of any age, who are poor surgical risks. It has been used for repair of pulmonic, aortic, and mitral stenosis.
27. c. Rationale: Repair of mitral or tricuspid valves has a lower operative mortality rate than does replacement and is becoming the surgical procedure of choice for these valvular diseases. Open repair is more precise than closed repair and requires cardiopulmonary bypass during surgery. All types of valve surgery are palliative, not curative, and patients require lifelong health care. Anticoagulation therapy is used for all valve surgery for at least a period of time postoperatively.
28. c. Rationale: Mechanical prosthetic valves require long-term anticoagulation, and this is a factor in making a decision about the type of valve to use for replacement. Patients who cannot take anticoagulant therapy, such as women of childbearing age or patients with a risk for hemorrhage, or patients who cannot be compliant with anticoagulation therapy may be candidates for the less durable biologic valves.
29. d. Rationale: The greatest risk to a patient who has an artificial valve is the development of endocarditis with invasive medical or dental procedures, and before any of these procedures, antibiotic prophylaxis is necessary to prevent infection. Health care providers must be informed of the presence of the valve and the anticoagulant therapy, but the most important factor is using antibiotic prophylaxis before invasive procedures.

Case Study

1. His age—incidence is higher in older adults; the invasive endoscopic cholecystectomy
2. Mitral valve prolapse
   Degenerative valve lesions:
      Calcification degeneration of a bicuspid aortic valve
      Senile calcification degeneration of a normal aortic valve
3. Stroke symptoms: embolization of vegetations to cerebral circulation with cerebral infarction
   Petechiae: occur as a result of fragmentation and embolization of vegetative lesions
   Systolic, crescendo-decrescendo murmur: aortic valve involvement
   Fever: infection; occurs in 90% of patients with infective endocarditis
4. It provided a route for introduction of bacteria into the bloodstream to trigger the infectious process.
5. Identification of the organism with blood cultures and appropriate IV antibiotic therapy; antipyretics to control fever; rest—with increase in activity after fever abates and if there are no symptoms of congestive heart failure; valve replacement if there is no response to antibiotic therapy
6. Preoperative prophylactic antibiotic therapy
7. *Nursing diagnoses:*
   - Hyperthermia related to infection
   - Impaired physical mobility related to hemiparesis/hemiplegia
   - Decreased cardiac output related to valvular insufficiency
   - Risk for impaired skin integrity related to immobility

   Collaborative problems:
   Potential complications: emboli; congestive heart failure

CHAPTER 37

1. d. Rationale: Regardless of the location, atherosclerosis is responsible for peripheral arterial disease (PAD) and is related to other cardiovascular disease and its risk factors, such as coronary artery disease and carotid artery disease. Venous thrombosis, venous stasis ulcers, and pulmonary embolism are diseases of the veins and are not related to atherosclerosis.
2. a. 2; b. 3; c. 1
3. c. Rationale: Although most abdominal aortic aneurysms are asymptomatic, on physical examination a pulsatile mass in the periumbilical area slightly to the left of the midline may be detected, and bruits may be audible with a stethoscope

placed over the aneurysm. Hoarseness and dysphagia may occur with aneurysms of the ascending aorta and the aortic arch. Severe back pain with flank ecchymosis is usually present on rupture of an abdominal aortic aneurysm, and neurologic loss in the lower extremities may occur from pressure of a thoracic aneurysm.

4. a. Rationale: A CT scan is the most accurate test to determine the diameter of the aneurysm and whether a thrombus is present. The other tests may also be used, but the CT yields the most descriptive results.
5. b. Rationale: Increased systolic blood pressure continually puts pressure on the diseased area of the artery, promoting its expansion. Small aneurysms can be treated by decreasing blood pressure, modifying atherosclerosis risk factors, and monitoring the size of the aneurysm. Anticoagulants are used during surgical treatment of aneurysms, but physical activity is not known to increase their size. Calcium intake is not related to calcification in arteries.
6. b. Rationale: Because atherosclerosis is a systemic disease, the patient with an AAA is likely to have cardiac, pulmonary, cerebral, and/or lower extremity vascular problems that should be noted and monitored throughout the perioperative period. Postoperatively, the blood pressure is balanced: high enough to keep adequate flow through the artery to prevent thrombosis but low enough to prevent bleeding at the surgical site.
7. a. secular; b. synthetic graft; c. all; d. iliac; e. endovascular graft; f. renal
8. b. Rationale: The blood pressure and peripheral pulses are evaluated every hour in the acute postoperative period to ensure that blood pressure is adequate and that extremities are being perfused. Blood pressure is kept within normal range—if it is too low, thrombosis of the graft may occur, and if it is too high, it may cause leaking or rupture at the suture line. Hypothermia is induced during surgery, but the patient is rewarmed as soon as the surgery is completed. Fluid replacement to maintain urine output at 100 ml/hr would increase the blood pressure too much.
9. c. Rationale: During repair of an ascending aortic aneurysm, blood supply to the carotid arteries may be interrupted, leading to neurologic complications manifested by a decreased level of consciousness and altered pupil responses to light, as well as changes in facial symmetry, speech, and movement of upper extremities. The thorax is opened for ascending aortic surgery, and shallow breathing, poor cough, and decreasing chest drainage are expected. Often, lower limb pulses are normally decreased or absent for a short period of time following surgery.
10. a. decreased or absent pulses in conjunction with cool, painful extremities below the level of repair; b. cardiac arrhythmias, chest pain; c. absent bowel sounds, abdominal distention, diarrhea, bloody stools; d. increased temperature, WBCs; surgical site inflammation or drainage; e. low urine output, increasing BUN and serum creatinine; f. decreased voluntary movement and sensation
11. c. Rationale: Patients are taught to palpate peripheral pulses to identify changes in their quality or strength, but rate is not a significant factor in peripheral perfusion. The color and temperature of the extremities are also important for patients to observe. The remaining statements are all true.
12. d. Rationale: The onset of an aortic dissection involving the distal, descending aorta is usually characterized by a sudden, severe, tearing pain in the back, and as it progresses down the aorta, the abdominal organs and lower extremities may begin to show evidence of ischemia. Aortic dissections of the ascending aorta and aortic arch may affect the heart and circulation to the head, with the development of murmurs, ventricular failure, and cerebral ischemia.
13. d. Rationale: Initial treatment for aortic dissection is to lower the BP and myocardial contractility to diminish the pulsatile forces in the aorta. The aorta is fragile after dissection, and surgery is delayed for as long as possible to allow time for blood to clot in the false lumen and for edema to decrease. Anticoagulants would prolong and intensify the bleeding, and blood is administered only if the dissection ruptures.
14. a. Rationale: Relief of pain is an indication that the dissection has stabilized, and it may be treated conservatively for an extended time with drugs that lower the blood pressure and decrease myocardial contractility. Surgery is usually indicated for dissections of the ascending aorta or if complications occur.
15. a. intermittent claudication; b. nonhealing ischemic ulcers, gangrene; c. 0.77, mild to moderate; d. rest
16. b. Rationale: Cilostazol (Pletal) is a type II phosphodiesterase inhibitor that inhibits platelet aggregation and increases vasodilation, significantly increasing pain-free walking distance. The other drugs are all antiplatelet agents used not only to prevent thrombus in diseased peripheral arteries but also to decrease the risk of MI, stroke, and other cardiovascular causes of death.
17. a. 4; b. 3; c. 6; d. 5; e. 1; f. 2

18. c. Rationale: Walking exercise increases oxygen extraction in the legs and improves skeletal muscle metabolism. The patient with PAD should walk at least 30 minutes a day, preferably twice a day. Exercise should be stopped when pain occurs and resumed when the pain subsides. Elevation of the limbs impairs arterial circulation, so the legs should be kept dependent. Feet should not be soaked because skin breakdown and maceration may occur. Nicotine in all forms causes vasoconstriction and must be eliminated.
19. d. Rationale: Peripheral arterial occlusive disease occurs as a result of atherosclerosis, and the risk factors are the same as for other diseases associated with atherosclerosis, such as coronary artery disease, cerebral vascular disease, and aneurysms. Major risk factors are hypertension, cigarette smoking, and hyperlipidemia. The risk for amputation is high in patients with severe occlusive disease, but it is not the best approach to encourage patients to make lifestyle modifications.
20. a. A; b. V; c. V; d. A; e. A; f. V; g. A; h. V; i. A; j. V; k. V
21. a. Rationale: Diminished blood perfusion to nerve tissue cells produces a neuropathy manifested by loss of both sensation and deep pain, and injuries to the extremity often go unnoticed. It is important to teach the patient to protect the feet and detect and prevent injuries to prevent breaks in the skin that can lead to infection and gangrene.
22. c. Rationale: Loss of palpable pulses and numbness and tingling of the extremity are indications of occlusion of the bypass graft and need immediate medical attention. Pain, redness, and serous drainage at the incision site are expected postoperatively, but decreasing ankle-brachial indices may indicate graft obstruction.
23. a. pain; b. pallor; c. pulselessness; d. paresthesia; e. paralysis; f. poikilothermia
24. a. R; b. B; c. R; d. B; e. R; f. R; g. B; h. R; i. B; j. R
25. a. damage of the endothelium; b. venous stasis; c. hypercoaguability; d. venous stasis; e. hypercoaguability; f. venous stasis
26. a. F, varicose veins; b. F, superficial vein; c.T; d. F, intermittent compression devices
27. d. Rationale: Prevention of emboli formation can be achieved by bed rest and limiting movement of the involved extremity until the clot is stable, inflammation has receded, and anticoagulation is achieved. Elevating the affected limb will promote venous return, but it does not prevent embolization, and dangling the legs promotes venous stasis and further clot formation.
28. a. 3; b. 3; c. 4; d. 2; e. 2; f. 1; g. 1; h. 4; i. 4
29. b. Rationale: Anticoagulant therapy with heparin or Coumadin does not dissolve clots but prevents propagation of the clot, development of new thrombi, and embolization, while lysis of the clot occurs through the action of the body's intrinsic fibrinolytic system or by the administration of fibrinolytic agents.
30. d. Rationale: Exercise programs for patients recovering from DVT should emphasize swimming and wading, which are particularly beneficial because of the gentle, even pressure of the water. Coumadin will not blacken stools, and if these occur, could be signs of GI bleeding. Dark green and leafy vegetables have high amounts of vitamin K and should not be increased during Coumadin therapy, but they do not need to be restricted. The legs must not be massaged because of the risk for dislodging any clots that may be present.
31. a. Rationale: During walking, the muscles of the legs continuously knead the veins, promoting movement of venous blood toward the heart, and walking is the best measure to prevent venous stasis. The other methods will help venous return, but they do not provide the benefit that ambulation does.
32. a. 4; b. 7; c. 1; d. 5; e. 8; f. 3; g. 9; h. 6; i. 2
33. b. Rationale: Although leg elevation, moist dressings, and topical antibiotics are useful in treatment of venous stasis ulcers, the most important factor appears to be extrinsic compression to minimize venous stasis, venous hypertension, and edema. Extrinsic compression methods include compression gradient stockings, elastic bandages, and Unna's boot.
34. a. Rationale: Until the physician is notified and specific orders for IV therapy, oxygen, and medications are received, the patient should be placed in a semi-Fowler's position to facilitate breathing, and the nurse should stay with the patient to explain the situation and provide emotional support. The legs should not be elevated, because increased venous return will increase right ventricular preload, and pulmonary circulation may be significantly obstructed by the emboli.
35. d. Rationale: A pulmonary angiogram, in which a contrast medium is used to visualize the pulmonary vasculature, is the most definitive diagnostic test to locate a pulmonary embolism. The pulmonary angiogram is an invasive test, requiring that a catheter inserted into the femoral or antecubital vein be threaded to the pulmonary artery. ECGs and chest x-rays are not specific

tools for diagnosing pulmonary embolism, and a perfusion lung scan is more useful in screening for pulmonary embolism and evaluating the effectiveness of medical management.

Case Study

1. Smoking history; history of atherosclerosis with coronary artery disease; age; sex
2. The primary etiology of an AAA is atherosclerotic plaquing that causes degenerative changes in the media lining of the aorta. The changes lead to loss of elasticity, weakening, and eventual dilation of the aorta. Trauma and infections and a possible genetic component are responsible for a small number of AAAs.
3. The severe back pain
   The shock symptoms: BP 88/68 mm Hg; cool, clammy extremities
4. The first priority is to control the bleeding, which will require immediate surgical repair of the aneurysm. Fatal hemorrhage is likely if the bleeding is not controlled.
5. The patient will most likely be taken to surgery from the emergency department, and emergency departments are not the most private or supportive environments. It is important for the nurse to provide privacy as much as possible and allow the patient and family to be together and ask questions as necessary. The nurse should also provide explanations of the procedures and interventions that are being implemented and be supportive during this critical time.
6. The only effective treatment for AAA is surgery, and the only way to prevent rupture is to surgically repair the aneurysm before it ruptures. Patients with AAAs should have close medical observation to detect increases in aneurysm size because when the aneurysm is twice normal aorta size, there is a high risk for rupture.
7. *Nursing diagnoses:*
   - Acute pain related to compression of internal structures with blood
   - Decreased cardiac output related to hypovolemia

   Collaborative problems:
   Potential complications: organ ischemia; hypovolemic shock; myocardial infarction

CHAPTER 38

1. a. parotid gland; b. submandibular gland; c. pharynx; d. trachea; e. esophagus; f. diaphragm; g. liver; h. hepatic flexure; i. transverse colon; j. ascending colon; k. ileum; l. cecum; m. ileocecal valve; n. vermiform appendix; o. anal canal; p. rectum; q. sigmoid colon; r. descending colon; s. stomach; t. splenic flexure; u. spleen; v. larynx; w. sublingual gland; x. tongue
   Inset: a. hepatic duct; b. liver; c. cystic duct; d. gallbladder; e. duodenum; f. pancreas; g. spleen
2. a. muscularis; b. longitudinal layer; c. circular layer; d. oblique layer; e. submucosa; f. mucosa; g. pyloric sphincter; h. duodenal bulb; i. duodenum; j. pylorus; k. rugae; l. serosa; m. body; n. fundus; o. lower esophageal sphincter
3. c. Rationale: The parasympathetic nervous system stimulates activity of the GI tract, increasing motility and secretions and relaxing sphincters to promote movement of contents. A drug that blocks this activity decreases secretions and peristalsis, slows gastric emptying, and contracts sphincters. The enteric nervous system of the GI tract is modulated by sympathetic and parasympathetic influence.
4. d. Rationale: Cholecystokinin is secreted by the duodenal mucosa when fats and amino acids enter the duodenum and stimulates the gallbladder to release bile to emulsify the fats for digestion. The bile is produced by the liver but stored in the gallbladder. Secretin is responsible for stimulating pancreatic bicarbonate secretion, and gastrin increases gastric motility and acid secretion.
5. d. Rationale: The stomach secretes intrinsic factor, necessary for cobalamin (vitamin B_{12}) absorption in the intestine. In removal of part or all of the stomach, cobalamin must be supplemented for life.
6. a. F, lower esophageal sphincter; b. T; c. F, parietal cells; d. T; e. F, conjugated (direct); f. T
7. a. 3; b. 5; c. 7; d. 8; e. 10; f. 9; g. 1; h. 4; i. 2; j. 6
8. a. Rationale: Bacteria in the colon synthesize vitamin K, needed for production of prothrombin by the liver; deaminate undigested or nonabsorbed proteins, producing ammonia, which is converted to urea by the liver; and reduce bilirubin in the bowel to urobilinogen. A reduction in normal flora bacteria by antibiotic therapy can lead to decreased vitamin K, resulting in decreased prothrombin and coagulation problems, but would result in decreased serum ammonia levels and

decreased serum urobilinogen. Bowel bacteria do not influence protein absorption.

9. c. Rationale: The ampulla of Vater is the site where the pancreatic duct and common bile duct enter the duodenum, and the opening and closing of the ampulla is controlled by the sphincter of Oddi. Because bile from the common bile duct is needed for emulsification of fat to promote digestion and pancreatic enzymes from the pancreas are needed for digestion of all nutrients, a blockage at this point would affect the digestion of all nutrients. Gastric contents pass into the duodenum through the pylorus or pyloric valve.
10. a. Conjugation and excretion of adrenal steroids, including aldosterone; b. Synthesis of albumin; c. Urea formation from ammonia; d. Conjugation of bilirubin to soluble bilirubin excreted in bile; e. Synthesis of prothrombin, fibrinogen, and other clotting factors; f. Synthesis of cholesterol; g. Conjugation and excretion of estrogen (and other gonadal steroids)
11. The bilirubin from hemoglobin is insoluble (unconjugated) and attached to albumin in the blood, removed by the liver and combined with glucuronic acid to become soluble (conjugated), and excreted in bile into the intestine. Bowel bacteria convert some of the bilirubin to urobilinogen; urobilinogen is absorbed into the blood; and a small amount of urobilinogen is excreted by the kidneys in urine, and the rest is removed by the liver and reexcreted in the bile.
12. d. Rationale: There is decreased tone of the lower esophageal sphincter with aging, and regurgitation of gastric contents back into the esophagus occurs, causing heartburn and belching. There is a decrease in hydrochloric acid secretion in aging. Jaundice and intolerance to fatty foods are symptoms of liver or gallbladder disease and are not normal age-related findings.
13. a. Excessive alcohol intake, smoking, exposure to hepatoxins, recent foreign travel
    b. Anorexia and weight loss, excessive weight gain, inadequate diet
    c. Change in bowel patterns, laxative/enema use, decreased fluid/fiber intake
    d. Weakness, fatigue, inability to procure and prepare food, inability to feed self
    e. Interruption of sleep with gastrointestinal symptoms
    f. Changes in taste or smell, use of pain medications, sensory problems that interfere with food preparation or intake
    g. Self-esteem and body image problems related to weight, symptoms affecting appearance
    h. Loss of employment because of chronic illness, altered relationships with others
    i. Anorexia, alcohol intake, decreased acceptance by sexual partner
    j. Gastrointestinal problems or symptoms induced by stress, depression
    k. Religious dietary restrictions, vegetarianism
14. c. Rationale: A thin white coating of the dorsum (top) of the tongue is normal. A red, slick appearance is characteristic of cobalamin deficiency, and scattered red, smooth areas on the tongue are known as geographic tongue. The uvula should remain in the midline while the patient is saying "Ahh."
15. b. Rationale: The pulsation of the aorta in the epigastric area is a normal finding. Bruits indicate abnormal blood flow, the liver is percussed in the right midclavicular line, and a normal spleen cannot be palpated.
16. c. Rationale: The pancreas is located in the left upper quadrant, the liver is in the right upper quadrant, the appendix is in the right lower quadrant, and the gallbladder is in the right upper quadrant.
17. a. Rationale: Borborygmi are loud gurgles (stomach growling) that indicate hyperperistalsis. The bell of the stethoscope is used to detect low-pitched sounds, and normal bowel sounds are relatively high-pitched. The bowel sounds become higher-pitched when the intestines are under tension, as in bowel obstructions. Absent bowel sounds may be reported only when no sounds are heard for 5 minutes in each quadrant.

18.

	(1) NPO	(2) Bowel	(3) Consent	(4) Allergy
UGI series	X			
Barium enema	X	X		
IV cholangiogram	X			X
Gallbladder ultrasound	X			
Hepatobiliary scintigraphy	X			
Upper GI endoscopy	X		X	
Colonoscopy	X	X	X	
Endoscopic retrograde cholangiopancreatography	X		X	

19. a. Rationale: Amylase is released by damaged pancreatic cells into the blood, and an elevation of the enzyme is important in diagnosing acute pancreatitis. Ultrasound and ERCP are not as specific as the serum amylase for pancreatitis. The serum gamma-glutamyl transpeptidase is elevated in liver and biliary tract disease.
20. c. Rationale: The AST level is elevated in liver disease, but it is important to note that it is also elevated in damage to the heart and lungs and is not a specific test for liver function. Measurement of most of the transaminases are nonspecific tests unless isoenzyme fractions are determined. Nervous system symptoms of hepatic encaphalopathy are related to elevated ammonia levels.
21. a. 1, 2; b. 6 (signs of peritonitis); c. 1; d. 3; e. 4; f. 5, 6; g. 4; h. 4; i. 2; j. 5

CHAPTER 39

1. a. protein: 120 g x 4 = 480 cal = 16% of 3000 cal
   fat: 160 g x 9 = 1440 cal = 48% of 3000 cal
   carbohydrate: 270 g x 4 = 1080 cal = 36% of 3000 cal
   b. protein: 63 g (0.8 g/kg body weight) = 252 cal
   fat: 100 g (30% of 3000 cal) = 900 cal
   carbohydrate: should be the balance—1848 cal = 462 g carbohydrate
   c. An average adult requires an estimated 20-35 calories/kg of body weight per day. In his case it would be between 1580 and 2450 calories per day (70 kg x 20 and 70 kg x 35).
   d. Increase breads, cereals, rice, and pasta as sources of complex carbohydrate to at least 11 servings a day
   Decrease meat and egg group to 3 servings a day to lower protein and fat
   Use 3 servings of milk group to lower fat intake
   Use all fats, oils, and sweets sparingly
2. a. T; b. F, vitamin B_{12} and iron; c. F, fat; d. F, Kwashiorkor
3. d. Rationale: In the United States, where protein intake is high and of good quality, protein-calorie malnutrition is most commonly secondary to problems of the gastrointestinal system. In developing countries, adequate food sources may not exist, the inhabitants may not be well educated about nutritional needs, and economic conditions can prevent purchase of balanced diets.
4. a. Carbohydrate stored in the liver and muscles in the form of glycogen is used and may be quickly depleted.
   b. Protein, primarily the amino acids alanine and glutamine, is converted to glucose for energy, and a negative nitrogen balance occurs.
   c. Body fat is mobilized and is used as the primary source of energy, conserving protein.
   d. Fat stores are usually depleted in 4 to 6 weeks, and body proteins are used because they are the only source of energy available.
5. c. Rationale: The sodium-potassium exchange pump uses 20% to 50% of all calories ingested. When energy sources are decreased, the pump fails to function, and sodium is left in the cell, and potassium remains in extracellular fluids. Hyperkalemia, as well as hyponatremia, occurs.

6. a. T; b. T; c. F, peripheral nervous system; d. T
7. a. xanthine bronchodilators; b. cholestyramine; c. warfarin; d. chlorpromazine and amitriptyline; e. phenytoin and barbiturates; f. monoamine oxidase inhibitors; g. erythropoietin
8. b. Rationale: In malnutrition, metabolic processes are slowed, leading to increased sensitivity to cold, slowed heart rate and cardiac output, and decreased neurologic function. Because of slowed GI motility and absorption, the abdomen becomes distended and protruding.
9. d. Rationale: Malnutrition that results from a decreased intake of food is most common in individuals with severe anorexia that decreases the desire to eat. Infections create a hypermetabolic state that increases nutritional demand, malabsorption causes loss of nutrients that are ingested, and draining decubitus ulcers are examples of disorders that cause both loss of protein and hypermetabolic states.
10. c. Rationale: Serum transferrin is a protein that is synthesized by the liver and used for iron transport and decreases when there is protein deficiency. An increase in the protein would indicate a more positive nitrogen balance with amino acids available for synthesis. Decreased lymphocytes and serum prealbumin are indicators of protein depletion, and an increased serum potassium shows continuing failure of the sodium-potassium pump.
11. d. Rationale: Anthropometric measurements that include mid-upper arm circumference and triceps skinfold measurements are good indicators of lean body mass and skeletal protein reserves and are valuable in evaluating persons who may have acute protein malnutrition. The other measurements do not specifically address muscle mass.
12. a. Rationale: The breakfast with the eggs provides 24 g of protein, compared with 14 g for the protein-fortified cream of wheat and milkshake breakfast. Whole milk instead of skim helps meet the calorie requirements. The toast breakfast has 10 g of protein, and the pancakes have about 6 g. The bacon is considered a fat rather than a meat serving.
13. d. Rationale: At a minimum of <92.5% (100 ÷ 108) desirable weight, the patient does not meet the criteria for nutritional risk of <80% of desired weight. But because she is somewhat underweight and relocation to a long-term care facility can significantly impact the eating habits of the older adult, the patient's nutritional status should be carefully monitored.
14. b. Rationale: Although calorie intake should be decreased in the older adult because of decreased activity and basal metabolic rate, the needs for specific nutrients, such as proteins and vitamins, is believed to be unchanged during aging.
15. a. Rationale: Socioeconomic conditions frequently have the greatest effect on the nutritional status of the healthy older adult. Limited income and social isolation can result in the "tea and toast" meals of the older adult.
16. a. Rationale: Standard nasogastric tubes are used for tube feedings for short-term feeding problems because prolonged therapy can result in irritation and erosion of the mucosa of the upper GI tract. Gastric reflux and the potential for aspiration can occur with both tubes that deliver fluids into the stomach. Both NG and gastrostomy tubes can become displaced and deprive the patient of the sensations associated with eating.
17. a. Position the patient with the head of the bed elevated 30 to 45 degrees.
    Following intermittent feedings, keep the head of the bed elevated for 30 to 60 minutes.
    Measure residual feeding to detect retention of solution in the stomach so that the stomach does not become overdistended.
    b. Start tube feedings with small amounts and low concentrations and gradually increase the amount and strength of the solution.
    Refrigerate opened solutions to prevent bacterial growth but warm them to room temperature before administration.
    c. Flush the tube with water before and after feedings and medication administration.
    In continuous feedings, flush the tube with water every 4 hours.
    d. Verify position before every feeding, or every 8 hours with continuous feedings, by checking that the pH of aspirate is less than 5.
    e. Refrigerate opened solutions.
    Do not hang more solution than will infuse in 8 hours, and discard any remaining at the end of 8 hours.
    Wash equipment for intermittent feedings after each use, and change tubing every 24 hours with continuous feedings.
18. a. Rationale: If the residual stomach contents are more than 200 ml, the next feeding is held for 1 hour, and then the residual volume is rechecked. The aspirate should be reinstilled because it contains gastric secretions in addition to the feeding that has not passed from the stomach.
19. a. PPN; b. CPN; c. CPN; d. PPN; e. PPN; f. PPN; g. CPN
20. c. Rationale: In malabsorption syndromes, foods that are ingested into the intestinal tract cannot be digested or absorbed, and tube feedings infused into the intestinal tract would also not be absorbed. All of the other conditions may be

treated with enteral or parenteral nutrition, depending on the patient's needs.

21. a. Refrigerate solutions until 30 minutes before use; dressing change to catheter site per institutional protocol; IV tubing change every 24 hours; antimicrobial filters on the IV line to be changed every 24 hours; solution in one bottle should not infuse more than 24 hours
    b. Start infusions slowly, gradually increasing rate for 24 to 48 hours; check capillary blood glucose levels every 4 to 6 hours; provide sliding-scale doses of insulin as prescribed; do not speed up infusion rates or remove infusion from infusion controllers/pumps; visually check the amount infused every 30 minutes to 1 hour
    c. Securely fasten catheter to IV tubing; if the tubing disconnects from the catheter, place the patient in Trendelenburg's position on the left side to trap "air" in right atrium and notify physician; monitor for signs of air embolus
22. a. Rationale: Bacterial growth occurs at room temperature in nutritional solutions; therefore solutions must not be infused longer than 24 hours. Remaining solution should be discarded. Speeding up the solution may cause hyperglycemia and should not be done.
23. a. Rationale: Proper placement of the tip of the central catheter for parenteral nutrition is in the superior vena cava. If the tip is in the right atrium, the hyperosmolar fluid and the catheter tip may cause erosions of the atrial tissue. Repositioning of the catheter is only done by the physician or specially trained nurses.
24. d. Rationale: When peripheral parenteral nutrition is being run concurrently with fat emulsions, the fat emulsion should be connected below the filter through a Y-injection site as close as possible to the injection site. A separate IV site is not necessary, but the fat emulsion should be administered through the special tubing provided by the manufacturer.
25. c. Rationale: Nausea and vomiting and fever occur when lipids are infused quickly. Symptoms of fat emboli include dyspnea, cyanosis, and chest and back pain. Fatty acid deficiency can occur with prolonged TPN that does not contain the essential fatty acids. Allergies to fat emulsions do occur but manifest as allergic reactions with urticaria, angioedema, and perhaps anaphylactoid reactions.
26. a. 31 kg/m^2, obesity; b. 0.88, overweight
27. a. Restrict dietary intake so that it is below energy requirements.
    b. A goal for weight loss must be set, and 1 to 2 pounds a week is realistic. A more rapid loss often causes skin and underlying tissue to lose elasticity and become flabby folds of tissue.
    c. Will confirm eating patterns and often point out bad eating habits that can be changed
    d. It is thought that metabolism is temporarily increased by eating, and more calories are used when several small meals a day are ingested.
    e. Alcohol is not permitted because it increases caloric intake and has low nutritional value.
    f. Exercise increases energy expenditure, decreases appetite, and is important in maintaining weight loss.
    g. Programs deemphasize the diet and focus on how and when the person eats, help modify eating habits, and may lead to more success in maintaining weight loss over time.
28. a. When reducing diets severely restrict carbohydrates, the body's glycogen stores become depleted within a few days. The glycogen normally binds to water in fat cells, and it is this water loss that causes weight loss in the first few days. Fat is not burned until the glycogen-water pool is depleted.
    b. Daily weighing is not recommended because of the frequent fluctuation from retained water (including urine) and elimination of feces. A weekly weight is a more reliable indicator of weight loss.
    c. Men are able to lose weight more quickly than are women because women have a higher percentage of metabolically less active fat.
    d. Plateau periods during which no weight is lost are normal occurrences during weight reduction and may last for several days to several weeks, but weight loss will resume if the prescribed weight reduction plan is continued.
29. b. Rationale: Medications are used only as adjuncts to diet and exercise programs in the treatment of obesity. Drugs do not cure obesity without changes in food intake and physical activity, and weight gain will occur when the medications are discontinued. The medications used work in a variety of ways to control appetite, but over-the-counter drugs are probably the least effective and most abused of the drugs.
30. a. 3; b. 1; c. 2; d. 2; e. 3; f. 3; g. 1
31. a. F, gynoid; b. T; c. T
32. d. Rationale: Sedatives can precipitate severe respiratory complications in morbidly obese patients because of preexisting hypoventilation caused by pressure on the diaphragm and reduced movement of the muscles of the chest wall. Antihypertensive drugs and hypoglycemic agents are often used to treat complications of obesity, and IV solutions do not pose a problem for the obese patient.

33. c. Rationale: Special considerations are needed for the care of the morbidly obese patient because most hospital units are not prepared with beds, chairs, blood pressure cuffs, and other equipment that will need to be used with the very obese patient. Consideration of all aspects of care should be made before implementing care for the patient, including extra time and perhaps assistance for positioning, physical assessment, and transferring the patient.
34. d. Rationale: If any medication is to be given intramuscularly to the obese patient, it is important to use a needle long enough to reach muscle tissue. This requires an extra-long (3 to 4 inches) or spinal needle. If a nasogastric tube present following gastric surgery for morbid obesity becomes blocked or needs repositioning, the physician should be notified. Ambulation is usually started in the evening of surgery, and additional help will be needed to support the patient. Respiratory function is promoted by keeping the head of the bed elevated at a 30-degree angle.
35. c. Rationale: Fluids and foods high in carbohydrates tend to promote diarrhea and symptoms of the dumping syndrome in patients with gastric bypass surgery. The diet generally should be high in protein and low in carbohydrates, fat, and roughage, and consist of six small feedings a day because of the small stomach size. Liquid diets are likely to be used for a longer time for the patient with a gastroplasty.
36. a. A; b. AB; c. A; d. B; e. A; f. AB; g. AB; h. A
37. c. Rationale: The potential life-threatening cardiac complications related to the hypokalemia are the most important considerations in the patient's care. The other nursing diagnoses are important considerations in the patient's care but do not pose the immediate risk that the hypokalemia does.

Case Study

1. Her position on the weight for height and body frame chart
   Food intake history
   Assessment of each body system
2. The chemotherapy and radiation have greatly increased nutritional need, but food intake is decreased because of side effects of cancer treatment, weakness may lead to inability to procure and prepare food, she lives alone and has no socialization with meals, and she has feelings of hopelessness about treatment for cancer.
3. Edema and possible ascites indicated by hypoalbuminemia
   Paleness of skin, mucous membranes indicated by her Hg and Hct
4. Liver damage with fatty infiltration
   Susceptibility to infection very high because of chemotherapy and radiation immunosuppression in addition to that of malnutrition
5. Foods that are easy to prepare
   How to add protein supplement or powdered milk to foods
   Decrease fluids with meals so that more calories are consumed
   Eat small multiple feedings that are of nutritional value
   Provide all instructions written in Spanish
6. *Nursing diagnoses:*
   - Imbalanced nutrition: less than body requirements related to anorexia and decreased food intake
   - Activity intolerance related to fatigue and weakness
   - Hopelessness related to belief that cancer therapy is ineffective
   - Risk for infection related to decreased host defense mechanisms

   Collaborative problems:
   Potential complications: liver failure; electrolyte imbalance

CHAPTER 40

1. a. F, parasympathetic nervous system; b. F, labyrinthine stimulation; c. T; d. F, metabolic alkalosis, hydrochloric acid; e. F, projectile vomiting
2. c. Rationale: The loss of gastric hydrochloric acid causes metabolic alkalosis and increase in pH; loss of potassium, sodium, and chloride; and loss of fluid, which increases the hematocrit.
3. a. Rationale: "Coffee-ground" vomitus indicates stomach bleeding where blood has been mixed with gastric acid, changing it to a dark brown color. Active bleeding in the lower esophagus usually produces bright red blood in vomitus. Yellow-greenish vomitus is characteristic of bile reflux or an obstruction below the ampulla of Vater, and a fecal odor to the vomitus is characteristic of a bowel obstruction.
4. d. Rationale: The patient with severe or persistent vomiting requires intravenous replacement of fluids and electrolytes until able to tolerate oral intake to prevent serious dehydration and electrolyte imbalances. Oral fluids are not given until vomiting has been relieved, and parenteral antiemetics are often not used until a cause of the

vomiting can be established. Nasogastric intubation may be indicated in some cases, but fluid and electrolyte replacement is the first priority.

5. c. Rationale: Water is the fluid of choice for rehydration by mouth. Very hot or cold liquids are not usually well tolerated, and although broth and Gatorade have been used for the patient with severe vomiting, the substances are high in sodium and should be administered with caution.
6. d. Rationale: Ondansetron (Zofran) is one of several serotonin antagonists that act both centrally and peripherally to reduce vomiting—centrally on the vomiting center in the brainstem and peripherally by promoting gastric emptying. Dronabinol (Marinol) is an orally active cannabinoid that causes sedation and has a potential for abuse and is used when other therapies are ineffective. Antihistamines used as antiemetics also cause sedation.
7. a. 4; b. 6; c. 2; d. 3; e. 1; f. 5; g. 3; h. 7; i. 4; j. 6; k. 2
8. c. Rationale: A positive history of use of tobacco and alcohol is the most significant etiologic factor in oral cancer. Excessive exposure to ultraviolet radiation from the sun is a factor in the development of cancer of the lip. Herpes simplex infections have not been associated with oral cancer, and difficulty swallowing and ear pain are symptoms of advanced oral cancer, not risk factors.
9. b. Rationale: Because surgical treatment of oral cancers involves extensive excision, a tracheostomy is usually performed with the radical dissections. The first goal of care is that the patient will have a patent airway. The other goals are appropriate but of lesser priority.
10. b. Rationale: Measures to assess and treat withdrawal from alcohol should be implemented with patients who have heavy use of this substance, because alcohol is a strong risk factor and withdrawal can be life-threatening. Nutritional needs may need to be addressed with tube feedings postoperatively, and pain medications may need to be increased because of cross-tolerance. Counseling about lifestyle changes is not a priority in the early postoperative course.
11. a. fatty foods; b. chocolate; c. alcohol; d. tea, coffee—also peppermint and spearmint
12. d. Rationale: Bethanechol is a cholinergic drug that increases lower esophageal sphincter tone and increases gastric emptying. Alginic acid reacts with sodium bicarbonate to form a viscous solution that acts as a mechanical barrier to reflux. Histamine H_2-receptor blockers decrease gastric acid production, and antacids neutralize hydrochloric acid.
13. c. Rationale: The use of blocks to elevate the head of the bed facilitates gastric emptying by gravity and is strongly recommended to prevent nighttime reflux. Small meals should be eaten frequently, but patients should not eat at bedtime or lie down for 2 to 3 hours after eating. Liquids should be taken between meals to prevent gastric distention with meals. Activities that involve increasing intraabdominal pressure, such as bending over, lifting, or wearing tight clothing, should be avoided.
14. c. Rationale: Following a fundoplication, it is most important to maintain patency of the nasogastric tube to prevent overdistention of the stomach and pressure on the suture line, and replacement of an obstructed tube can perforate the surgical repair. Monitoring for return of peristalsis and assessment of the abdominal wounds are common postoperative interventions but are not related to disruption of the surgical site. Positioning on the right side is not indicated following surgical repair of a hiatal hernia.
15. c. Rationale: Dysphagia, occurring with meats, then soft foods, and eventually liquids, is the most common symptom of esophageal cancer and is often pronounced by the time the patient seeks medical attention. The patient frequently has poor nutritional status because of the inability to ingest adequate amounts of food before surgery. Fluid volume deficit could occur, but this is a late finding in comparison with inadequate food intake.
16. b. Rationale: Following esophageal surgery, the patient should be positioned in a semi-Fowler's or Fowler's position to prevent reflux and aspiration of gastric sections. Nasogastric drainage is expected to be bloody for 8 to 12 hours postoperatively. Abdominal distention is not a major concern following esophageal surgery, and even though the thorax may be opened during the surgery, clear breath sounds should be expected in all areas of the lungs.
17. a. 2; b. 5; c. 3; d. 1; e. 4
18. a. acute; b. autoimmune atrophic; c. laparoscopy; d. *Heliobacter pylori*; e. intrinsic factor; f. H_2R blocker, bismuth
19. a. Rationale: A bland diet with six small meals a day is recommended to help control the symptoms of gastritis. Nonsteroidal antiinflammatory drugs are often as irritating to the stomach as aspirin and should not be used in the patient with gastritis. Antacids are often used for control of symptoms but have the best neutralizing effect if taken after meals, and alcohol and caffeine should be entirely eliminated because they may precipitate gastritis.

20. a. Arterial blood that has not been in contact with gastric secretions, as in esophagel or oral bleeding
    b. Blood that has been in the stomach for some time and has reacted with gastric secretions
    c. Slow bleeding from an upper gastrointestinal (GI) source when blood passes through the GI tract and is digested
    d. Bleeding that has been of short duration and blood has not passed through the GI tract
21. a. 4; b. 8; c. 1; d. 7; e. 6; f. 2; g. 5; h. 3
22. a. Rationale: Although all of the interventions may be indicated when a patient has upper GI bleeding, the first nursing priority is to perform a physical assessment of the patient's condition, with emphasis on blood pressure, pulse, and peripheral perfusion to determine the presence of hypovolemic shock.
23. d. Rationale: Octreotide is a somatostatin analog that has been shown to reduce upper GI bleeding and inhibit the release of GI hormones such as gastrin, thereby decreasing hydrochloric acid secretions. Ranitidine is a histamine H_2-receptor blocker that decreases acid secretion, and omeprazole inhibits the pump necessary for the secretion of hydrochloric acid. Vasopressin has a vasoconstriction action useful in controlling upper GI bleeding.
24. b. Rationale: All over-the-counter drugs should be avoided because their contents may include drugs that are contraindicated because of the irritating effects on the gastric mucosa. Patients are taught to test suspicious vomitus or stools for occult blood, but all stools do not need to be tested. Antacids cannot be taken with all medications because they prevent the absorption of many drugs. Misoprostol is used to protect the gastric mucosa in patients who must take NSAIDs for other conditions because it inhibits acid secretion stimulated by NSAIDs.
25. a. Rationale: The patient's BUN is usually elevated with a significant hemorrhage because blood proteins are subjected to bacterial breakdown in the GI tract. With control of bleeding, the BUN will return to normal. During the early stage of bleeding, the hematocrit is not always a reliable indicator of the amount of blood lost or the amount of blood replaced and may be falsely high or low. A urinary output of 25 ml/hr indicates impaired renal perfusion and hypovolemia, and a urine specific gravity of 1.030 indicates concentrated urine typical of hypovolemia.
26. b. Rationale: Because the patient who requires regular administration of NSAIDs, such as naproxen or diclofenac, is at great risk for GI bleeding, substituting the newer NSAID COX-2 inhibitors, such as rofecoxib or celecoxib, may decrease GI side effects. Famotidine and nizatidine are both H_2R blockers that could be used to decrease gastric acidity, and misoprostol could be used with the NSAIDS to inhibit acid secretion.
27. a. D; b. G; c. B; d. D; e. B; f. G; g. G; h. D; i. B; j. D; k. G; l. G; m. B; n. D
28. a. 3; b. 5; c. 1; d. 6; e. 2; f. 4
29. a. Rationale: The ultimate damage to the tissues of the stomach and duodenum, precipitating ulceration, is acid back-diffusion into the mucosa. The gastric mucosal barrier is protective of the mucosa, but without the acid environment and damage, ulceration does not occur. Ammonia formation by *H. pylori* and release of histamine impair the barrier but are not directly responsible for tissue injury.
30. b. Rationale: Back pain is a common manifestation of ulcers located on the posterior aspect of the duodenum and is important for nurses to keep in mind during assessment of the patient, because the more typical epigastric burning and pain may not be present. Duodenal ulcers are more often relieved by food than are gastric ulcers, and when epigastric discomfort occurs, it is lower than that of gastric ulcers. Eating stimulates gastric acid production, increasing discomfort for patients with gastric ulcers, while the pain of duodenal ulcers usually occurs several hours after eating.
31. a. Rationale: Fiberoptic endoscopy is an important procedure used for locating and diagnosing any disorder of the upper GI tract, including peptic ulcers, gastritis, esophageal disorders, gastric cancer, and bleeding. Endoscopy is the most reliable test because of the ability to directly visualize and biopsy tissue. Serologic testing for *H. pylori* and analysis of gastric secretions may help identify precipitating factors related to ulceration.
32. c. Rationale: There is no specific diet used for treatment of peptic ulcers, and patients are encouraged to eat as normally as possible, eliminating foods that cause discomfort or pain. Eating six meals a day prevents the stomach from being totally empty and is also recommended. Caffeine and alcohol should be eliminated from the diet because they are known to cause gastric irritation, and milk and milk products should be used because milk can neutralize gastric acidity and contains prostaglandins and growth factors protective of the GI mucosa.
33. a. Remove stimulation for HCl acid and pepsin secretion by keeping stomach empty
    b. Stop spillage of gastrointestinal contents into the peritoneal cavity
    c. Remove excess fluids and undigested food from the stomach

34. a. 0800, 1030, 1300, 1600, 1900, 2200; b. 2100; c. 0600, 1100, 1700, 2100
Sucralfate should be given on an empty stomach, necessitating administration of the midmorning dose of antacids at least 30 minutes before the prelunch dose of sucralfate and the bedtime dose of antacids 1 hour after the sucralfate. Although newer histamine H_2-receptor blockers can be given with antacids, administration of cimetidine and ranitidine should be separated from antacids by at least an hour. Sucralfate binds a number of drugs, including cimetidine, but can be given with ranitidine.
35. a. 3; b. 6; c. 4; d. 2; e. 7; f. 3; g. 1; h. 5; i. 3; j. 7; k. 1
36. c. Rationale: Increased vagal stimulation from emotional stress causes hypersecretion of hydrochloric acid, and stress reduction is an important part of the patient's management of peptic ulcers, especially duodenal ulcers. If side effects to medications develop, the patient should notify the health care provider before altering the drug regimen. Although effective treatment will promote pain relief in several days, the treatment regimen should be continued until there is evidence that the ulcer has completely healed. Interchanging brands and preparations of antacids and histamine H_2-receptor blockers without checking with health care providers may cause harmful side effects, and patients should take only prescribed medications.
37. c. Rationale: Perforation of an ulcer causes sudden, severe abdominal pain that is often referred to the shoulder, accompanied by a rigid, boardlike abdomen and other signs of peritonitis. Vomiting of blood indicates hemorrhage of an ulcer, and gastric outlet obstruction is characterized by projectile vomiting of undigested food, hyperactive stomach sounds, and upper abdominal swelling.
38. a. Rationale: If symptoms of gastric outlet obstruction, such as nausea, vomiting, and stomach distention, occur while the patient is on NPO status or has a nasogastric tube, the patency of the NG tube should be suspected. A recumbent position should not be used in a patient with an outlet obstruction because it increases abdominal pressure on the stomach, and vital sign and circulatory status assessment are important if hemorrhage or perforation is suspected. Deep breathing and relaxation may help some patients with nausea but not when stomach contents are obstructed from flowing into the small intestine.
39. d. Rationale: Abdominal pain that causes the knees to be drawn up and shallow, grunting respirations in a patient with peptic ulcer disease are characteristic of perforation, and the nurse should assess the patient's vital signs and abdomen before notifying the physician. Irrigation of the NG tube should not be performed because the additional fluid may be spilled into the peritoneal cavity, and the patient should be placed in a position of comfort—usually on the side with the head slightly elevated.
40. a. 3; b. 4; c. 2; d. 1
41. d. Rationale: Because there is no sphincter control of food taken into the stomach following a Billroth procedure, concentrated food and fluid move rapidly into the small intestine, creating a hypertonic environment that pulls fluid from the bowel wall into the lumen of the intestine, reducing plasma volume and distending the bowel. Postprandial hypoglycemia occurs when the concentrated carbohydrate bolus in the small intestine results in hyperglycemia and the release of excessive amounts of insulin into the circulation, resulting in symptoms of hypoglycemia.
42. a. Rationale: Dietary control of dumping syndrome includes small, frequent meals with low carbohydrate content and elimination of fluids with meals. The patient should also lie down for 30 to 60 minutes after meals. These measures help delay stomach emptying, preventing the rapid movement of a high-carbohydrate food bolus into the small intestine.
43. d. Rationale: If the patient's nasogastric tube becomes obstructed following a gastrectomy with an intestinal anastomosis, gastric secretions may put a strain on the sutured anastomosis and cause serious complications. Because of the danger of perforating the gastric mucosa or disrupting the suture line, the nurse should notify the physician if the tube needs to be repositioned or replaced.
44. a. Rationale: Although no single causative agent of gastric cancer has been identified, it is known that the person with achlorhydria or pernicious anemia is more likely to develop gastric cancer than is the person with normal gastric acid production. Other possible risk factors include alcohol intake; genetics; a diet of smoked, highly salted, or spiced foods; *H. pylori* infection; and chronic irritation. Peptic ulcer disease, smoking, and acute gastritis are not known to be associated with gastric cancer.
45. d. Rationale: Anorexia with weight loss, nausea, vomiting, and hematemesis, and anemia and melena may occur in patients with either peptic ulcers or gastric cancer, and antacids and antisecretory agents may also relieve early symptoms of gastric cancer. However, when epigastric pain has been controlled with ingestion of foods, fluids, or antacids for a period of time but becomes

worse regardless of interventions, gastric cancer should be suspected.

46. d. Rationale: A total gastrectomy removes the gastric cells responsible for secreting intrinsic factor necessary for absorption of cobalamin, and lifelong intramuscular or intranasal administration of cobalamin is necessary to prevent the development of pernicious anemia. Wound healing is usually impaired in the patient with a total gastrectomy performed for gastric cancer because of impaired nutritional status before surgery. Following a total gastrectomy, the patient also requires diet modifications as a result of dumping syndrome and postprandial hypoglycemia. Peptic ulcers are not a common finding after total gastrectomy.
47. b. Rationale: Food poisoning caused by *E. coli* is characterized by profuse diarrhea, abdominal cramping, and bloody stools and is most often associated with contaminated beef, especially ground beef. Salmonella contamination most often occurs with poultry, staphylococcal infections occur with milk and salad dressings, and botulism occurs with fish and low-acid canned products.

Case Study

1. Infiltration of the gastric wall by a tumor causes epigastric discomfort, while growth of the tumor into the gastric lumen can cause anorexia and weight loss. Release of substances by cancer cells also contribute to anorexia, nausea, and vomiting. Nausea and vomiting may also be caused if the tumor obstructs the gastric outlet. Fatigue and other symptoms of anemia occur because of chronic blood loss as the lesion erodes through the mucosa.
2. Malnutrition is indicated in Mrs. E. by weight loss, decreased hemoglobin and hematocrit, decreased serum albumin, skin changes and discoloration, and her emaciated appearance.
3. Other factors that may contribute to malnutrition in Mrs. E. include the increased metabolic demands of tumor cells; responses to radiation therapy, such as vomiting, stomatitis, esophagitis, diarrhea, and decreased bone marrow function; and perhaps pernicious anemia resulting from the achlorhydria common with gastric cancer.
4. Malnourished patients do not respond well to radiation therapy, and normal cells do not recover from radiation damage when malnutrition is present. Depletion of protein stores also places Mrs. E. at risk for impaired immune function.
5. A plan for Mrs. E. and her family should include the following:
   - Increasing nutrition with bland, warm, high-calorie, high-protein foods; small, frequent feedings; and nutritional supplements as tolerated
   - Skin care for radiation therapy
   - Anticipatory planning for pain relief and continuing care as she becomes more impaired
   - Discussion of feelings and concerns of Mrs. E. and her family with explanations of realistic expectations of outcome of her condition
6. In responding to Mrs. E., the nurse should provide accurate information in a way that will decrease her stress and promote her decision-making and coping skills. It is important to tell her that while it is unlikely she will recover from her cancer, the radiation treatment can help shrink the tumor mass and improve her nutritional status and promote a feeling of well-being. She should be told that her family and health care providers will help her function effectively as long as possible.
7. *Nursing diagnoses:*
   - Imbalanced nutrition: less than body requirements related to inability to ingest, digest, and absorb nutrients
   - Fatigue related to anemia and effects of radiation therapy
   - Activity intolerance related to generalized weakness
   - Impaired skin integrity related to malnutrition and radiation therapy
   - Risk for ineffective management of therapeutic regimen related to lack of knowledge regarding disease progression

   Collaborative problems:
   Potential complications: sepsis related to immunosuppression; negative nitrogen balance; organ failure

CHAPTER 41

1. a. 3; b. 1; c. 2; d. 1; e. 3; f. 2; g. 1; h. 1; i. 2
2. d. Rationale: Antiperistaltic agents, such as loperamide and paregoric, should not be used in infectious diarrhea because of the potential of prolonging exposure to the infectious agent. Demulcent agents may be used to coat and protect mucous membranes in these cases. The other options are all appropriate measures to use in cases of infectious diarrhea.

3. d. Rationale: The first interventions to establish bowel regularity include promoting bowel evacuation at a regular time each day, preferably by placing the patient on the bedpan, using a bedside commode, or walking the patient to the bathroom. To take advantage of the gastrocolic reflex, an appropriate time is 30 minutes after the first meal of the day or at the patient's usual individual timing. Perianal pouches are used to protect the skin only when regularity cannot be established, and evacuation suppositories are also used only if other techniques are not successful.
4. All of the following factors indicate causes of constipation that are responsive to nursing intervention:
   a. Ignoring the urge to defecate causes the muscles and mucosa in the rectal area to become insensitive to the presence of feces, and drying of the stool occurs. The urge to defecate is decreased, and stool becomes more difficult to expel.
   b. Diverticulosis is seen in individuals with low fiber intake, small stool mass, and development of hard stool.
   c. A belief that one must have a daily bowel movement may lead to chronic laxative use and chronic dilation and loss of tone in the colon.
   d. Hemorrhoids are the most common complication of chronic constipation, caused by straining to pass hardened stool. The straining may cause problems in patients with hypertension.
   e. Increased fiber intake without increasing fluids may predispose the patient to impaction or obstruction.
5. c. Rationale: Of the foods listed, dried beans contain the highest amount of dietary fiber and are an excellent source of soluble fiber. Bran and berries also have large amounts of fiber.
6. d. Rationale: Enemas are fast-acting and are beneficial in the immediate treatment of acute constipation but should be limited in their use. Soapsuds enemas should be avoided because they may lead to inflammation of colon mucosa. Stimulant cathartics irritate the entire intestinal tract and lead to cramping, while stool softeners have a prolonged action, taking up to 72 hours for an effect.
7. a. Rationale: The patient with an acute abdomen may have significant fluid or blood loss into the abdomen, and evaluation of blood pressure and heart rate should be the first intervention, followed by assessment of the abdomen and the nature of the pain. Analgesics are usually withheld until a diagnosis can be determined, so that symptoms are not masked.
8. a, c, d, f
9. c. Rationale: Adequately functioning nasogastric suction should prevent nausea and vomiting because stomach contents are continuously being removed. The first intervention in this case is to check the amount and character of the recent drainage and check the tube for patency. Decreased or absent bowel sounds are expected after a laparotomy, and the Jackson-Pratt only drains fluid from the tissue of the surgical site. Antiemetics may be given if the NG tube is patent, because anesthetic agents may cause nausea.
10. d. Rationale: The patient is experiencing paralytic ileus, or impaired peristalsis, which almost always occurs as a result of anesthetic agents and manipulation of the bowel during surgery. Nasogastric tubes help remove gas and secretions from the stomach but do not prevent the impaired motility of the intestines. Passing flatus or having a bowel movement indicates that the bowel has resumed peristaltic activity.
11. a. Rationale: The abdominal pain and distention that occur from the decreased motility of the bowel should be treated with increased ambulation and frequent position changes to increase peristalsis. If the pain is severe, cholinergic drugs, rectal tubes, or application of heat to the abdomen may be ordered. Assessment of bowel sounds is not an intervention to relieve the pain, and a high Fowler's position is not indicated. Narcotics may still be necessary for pain control, and motility can be increased by other means.
12. d. Rationale: A high-fiber diet will help control symptoms of both diarrhea and constipation in the patient with IBS. Diagnosis of IBS is made by elimination of other problems, and there are established criteria for diagnosis. Although IBS can be precipitated and aggravated by stress and emotions, it is not a totally psychogenic illness. Medications are available but usually used as a last resort because of side effects.
13. a. Rationale: The patient is having symptoms of an acute abdomen and should be evaluated by a physician immediately. The patient's age, location of pain, and other symptoms are characteristic of appendicitis. Heat application and laxatives should not be used in patients with undiagnosed abdominal pain because they may cause perforation of the appendix or other inflammations. Fluids should not be taken until vomiting is controlled, nor should they be taken in the event that surgery may be performed.
14. a. T; b. F, perforation with peritonitis; c. F, McBurney's point; d. T; e. T

15. c. Rationale: With such abdominal trauma as a gunshot or stab wound that perforates the bowel, the major bacterial contamination results from spillage of bowel contents into the peritoneal cavity. Fluid and blood do accumulate in the peritoneum but are generally sterile unless bacteria are present from other sources.
16. a. B; b. UC; c. CD; d. B; e. UC; f. CD; g. UC; h. B; i. UC; j. B; k. CD; l. B; m. B; n. CD
17. a. decreased hemoglobin, hematocrit; b. hypoalbuminemia; c. decreased Na, K, Mg, Cl, and bicarbonate; d. elevated WBC
18. c. Rationale: Ulcerative colitis and Crohn's disease have many of the same extraintestinal symptoms, including erythema nodosum and arthritis, as well as uveitis, conjunctivitis, and gallstones. However, osteoporosis and peptic ulcer disease are specific to ulcerative colitis, and gluten intolerance is more commonly seen in Crohn's disease.
19. a. 2; b. 1; c. 4; d. 6; e. 3; f. 1; g. 5; h. 2; i. 1; j. 4; k. 1
20. a. Rationale: The initial procedure for a total colectomy and ileal reservoir includes a colectomy, rectal mucosectomy, ileal reservoir construction, ileoanal anastomosis, and a temporary ileostomy. The ileostomy is closed in the second surgery after healing from the first surgery is complete. A loop ileostomy is the most common temporary ileostomy, and it is opened the first or second day postoperatively. A rectal tube to suction is not indicated in any of the surgical procedures for ulcerative colitis. A catheter placed in an ileostomy stoma would be expected following a total proctocolectomy with a continent ileostomy (Kock pouch), while a permanent ileostomy stoma would be expected following a total proctocolectomy with a permanent ileostomy.
21. a. Rationale: Initial output from a newly formed ileostomy may be as high as 1500 to 2000 ml/day, and intake and output must be accurately monitored for fluid and electrolyte imbalance. Ileostomy bags may need to be emptied every 3 to 4 hours, but the appliance should not be changed for several days unless there is leakage onto the skin. A terminal ileum stoma is permanent, and the entire colon has been removed. A return to a normal, presurgical diet is the goal for the patient with an ileostomy, with restrictions based only on the patient's individual tolerances.
22. b. Rationale: Elemental diets are enteral feedings that are high in calories and nutrients, lactose-free, fat- and residue-free, and absorbed in the proximal small intestine, which allows distal bowel rest. High-fat diets are contraindicated in Crohn's disease because of the loss of absorbing mucosa and altered bile salt metabolism and absorption, and lactose found in milk may not be adequately absorbed because of lactase deficiency.
23. a. Rationale: Signs of malnutrition include pallor from anemia, hair loss, bleeding, cracked gingivae, and muscle weakness, which support a nursing diagnosis that identifies impaired nutrition. Diarrhea may contribute to malnutrition but is not a defining characteristic. Anorectal excoriation and pain relate to problems with skin integrity, and the hypotension relates to problems with fluid deficit.
24. a. 3; b. 4; c. 5; d. 2; e. 6; f. 1
25. d. Rationale: The increased pressure of fluids and secretions retained in the bowel during an obstruction causes an increase in capillary permeability and extravasation of fluids and electrolytes into the peritoneal cavity, resulting in a severe reduction in circulating blood volume and hypovolemic shock. Secretion of intestinal fluids is increased by the distention occurring with bowel obstruction, and persistent copious vomiting occurs with upper small bowel obstruction. Although bleeding can occur from a necrotic strangulation, it is uncommon and a late event.
26. a. F, upper small bowel obstruction; b. T; c. T; d. F, metabolic acidosis; e. F, strangulated; f. F, mechanical obstruction; g. F, small bowel
27. b. Rationale: Mouth care is critical in the patient who has a nasointestinal tube, because of vomiting and fecal taste and odor as well as mouth breathing, and should be done very frequently. The patient is NPO with a nasointestinal tube and cannot have ice chips. The tube may be checked for patency, but irrigation is only performed as ordered. A patient with a nasointestinal tube should lie on the right side initially and then be turned every 2 hours to assist in passage of the tube through the small bowel.
28. c. Rationale: Although all polyps are abnormal growths, the most common type of polyps (hyperplastic) is nonneoplastic as are several other types of polyps. However, adenomatous polyps are characterized by neoplastic changes in the epithelium, and most colorectal cancers appear to arise from these polyps. Only patients with a family history of familial adenomatous polyposis have close to a 100% lifetime risk of developing colorectal cancer.
29. d. Rationale: Cancers of the right side of the colon (ascending) are usually asymptomatic and cannot be felt or visualized with digital examination or sigmoidoscopy. An annual test for occult blood is the best way to screen for tumors in this

area of the bowel. Serum carcinoembryonic antigen (CEA) is not specific for colon cancer and is used most effectively in following the progress of a patient after surgery for cancer.

30. a. Rationale: A high-calorie, high-fat diet is the most important environmental factor associated with development of colon cancer, and smoking, alcohol, or other environmental agents are not known to be related to colorectal cancer.
31. An abdominal incision is made, and the proximal sigmoid colon is brought through the abdominal wall and formed into a colostomy. The patient is repositioned, a perineal incision is made, and the distal sigmoid colon, rectum, and anus are removed through the perineal incision.
32. b. Rationale: A normal new colostomy stoma should appear rose to brick red, have mild to moderate edema, and have a small amount of bleeding or oozing of blood when touched. A purplish stoma indicates inadequate blood supply and should be reported. The colostomy will not have any fecal drainage for 2 to 4 days, but there may be some earlier mucus or serosanguineous drainage. Bowel sounds after extensive bowel surgery will be diminished or absent.
33. d. Rationale: Sexual dysfunction may result from an abdominal-perineal resection, but the nurse should discuss with the patient that different nerve pathways affect erection, ejaculation, and orgasm and that a dysfunction of one does not mean total sexual dysfunction and also that an alteration in sexual activity does not have to alter sexuality. Simple reassurance of desirability and ignoring concerns about sexual function do not help the patient regain positive feelings of sexuality.
34. a. liquid to semiliquid, constant, extremely irritating to skin, less odor than colostomy
    b. formed, may be able to be regulated with irrigation, least irritating
    c. semiformed, irregular, irritating to skin, foul odor
35. b. Rationale: A nursing diagnosis of disturbed body image is characterized by patients' comments that express shame or an altered image of themselves because of a change in appearance. Although this patient does not yet have the knowledge to care for the colostomy, the primary problem is that the patient cannot or will not yet learn because the colostomy is not acceptable to his image of himself.
36. b. Rationale: Following infusion of the fluid into the stoma, the solution and feces will take about 30 to 45 minutes to return, and the patient can plan to read or perform other quiet activities during the wait time. Between 500 and 1000 ml of warm tap water should be used, a cone tip on the end of the tubing prevents bowel damage that could occur if a stiff plastic catheter is used, and the fluid should be elevated about 18 to 24 inches above the stoma, or about shoulder level, to prevent too-rapid infusion of the solution.
37. c. Rationale: Formation of diverticula is common when decreased bulk of stool, combined with a more narrowed lumen in the sigmoid colon, causes high intraluminal pressures that result in saccular dilation or outpouching of the mucosa through the muscle of the intestinal wall. To prevent the high intraluminal pressure, fecal volume should be increased with use of high-fiber diets and bulk laxatives, such as psyllium hydrophilic mucilloid (Metamucil). Anticholinergic drugs are used only during an acute episode of diverticulitis, and the lesions are not premalignant.
38. a. Rationale: The inflammation and infection of diverticula cause small perforations with spread of the inflammation to the surrounding area in the intestines. Abscesses may form, or complete perforation with peritonitis may occur. Systemic antibiotic therapy is often used, but medicated enemas would increase intestinal motility and increase the possibility of perforation, as would the application of heat. Surgery is indicated when it is necessary to drain abscesses or to resect an obstructing inflammatory mass.
39. a. 6; b. 4; c. 1; d. 5; e. 2; f. 3
40. b. Rationale: Scrotal edema is a common and painful complication after an inguinal hernia repair and can be relieved in part by application of ice and elevation of the scrotum with a scrotal support. Heat would increase the edema and the discomfort, and a truss is used to keep unrepaired hernias from protruding. Coughing is discouraged postoperatively because it increases intraabdominal pressure and stress on the repair site.
41. b. Rationale: The most common type of malabsorption syndrome is lactose intolerance, and it is managed by restricting the intake of milk and milk products. Antibiotics are used in cases of bacterial infections that cause malabsorption, pancreatic enzyme supplementation is used for pancreatic insufficiency, and restriction of gluten is necessary for control of adult celiac disease (nontropical sprue, celiac sprue, gluten-induced enteropathy).
42. c. Rationale: Short bowel syndrome results from extensive resection of portions of the small bowel and would occur if a patient had an extensive resection of the ileum. The other conditions primarily affect the large colon and result in fewer and less severe symptoms.
43. a. 5; b. 4; c. 2; d. 1; e. 3

44. d. Rationale: Warm sitz baths provide comfort, healing, and cleaning of the area following all anorectal surgery and may be done three or four times a day for 1 to 2 weeks. Stool softeners may be ordered for several days postoperatively to help keep stools soft for passage, but laxatives may cause irritation and trauma to the anorectal area and are not used postoperatively. Early passage of a bowel movement, although painful, is encouraged to prevent drying and hardening of stool resulting in an even more painful bowel movement.

Case Study

1. Changes in bowel patterns with alternating constipation and diarrhea; changes in stool caliber with ribbon or pencil stools; rectal bleeding; sensation of incomplete evacuation
2. Assess drains placed in the wound and the type and amount of drainage; assess the incision for suture integrity and signs and symptoms of wound infection; assess drainage from the wound for amount, color, and characteristics; warm sitz baths at 100.4° to 106° F for 10 to 20 minutes three to four times a day; pressure-reducing chair cushions for comfort
3. To be able to manage care independently; have normal skin integrity; adjust to altered body image
4. It appears that Mr. D. is depersonalizing the stoma and, to preserve his body image, is seeing it as something separate from himself with a name and personality of its own.
5. Anxiety, ineffective coping, fear—all may influence his tolerance to pain
6. Care of the perineal wound; importance of fluids and diet; care for colostomy, including skin care, odor control, supplies needed, and where to obtain supplies; signs and symptoms of complications to report and when to seek medical care; name and contact for enterostomy nurse; name and address of ostomy association
7. *Nursing diagnoses:*
   - Disturbed body image related to presence of stoma
   - Acute pain related to surgical incisions and inadequate pain-control measures
   - Risk for impaired skin integrity related to stoma drainage and open perineal wound

   Collaborative problems:
   Potential complications: perineal infection; stomal necrosis, retraction, prolapse, obstruction

CHAPTER 42

1. a. obstructive; conjugated (direct)
   b. increased breakdown of RBCs; unconjugated (indirect)
   c. hepatocellular; both conjugated and unconjugated
2. a. 3; b. 5; c. 4; d. 2; e. 3; f. 1; g. 2; h. 1; i. 5; j. 1
3. a. HBsAg, Anti-HBs; b. HBeAg, Anti-HBe; c. HBcAg, Anti-HBc IgM and Anti-HBc IgG
4. a. HBV DNA; b. Anti-HBs; c. Anti-HBc IgG; d. HbsAg; e. Anti-HAV IgM, Anti-HAV IgG; f. Anti-HDV; g. Anti-HCV; h. HVC RNA; i. Recombinant immunoblot assay (RIBA)
5. d. Rationale: The systemic manifestations of rash, angioedema, arthritis, fever, and malaise in viral hepatitis are caused by the activation of the complement system by circulating immune complexes. Liver manifestations include jaundice from hepatic cell damage and cholestasis, as well as anorexia perhaps caused by toxins produced by the damaged liver. Impaired portal circulation usually does not occur in uncomplicated viral hepatitis but would be a liver manifestation.
6. c. Rationale: Preicteric symptoms occur before the onset of jaundice and include a variety of gastrointestinal symptoms as well as discomfort and heaviness in the upper right quadrant of the abdomen. Pruritus, dark urine, and light-colored stools occur with the onset of jaundice in the icteric phase.
7. d. Rationale: Although fulminant hepatitis can occur with hepatitis A and hepatitis C, it is more common in hepatitis B, especially in hepatitis B infection accompanied by infection with HDV.
8. a. hepatitis B vaccine (Recombivax HB or Engerix-B)
   b. hepatitis B immune globulin (HBIg) *and* hepatitis B vaccine
9. d. Rationale: Individuals who have been exposed to hepatitis A through household contact or foodborne outbreaks should be given immune globulin within 1 to 2 weeks of exposure to prevent or modify the illness. Hepatitis A vaccine is used to provide preexposure immunity to the virus and is indicated for individuals at high risk for hepatitis A exposure. Although hepatitis A can be spread by sexual contact, the risk is higher for transmission with the oral-fecal route.
10. a. Rationale: No specific drugs are effective in treating acute viral hepatitis, although supportive drugs, such as antiemetics, sedatives, or antipruritics, may be used for symptom control. Antiviral agents, such as lamivudine or ribavirin, and α-interferon may be used for treating chronic

hepatitis B or C but are effective in only 20% to 25% of patients.

11. b. Rationale: The patient with hepatitis B is infectious for 4 to 6 months, and precautions to prevent transmission through percutaneous and sexual contact should be maintained until tests for HbsAg are negative. Close contact does not have to be avoided, but close contacts of the patient should be vaccinated. Alcohol should not be used for at least a year, and rest with increasing activity during convalescence is recommended.
12. a. Rationale: Adequate nutrition is especially important in promoting regeneration of liver cells, but the anorexia of viral hepatitis is often severe, requiring creative and innovative nursing interventions. Strict bed rest is not usually required, and the patient usually has only minor discomfort with hepatitis. Diversional activities may be required to promote psychologic rest but not during periods of fatigue.
13. c. Rationale: Immunosuppressive agents are indicated in hepatitis associated with immune disorders in order to decrease liver damage caused by autoantibodies. Autoimmune hepatitis is similar to viral hepatitis in presenting signs and symptoms and may become chronic and lead to cirrhosis.
14. a. 3; b. 4; c. 1; d. 2; e. 1; f. 2; g. 3
15. a. 5; b. 3; c. 6; d. 3; e. 7; f. 8; g. 2; h. 4; i. 3; j. 1
16. a. Scarring and nodular changes in liver lead to compression of the veins and sinusoids, causing resistance of blood flow through the liver from the portal vein.
    b. Development of collateral channels of circulation in inelastic, fragile esophageal veins.
17. a. liver lymphatics, liver tissue, intestinal vasculature
    b. decreased liver production of albumin
    c. decreased, decreased, decreased
    d. decreased, aldosterone, ADH
    e. peripheral edema
    f. aldosterone
    g. hypoalbuminemia, hypokalemia (from hyperaldosteronism)
18. b. Rationale: Serum bilirubin, both direct and indirect, would be expected to be increased in cirrhosis. Serum albumin and cholesterol are decreased, and liver enzymes, such as AST, ALT, SGPT, and GTT, are elevated.
19. a. Helps promote diuresis and fluid excretion
    b. Increases plasma colloid osmotic pressure and maintains intravascular volume and kidney perfusion
    c. Increase fluid loss through the kidneys and mobilize peritoneal fluid; spironolactone blocks effects of the excess aldosterone
    d. Decrease intake of fluid-retaining sodium
    e. Temporary measure to relieve impaired respiration or pain of severe ascites
    f. Shunts peritoneal fluid from the abdomen to the venous system, decreasing ascites and improving hemodynamic factors.
20. d. Rationale: Early signs of this neurologic condition include euphoria, depression, apathy, irritability, confusion, agitation, drowsiness, and lethargy. Loss of consciousness is usually preceded by asterixis, disorientation, hyperventilation, hypothermia, and alterations in reflexes. Increasing oliguria is a sign of hepatorenal syndrome.
21. a. Reduction of ammonia formation in the bowel by limiting protein intake
    b. Reduction of ammonia formation by decreasing absorption of ammonia from bowel
    c. Reduction of ammonia formation by reducing bacterial flora that produce ammonia
    d. Reduction of ammonia formation by removing red blood cells as a source of protein
22. a. Rationale: Although there are many physical changes in the appearance of the patient with cirrhosis, the presence of jaundice and ascites is often the most distressing to the patient. Pruritus and decreased sensory perception do not commonly affect body image, and alopecia and periorbital edema are not manifestations of cirrhosis.
23. d. Rationale: The patient with advanced, complicated cirrhosis requires a high-calorie, high-carbohydrate diet with protein and sodium restrictions. Fat is not limited unless it promotes early satiety. The tomato sandwich with low-protein bread and salt-free butter best meets these requirements. Rough foods, such as popcorn, may irritate the esophagus and stomach and lead to bleeding. Peanut butter is high in sodium and protein, and canned chicken noodle soup is very high in sodium.
24. d. Rationale: Ascites causes pressure on the diaphragm and reduces lung volume, and patients should be positioned in a semi-Fowler's or Fowler's position to relieve the pressure on the diaphragm. A paracentesis is not performed unless there is severe respiratory distress from the ascites, because the fluid rapidly reaccumulates. Coughing and deep breathing should be performed but do not relieve the pressure, nor does oxygen administration.
25. c. Rationale: Bleeding esophageal varices are a medical emergency and involve treatment with IV vasopressin and nitroglycerin, endoscopic sclerotherapy, shunt therapy and, rarely, balloon tamponade, in addition to measures to replace blood loss. During an episode of bleeding, man-

agement of the airway and prevention of aspiration of blood are critical factors. Occult blood as well as fresh blood from the GI tract would be expected and is not tested. Vasopressin and nitroglycerine cause a decreased heart rate. Portal shunting surgery is performed for esophageal varices but not during an acute hemorrhage.

26. d. Rationale: By shunting fluid sequestered in the peritoneum into the venous system, pressure on esophageal veins is decreased, and more volume is returned to the circulation, improving cardiac output and renal perfusion. However, because ammonia is diverted past the liver, hepatic encephalopathy continues. These procedures do not prolong life or promote liver function.
27. c. Rationale: Abstinence from alcohol is very important in alcoholic cirrhosis and may result in improvement if started when liver damage is limited. Although further liver damage may be reduced by rest and nutrition, most changes in the liver cannot be reversed. Exercise does not promote portal circulation, and very moderate exercise is recommended. Acetaminophen should not be used by the patient with liver disease, because it is potentially hepatotoxic.
28. c. Rationale: Because the prognosis for cancer of the liver is poor, and treatment is largely palliative, supportive nursing care is appropriate. The patient exhibits clinical manifestations of liver failure as seen in any patient with advanced liver failure. Whether the cancer is primary or metastatic, there is usually a poor response to chemotherapy, and surgery is indicated only in the few patients that have localization of the tumor to one portion of the liver.
29. d. Rationale: Liver transplantation is indicated for patients with cirrhosis, as well as for many adults and children with other irreversible liver diseases. Although physicians make the decisions regarding the patient's qualifications for transplant, nurses should be knowledgeable about the indications for transplantation and be able to discuss the patient's questions and concerns related to transplantation. Rejection is less of a problem in liver transplants than in kidney or heart transplantation.
30. a. 2; b. 5; c. 3; d. 1; e. 4
31. c. Rationale: The predominant symptom of acute pancreatitis is severe, deep abdominal pain that is usually located in the left upper quadrant but may be in the midepigastrium. Bowel sounds are decreased or absent, temperature is elevated only slightly, and the patient has hypovolemia and may manifest symptoms of shock.
32. b. Rationale: Although serum lipase levels and urinary amylase levels are increased, an increased serum amylase level is the criterion most commonly used to diagnose acute pancreatitis. Renal clearance of amylase that is higher than the clearance of creatinine is also found in acute pancreatitis.
33. c. Rationale: Pancreatic rest and suppression of secretions are promoted by preventing any gastric contents from entering the duodenum, which would stimulate pancreatic activity. Surgery is not indicated for acute pancreatitis but may be used to drain abscesses or cysts. An ERCP pancreatic sphincterotomy may be performed when pancreatitis is related to gallstones. Pancreatic enzymes are necessary in chronic pancreatitis if a deficiency in secretion occurs.
34. b. Rationale: Food and fluid intake stimulates gastric secretions, which in turn will stimulate pancreatic secretions, so patients are always initially on NPO status. Drugs to reduce gastric secretions, such as H_2R blockers and proton pump inhibitors, may be used but have not been found to be effective in controlling pancreatic secretion. Antispasmotics may help relieve pain, but antibiotics are not indicated unless infection is present.
35. c. Rationale: Positions that flex the trunk and draw the knees up to the abdomen help relieve the pain of acute pancreatitis, and positioning the patient on the side with the head elevated decreases abdominal tension. Diversional techniques are not as helpful as positioning in controlling the pain. The patient is usually NPO because food intake increases the pain and inflammation. Bed rest is indicated during the acute attack because of hypovolemia and pain.
36. c. Rationale: Sodium restriction is not indicated for patients recovering from acute pancreatitis, but the stools should be observed for steatorrhea, indicating that fat digestion is impaired, and glucose levels should also be monitored for indication of impaired beta-cell function. Alcohol is a primary cause of pancreatitis and should not be used.
37. c. Rationale: Chronic damage to the pancreas causes pancreatic exocrine and endocrine insufficiency, resulting in a deficiency of digestive enzymes and insulin. Malabsorption and diabetes often result. Abstinence from alcohol is necessary in both types of pancreatitis, as is a high-carbohydrate, high-protein, and low-fat diet. Although abdominal pain is a major manifestation of chronic pancreatitis, more commonly a heavy, gnawing feeling occurs.
38. a. Rationale: Pancreatic extracts are given with meals and food so that enzymes are available for digestion of the nutrients. The enzymes should

not be dissolved in water, nor are they available in liquid form. The effectiveness of the enzyme replacement is monitored by observing for steatorrhea.

39. b. Rationale: Major risk factors for pancreatic cancer are believed to be cigarette smoking, high-fat diet, diabetes, and exposure to benzidine and coke. It is not associated with alcohol intake, as pancreatitis is.
40. a. duodenum; b. gallbladder; c. distal stomach; d. distal common bile duct; e. proximal pancreas; f. pancreatic duct to jejunum; g. common bile duct to jejunum; h. stomach to jejunum
41. a. T; b. F, cholesterol; c. T; d. F, cholelithiasis; e. T
42. a, c, d, g, h
43. a. Obstruction of the common duct prevents bile drainage into the duodenum, with congestion of bile in the liver and subsequent absorption into the blood
    b. Absence of bile in the intestines
    c. Soluble bilirubin in the blood excreted into the urine
    d. Absence of bile salts in duodenum, preventing fat emulsion and digestion
    e. Contraction of the inflamed gallbladder and obstructed ducts, stimulated by cholecystokinin when fats enter the duodenum
44. a. Rationale: Ultrasonography is 90% to 95% accurate in detecting gallstones and is a noninvasive procedure. It is especially useful for patients with contrast-medium allergies but is used for the majority of all patients. Liver function tests will be elevated if liver damage has occurred but do not indicate gallbladder disease. An IV cholangiogram uses radiopaque dye to outline the gallbladder and the ducts.
45. a. Prevent gallbladder stimulation by food or fluids moving into the duodenum.
    b. Meperidine causes less spasm in the bile ducts than do other opiates.
    c. Inflammation of the gallbladder may be caused by bacterial infection or lead to bacterial colonization.
    d. Counteract smooth muscle spasms of the bile ducts.
46. a. 2; b. 1; c. 3; d. 4
47. d. Rationale: Removal of the gallbladder will prevent further stone formation and inflammation of the gallbladder and is the preferred treatment of choice for most patients. The laparoscopic approach is performed about 85% of the time. A cholecystostomy is usually an emergency procedure in which an incision is made into the gallbladder to remove stones; a choledocholithotomy is an incision into the common bile duct to remove stones; a cholecystoduodenostomy is an anastomosis between the gallbladder and duodenum to relieve obstruction at the distal common duct.
48. c. Rationale: The laparoscopic cholecystectomy requires four small abdominal incisions to visualize and remove the gallbladder, and the patient has small dressings placed over these incisions. The patient with an incisional cholecystectomy is usually hospitalized 3 to 5 days, while the laparoscopic procedure allows same-day or next-day discharge with return to work in 2 to 3 days. A T-tube is placed in the common bile duct after exploration of the duct during an incisional cholecystectomy.
49. c. Rationale: After removal of the gallbladder, bile drains directly from the liver into the duodenum, and a low-fat diet is recommended until adjustment to this change occurs. Most patients tolerate a regular diet with moderate fats but should avoid excessive fats, as large volumes of bile previously stored in the gallbladder are not available, and steatorrhea could occur with a large fat intake.
50. b. Rationale: The high abdominal incision makes the patient reluctant to take deep breaths, and adequate pain relief will enable the patient to cough, deep breathe, and move about, preventing postoperative complications. Positioning the patient on the operative side is more likely to increase pain.
51. a. Rationale: The T-tube drains bile from the common bile duct until swelling from trauma has subsided and bile can freely enter the duodenum. The tube is placed to gravity drainage and should be kept open and free from kinks to prevent bile from backing up into the liver. The tube is not normally irrigated.
52. c. Rationale: Bile-colored drainage or pus from any incision may indicate an infection and should be reported to the physician immediately. The bandages on the puncture sites should be removed the day after surgery, followed by bathing or showering. Referred shoulder pain is a common and expected problem following laparoscopic procedures, when carbon dioxide used to inflate the abdominal cavity is not readily absorbed by the body. Nausea and vomiting are not expected postoperatively and may indicate damage to other abdominal organs and should be reported to the physician.

creatic
es in
nd the
elf, a
ated
pancreas and
ospholipase. Elastase
by dissolving the elastic
ssels, and phospholipase A
is. The pancreas may be merely
come necrotic.
lbladder disease
d urinary amylase are elevated,
release of these enzymes into the
blood circulating through the pancreas. The WBC count is high, indicating marked inflammation. The blood glucose level is elevated, indicating impairment of insulin production and release by the beta cells. The decreased calcium indicates hypocalcemia, a sign of severe pancreatitis.

4. Hypocalcemia occurs in part because calcium combines with fatty acids released during fat necrosis of the pancreas. The nurse should observe for symptoms of tetany, such as jerking, irritability, muscular twitching, and positive Chvostek's and Trousseau's signs. Numbness or tingling around the lips and in the fingers is an early indicator of hypocalcemia.
5. The pain is usually located in the upper left quadrant but may be in the midepigastric area and frequently radiates to the back. It has a sudden onset and is described as severe, deep, piercing, and continuous. It is aggravated by eating and often begins when the patient is recumbent. It is not relieved by vomiting and may be accompanied by flushing, cyanosis, and dyspnea.
6. Hypovolemia, shock, and the local complications of pseudocysts and abscesses
7. Meperidine—for pain relief with minimal stimulation of the pancreatic ducts
   Ranitidine—to decrease hydrochloric acid production by the stomach, because the hydrochloric acid stimulates pancreatic activity
8. NPO status and suction with a nasogastric tube prevent gastric contents from entering the duodenum and stimulating pancreatic secretion.
9. *Nursing diagnoses:*
   - Acute pain related to distention of the pancreas and peritoneal irritation
   - Deficient fluid volume related to nausea, vomiting, NG suction, restricted oral intake
   - Impaired oral mucous membrane related to NG tube and NPO status
   - Imbalanced nutrition: less than body requirements related to dietary restrictions, nausea and vomiting, impaired digestion

   Collaborative problems:
   Potential complications: hypovolemia/shock; hypocalcemia; hyperglycemia; fluid and electrolyte imbalance

CHAPTER 43

1. a. adrenal gland; b. right renal artery; c. right renal vein; d. vena cava; e. bladder; f. urethra; g. ureter; h. aorta; i. kidney; j. pyramid; k. papilla; l. renal pelvis; m. ureter; n. cortex; o. medulla; p. major calyx; q. minor calyx; r. fibrous capsule
2. a. 4; b. 1; c. 2; d. 3; e. 1; f. 5; g. 2; h. 5; i. 5; j. 2; k. 5
3. a. T; b. F, regulate the volume and composition of extracellular fluid; c. T; d. F, high, ADH; e. T
4. a. Rationale: Renin is released in response to decreased arterial blood pressure, renal ischemia, ECF, depletion, and other factors affecting blood supply to the kidney. It is the catalyst of the renin-angiotensin-aldosterone system, which raises blood pressure when stimulated. ADH is secreted by the posterior pituitary in response to serum hyperosmolality and low blood volume. Aldosterone is secreted within the renin-angiotensin system only after stimulation by angiotensin II, and kidney prostaglandins lower blood pressure by causing vasodilation.
5. a. Rationale: Erythropoietin is released when the oxygen tension of the renal blood supply is low and stimulates production of red blood cells in the bone marrow. Hypotension causes activation of the renin-angiotensin-aldosterone system, as well as release of ADH. Hyperkalemia stimulates the release of aldosterone from the adrenal cortex, and fluid overload does not directly stimulate factors affecting the kidney.
6. a. ureteropelvic junction and ureterovesical junction; b. ureterovesical junction; c. 200 to 250; d. 600 to 1000; e. urothelium
7. a. Rationale: The short urethra of women allows for easier ascension and colonization of bacteria in the bladder than occurs in men. Relaxation of pelvic floor muscles may contribute to stress and urge incontinence but is not associated with urinary tract infections. The bladder capacity of men and women is the same, and the muscular support at the rhabdosphincter in men increases the risk for stricture at this point.
8. d. Rationale: The decreased ability to concentrate urine results in an increased volume of dilute urine, which does not maintain the usual diurnal

elimination pattern. A decrease in bladder capacity also contributes to nocturia, but decreased bladder muscle tone results in urinary retention. Decreased renal mass decreases renal reserve, but function is generally adequate under normal circumstances.

9. a. Smoking history, history of exposure to carcinogenic and nephrotoxic chemicals; family history of kidney disease, geographic residence
   b. Low fluid intake or loss of fluids, high calcium and purine intake, coffee intake, weight gain secondary to fluid retention
   c. Change in appearance and amount of urine, change in urinary patterns, necessary assistance in emptying bladder
   d. Change in energy level, sedentary lifestyle, urine leakage during activity
   e. Sleep deprivation from nocturia
   f. Pain in flank, groin, suprapubic area, dysuria, absence of pain with other urinary symptoms; cognitive impairment affecting continence
   g. Decreased self-esteem and body image because of urinary problems
   h. Problems maintaining job and social relationships
   i. Change in sexual pleasure or performance
   j. Withdrawal or ineffective coping with incontinence or urinary problem
   k. Any treatment decisions that are affected by value system
10. c. Rationale: To assess for kidney tenderness, the nurse strikes the fist of one hand over the dorsum of the other hand at the posterior costovertebral angle. The upper abdominal quadrants and costovertebral angles are auscultated for vascular bruits in the renal vessels and aorta, and an empty bladder is not palpable. The kidneys are palpated through the abdomen, with the patient supine.
11. a. 8; b. 6; c. 9; d. 10; e. 5; f. 1; g. 2; h. 12; i. 7; j. 11; k. 4; l. 3
12. b. Rationale: Bacteria in warm urine specimens multiple rapidly, and false or unreliable bacterial counts may occur with old urine. Glucose, specific gravity, and white blood cells do not change in urine specimens, but pH becomes more alkaline, RBCs are hemolyzed, and casts may disintegrate.
13. b. Rationale: Cloudiness from a fresh urine specimen, WBC count above 5/hpf, and presence of casts are all indicative of urinary tract infection, and pH is usually elevated because bacteria split the urea in urine into alkaline ammonia. Cloudy, brown urine usually indicates hematuria or the presence of bile, while colorless urine is usually very dilute. Option "a" is normal.
14. a. Rationale: A urine specific gravity of 1.002 is low, indicating dilute urine and the excretion of excess fluid caused by diuretics. Normal urine specific gravity is 1.003 to 1.030. A high specific gravity indicates concentrated urine that would be seen in dehydration.
15. d. Rationale: During a renal arteriogram, a catheter is inserted most commonly at the femoral artery, and following the procedure the patient is positioned with the affected leg extended with a pressure dressing applied. Peripheral pulse monitoring is essential to detect the development of thrombi around the insertion site, which may occlude blood supply to the leg. Gross bleeding in the urine is a complication of a renal biopsy. Allergy to the contrast medium should be established before the procedure, but the medium can be nephrotoxic, and renal function should be monitored after the procedure.
16. b. Rationale: The BUN is increased in renal problems but may also be increased when there is rapid or extensive tissue damage from other causes. Serum creatinine is more specific to renal function and does not vary with other tissue damage.
17. d. Rationale: The rate at which creatinine is cleared from the blood and eliminated in the urine approximates the glomerular filtration rate and is the most specific test of renal function. The renal scan is useful in showing the location, size, and shape of the kidney and general blood perfusion.
18. a. Impaired conversion of inactive vitamin D to active vitamin D results in poor calcium absorption from the bowel, resulting in a hypocalcemia.
    b. Loss of cells that produce erythropoietin results in no stimulation of bone marrow to produce red blood cells.
    c. This serum creatinine level is high, indicating the loss of tubular secretion (passage of substances from the blood into the tubule) by the kidney.
19. b. Rationale: Bleeding from the kidney following a biopsy is the most serious complication of the procedure, and urine must be examined for both gross and microscopic blood, in addition to vital signs and hematocrit levels being monitored. Following a cystoscopy the patient may have burning with urination, and warm stiz baths may be used. Urinary infections are a complication of any procedure requiring instrumentation of the bladder.
20. a. 5; b. 6; c. 8; d. 9; e. 7; f. 4; g. 3; h. 1; i. 6; j. 3; k. 2; l. 3; m. 7

CHAPTER 44

1. a. 4; b. 6; c. 8; d. 3; e. 1; f. 2; g. 7; h. 5
2. d. Rationale: The older adult woman has the most risk factors for urinary tract infection: age, female, hospitalization, neurogenic bladder, and instrumentation. The younger male has one risk factor: presence of calculi. The pregnant female has three risk factors: female, pregnancy, and possible previous injury. The older male has two risk factors: age and urinary retention.
3. c. Rationale: The usual classic symptoms of UTI are often absent in older adults who tend to experience nonlocalized abdominal pain rather than dysuria and suprapubic pain. They also may experience cognitive impairment characterized by confusion or decreased level of consciousness.
4. d. Rationale: Unless a patient has a history of recurrent UTIs or a complicated UTI, TMP-SMX or nitrofurantoin (Macrodantin) is usually used to empirically treat an initial UTI without a culture and sensitivity or other testing. Asymptomatic bacteriuria does not justify treatment, but symptomatic UTIs should always be treated.
5. b. Rationale: Voiding before and after sexual intercourse helps wash from the urinary tract bacteria that are milked into the urethra from the vagina and perineum during intercourse. The bladder should be emptied at least every 2 to 3 hours. Fluid intake should be increased to about 2000 ml/day without caffeine, alcohol, citrus juices, and chocolate drinks because they are potential bladder irritants. Cleaning the urinary meatus with an antiinfective agent after voiding will irritate the meatus, but the perineal area should be wiped from front to back after urination and defecation to prevent fecal contamination of the meatus.
6. c. Rationale: Ascending infections from the bladder to the kidney are prevented by the normal anatomy and physiology of the urinary tract unless a preexisting condition, such as bladder tumors, prostatic hyperplasia, strictures, or stones, is present. Resistance to antibiotics and failure to take a full prescription of antibiotics for a UTI usually result in relapse or reinfection of lower urinary tract infections.
7. a. Rationale: Systemic symptoms of fever and chills with leukocytosis and nausea and vomiting are more common in pyelonephritis than in cystitis, and local symptoms of bladder involvement may or may not be present. Either patient may have a knowledge deficit regarding prevention of recurrence.
8. a. F, chronic; b. T; c. T; d. F, urine culture; e. T
9. d. Rationale: The symptoms of interstitial cystitis imitate those of an infection of the bladder, but the urine is free of infectious agents. Unlike a bladder infection, the pain with interstitial cystitis increases as urine collects in the bladder and is temporarily relieved by urination. Acidic urine is very irritating to the bladder in interstitial cystitis, and the bladder is small, but urinary retention is not common.
10. b. Rationale: Calcium glycerophosphate (Prelief) alkalinizes the urine and can help relieve the irritation from acidic foods. A diet low in acidic foods is recommended, and if a multivitamin is used, high-potency vitamins should be avoided because these products may irritate the bladder. A voiding diary is useful in diagnosis but does not need to be kept indefinitely.
11. d. Rationale: Glomerulonephritis is not an infection but rather an antibody-induced injury to the glomerulus, where either autoantibodies against the glomerular basement membrane directly damage the tissue, or antibodies reacting with nonglomerular antigens are randomly deposited as immune complexes along the glomerular basement membrane. Prior infection by bacteria or viruses may stimulate the antibody production but is not present or active at the time of glomerular damage.
12. a. GFR; b. GBM; c. GBM; d. GFR; e. GFR; f. GFR
13. d. Rationale: An elevated BUN indicates that the kidneys are not clearing nitrogenous wastes from the blood, and protein may be restricted until the kidney recovers. Proteinuria indicates loss of protein from the blood and may indicate a need for increased protein intake. Hypertension is treated with sodium and fluid restriction, diuretics, and antihypertensive drugs. The hematuria is not specifically treated.
14. a. Rationale: Most patients recover completely from APSGN with supportive treatment. Chronic glomerulonephritis that progresses insidiously over years and rapidly progressive glomerulonephritis that results in renal failure within weeks or months occurs in only a few patients with APSGN. In Goodpasture's syndrome, antibodies are present against both the glomerular basement membrane and the alveolar basement membrane of the lungs, and dysfunction of both kidney and lung is present.
15. c. Rationale: The massive proteinuria that results from increased glomerular membrane permeability in nephrotic syndrome leaves the blood without adequate proteins (hypoalbuminemia) to create an oncotic colloidal pressure to hold fluid in the vessels. Without oncotic pressure, fluid moves

into the interstitium, causing severe edema. Hypercoagulability occurs in nephrotic syndrome but is not a factor in edema formation, and glomerular filtration rate is not necessarily affected in nephrotic syndrome.

16. c. Rationale: Both humoral and cellular immune responses are altered in nephrotic syndrome, and infection is a serious complication. Skin integrity is at risk from massive edema, and hypercoagulability increases the risk for thrombosis. The elevated serum cholesterol level characteristic of nephrotic syndrome results from increased hepatic synthesis and not dietary intake.
17. a. proteinuria and nephrotic syndrome; b. HIV-associated nephropathy; c. acute renal failure
18. a. 7; b. 4; c. 1; d. 5; e. 9; f. 2; g. 6; h. 3; i. 8
19. c. Rationale: Because crystallization of stone constituents can precipitate and unite to form a stone when in supersaturated concentrations, one of the best ways to prevent stones of any type is by drinking adequate fluids to keep the urine dilute and flowing, which is an output of about 2 L of urine a day. Sedentary lifestyle is a risk factor for renal stones, but exercise also causes fluid loss and a need for additional fluids. Protein foods high in purine should be restricted only for the small percentage of patients with stones that are uric acid, and although urinary tract infections contribute to stone formation, prophylactic antibiotics are not indicated.
20. a. 3; b. 5; c. 2; d. 1; e. 3; f. 4; g. 5; h. 1; i. 3; j. 4
21. c. Rationale: A classic sign of the passage of a calculus down the ureter is intense, colicky back pain that may radiate into the testicles, labia, or groin and may be accompanied by mild shock with cool, moist skin. Stones obstructing a calyx or at the ureteropelvic junction may produce dull costovertebral flank pain, and large bladder stones may cause bladder fullness and lower obstructive symptoms. Many patients with renal stones do not have a history of chronic urinary tract infections.
22. d. Rationale: Currently it is believed that high dietary calcium intake may actually lower the risk for renal stones by reducing the urinary excretion of oxalate, and oxalate-rich foods should be limited to reduce oxalate excretion. Foods high in oxalate include spinach, rhubarb, asparagus, cabbage, and tomatoes in addition to chocolate, coffee, and cocoa. Milk, milk products, dried beans, and dried fruits are high sources of calcium, and organ meats are high in purine, which contributes to uric acid lithiasis.
23. b. Rationale: A high fluid intake maintains a dilute urine, which decreases bacterial concentration in addition to washing stone fragments and expected blood through the urinary system following lithotripsy. Moist heat to the flank may be helpful to relieve muscle spasms during renal colic, and all urine should be strained in patients with renal stones but to collect and identify stone composition.
24. a. T; b. F, antihypertensives; c. F, hypertension; d. F, anticoagulants; e. T
25. b. Rationale: Adult polycystic kidney disease is an inherited autosomal dominant disorder that often manifests after the patient has children, but the children should receive genetic counseling regarding their life choices. The disease progresses slowly, eventually causing progressive renal failure. Hereditary medullary cystic disease causes poor concentration ability of the kidneys, and Alport's syndrome is a hereditary nephritis that is associated with deafness and deformities of the optic lens.
26. a. 2; b. 3; c. 5; d. 1; e. 4
27. a. Rationale: Both cancer of the kidney and cancer of the bladder are associated with smoking. A family history of renal cancer is a risk factor for kidney cancer, and cancer of the bladder has been associated with use of phenacetin-containing analgesics and recurrent upper urinary tract infections.
28. c. Rationale: There are no early characteristic symptoms of cancer of the kidney, and gross hematuria, flank pain, and a palpable mass do not occur until the disease is advanced. The treatment of choice is a radical nephrectomy and can be successful in early disease. Small renal tumors can be detected with CT scans and MRI. The most common sites of metastases are the lungs, liver, and long bones.
29. b. Rationale: Sitz baths following local bladder surgery promote muscle relaxation and reduce urinary retention. Fluids should be increased to dilute blood in the urine and prevent clots. Irritative bladder symptoms most commonly occur with local instillation of chemotherapeutic agents, and urinary catheterization is not usually necessary with laser photocoagulation.
30. a. 2; b. 1; c. 1; d. 4; e. 2; f. 1; g. 5; h. 3; i. 4; j. 2; k. 3; l. 1
31. a. Stress and urge; increase urethral tone and suppleness
    b. Urge; relaxes bladder tone and increases sphincter tone, decreasing unwanted contractions
    c. Overflow and reflex; relax spastic bladder neck, preventing retention
    d. Stress; increase urethral tone and resistance

32. c. Rationale: Pelvic floor exercises (Kegel exercises) increase the tone of the urethral sphincters and should be done in sets of 10 or more contractions four to five times a day. Frequent bladder emptying is recommended for patients with urge incontinence and an increase in pressure on the bladder for overflow incontinence. Absorptive perineal pads should only be a temporary measure because long-term use discourages continence and can lead to skin problems.
33. c. Rationale: All urinary catheters in hospitalized patients pose a very high risk for infection, especially antibiotic-resistant, nosocomial infections, and scrupulous aseptic technique is essential in the insertion and maintenance of all catheters. Routine irrigations are not performed. Cleaning the insertion site with soap and water should be performed for urethral and suprapubic catheters, but application of antimicrobial ointments is controversial, and site care for other catheters may require special interventions. Turning the patient to promote drainage is recommended only for suprapubic catheters.
34. b. Rationale: Output from ureteral catheters must be monitored every 1 to 2 hours because an obstruction will cause overdistention of the kidney pelvis and renal damage. The renal pelvis only has a capacity of 3 to 5 ml, and if irrigation is ordered, no more than 5 ml of sterile saline is used. The patient with a ureteral catheter is usually kept on bed rest until specific orders for ambulation are given. Suprapubic tubes may be milked to prevent obstruction of the catheter by sediment and clots.
35. b. Rationale: A nephrectomy incision usually is in the flank, just below the diaphragm, and occasionally the 12th rib is removed. Although the patient is reluctant to breathe deeply because of incisional pain, the lungs should be clear. Decreased sounds and shallow respirations are abnormal and would require intervention.
36. a. 2; b. 3; c. 1; d. 4
37. d. Rationale: Urine drains continuously from an ileal conduit, and the drainage bag must be emptied every 2 to 3 hours and measured to ensure adequate urinary output. With an ileal conduit, mucus is present in the urine because it is secreted by the ileal segment as a result of the irritating effect of the urine, but the surgery causes paralytic ileus, and the patient will be NPO for several days postoperatively. Fitting for a permanent appliance is not done until the stoma shrinks to its normal size in several weeks. Self-catheterization is performed when patients have formation of a continent Kock pouch.
38. b. Rationale: Because the stoma continuously drains urine, a wick formed of a rolled-up 4 x 4 gauze is held against the stoma to absorb the urine while the skin is cleaned and a new appliance is attached. The skin is cleaned with warm water only, because soap and other agents cause drying and irritation, and clean, not sterile, technique is used. The appliance should be left in place as long as possible before it loosens and allows leakage onto the skin, perhaps up to 14 days.

Case Study

1. The Jewett-Strong-Marshall classification of bladder cancer identifies the tumor as superficial (CIS, O, A), invasive (B1, B2, C), or metastatic (D1 through D4). The A classification for Mr. G. indicates that the tumor is superficial with submucosal involvement. The TNM grading system indicates the characteristics of the tumor (T), the nodal involvement (N), and the presence of distant metastasis (M). (See Chapter 15 for TNM classification.)
2. The drug will be instilled into the bladder and needs to be retained for about 2 hours. His position will be changed about every 15 minutes to ensure that the drug comes into maximum contact with all areas of the bladder, especially the dome. He may have irritative symptoms, such as frequency, urgency, and bladder spasms, in addition to hematuria during the weeks of treatment. BCG therapy may cause flulike symptoms or systemic infection, but the usual side effects of cancer chemotherapy are not experienced with BCG therapy or with intravesical chemotherapy. BCG stimulates the immune system rather than directly destroying cancer cells.
3. Stop smoking—it is the only significant risk factor in his history.
4. Follow-up is essential to evaluate the effectiveness of the treatment and detect any new tumors while they are in a superficial stage.
5. A cystectomy with urinary diversion would be indicated.
6. *Nursing diagnoses:*
   - Anxiety related to unknown outcome
   - Impaired urinary elimination related to effects of treatment
   - Acute pain related to effects of treatment
   - Risk for infection related to effects of treatment

   Collaborative problem:
   Potential complication: bladder injury

CHAPTER 45

1. a. 1; b. 3; c. 1; d. 3; e. 2; f. 1; g. 3; h. 2; i. 3; j. 1; k. 2; l. 1
2. a. renal ischemia; nephrotoxic injury
   b. basement membrane; tubular epithelium
   c. tubular epithelium; tubules
   d. basement membrane
3.

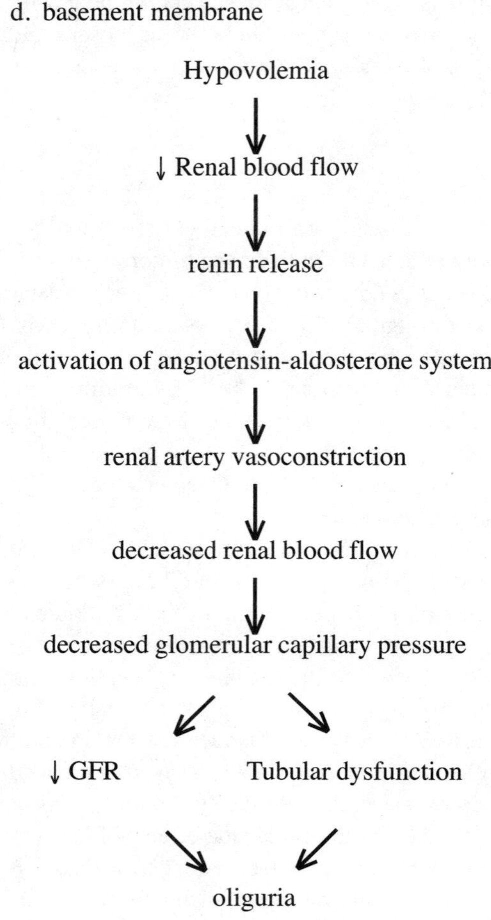

4.

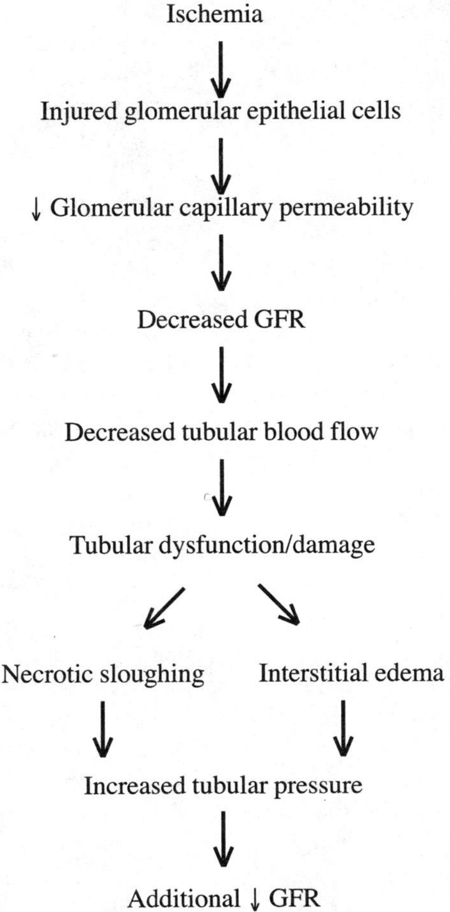

5. d. Rationale: In prerenal oliguria, the oliguria is caused by a decrease in circulating blood volume, and there is no damage yet to the renal tissue. It can potentially be reversed by correcting the precipitating factor, such as fluid replacement for hypovolemia. Prerenal oliguria is characterized by urine with a high specific gravity and a low sodium concentration, while oliguria of intrarenal failure is characterized by urine with a low specific gravity and a high sodium concentration. Malignant hypertension causes damage to renal tissue and intrarenal oliguria.
6. b. Rationale: A urine specific gravity that is consistently 1.010 and a urine osmolality of about 300 mOsm/kg is the same specific gravity and osmolality as plasma and indicates that tubules are damaged and not able to concentrate urine. Hematuria is more common with postrenal damage, and tubular damage is associated with a high sodium concentration (>40 mEq/L).
7. a. Rationale: Metabolic acidosis occurs in ARF because the kidneys cannot synthesize ammonia needed to excrete H^+, resulting in an increased acid load. Sodium is lost in urine because the kidneys cannot conserve sodium, and impaired excretion of potassium results in hyperkalemia. Bicarbonate is normally generated and reabsorbed by the functioning kidney to maintain acid-base balance.
8. a. Rationale: The normal BUN/creatinine ratio of 10:1 is increased in renal failure caused by conditions in which there is markedly increased catabolism, or breakdown of tissue, such as in severe injury, infections, fever, or GI bleeding. The BUN is quite high in this case in comparison with the mild elevation of serum creatinine.
9. c. Rationale: The BUN and creatinine levels remain high during the oliguric and diuretic phases of acute renal failure. The recovery phase begins when the glomerular filtration returns to a rate at which BUN and creatinine stabilize and then decrease. Urinary output of 3 to 5 L/day, decreasing sodium and potassium levels, and fluid weight loss are characteristic of the diuretic phase of ARF.
10. d. Rationale: Hyperkalemia is a potentially life-threatening complication of ARF in the oliguric phase. Muscle weakness and abdominal cramping are signs of the neuromuscular impairment that occurs with hyperkalemia, in addition to cardiac

conduction abnormalities of peaked T wave, prolonged PR interval, prolonged QRS interval, and depressed ST segment. Urine output of 300 ml/day is expected during the oliguric phase, as is the development of peripheral edema.

11. a. F, infection; b. T; c. F, 600; d. F, sodium and potassium serum levels; e. T
12. a. Potassium above 6 mEq/L with cardiac changes; b. Bicarbonate level of 14 mEq/L, indicating metabolic acidosis; c. Change in mental status
13. b. Rationale: During acidosis, potassium moves out of the cell in exchange for H^+ ions, increasing the serum potassium level. Correction of the acidosis with sodium bicarbonate will help lower the potassium levels. A decrease in pH and the bicarbonate and $PaCO_2$ levels would indicate worsening acidosis.
14. b. Rationale: Stages of chronic kidney disease are based on the glomerular filtration rate and/or the presence of kidney damage over a period of 3 months. No specific markers of urinary output, azotemia, or urine output classify the degree of chronic kidney disease.
15. c. Rationale: The creatinine clearance test is used to approximate the glomerular filtration rate, and when the GFR is between 30 and 59 ml/min, moderate chronic kidney disease exists.
16. a. Yellowish discoloration; retention of urinary chromogens
    Pallor; anemia of decreased erythropoiesis, folic acid deficiency
    Uremic frost; urea crystallization on skin with very high BUN levels
    Excoriations; Pruritis caused scratching from calcium-phospate deposition in the skin
    b. Hypertension; sodium retention and fluid overload, increased renin production
    Pericardial friction rub; uremic pericarditis
    Peripheral edema; sodium and fluid retention
    c. Kussmaul's respiration; respiratory compensation of metabolic acidosis
    Dyspnea; pulmonary edema of congestive heart failure and fluid overload
    Pleural friction rub; uremic pleuritis
    d. Mucosal ulcerations; increased ammonia from bacterial breakdown of urea
    Anorexia, nausea, vomiting; irritation of the GI tract from urea
    Diarrhea; hyperkalemia and hypocalcemia
    Urine odor of breath; high urea content of the blood
    e. General CNS depression; high urea content of the blood
    Coma and convulsions; high urea content of the blood
17. a. increased BUN; b. increased creatinine; c. increased glucose; d. decreased RBC; e. increased VLDL; f. increased LDL; g. decreased HDL; h. decreased T_3; i. decreased T_4; j. decreased fibrinogen; k. decreased factor VIII; l. increased phosphorus; m. decreased calcium; n. increased potassium
18. c. Rationale: The calcium-phosphorus imbalances that occur in chronic kidney disease result in osteomalacia, osteitis fibrosa, and metastatic deposits of calcium phosphate, but pathologic fractures are most likely to occur from the osteomalacia resulting from hypocalcemia, which occurs from a deficiency of active vitamin D. Aluminum accumulation is also believed to contribute to the osteomalacia. Osteitis fibrosa involves replacement of calcium in the bone with fibrous tissue and is primarily a result of elevated levels of parathyroid hormone resulting from hypocalcemia.
19. b. Rationale: Conservative management of the patient with renal insufficiency with an elevated potassium level would include a dietary potassium restriction of 2–3 g (51 to 76 mEq), a protein restriction of 0.6 to 0.8 g/kg (42 to 56 g for this patient), and moderate (2–3 g) restriction of sodium unless there is marked edema or hypertension. Breads and cereals are not allowed in unrestricted amounts, because they contain protein.
20. b. Rationale: The peritoneal membrane is permeable to plasma proteins, amino acids, and polypeptides, and protein may be lost at a rate of 9 to 12 g per day into the dialysate fluid, necessitating an increased amount of protein for the patient progressing from renal insufficiency to peritoneal dialysis. Amounts of fats, carbohydrates, and calories are determined by ideal body weight.
21. d. Rationale: A patient with chronic kidney disease may have unlimited intake of sugars and starches (unless the patient is diabetic), and hard candy is an appropriate snack and may help relieve the metallic and urine taste common in the mouth. Raisins are a high-potassium food, pickled foods have high sodium contents, and ice cream contains protein.
22. a. 3; b. 1; c. 4; d. 2; e. 1; f. 4; g. 2; h. 1
23. a. F, folic acid; b. F, uremia; c. T; d. F, meperidine (Demerol)
24. c. Rationale: The most common causes of chronic kidney disease in the United States are hypertension and diabetes mellitus. The nurse should obtain information on long-term health problems that are related to kidney disease. The other disorders are not closely associated with renal disease.

25. b. Rationale: A daily weight gain of 4 lb (2 kg) indicates fluid retention and in the patient with kidney disease could indicate early failure. Proteinuria is not a reliable test for kidney tubular damage and is not performed by the patient, and weights are used rather than I&O to evaluate fluid balance. Patients are taught to weigh daily, take daily blood pressures, and be able to identify signs and symptoms of edema, hyperkalemia, and hypocalcemia. Calcium-based phosphate binders should be taken with meals.
26. c. Rationale: A patient on hemodialysis will continue to have dietary and fluid restrictions that the machine cannot compensate for, and the patient needs additional teaching regarding her therapeutic regimen. The other nursing diagnoses are not supported with defining characteristics.
27. a. HD; b. PD; c. HD; d. PD; e. PD; f. PD; g. HD; h. HD; i. PD
28. d. Rationale: Glucose is added to dialysate fluid to create an osmotic gradient across the membrane in order to remove excess fluid from the blood. The glucose content is so high in peritoneal dialysate that as much as 100 to 150 g per day may be absorbed via the peritoneum, increasing triglyceride levels and creating hyperinsulinism. The dialysate fluid has no potassium so that potassium will diffuse into the dialysate from the blood and usually contains higher calcium to promote its movement into the blood. Dialysate sodium is usually less than or equal to blood to prevent sodium and fluid retention.
29. a. fill, dwell, drain; b. 2; c. automated
30. b. Rationale: Peritonitis is a common complication of peritoneal dialysis and may require catheter removal and termination of dialysis. Infection occurs from contamination of the dialysate or tubing or from progression of exit-site or tunnel infections, and strict sterile technique must be used by health professionals as well as the patient to prevent contamination. Too-rapid infusion may cause shoulder pain, and pain may be caused if the catheter tip touches the bowel. Difficulty breathing, atelectasis, and pneumonia may occur from pressure of the fluid on the diaphragm, which may be prevented by elevating the head of the bed and promoting repositioning and deep breathing.
31. a. Rationale: Because the dialysate glucose is absorbed through the peritoneum, diabetics especially have difficulty with blood glucose control and hypertriglyceridemia, which can lead to vascular disease and complicate existing kidney disease.
32. a. 3; b. 2; c. 1; d. 3; e. 1; f. 2
33. d. Rationale: A more permanent, soft, flexible Silastic double-lumen catheter is being used for long-term access when other forms of vascular access have failed. Femoral vein catheters may only remain in place for up to 1 week and subclavian catheters for 1 to 3 weeks. When the vessels of the extremity have already been used for grafts and are needed for additional permanent access, an external access shunt is not used.
34. a. Rationale: While patients are undergoing hemodialysis, they can perform quiet activities that do not require the limb that has the vascular access. Blood pressure is monitored frequently, and the dialyzer monitors dialysis function, but cardiac monitoring is not indicated. The hemodialysis machine continuously circulates both the blood and the dialysate past the semipermeable membrane in the machine. Graft and fistula access involve the insertion of two needles into the site to remove and return blood to the dialyzer.
35. b. Rationale: A patent AV graft creates turbulent blood flow that can be assessed by listening for a bruit or palpated for a thrill as the blood passes through the graft. Assessment of neurovascular status in the extremity distal to the graft site is important to determine that the graft does not impair circulation to the extremity, but neurovascular status does not indicate whether the graft is open.
36. c. Rationale: A complication of hemodialysis, especially in initial treatment, is disequilibrium syndrome, which is caused by too-rapid removal of urea and other solutes from the blood, leaving a high concentration of the solutes in the cerebrospinal fluid and brain. The higher concentration pulls fluid into these areas, causing cerebral edema and the related symptoms. Loss of blood can occur from heparin use and loss into the dialyzer, and hypotension frequently occurs from fluid loss during dialysis, but the symptoms relate to hypovolemia rather than increased intracranial pressure. Muscle cramps result from neuromuscular hypersensitivity not related to disequilibrium syndrome.
37. d. Rationale: Continuous renal replacement therapy is indicated for the patient with acute renal failure as an alternative or adjunct to hemodialysis to slowly remove solutes and fluid in the hemodynamically unstable patient. It is especially useful for treatment of fluid overload, but hemodialysis is indicated for treatment of hyperkalemia, pericarditis, or other serious effects of uremia.

38. d. Rationale: Extensive vascular disease is a contraindication of renal transplantation, primarily because adequate blood supply is essential to health of the new kidney and circulation of immunosuppressive drugs. Other contraindications include disseminated malignancies, refractory or untreated cardiac disease, chronic respiratory failure, chronic infection, or unresolved psychosocial disorders. Coronary artery disease may be treated with bypass surgery before transplantation, and transplantation can relieve hypertension. Hepatitis B or C infection is not a contraindication.
39. b. Rationale: The best possible match between donor and recipient for transplant includes ABO compatibility, HLA-A, HLA-B, and HLA-DR loci match (six antigens) and a negative antibody crossmatch indicating that there are no preformed cytotoxic antibodies to the donated kidney. (See Chapter 13.) Although ABO blood incompatibility and a positive antibody crossmatch can be managed in living donor transplants, they complicate the procedure.
40. a. Rationale: Fluid and electrolyte balance is critical in the transplant recipient patient, especially because diuresis often begins soon after surgery. Fluid replacement is adjusted hourly, based on kidney function and output. Urine-tinged drainage on the abdominal dressing may indicate leakage from the ureter implanted into the bladder, and the physician should be notified. The donor patient has a flank incision where the kidney was removed; the recipient patient has an abdominal incision where the kidney was placed in the iliac fossa. The urinary catheter is usually used for 2 to 3 days to monitor urine output and kidney function.
41. b. Rationale: Gradual occlusion of the renal blood vessels with signs of increasing renal insufficiency is characteristic of chronic rejection. Recurrence of the original kidney disease may occur, but this is not a rejection problem. Acute rejection occurs when kidney tissue is attacked by T-cytotoxic lymphocytes, and hyperacute rejection occurs when the kidney is damaged by immediate attack by preformed antibodies.
42. b. Rationale: Fever, pain at the site, increasing blood pressure with weight gain, and laboratory findings consistent with renal insufficiency are symptoms of acute rejection. The other symptoms may be caused by side effects of immunosuppressant agents.

Case Study

1. T-cytotoxic lymphocytes recognize the kidney as foreign tissue and attack it, setting in process the inflammatory and complement systems. It usually occurs 4 days to 4 weeks after the transplant, but it may occur later, and it is not uncommon to have at least one rejection episode.
2. All of the laboratory results are abnormal, except potassium at high normal, and are typical of renal insufficiency that occurs during acute rejection:
   - Serum creatinine—decreased excretory function of tubules
   - BUN—decreased ability of the kidney to excrete urea
   - Glucose—insulin resistance occurs in chronic renal failure from unknown cause; may also be increased by corticosteroid therapy
   - Potassium—decreased ability of the kidney to excrete potassium
   - Bicarbonate—impaired generation and reabsorption by the kidney as it is being used to buffer acid load

   Nursing care includes monitoring for central nervous system depression and skin and oral mucus breakdown from high urea; monitoring capillary blood glucose and administering insulin to keep glucose within normal range; and monitoring for increasing weakness and cardiac changes related to hyperkalemia and for symptoms of metabolic acidosis, such as Kussmaul's respiration.
3. Immunosuppressive therapy: designed to reduce proliferation and action of T-cytotoxic lymphocytes that are responsible for acute rejection
   - Muromonab-CD3 (Orthoclone OKT3) is a monoclonal antibody that binds to CD3 receptors on lymphocytes and lyses the cells; is given IV to reverse acute rejection
   - Mycophenolate mofetil (Cellcept) is an antimetabolite that inhibits purine synthesis and suppresses proliferation of T and B cells.
   - Methylprednisolone (Solu-Medrol) is a corticosteroid that inhibits cytokine production and T-cell activation.
   - Tacrolimus (Prograf) is a calcineurin inhibitor that prevents production and release of IL-2, IL-4, and α-interferon, in addition to inhibiting production of T-cytotoxic lymphocytes.

   Supportive therapy: designed to control the symptoms produced by renal insufficiency
   - Furosemide is a loop diuretic that is not influenced by glomerular filtration rate and is used to promote sodium, potassium, and fluid loss through the kidney; helps to relieve hypervolemia and hypertension

- Nifedipine is a calcium channel blocker that reduces cardiac output to control blood pressure.
- Sodium bicarbonate helps control the metabolic acidosis of renal insufficiency and replaces that which is not produced or reabsorbed by the kidney.
- Insulin controls the hyperglycemia resulting from insulin resistance.

4. Many side effects may occur from immunosuppressive therapy, but the most common to all is decreased resistance to infection and increased incidence of cancer because of depression of T-cytotoxic lymphocytes.
   - Muromonab-CD3 causes fever, tachycardia, infections, headache, vomiting, chills, joint and muscle pain, and diarrhea.
   - Mycophenolate mofetil causes gastrointestinal toxicity, leukopenia, and thrombocytopenia.
   - As a corticosteroid, methylprednisolone causes cushingoid syndrome, with sodium and water retention, redistribution of fat, muscle weakness with protein wasting, hyperglycemia, and osteoporosis.
   - Tacrolimus is nephrotoxic and neurotoxic with headaches, seizures, and tremors; nausea and vomiting; hyperglycemia; hypertension; and hair loss.
5. Increased risk for infections, malignancies; chronic liver disease; increased risk for atherosclerosis with coronary artery disease a major cause of death; joint necrosis from chronic steroid therapy; psychologic adjustment—constant fear of rejection and wondering how long the transplant will last; depression if there is failure and a return to dialysis
6. *Nursing diagnoses:*
   - Excess fluid volume related to inability of kidney to excrete fluid
   - Anticipatory grieving related to threat of loss of kidney
   - Disturbed sensory perception related to CNS changes induced by uremic toxins and immunosuppressive drugs
   - Risk for infection related to suppressed immune system

   Collaborative problems:

   Potential complications: hypertension; hyperkalemia with cardiac arrhythmias; hyperglycemia; metabolic acidosis

CHAPTER 46

1. a. hypothalamus; b. pituitary; c. parathyroids; d. thyroid; e. thymus; f. adrenals; g. pancreatic islets; h. ovaries; i. testes
2. a. 3; b. 8; c. 6; d. 1; e. 10; f. 1; g. 3; h. 1; i. 5; j. 1; k. 3; l. 1; m. 7; n. 9; o. 1; p. 2
3. a. T; b. F, growth hormone, T_3/T_4 or cortisol; c. T; d. F, false low; e. F, thyroid hormones; f. T; g. F, thyroid gland and adrenal cortex (also gonads); h. T; i. F, steroid hormones
4. a. 3, 2; b. 1, 4; c. 13, 14; d. 6, 5; e. 9, 10; f. 11, 12; g. 8, 7; h. 10, 9; i. 7, 8
5. b. Rationale: ADH release is controlled by the osmolality of the blood, and as the osmolality rises, ADH is released from the posterior pituitary gland and acts on the kidney to cause reabsorption of water from the kidney tubule, resulting in more dilute blood and more concentrated urine. Aldosterone, the major mineralocorticoid, causes sodium reabsorption from the kidney and potassium excretion. Calcium levels are not a factor in serum osmolality.
6. d. Rationale: Parathormone, or parathyroid hormone, is responsible for maintaining adequate serum calcium levels and raises calcium levels by stimulating calcium resorption from the bone, absorption from the intestines, and retention by the kidney. Calcitonin secreted by the thyroid gland has the opposite effect. TSH and aldosterone are not involved in calcium balance.
7. d. Rationale: Atrial natriuretic hormone is secreted in response to high blood volume and high serum sodium levels and has an inhibiting effect on ADH and the renin-angiotensin-aldosterone system, effects of which would make the blood volume even higher. Glucagon secretion inhibits insulin secretion, but insulin does not inhibit glucagon. The relationship between cortisol and insulin is indirect—cortisol raises blood glucose levels, and insulin secretion is stimulated by the high glucose levels. Testosterone and estrogen have no reciprocal action, and both are secreted by the body in response to tropic hormones.
8. d. Rationale: Usually insulin and glucagon function in a reciprocal manner, except after a high-protein, carbohydrate-free meal, in which both hormones are secreted. Glucagon increases gluconeogenesis, and insulin causes target tissue to accept the amino acids for protein synthesis.
9. b. Rationale: The mineralocorticoid effects of cortisol causes sodium retention and potassium excretion from the kidney, resulting in hypokalemia. Because water is reabsorbed with the sodium, serum sodium remains normal. In its

effect on glucose and fat metabolism, cortisol causes an elevation in blood glucose, as well as increases in free fatty acids and triglycerides.

10. a. Rationale: Hypokalemia inhibits aldosterone release as well as insulin release. These are the major hormones hypokalemia affects.
11. b. Rationale: Many symptoms of hypothyroidism, such as fatigue, mental impairment, dry skin, and constipation, that would be apparent in younger persons are attributed to general aging in the older adult, thus going unrecognized as a treatable condition.
12. c. Rationale: Assessment of the endocrine system is often difficult because hormones affect every body tissue and system, causing great diversity in the signs and symptoms of endocrine dysfunction. Weight loss, fatigue, and depression are signs that may occur with many different endocrine problems, but goiter, exophthalmos, and the three "polys" are specific findings of endocrine dysfunction.
13. a. Decreased energy level in relation to past; family history of similar problem
    b. Changes in appetite and weight, difficulty swallowing; changes in hair distribution, color, and texture; skin changes; hot and cold intolerances
    c. Increased thirst with frequent urination; kidney stones; frequent defecation or constipation
    d. Decrease in previous activity levels; apathy
    e. Sleep disturbances, nightmares, sweating, nocturia, insomnia or excessive sleep
    f. Memory deficits, depression, inability to concentrate; visual disturbances or exophthalmos
    g. Changes in body appearance and self-perception
    h. Changes in ability to maintain usual roles
    i. Menstrual irregularity and infertility; history of large babies; male sexual dysfunction; changes in secondary sex characteristics
    j. perception of stress in life and usefulness of previous coping mechanisms, changes in response to stress
    k. commitment to lifestyle changes, value of health
14. c. Rationale: In the patient with thyroid disease, palpation can cause the release of thyroid hormone into circulation, increasing the patient's symptoms and potentially causing a thyroid storm. Examination should be deferred to a more experienced clinician if possible. Pressure should not be so great as to damage the cricoid cartilage or laryngeal nerve, and if the thyroid is palpated correctly, the carotid arteries are not compressed.
15. a. parathyroid; b. adrenal; c. thyroid; d. excessive; e. thyroid; f. growth; g. adrenal; h. thyroid
16. a. Rationale: Endocrine disorders related to hormone secretion from glands that are stimulated by tropic hormones can be caused by a malsecretion of the tropic hormone or malsecretion of the target gland. If the problem is in the target gland, it is known as a primary endocrine disorder, and a problem with tropic hormone secretion is known as a secondary endocrine disorder. Serum levels of tropic hormones can illustrate the status of the negative feedback system in relation to target organ hormone levels. If a target organ produces low amounts of hormone, tropic hormones will be increased; if a target organ is overproducing hormones, tropic hormones will be low or undetectable.
17. b. Rationale: Normal secretion and action of insulin will usually result in fasting levels of glucose in 2 to 3 hours following carbohydrate ingestion, but to ensure that the level is a fasting level, a minimum of 4 hours should be allowed. Water may be taken, however, and does not affect the glucose level.
18. a. 4; b. 1; c. 5; d. 8; e. 3; f. 7; g. 6; h. 2

CHAPTER 47

1. d. Rationale: Insulin is an anabolic hormone, responsible for growth, repair, and storage, and facilitates movement of amino acids into cells, synthesis of protein, storage of glucose as glycogen, and deposition of triglycerides and lipids as fat into adipose tissue. Glucagon is responsible for hepatic glycogenolysis and gluconeogenesis, and fat is used for energy when glucose levels are depleted.
2. a. skeletal muscle, adipose; b. proinsulin c-peptides; c. cortisol and epinephrine; d. type 1
3. a. 2; b. 2; c. 2; d. 1; e. 1; f. 2; g. 1; h. 2; i. 2
4. a. High glucose levels cause loss of glucose in urine with osmotic diuresis; b. Thirst caused by fluid loss of polyuria; c. Cellular starvation from lack of glucose and use of fat and protein for energy
5. d. Rationale: Type 2 diabetes has a strong genetic influence, and offspring of parents who both have type 2 diabetes have a 15% to 45% chance of developing diabetes. While type 1 diabetes is associated with genetic susceptibility related to HLAs, offspring of parents who both have type 1 diabetes have only a 6% to 9% chance of developing the disease. Lower risk factors for type 2 diabetes include obesity, Native American, Hispanic, African American, and age over 55 years.
6. c. Rationale: Insulin resistance syndrome is a cluster of abnormalities that include elevated

insulin levels, hypertension, elevated triglycerides and low-density lipoproteins (LDL), and decreased high-density lipoproteins (HDL). These abnormalities greatly increase the risk for cardiovascular disease associated with diabetes that can be prevented or delayed with weight loss and regular physical activity.

7. d. Rationale: The patient has marked hyperglycemia but has not developed an acidosis, indicating that he probably has type 2 diabetes. Type 2 diabetes may be treated with diet and weight loss, oral hypoglycemics, or insulin, depending on the patient's response to treatment.
8. c. Rationale: On at least two testings, diabetes is diagnosed with a random plasma glucose over 200 mg/dl, a fasting plasma glucose over 126 mg/dl, or a 2-hour oral glucose tolerance test over 200 mg/dl using a glucose load of 75 gm. Any of the three types of testing may be used, but the fasting plasma glucose test is preferred.
9. c. Rationale: Impaired glucose tolerance exists when a 2-hour plasma glucose level is higher than normal but lower than that level diagnostic for diabetes (between 140 mg/dl and 200 mg/dl). Impaired fasting glucose exists when fasting glucose levels are greater than the normal of 110 mg/dl but less than the 126 mg/dl diagnostic of diabetes. Both conditions are risk factors for development of diabetes and cardiovascular disease.
10. c. Rationale: U100 insulin must be used with a U100 syringe, but for those using low doses of insulin, syringes are available that have increments of 1 unit instead of 2 units. Errors can be made in dosing if patients switch back and forth between different sizes of syringes. Aspiration before injection of the insulin is not recommended, nor is the use of alcohol to clean the skin. Because the rate of peak serum concentration varies with the site selected for injection, injections should be rotated within a particular area, such as the abdomen.
11. c. Rationale: A split-mixed dose of insulin requires that the patient adhere to a set meal pattern to provide glucose for the action of the insulins, and a bedtime snack is usually required when patients take a long-acting insulin late in the day to prevent nocturnal hypoglycemia. Hypoglycemia is most likely to occur with this dose late in the afternoon and during the night. When premixed formulas are used, flexible dosing based on glucose levels is not recommended.
12. d. Rationale: Lispro is a rapid-acting insulin that has an onset of action of 5-15 minutes and should be injected at the time of the meal to within 15 minutes of eating. Regular insulin is short-acting with an onset of action in 30 to 60 minutes following administration and should be given 30 to 45 minutes before meals.
13. a. Rationale: When mixing regular with a longer-acting insulin, regular insulin should always be drawn into the syringe first to prevent contamination of the regular insulin vial with longer-acting insulin additives. Air is added to the NPH vial, then air is added to the regular vial, and the regular insulin is withdrawn, bubbles are removed, and the dose of NPH is withdrawn.
14. d. Rationale: Insulin glargine (Lantus), a long-acting insulin that is continuously released with no peak of action, cannot be diluted or mixed with any other insulin or solution. Mixed insulins should be stored needle-up in the refrigerator and warmed before administration. Currently used bottles of insulin can be kept at room temperature.
15. a. Rationale: Insulin pumps provide tight glycemic control by continuous subcutaneous insulin infusion based on the patient's basal profile, with bolus doses at mealtime at the patient's discretion. Intensive insulin therapy consists of several daily insulin injections with dosage based on frequent self-monitoring of blood glucose. Errors in insulin dosing and complications of insulin therapy are still potential risks with intensive insulin therapy or insulin pumps.
16. c. Rationale: The patient's elevated glucose on arising may be the result of either dawn phenomenon or Somogyi effect, and the best way to determine whether the patient needs more or less insulin is by monitoring the glucose at bedtime, between 2 and 4 a.m., and on arising. If predawn levels are below 60 mg/dl, the insulin dose should be reduced, but if the 2-to-4-a.m. blood glucose is high, the insulin should be increased.
17. a. 5; b. 2; c. 1; d. 1; e. 2; f. 4; g. 1; h. 3; i. 3; j. 4; k. 4
18. c. Rationale: If they only have to take a pill for glycemic control, many patients take their diabetes casually and do not consider it the serious condition it is. Hypoglycemic episodes are more prolonged when they occur as the result of oral agents but do not occur as often as in patients with insulin use. Blood glucose monitoring is usually performed bid in patients taking oral agents, and both insulin and OAs interact with a variety of other drugs that may alter their actions.
19. a. Rationale: The body requires food at regularly spaced intervals throughout the day, and omission or delay of meals can result in hypoglycemia, especially for the patient taking insulin or oral hypoglycemic agents. Weight loss may be recommended in type 2 diabetes if the individual is

overweight, but many patients with type 1 diabetes are thin and require an increase in caloric intake. Less than 10% of total calories should be from saturated fats, and simple sugar should be limited but moderate amounts can be used if counted as a part of total carbohydrate intake.

20. b. Rationale: Maintenance of as near-normal blood glucose levels as possible and achievement of optimal serum lipid levels with dietary modification are believed to be the most important factors in preventing both short-term and long-term complications of diabetes. There is no specific "diabetic diet," and use of dietetic foods is not necessary for diabetes control. Most diabetics eat three meals a day, and some require a bedtime snack for control of nighttime hypoglycemia. A reasonable weight, which may or may not be an ideal body weight, is also a goal of nutritional therapy.
21. b. Rationale: During exercise, a diabetic needs both adequate glucose, to prevent exercise-induced hypoglycemia, and adequate insulin because counterregulatory hormones are produced during the stress of exercise and may cause hyperglycemia. Exercise after meals is best, but a 10- to 15-g carbohydrate snack may be taken if exercise is performed before meals or if exercise is prolonged. Blood glucose levels should be monitored before, during, and after exercise to determine the effect of exercise on the levels.
22. c. Rationale: Cleaning the puncture site with alcohol is not necessary and may interfere with test results and lead to drying and splitting of the fingertips. Washing the hands with warm water is adequate cleaning and promotes blood flow to the fingers. Blood flow is also increased by holding the hand down. Punctures on the side of the finger pad are less painful. SMBG should be performed before and after exercise.
23. c. Rationale: Important goals in diabetes education are enabling the patient to become the most active participant in care and promoting self-management to the ability of the individual patient. Patients who actively manage their diabetes care have better outcomes than those who do not. Management of diabetes includes not only the patient but also health care providers to teach and support the patient. Not all patients with diabetes are capable of self-management, and family members may be involved in these cases.
24. b. Rationale: The American Diabetes Association recommends that testing for type 2 diabetes with an FPG should be considered in all individuals at the age of 45 and above, and if normal, it should be repeated every 3 years. Testing for immune markers of type 1 diabetes is not recommended. Testing at a younger age or more frequently should be done for those members of a high-risk ethnic population, including African Americans, Hispanics, Native Americans, Asian Americans, and Pacific Islanders.
25. a. Rationale: During minor illnesses, the patient with diabetes should continue drug therapy and food intake. Insulin is important because counterregulatory hormones may raise blood glucose during the stress of illness, and food or a carbohydrate liquid substitution is important because during illness the body requires extra energy to deal with the stress of the illness. Blood glucose monitoring should be done every 4 hours, and the health care provider should be notified if the level is more than 250 mg/dl (13.9 mmol/L) or if fever, ketonuria, or nausea and vomiting occur.
26. c. Rationale: When insulin is insufficient and glucose cannot be used for cellular energy, the body releases and breaks down stored fats and protein to meet energy needs. Free fatty acids from stored triglycerides are released and metabolized in the liver in such large quantities that ketones are formed. Ketones are acidic and alter the pH of the blood, causing acidosis. Osmotic diuresis occurs as a result of loss of both glucose and ketones in the urine.
27. a. 5; b. 6; c. 2; d. 7; e. 4; f. 3; g. 8; h. 1
28. a. Kussmaul's respirations; b. ketonuria; c. sweet, fruity odor to breath; d. decreased arterial pH (acidosis); e. ketonemia
29. c. Rationale: The management of DKA is similar to that of HHNS except that HHNS requires greater fluid replacement because of the severe hyperosmolar state. Bicarbonate is not usually given in DKA to correct acidosis unless the pH is less than 7.0, because administration of insulin will reverse the abnormal fat metabolism. Total body potassium deficit is high in both conditions, requiring potassium administration, and in both conditions, glucose is added to IV fluids when blood glucose levels fall to 250 mg/dl (13.9 mmol/L).
30. c. Rationale: During the acute phase of HHNS, polyuria is present because of osmotic diuresis, but as fluid continues to be lost and hypovolemia occurs, decreased renal perfusion with oliguria and anuria follows. Vital signs will indicate hypovolemia, but CVP will be decreased. Depressed ST segment and T waves on cardiac monitoring are signs of hypokalemia. Rapid, deep breathing is characteristic of a metabolic acidosis and is found in DKA.
31. a. 1; b. 3; c. 2; d. 1; e. 2; f. 1; g. 2; h. 3
32. b. Rationale: If a diabetic patient is unconscious, immediate treatment for hypoglycemia must be given to prevent brain damage, and 1 mg of

glucagon should administered IM or SC. If the unconsciousness has another cause, such as ketosis, the rise in glucose caused by the glucagon is not as dangerous as the low glucose level. Following administration of the glucagon, the patient should be transported to a medical facility for further treatment and evaluation. Insulin is contraindicated without knowledge of the patient's glucose level, and oral carbohydrate cannot be given when patients are unconscious.

33. a. Rationale: Blood glucose levels of 80 to 90 mg/dl (4.4 to 5 mmol/L) are within the normal range and are desired in the patient with diabetes, even following a recent hypoglycemic episode. Hypoglycemia is often caused by a single event, such as skipping a meal or taking too much insulin or vigorous exercise, and once corrected, normal control should be maintained.
34. b. Rationale: The development of atherosclerotic vessel disease seems to be promoted by the altered lipid metabolism common to diabetes, and although tight glucose control may help delay the process, it does not prevent it completely. Atherosclerosis in diabetics does respond somewhat to reduction in general risk factors as it does in nondiabetics, and reduction in fat intake, control of hypertension, abstention from smoking, maintainence of a normal weight, and regular exercise should be carried out by diabetics.
35. a. 3; b. 1; c. 2; d. 1; e. 4; f. 1; g. 4; h. 2; i. 1; j. 3; k. 2
36. d. Rationale: Complete or partial loss of sensitivity of the feet is common with peripheral neuropathy of diabetes, and diabetics may suffer foot injury and ulceration without ever having pain. Feet must be inspected during daily care for any cuts, blisters, swelling, or reddened areas.
37. a. Rationale: Because the clinical manifestations of long-term complications of diabetes take 10 to 20 years to develop, and because tight glucose control in the older patient is associated with an increased frequency of hypoglycemia, the goals for glycemic control are not as rigid as in the younger population. Treatment is indicated, and insulin may be used if the patient does not respond to OAs. The patient's needs, rather than age, determine the responsibility of others in care.

Case Study

1. The hypoglycemia may have been prevented by taking time to eat breakfast and perhaps increasing food intake in anticipation of strenuous exercise. She also should have checked her glucose level before exercising.
2. *Sympathetic response to hypoglycemia:*
   Weakness, nervousness, tremor
   Vasoconstriction with pallor, numbness, coldness, headache, tachycardia
   Brain neuroglycopenia:
   Confusion, slurred speech, unsteady gait
3. The hypoglycemia should be treated with a fast-acting carbohydrate—120 to 180 ml of orange juice or regular soda, five or six hard candies, or 8 ounces of low-fat milk.
   Repeat the carbohydrate in 10 to 15 minutes if symptoms are still present or if blood glucose remains below 70 mg/dl (3.9 mmol/L).
   When glucose is greater than 70 mg/dl, a regularly scheduled meal or snack of complex carbohydrate and protein should be eaten.
   The blood glucose should be checked again about 45 minutes after treatment to ensure that the hypoglycemia does not recur.
4. How to recognize situations that lead to hypoglycemia; review the effects of exercise on glucose levels and the need for both adequate glucose and insulin
5. Monitor her blood glucose before, during, and after exercise; increase dietary intake before exercise; maintain insulin doses; exercise 60 to 90 minutes after meals; carry simple carbohydrates to take at first symptoms
6. *Nursing diagnoses:*
   Ineffective therapeutic regimen management related to noncompliance with recommended regimen
   Collaborative problems:
   Potential complications: brain damage, coma, seizures, death

CHAPTER 48

1. d. Rationale: A normal response to growth hormone (GH) secretion is stimulation of the liver to produce somatomedin C, or insulin-like growth factor-1 (IGF-1), which stimulates growth of bones and soft tissues. The increased levels of somatomedin C normally inhibit growth hormone, but in acromegaly, the pituitary gland secretes GH despite elevated IFG-1 levels. When both GH and IGF-1 levels are increased (IGF-1 levels >300 ng/ml), overproduction of growth hormone is confirmed. GH also causes elevation of blood glucose, and normally GH levels fall during an oral glucose challenge but do not in acromegaly.
2. c. Rationale: The increased production of growth hormone in acromegaly causes an increase in thickness and width of bones and enlargement of soft tissues, resulting in marked changes in facial

features, oily and coarse skin, and speech difficulties. Height is not increased in adults with growth hormone excess because the epiphyses of the bones are closed, and infertility is not a common finding because growth hormone is usually the only pituitary hormone involved in acromegaly.

3. d. Rationale: A transsphenoidal hypophysectomy involves entry into the sella turcica through an incision in the upper lip and gingiva into the floor of the nose and the sphenoid sinuses. Postoperative clear nasal drainage with glucose content indicates CSF leakage from an open connection to the brain, putting the patient at risk for meningitis. After surgery, the patient is positioned with the head elevated to avoid pressure on the sella turcica, coughing and straining are avoided to prevent increased intracranial pressure and CSF leakage, and although mouth care is required q4hr, toothbrushing should not be performed, because injury to the suture line may occur.
4. a. F, lower the levels; b. F, smaller; c. T; d. F, hypersecretion; e. T
5. a. cortisol; b. thyroid; c. vasopressin/ADH analog; d. growth hormone; e. sex hormones: testosterone; FSH and LH if fertility is desired; estrogen/progesterone if fertility is not an issue

6.

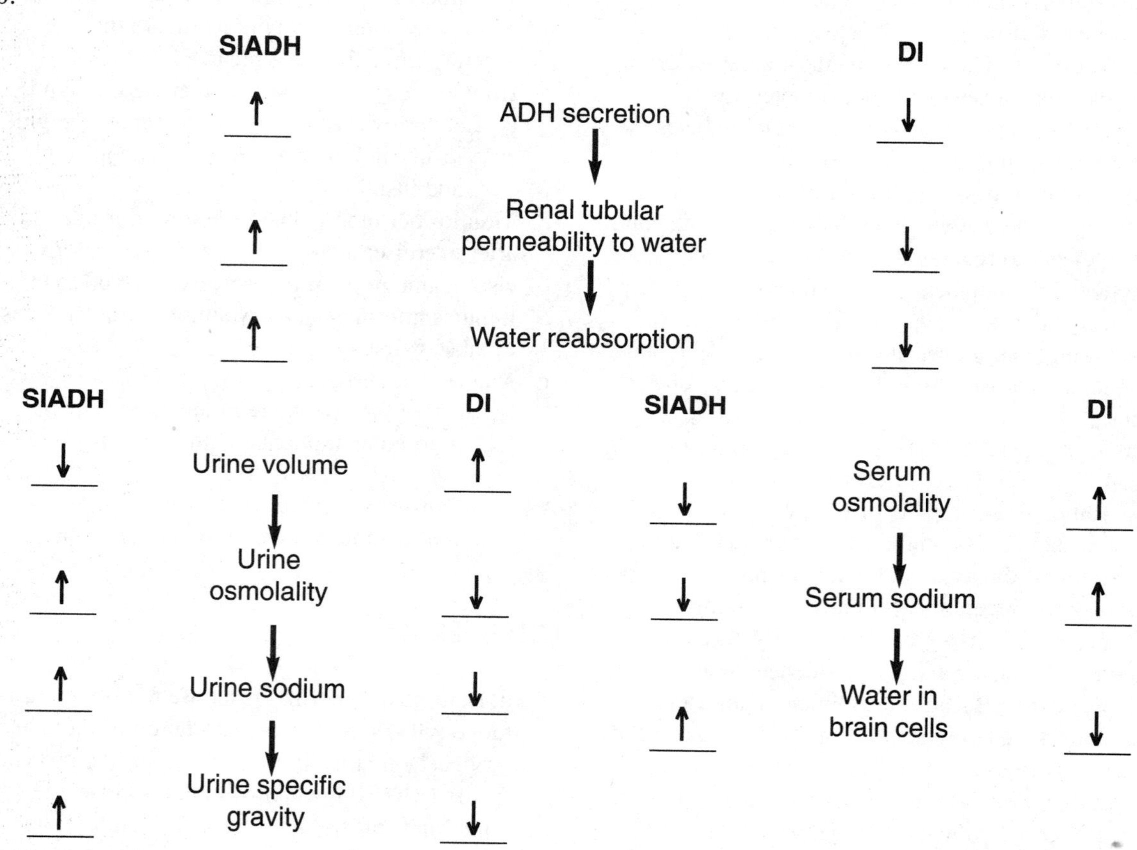

7. a. Rationale: The patient with SIADH has marked dilutional hyponatremia and should be monitored for decreased neurologic function and convulsions every 2 hours. ADH release is reduced by keeping the head of the bed flat to increase left atrial filling pressure, and sodium intake is supplemented because of the hyponatremia and sodium loss caused by diuretics. A reduction in blood pressure indicates a reduction in total fluid volume and is an expected outcome of treatment.
8. b. Rationale: The patient with SIADH has water retention with hyponatremia, decreased urine output, and concentrated urine with high specific gravity. Improvement in the patient's condition is reflected by increased urine output, normalization of serum sodium, and more water in the urine, decreasing the specific gravity.
9. d. Rationale: A patient with diabetes insipidus has a deficiency of ADH with excessive loss of water from the kidney, hypovolemia, hypernatremia, and dilute urine with a low specific gravity. When vasopressin is administered, the symptoms are reversed, with water retention, decreased urinary output that increases urine osmolality, and an increase in blood pressure.
10. c. Rationale: Normal urine specific gravity is 1.003 to 1.030, and urine with a specific gravity of 1.002 is very dilute, indicating that there continues to be excessive loss of water and that treatment of diabetes insipidus is inadequate. Headache, weight gain, and oral intake greater than urinary output are signs of volume excess that occur with overmedication. Nasal irritation and nausea may also indicate overdosage.
11. b. Rationale: In nephrogenic diabetes insipidus, the kidney is unable to respond to ADH, so vasopressin or hormone analogs are not effective. Thiazide diuretics slow the glomerular filtration rate in the kidney and produce a decrease in urine output. Low-sodium diets (<3 gm/day) are also thought to decrease urine output. Fluids are not restricted, because the patient could become easily dehydrated.
12. a. T; b. F, Graves' disease; c.T; d. F, decreased TSH level, 25% to 95%; e. F, inhibit, to be avoided
13. d. Rationale: The antibodies present in Graves' disease that attack thyroid tissue cause hyperplasia of the gland and stimulate TSH receptors on the thyroid and activate the production of thyroid hormones, creating hyperthyroidism. The disease is not directly genetic, but individuals appear to have a genetic susceptibility to become sensitized to develop autoimmune antibodies. Goiter formation from insufficient iodine intake is usually associated with hypothyroidism.
14. c. Rationale: A hyperthyroid crisis results in marked manifestations of hyperthyroidism, with severe tachycardia, heart failure, shock, hyperthermia, agitation, nausea, vomiting, diarrhea, delirium, and coma. Although exophthalmos may be present in the patient with Graves' disease, it is not a significant factor in hyperthyroid crisis. Hoarseness and laryngeal stridor are characteristic of the tetany of hypoparathyroidism, and lethargy progressing to coma is characteristic of myxedema coma, a complication of hypothyroidism.
15. a. 2; b. 4; c. 2; d. 1; e. 1; f. 2; g. 3; h. 1; i. 4; j. 2; k. 4
16. a. Risk for injury: corneal ulceration related to inability to close eyelids
    b. Imbalanced nutrition: less than body requirements related to hypermetabolism
    c. Disturbed body image related to change in body appearance
    d. Activity intolerance related to fatigue and dyspnea
17. a. Rationale: To prevent strain on the suture line postoperatively, the head must be manually supported while turning and moving in bed, but range-of-motion exercises for the head and neck are also taught preoperatively to be gradually implemented after surgery. There is no contraindication for coughing and deep breathing, and they should be carried out postoperatively. Tingling around the lips or fingers is a sign of hypocalcemia, which may occur if the parathyroid glands are inadvertently removed during surgery, and should be reported immediately.
18. a. Needed in case airway obstruction occurs because of vocal cord paralysis from recurrent laryngeal nerve damage during surgery or laryneal stridor occurs with tetany
    b. Needed in case hypocalcemia occurs from parathyroid gland removal or damage during surgery, resulting in tetany
    c. In case of airway obstruction, laryngeal stridor or edema around trachea
19. c. Rationale: When a patient has had a subtotal thyroidectomy, thyroid replacement therapy is not given, because exogenous hormone inhibits pituitary production of TSH and delays or prevents the restoration of thyroid tissue regeneration. However, the patient should avoid goitrogens, foods that inhibit thyroid, such as soybeans, turnips, rutabagas, and peanut skins. Regular exercise stimulates the thyroid gland and is encouraged. Salt water gargles are used for dryness and irritation of the mouth and throat following radioactive iodine therapy.
20. a. 4; b. 3; c. 1; d. 5; e. 6; f. 2

21. d. Rationale: Both Graves' disease and Hashimoto's thyroiditis are autoimmune disorders that eventually destroy the thyroid gland, leading to primary hypothyroidism. Thyroid tumors most often result in hyperthyroidism. Secondary hypothyroidism occurs as a result of pituitary failure, and iatrogenic hypothyroidism results from thyroidectomy or radiation of the thyroid gland.
22. a. R/T depression and altered metabolism; AMB excessive sleeping, no relief of somnolence, altered sleep stages
    b. R/T hypometabolism; AMB weight gain, myxedema facies
    c. R/T diminished cerebral blood flow secondary to decreased cardiac output; AMB forgetfulness, memory loss, personality changes, stupor
    d. R/T decreased metabolic rate and mucin deposits in joints; AMB fatigue, weakness, muscular aches and pains
23. d. Rationale: Hypothyroidism affects the heart in many ways, causing cardiomyopathy, coronary atherosclerosis, bradycardia, pericardial effusions, and weakened cardiac contractility. When thyroid replacement therapy is started, myocardial oxygen consumption is increased, and the resultant oxygen demand may cause angina, cardiac arrhythmias, and heart failure. It is important to monitor patients with compromised cardiac status when starting replacement therapy.
24. b. Rationale: Because of the mental sluggishness, inattentiveness, and memory loss that occur with hypothyroidism, it is important to provide written instructions and repeat information when teaching the patient. Caloric intake can be increased when drug therapy is started, because of an increased metabolic rate, and replacement therapy must be taken for life. Although most patients return to a normal state with treatment, cardiovascular conditions and psychoses may persist.
25. a. 1; b. 2; c. 1; d. 1; e. 1; f. 2; g. 2; h. 1; i. 2; j. 1
26. b. Rationale: A high fluid intake is indicated in hyperparathyroidism to dilute the hypercalcemia and flush the kidneys so that calcium stone formation is reduced. Seizures are not associated with hyperparathyroidism, but impending tetany of hypoparathyroidism can be noted with Trousseau's phenomenon and Chvostek's sign. The patient with hyperparathyroidism is at risk for pathologic fractures due to decreased bone density, but mobility is encouraged to promote bone calcification.
27. b. Rationale: Rebreathing in a paper bag promotes carbon dioxide retention in the blood, which lowers pH and creates an acidosis. An acidemia enhances the solubility and ionization of calcium, increasing the proportion of total body calcium available in physiologically active form and relieving the symptoms of hypocalcemia. Saline promotes calcium excretion, as does furosemide. Phosphate levels in the blood are reciprocal to calcium, and an increase in phosphate promotes calcium excretion.
28. c. Rationale: The hypocalcemia that results from parathyroid hormone deficiency is controlled with calcium and vitamin D supplementation and possibly oral phosphate binders. Replacement with PTH is not used, because of antibody formation to PTH, the need for parenteral administration, and cost. Milk products, although good sources of calcium, also have high levels of phosphate, which reduce calcium absorption. Whole grains and foods containing oxalic acid also impair calcium absorption.
29. a. Rationale: The effects of glucocorticoid excess include weight gain from accumulation and redistribution of adipose tissue, sodium and water retention, glucose intolerance, protein wasting, loss of bone structure, loss of collagen, and capillary fragility. Clinical manifestations of corticosteroid deficiency include hypotension, dehydration, weight loss, and hyperpigmentation of the skin.
30. c. Rationale: Electrolyte changes that occur in Cushing syndrome include sodium retention and potassium excretion by the kidney, resulting in a hypokalemia, which may lead to cardiac arrhythmias or arrest. Hypotension, hypoglycemia, and decreased cardiac strength and output are characteristic of adrenal insufficiency.
31. c. Rationale: Although the patient with Cushing syndrome has excess corticosteroids, removal of the glands and the stress of surgery require that high doses of cortisone be administered postoperatively for several days. The nurse should monitor the patient postoperatively to detect whether large amounts of hormones were released during surgical manipulation and to ensure that healing is satisfactory.
32. c. Rationale: Vomiting and diarrhea are early indicators of addisonian crisis, and fever indicates an infection, which is causing additional stress for the patient. Treatment of a crisis requires immediate glucocorticoid replacement, and IV hydrocortisone, fluids, sodium, and glucose are necessary for 24 hours. Addison's disease is a primary insufficiency of the adrenal gland, and ACTH is not effective, nor would vasopressors be effective with the fluid deficiency of Addison's. Potassium levels are increased in Addison's disease, and KCl would be contraindicated.

33. a. Rationale: Confusion, irritability, disorientation, or depression is often present in the patient with Addison's disease, and a positive response to therapy would be indicated by a return to alertness and orientation. Other indications of response to therapy would be a decreased urinary output, decreased serum potassium, and increased serum sodium and glucose. The patient with Addison's would be very dehydrated and volume-depleted and would not have pulmonary edema.
34. b. Rationale: A weight reduction in the patient with Addison's disease may indicate a fluid loss and a dose of replacement therapy that is too low, rather than too high. Patients with Addison's disease are taught to take two to three times their usual dose of steroids if they become ill, have teeth extracted, or engage in rigorous physical activity and should always have injectable hydrocortisone available if oral doses cannot be taken. Because vomiting and diarrhea are early signs of crisis and because fluid and electrolytes must be replaced, patients should notify their physician if these symptoms occur.
35. a. Sodium and fluid retention because of mineralocorticoid effect; b. GI irritation with increase in secretion of pepsin and hydrochloric acid; c. Corticosteroid-induced osteoporosis; d. Glucose intolerance with hyperglycemia; e. Hypokalemia because of mineralocorticoid effect; f. Inhibition of inflammation and immune response; may reactivate latent TB
36. c. Rationale: Taking corticosteroids on an alternate-day schedule for pharmacologic purposes is less likely to suppress ACTH production from the pituitary and prevent adrenal atrophy. Normal adrenal hormone balance is not maintained during glucocorticoid therapy, because excessive exogenous hormone is used.
37. a. Rationale: Hyperaldosteronism is an excess of aldosterone, which is manifested by sodium and water retention and potassium excretion. Furosemide is a potassium-wasting diuretic that would increase the potassium deficiency. Aminoglutethimide blocks aldosterone synthesis; amiloride is a potassium-sparing diuretic; and spironolactone blocks mineralocorticoid receptors in the kidney, increasing excretion of sodium and water and retention of potassium.
38. b. Rationale: A pheochromocytoma is a catecholamine-producing tumor of the adrenal medulla, which may cause severe, episodic hypertension; severe, pounding headache; and profuse sweating. Monitoring for a dangerously high blood pressure before surgery is critical, as is monitoring for blood pressure fluctuations during medical and surgical treatment.

Case Study

1. All of the blood tests are altered because of the effect of glucocorticoids:
   - Elevated glucose—increased gluconeogenesis by liver and induced insulin resistance
   - Elevated WBC—granulocytosis
   - Decreased lymphocytes—lymphocytopenia
   - Increased RBC—polycythemia
   - Decreased K—increased mineralocorticoid effect causing sodium retention and potassium excretion
2. There are several causes of Cushing syndrome:
   - ACTH-secreting pituitary tumor is the most common cause of endogenous Cushing syndrome
   - Adrenal tumors
   - Ectopic ACTH production by tumors outside the hypothalamic-pituitary-adrenal axis
   - The pathophysiology of Cushing syndrome reflects an excess of normal glucocorticoid and mineralocorticoid activity, an exaggeration of normal functions.
3. ACTH levels: high or normal levels of ACTH indicate ACTH-dependent Cushing or a tumor of the pituitary gland; low or undetectable levels of ACTH indicate an adrenal or ectopic cause.
4. Pituitary cause—transsphenoidal hypophysectomy; adrenal cause—adrenalectomy; ectopic cause—removal if possible
5. A medical adrenalectomy involves treatment with mitotane (Lysodren), a drug that suppresses cortisol production, alters peripheral metabolism of steroids, and decreases plasma and urine steroid levels by actually killing adrenocortical cells.
6. Major nursing responsibilities are included in the following list:
   Assessment of signs and symptoms of hormone toxicity:
   - Vital signs q4hr
   - Daily weights
   - Glucose monitoring
   - Changes in mental status

   Assessment for complications:
   - Signs and symptoms of infection, such as pain or purulent drainage, because fever and inflammation may be minimal or absent
   - Signs and symptoms of thromboembolic phenomena, such as chest pain, dyspnea, tachypnea
   - Signs and symptoms of bone pain or limitations in motion, indicating pathologic fractures
   - Signs and symptoms of nephrolithiasis from increased calcium excretion

Preoperative preparation:
- Instruction about exercises, coughing, and deep breathing
- Explanations about early monitoring for circulatory instability
- Explanations about hormone replacement

7. *Nursing diagnoses:*
   - Risk for infection related to suppression of inflammation and immune function
   - Risk for injury related to osteoporosis
   - Risk for impaired skin integrity related to edema and altered skin fragility
   - Disturbed body image related to altered physical appearance

   Collaborative problems:
   Potential complications: thromboembolism; cardiac arrhythmias; pathologic fractures; nephrolithiasis; diabetes mellitus; hypertensive crisis

CHAPTER 49

1. a. ureter; b. urinary bladder; c. ductus deferens; d. corpus cavernosum; e. corpus spongiosum; f. urethra; g. penis; h. glans; i. scrotum; j. testis; k. epididymis; l. anus; m. Cowper's gland; n. rectum; o. prostate gland; p. ejaculatory duct; q. seminal vesicle; r. ureter; s. posterior cul-de-sac; t. cervix; u. fornix of vagina; v. anus; w. vagina; x. labia majora; y. labia minora; z. urethra; aa. clitoris; ab. symphysis pubis; ac. urinary bladder; ad. anterior cul-de-sac; ae. fundus of uterus; af. round ligament; ag. body (corpus) of uterus; ah. fallopian tube
2. a. prepuce; b. labia minora; c. vagina; d. vestibule; e. perineum; f. anus; g. labia majora; h. urethra; i. clitoris; j. mons pubis; k. pectoralis major muscle; l. alveoli; m. areola; n. nipple
3. a. 3; b. 6; c. 2; d. 7; e. 1; f. 8; g. 4; h. 5
4. a. 4; b. 8; c. 6; d. 7; e. 3; f. 2; g. 1; h. 5
5. a. T; b. F, fallopian tube; c. F, squamocolumnar junction; d. T; e. F, 1 year
6. a. 2; b. 8; c. 6; d. 1; e. 5; f. 7; g. 4; h. 3; i. 6; j. 8; k. 1; l. 6; m. 5; n. 2
7. a. 2; b. 1; c. 2; d. 1; e. 3; f. 1; g. 1; h. 1
8. a. Rationale: Decreased estrogen levels during menopause lead to atrophy of the vaginal epithelium with vaginal dryness, which may cause dyspareunia. Menopause does cause such changes as atrophy of secondary sex characteristics, vasomotor instability, and increased incidence of osteoporosis, but sexual response is often increased when the threat of pregnancy is eliminated. The use of hormone replacement therapy is controversial, and other methods can be used to reduce the uncomfortable effects of menopause.
9. b. Rationale: Age-related changes in sexual function in males include a need for increased stimulation for an erection, decreased need to ejaculate, and a possible decreased response to sexual stimuli. There is a decreased ability to attain an erection, but it is not related to prostatic changes. A negative social attitude toward sexuality in older adults also affects the sexual activity of people in this age group.
10. c. Rationale: Information related to menstrual history is usually nonthreatening and is a good place to begin an interview about reproductive function before asking about more sensitive issues, such as sexual practices, drugs that affect sexual function, or sexually transmitted diseases.
11. a. Potential congenital anomalies if rubella occurs during first trimester of pregnancy
    b. Increased sterility in young men with mumps, because of testicular atrophy secondary to orchitis
    c. Impotence and retrograde ejaculation in male diabetics, in addition to erectile problems from neuropathies
    d. Many may cause impotence in men
12. a. Lack of Pap smears, breast self-examination, prostate examinations, or testicular self-examination; smoking, alcohol, and caffeine use; family history of breast disease and reproductive cancers
    b. History of anorexia nervosa, decreased calcium intake
    c. Urge and stress incontinence; difficulty in urinating in males; bladder infections
    d. Fatigue and activity intolerance related to menorrhagia
    e. Sleep interruption related to hot flashes and sweating; nocturia
    f. Pelvic pain; dyspareunia
    g. Changes in self-concept related to sexuality and aging
    h. Occupational hazards related to sexual functioning and reproductive capacity; dysfunctional roles and relationships with others
    i. Recent changes in sexual practices; dissatisfaction with sexual expression; reproductive problems that affect sexual satisfactions; changes in menstrual patterns; multiple sexual partners; no protection against sexually transmitted diseases
    j. STD effect on sex partners; stress of sexual problems; infertility
    k. Conflict between value system and treatment; abortion issues; infertility issues
13. d. Rationale: The prostate is palpated through the wall of the rectum with a digital rectal exam. Inguinal hernias are detected by palpating the

inguinal ring while the patient bears down, and scrotal palpation is done to detect testicular masses or tumors. No specific conditions are indicated by enlargement at the base of the penis.

14. a. Rationale: A decrease in the size of the penis is a normal finding in the older male. Loss of pubic hair is not normal, nor is any enlargement of the breasts. The normally darker color of the scrotum does not change with aging.
15. d. Rationale: The presence of dimpling or retractions can be observed by having the patient put her arms at her sides and over her head, lean forward, and press the hands on the hips. Lying down with the arm over the head flattens the breast for better palpation for lumps or thickness that can be felt with systematic palpation. Compressing the nipple is done to assess for drainage or galactorrhea.
16. d. Rationale: A diamond pubic hair distribution is characteristic of males and is abnormal in females. A small amount of clear vaginal discharge is normal in females, as are episiotomy scars in a woman who has had children. Skene's ducts should be nonpalpable.
17. b. Rationale: Pap smears are more accurate if they are performed at midcycle or during the secretory phase of the menstrual cycle because there is a greater likelihood that abnormal cells will be detected at this time. Douching should not be done for 24 hours before the examination, but sexual intercourse is not contraindicated.
18. a. 5; b. 4; c. 9; d. 7; e. 3; f. 1; g. 2; h. 8; i. 6
19. b. Rationale: The risk for bleeding is increased following a D&C because the endometrial lining is scraped and injury to the uterus may occur. The nurse should closely assess the amount of bleeding with frequent pad checks the first 24 hours. Infection following D&C is uncommon, and the urinary system is not affected.
20. a. Rationale: A culdoscopy involves insertion of an endoscope through an incision made through the posterior fornix of the cul-de-sac and requires surgical anesthesia, as does removal of cervical tissue during a conization. A D&C, laparoscopy, and breast biopsy are also operative procedures requiring surgical anesthesia, but colposcopy, contrast mammography, and endometrial biopsies do not require surgical anesthesia.
21. a. Rationale: A Huhner test (or Sims-Huhner) involves examination of a mucus sample of the cervix within 2 to 8 hours after intercourse to determine the number and mobility of sperm in the cervical mucus. A semen analysis is a simple examination of semen for the number, mobility, and structure of sperm. An endometrial biopsy provides a sample of endometrium to evaluate its changes under the influence of progesterone, and a hysterosalpingogram is a contrast x-ray of the uterine cavity and fallopian tubes.

CHAPTER 50

1. d. Rationale: The importance of performing breast self-examination (BSE) arises from the fact that early detection and treatment of breast cancer are the most significant factors in survival rates, and between BSE and regular mammography, most palpable and nonpalpable masses can be identified early enough for successful treatment. Most palpable breast lesions are discovered by women themselves, which is an important tool in early detection, but it must be followed by treatment. The role of BSE in reducing mortality from breast cancer in women under the age of 50 is controversial.
2. a. Monthly BSE over the age of 20; b. CBE every 3 years between the ages of 20 and 39; every year thereafter; c. Annual screening mammogram every year starting at the age of 40
3. c. Rationale: One of the major reasons women do not examine their breasts regularly is because of a lack of confidence in BSE skill, and a teaching program should include allowing time for women to use models to identify problems and perform a return demonstration of the examination on themselves. Fear and denial often interfere with BSE even when women know the perceived risk for cancer is high, know the statistics, and know they should seek medical care if an abnormality is detected.
4. d. Rationale: A definitive diagnosis of breast cancer can be made only by a histologic examination of biopsied tissue. A stereotactic core biopsy is as reliable as an open surgical biopsy and has the advantages of decreased length of time for the procedure and recovery and reduced cost. A limitation of fine-needle aspiration is that if negative results are found, more definite biopsy procedures are required.
5. d. Rationale: Most breast lesions are benign, and many mobile cystic lesions change in response to the menstrual cycle, while most malignant tumors do not. Caffeine has been associated with fibrocystic changes in some women, but research has not established caffeine as a cause of breast pain or cysts. Questions regarding a patient's last mammogram or family history are not closely related to the nurse's findings.
6. b. Rationale: Fibrocystic changes make breasts difficult to examine because of fibrotic changes and multiple lumps. A woman with this condition should be familiar with the characteristic changes

in her breasts and monitor them closely for new lumps that do not respond in a cyclic manner over 1 to 2 weeks. Estrogen antagonizes the condition, and fibrocystic changes are not precancerous.

7. a. 6; b. 3; c. 1; d. 2; e. 7; f. 5; g. 4; h. 6; i. 2; j. 4; k. 7; l. 3; m. 1
8. b. Rationale: After the age of 60, the incidence of breast cancer increases dramatically, and advanced age is the highest risk factor for females. Obesity is a contributing factor for breast cancer, but fibrocystic breast changes are neither a precursor of cancer nor a known risk factor for cancer. Only about 5% to 10% of women with breast cancer may have a BRCA1 or 2 gene, specific genetic abnormalities that contribute to the development of breast cancer.
9. b. Rationale: On palpation, malignant lesions are characteristically hard, irregularly shaped, poorly delineated, nontender, and nonmobile, and the most common site is the upper outer quadrant of the breast. A fibroademona is firm, defined, and mobile, while fibrocystic lesions are usually large, tender, moveable masses found throughout the breast tissue. A painful, immobile mass under a reddened area of skin is most typical of a local abscess.
10. a. Rationale: Axillary lymph node status is one of the most important prognostic factors in primary breast cancer, and the more nodes that are involved, the higher the risk for relapse or metastasis. Aneuploid DNA tumor content indicates that cells have abnormally high or low DNA content in comparison with normal cells and is associated with tumor aggressiveness. Cells in S-phase have a higher risk for recurrence and can produce earlier cancer death. Hormone receptor-negative tumors are usually poorly differentiated histologically, frequently recur, and usually unresponsive to hormonal therapy.
11. d. Rationale: Even with negative axillary lymph nodes, recurrence occurs in 30% to 35% of patients with breast cancer, illustrating that although most metastases occur through the lymphatic chains, metastasis can occur without invading the axillary nodes. Recurrence may be local or regional, with distant metastases most commonly to bone, lung, brain, and liver.
12. b. Rationale: Either treatment choice is indicated for women with early-stage breast cancer because the 10-year survival rate with lumpectomy with radiation is about the same as that with modified radical mastectomy. Each procedure has advantages and disadvantages that the patient must consider in making an informed choice, and the nurse should make that information available to the patient to assist in decision making.
13. d. Rationale: Axillary lymph node dissection is almost always performed regardless of the treatment option selected, because of its value in prognosis and decision making regarding adjuvant therapy. A lumpectomy, or breast conservation surgery, is followed by radiation therapy to the entire breast, and the use of chemotherapy or hormone therapy depends on the characteristics of the tumor and evidence of metastases.
14. a. Adjunct to surgery; b. Palliative; c. High-dose brachytherapy; d. Primary; e. Adjunct to surgery; f. High-dose brachytherapy
15. d. Rationale: Because micrometastases have probably occurred even in stage I disease, making breast cancer a systemic disease at the time of diagnosis, and because premenopausal women, especially with hormone receptor-negative tumors, are known to be at higher risk for recurrent or metastatic disease, systemic chemotherapy is recommended even when no evidence of node involvement is found.
16. c. Rationale: Tamoxifen is an antiestrogen agent that blocks the estrogen-receptor sites of malignant cells and is the usual first choice of treatment in postmenopausal women with hormone receptor-positive tumors, with or without nodal involvement. Tamoxifen reduces the risk for recurrent breast cancer and also that for new primary tumors. The side effects of the drug are minimal and are those commonly associated with decreased estrogen.
17. c. Rationale: As early as in the recovery room following a modified radical mastectomy, the patient should start flexing and extending the fingers and wrist of the affected arm with daily increases in activity. Postoperative mastectomy exercises, such as hair care, wall climbing with the fingers, and shoulder rotation and extension, are instituted gradually to prevent disruption of the wound.
18. b. Rationale: Removal of the axillary lymph nodes impairs lymph drainage from the affected arm and predisposes the patient to infection of the arm. The arm must be protected from even minor trauma, and blood pressure, venipunctures, and injections should not be done on the arm. The arm should never be dependent, even during sleep, and should be elevated to promote lymph drainage.
19. c. Rationale: The Reach to Recovery program consists of volunteers who are all women who have had breast cancer and can answer questions about what to expect at home, how to tell people about the surgery, and what prosthetic devices are available. It is a valuable resource for patients who have breast cancer and should be used if

available in the community. If a volunteer is not available, the nurse is responsible for assisting the patient in the same manner. Although the nurse should stress the importance of wearing a prosthesis, a permanent prosthesis cannot be used until healing is complete and inflammation is resolved.

20. b. Rationale: It is most important for the patient planning a mammoplasty that she have a realistic idea about what the surgery can accomplish and about possible complications. Currently surgery cannot restore nipple sensation or erectility, and the breast will not fully resemble its premastectomy appearance, but the outcome is usually more acceptable than the mastectomy scar. The woman's motives for breast reconstruction should not be questioned. There have been allegations of immune-related diseases associated with the use of silicone gel implants only, and these implants are currently off the market while FDA-mandated research on the effects of the implants is being conducted.
21. a. Rationale: When an expander is used to stretch the skin and muscle at the mastectomy site, the expander is gradually increased in size by weekly injections of water or saline until the site is large enough to hold an implant. The placement of the expander can be at the time of mastectomy or at a later date. A musculocutaneous flap procedure is a type of reconstruction using the patient's own tissue. The nipple of the affected breast is removed at mastectomy, and a new nipple can be reconstructed after breast reconstruction from various normal tissues.

Case Study

1. It is likely that micrometastases to distant sites have occurred at the time of the diagnosis of breast cancer even in stage I disease and almost certainly in stage III disease, supporting indications for systemic treatment of the cancer following local surgical treatment. Breast cancer is one of the solid tumors that is most responsive to chemotherapy, and destruction or control of tumor cells that have spread to distant sites is the goal of systemic chemotherapy.
2. a. cyclophosphamide [C]:
   alkylating agent, cell-cycle nonspecfic
   Side effects: myelosuppression, nausea and vomiting, alopecia, hemorrhagic cystitis

   b. doxorubicin:
   antitumor antibiotic, cell-cycle nonspecfic
   Side effects: myelosuppression, mucositis, nausea and vomiting, alopecia, cardiotoxicity

   c. 5-fluorouracil:
   antimetabolite, cell-cycle specific
   Side effects: myelosuppression, mucositis, nausea and vomiting, alopecia, photosensitivity
3. Teach Mrs. T. to perform the following activities as necessary:

   Myelosuppression:
   - Monitor her temperature every day.
   - Report any chilling; sore throat; cough; or rectal, urinary, or chest pain.
   - Keep the venous access catheter site clean and dry.
   - Avoid crowds and anyone with communicable diseases.
   - Wash her hands after toileting and before eating.
   - Report any bleeding, serious bruising, or persistent headaches.
   - Avoid using aspirin products.
   - Examine her mouth daily for blood-filled lesions.
   - Guard against bumping and other injury that may cause bleeding.

   Mucositis:
   - Examine her mouth daily for bleeding, redness, or ulcers.
   - Use a mouthwash of baking soda or salt water every 2 hours as needed.
   - Use a soft-bristled toothbrush or sponge-tipped applicators for oral care.
   - Avoid hot, spicy, acidic foods and alcohol and tobacco.
   - Drink water frequently during the day.

   Nausea and vomiting:
   - Use antiemetic medications as prescribed.
   - Use small frequent meals that include bland, lukewarm, high-calorie, high-protein foods, and use liquid nutritional supplements if necessary.
   - Avoid strong odors and sights that increase nausea.
   - Eat and drink slowly.
   - Use gum, tea, or any food that stimulates salivation without causing nausea.

   Alopecia:
   - Select a wig and begin to wear it before hair loss begins.
   - Wear a scarf or turban to conceal hair loss.
   - Use a mild, protein-based shampoo and hair conditioner every 4 to 7 days to avoid drying remaining hair.
   - Avoid excessive shampooing, brushing, and combing of hair.
   - Avoid use of curling irons, curlers, blow dryers, and hair spray.

4. An estrogen receptor-positive tumor is estrogen-dependent, and estrogen can promote growth of these breast cancer cells. Hormone receptor-positive cells usually are well differentiated, have low proliferative indices, and DNA content equal to that of normal cells. Drugs, such as tamoxifen, that block the estrogen receptor site of malignant cells can cause tumor regression and are widely used to treat recurrent or metastatic cancer that is estrogen-dependent.
5. The nurse should:
   - assist the patient to develop a positive but realistic attitude.
   - help her identify sources of support and strength to her.
   - encourage her to verbalize her guilt and anger and fears about her diagnosis and the impact it is having on her life.
   - promote open communication between the patient and her husband.
   - provide accurate and complete answers to her questions about her disease.
   - offer information about community resources and local support groups.
6. Fear, denial, and embarrassment are common reasons that women do not perform BSE or have a mammogram, and a lack of practice and skill at breast examination undermines their confidence in performing the exam. Denial was probably a big factor for Mrs. T. in view of the value of her breasts in her relationship with her husband.
7. Teach Mrs. T. that she will need follow-up for the rest of her life at regular intervals. She should expect to have a professional examination every 3 months for 2 years, every 6 months for the next 3 years, and then annually thereafter. She should be taught to perform breast self-examination of both breasts every month and informed that recurrence of breast cancer is most likely to happen.
8. *Nursing diagnoses:*
   - Ineffective therapeutic regimen management related to lack of compliance and information regarding breast cancer surveillance
   - Ineffective coping related to reported feelings of guilt and perceived expectations of husband
   - Impaired physical mobility related to decreased arm and shoulder mobility

   Collaborative problems:

   Potential complications: vascular access catheter displacement or infection; hyperuricemia; bleeding; septicemia; tumor recurrence

CHAPTER 51

1. a. Rationale: Although there are many factors that relate to the current STD rates, one major factor is the high use of oral contraceptives, long-acting parenteral contraceptives, and IUDs for contraception. The condom, both male and female, provides a barrier to microorganisms causing STDs and is the only contraceptive device that is prophylactic in regard to STDs. Oral contraceptives provide a more favorable environment for growth of organisms that cause STDs, and while IUDs and parenteral long-acting contraceptives, such as Norplant and Depo-Provera, are not known to increase risk for STDs, they do not provide protection against the diseases.
2. a. 3; b. 4; c. 1; d. 5; e. 2
3. d. Rationale: An established diagnosis of gonorrhea is treated with both ceftriaxone and doxycycline or tetracycline—ceftriaxone for resistant strains of *N. gonorrhoeae* and doxycycline because of the high frequency of chlamydial infections coexisting with gonorrhea. Gram-stain smears are not useful in diagnosing gonorrhea in women, because the female GU tract normally harbors a large number of organisms that resemble *N. gonorrhoeae*, and cultures must be performed to diagnose the disease in women. Penicillin G is used to treat syphilis, and although gonorrhea may lead to PID, its diagnosis would not necessarily indicate the patient had PID.
4. a. Rationale: Upward extension of gonorrhea or chlamydia commonly causes salpingitis and pelvic inflammatory disease, which can cause adhesions and fibrous scarring, leading to tubal abnormalities and tubal pregnancies and infertility. Disseminated gonococcal infection is rare, and endocarditis and aneurysms are associated with syphilis.
5. a. S; b. T; c. T; d. P; e. T; f. S; g. L; h. T; i. S; j. T
6. c. Rationale: Many other diseases or conditions may cause false-positive tests on nontreponemal VDRL or RPR tests, and additional testing is needed before a diagnosis is confirmed or treatment administered. Positive results on these tests should be confirmed by specific treponemal tests, such as the FTA-ABS test or the MHA test, to rule out other causes. Analysis of CSF is used to diagnose asymptomatic neurosyphilis.
7. d. Rationale: The risk factors of drug abuse and sexual promiscuity are found in patients with both syphilis and HIV infection, and persons at highest risk for acquiring syphilis are also at high risk for acquiring HIV. Syphilitic lesions on the genitals enhance HIV transmission. Also, HIV-

infected patients with syphilis appear to be at greatest risk for CNS involvement and may require more intensive treatment with penicillin to prevent this HIV complication.

8. b. Rationale: Although chlamydial infections may cause cervicitis and urethritis in women, it is more common for symptoms to be absent or minor in most infected women. The absence of symptoms necessitates screening of asymptomatic individuals at risk with nonculture tests, such as direct fluorescent antibody (DFA), or enzyme immunoassay (EIA) tests to identify and treat the disease.
9. b. Rationale: Notification and treatment of sex partners are necessary to prevent recurrence and the ping-pong effect of passing STDs between partners. Tetracycline is prescribed qid for 7 to 10 days, and although alcohol may cause more urinary irritation in the patient with chlamydia, it will not interfere with treatment.
10. c. Rationale: Gonorrhea and chlamydia have very similar symptoms in males, and chlamydial infections in men are diagnosed by excluding gonorrhea. When Gram-stain smears and cultures for *N. gonorrhoeae* are negative, a diagnosis of NGU-*Chlamydia* infection is made.
11. a. F, oral or genital lesions; b. T; c. F, decrease recurrences; d. F, sexual contact should be avoided; e. T
12. d. Rationale: The human papillomavirus is responsible for causing genital warts, which manifest as discrete single or multiple white to gray warts that may coalesce to form large cauliflower like masses on the vulva, vagina, cervix, and perianal area. Purulent vaginal discharge is associated with gonorrhea or chlamydia, painful perineal vesicles and ulcerations are characteristic of genital herpes, and a chancre of syphilis is a painless indurated lesion on the vulva, vagina, lips, or mouth.
13. a. Rationale: There is a strong association of genital warts to the development of dysplasia and neoplasia of the genital tract, especially when lesions involve the cervix, introitus, and perianal and intraanal mucosa of women or the penis and perianal and anal mucosa of men. Regular Pap smears in women are critical in detecting early malignancies of the cervix. Oral acyclovir is used to treat HSV-2, but topical use has no value in treating sexually transmitted viral diseases. Sexual partners of patients with HPV should be examined and treated, but because treatment does not destroy the virus, condoms should always be used during sexual activity. Genital warts often grow more rapidly during pregnancy, but pregnancy is not contraindicated.
14. c. Rationale: Although gonorrhea and syphilis rank first and third, respectively, as the most common reportable communicable diseases in the United States, chlamydial infections are not required to be reported and are the most prevalent bacterial STD in the United States today, with an estimated 3 million cases occurring annually. Because genital warts infection also is not a reportable disease in most states, its incidence is difficult to determine, but it is estimated that 20 million people are currently infected with HPV.
15. a. Treatment with parenteral penicillin will cure both the mother and fetus; b. Erythromycin or silver nitrate required to the eyes of all newborns; c. C-section if mother has active lesions; d. Erythromycin treatment during pregnancy; cesarean section if active at labor; e. May be spread to newborn by direct contact; cesarean section not routine unless massive warts block the birth canal
16. a. Rationale: Although sexual abstinence is the most certain method of avoiding all sexually transmitted diseases, it is not usually a feasible alternative, and a condom with spermicidal jelly is the next best protection. STDs may be spread with oral-anal intercourse. Conscientious hand washing and voiding after intercourse are positive hygienic measures that will help prevent secondary infections but will not prevent STDs.
17. a. Rationale: STDs that can be treated with a single dose or short course of antibiotic therapy often lead to a casual attitude about the outcome of the disease, which leads to noncompliance with instructions and delays in treatment. This is particularly true of diseases that initially show few distressing or uncomfortable symptoms, such as syphilis.

Case Study

1. The nurse should tell Jack that he must tell his fiancée the truth about the sexual encounter and that it is most important for her to be evaluated for the disease. She may have the disease without symptoms, yet be at risk for development of PID and infertility as a result of the gonorrhea. The nurse may offer a counseling referral, if necessary, for them to work through problems in their relationship.
2. Females often do not have any symptoms, but she could have a vaginal discharge, dysuria, urinary frequency, or changes in her menstrual patterns.
3. In Jack, diagnosis can be confirmed by a positive Gram's-stain smear of urethral drainage; in Ann, a positive culture of cervical secretions or of the urethra, anus, or oropharynx is necessary for confirmation of diagnosis.

4. Support and counseling may be needed from the nurse, and the couple should be assisted to verbalize their feelings and concerns. Active listening with a nonjudgmental attitude is important. Referral for professional counseling may be indicated.
5. Ceftriaxone IM in a single dose and doxycycline bid or tetracycline qid for 7 to 10 days is the recommended treatment for gonorrhea with a possible concurrent chlamydial infection. Because chlamydial infections are closely associated with gonococcal infections, both infections are usually treated concurrently even without diagnostic evidence.
6. Men: prostatitis, urethral strictures, and sterility from orchitis or epididymitis
   Women: PID, Bartholin's abscess, ectopic pregnancy, infertility from tubal stricture
   Both men and women may develop disseminated gonococcal infection.
7. *Nursing diagnoses:*
   - Anxiety related to impact of condition on relationships and disease outcomes
   - Disturbed body image related to symptoms associated with gonorrhea
   - Risk for infection related to failure to practice precautionary measures

   Collaborative problems:
   Potential complication: infertility

CHAPTER 52

1. a. Rationale: The initial visit of a couple seeking assistance with infertility includes a history and physical for both partners, testing for medical problems and STDs, a cervical Pap smear, possible semen analysis, and instruction for at-home ovulation testing. A discussion of possible future testing options and cost is also done. If the couple decides to continue with treatment, further visits will include more intensive evaluation, including postcoital testing, a hysterosalpingogram, pelvic ultrasound, and midluteal progesterone/prolactin levels.
2. b. Rationale: To determine the time of ovulation by body temperature, the woman must take and graph her temperature on awakening before any activity, noting any illness or variation in normal patterns. The increase in estrogen as ovulation approaches causes a temperature drop. When ovulation occurs, progesterone is produced and causes a sharp rise in temperature. Using basal body temperature to dictate the timing of sexual intercourse for conception is stressful and may decrease sexual performance and also the possibility of pregnancy. Anovulation can be detected, but it is primarily treated with hormone agents.
3. d. Rationale: Infertility and treatment of infertility frequently result in great emotional and financial stress for a couple, and participation in a support group for infertile couples, as well as individual therapy, are recommended. Many infertile couples cannot be successfully treated, and the cause of infertility can be female, male, or combined. Although the cost of treatment of infertility can be high, expenses should be realistically explained at each step of the treatment so that couples can make realistic decisions and plans.
4. c. Rationale: In the presence of a confirmed pregnancy, uterine cramping with vaginal bleeding is the most important sign of spontaneous abortion. Other conditions causing vaginal bleeding, such as an incompetent cervix, do not usually cause cramping. There is no evidence that any medical treatment improves the outcome for spontaneous abortion. Blood loss can be significant, and the loss of the pregnancy may cause long-term grieving. D&C is usually performed after the abortion to minimize blood loss and reduce the chance of infection.
5. d. Rationale: Mifepristone (RU 486) works by blocking progesterone, the hormone that supports pregnancy, and is effective within the first 49 days of pregnancy. Methotrexate is a chemotherapeutic agent that is toxic to trophoblastic tissue. Both of these agents are administered with misoprostol (Cytotec) to produce uterine contractions that expel the products of conception.
6. d. Rationale: PMS is diagnosed when other possible causes for symptoms have been eliminated and is based on a symptom diary that indicates the same symptoms during the luteal phase for two or three consecutive menstrual cycles. Oral contraceptives may be used to control the symptoms of PMS by suppressing ovulation, and although progesterone may also relieve the symptoms of PMS, its effectiveness is not associated with the diagnosis of PMS. There are no laboratory findings that account for the premenstrual symptoms.
7. c. Rationale: Limitation of salt, refined sugar, and caffeine in the diet has been shown to decrease the PMS symptoms of abdominal bloating, increased appetite, and irritability. Exercise is encouraged because it increases release of endorphins, elevating mood, and also has a tranquilizing effect on muscular tension. Estrogen is not used during the luteal phase, but progesterone may be tried. Vitamin B6 and foods high in tryptophan may promote serotonin production, which improves symptoms.
8. c. Rationale: The release of excess prostaglandin F_2 alpha (PGF_2 alpha) from the endometrium at the time of menstruation or increased sensitivity

to the prostaglandin is responsible for symptoms of primary dysmenorrhea, and drugs that inhibit prostaglandin production and release, such as NSAIDs, are effective in many patients with primary dysmenorrhea. Oral contraceptives are also used for primary dysmenorrhea to suppress ovulation and the associated production of prostaglandins.

9. a. 3; b. 1; c. 3; d. 4; e. 2; f. 4; g. 1
10. c. Rationale: When ovulation does not occur, estrogen continues to be unopposed by progesterone, and excessive build-up of the endometrium occurs. To prevent the risk of endometrial cancer by the build-up of the endometrium or to prevent menorrhagia from an unstable endometrium, progesterone or birth control pills are prescribed to ensure that the patient's endometrial lining will be shed at least four to six times a year. Balloon therapy to treat menorrhagia is contraindicated in women desiring future fertility.
11. b. Rationale: Ectopic pregnancy is a life-threatening condition, and if the fallopian tube ruptures, profuse bleeding can lead to hypovolemic shock. All of the interventions are indicated, but the priority should be monitoring the vital signs and pain for evidence of bleeding.
12. a. F, postmenopausal; b. F, estrogen (FSH levels rise); c. T; d. T; e. T
13. *Benefits:*
    - Control of vasomotor symptoms
    - Relief of atrophic vaginal changes
    - Decreased atrophic changes of urinary system (stress, urge incontinence)
    - Decreased osteoporosis

    Risks:
    - Endometrial cancer
    - Breast cancer
    - Cardiovascular disease (myocardial infarction, stroke)
    - Hyperlipidemia
14. d. Rationale: Regular aerobic, weight-bearing exercises will help prevent both osteoporosis and cardiovascular disease and should be maintained by all postmenopausal women, regardless of hormone therapy status. The diet should be high in complex carbohydrates and vitamin B complex. Calcium intake for women not using HRT should be 1500 mg daily with adequate vitamin D. Vitamin E may be used to decrease the intensity of hot flashes, but this is not a serious menopausal symptom.
15. c. Rationale: Phytoestrogens from plant sources have been shown to be effective in reducing menopausal symptoms. Soy, black cohosh, and dong quai may all decrease hot flashes and improve cardiovascular health, but soy products have almost no ill effects and appear to be very effective in many women. Valerian is used for a tranquilizing effect.
16. b. Rationale: Sexual assault is an act of violence, and the first priority of care for the patient should be assessment and treatment of serious injuries involving extragenital areas, such as fractures, subdural hematomas, cerebral concussions, and intraabdominal injuries. All of the other options are correct, but treatment for shock and urgent medical injuries is the first priority.
17. a. Rationale: Specific informed consent must be obtained from the rape victim before any examination can be made or rape data collected. Following consent the patient is advised not to wash, eat, drink, or urinate before the examination so that evidence can be collected for medicolegal use. Prophylaxis for STDs, hepatitis B, and tetanus is administered following examination, and follow-up testing for pregnancy and HIV is done in several weeks.
18. a. 2; b. 1; c. 1; d. 4; e. 3; f. 1; g. 2; h. 1; i. 4
19. a. Rationale: *Gardnerella vaginalis* infection is a bacterial vaginosis that is sexually transmitted, and almost always both partners are infected. Successful treatment of the condition requires oral treatment with metronidazole (Flagyl) or clindamycin (Cleocin) for both partners. Minipads may be used to contain vaginal secretions, but they do not prevent reinfection.
20. b. Rationale: Sexual activity with multiple partners increases the risk for PID, and there is often a history of an acute infection of the lower genital tract caused by gonococcal or chlamydial microorganisms. The only significant contraceptive issue related to PID is that condom use will help prevent sexually transmitted diseases that may lead to PID.
21. b. Rationale: Bed rest in a semi-Fowler's position promotes drainage of the pelvic cavity by gravity and may prevent the development of abscesses high in the abdomen. Coitus, douching, and tampon use should be avoided to prevent spreading infection upward from the vagina, although frequent perineal care should be done to remove infectious drainage.
22. b. Rationale: The risk for infertility following PID is high, and the nurse should allow time for the patient to express her feelings, clarify her concerns, and begin problem solving with regard to the outcomes of the disease. Responses that do not allow for discussion of feelings and concerns or that tell the patient how she should feel or what she should worry about are not therapeutic.

23. a. F, endometriosis; b. F, endometriosis and uterine leiomyoma; c. T; d. T; e. F, pseudomenopause; f. F, metrorrhagia; g. T
24. b. Rationale: A stage O Pap smear indicates cancer in situ that is confined to the epithelial layer of the cervix and requires treatment. While the Bethesda system reports nonmalignant changes in cervical cells, the international classification of clinical stages of cervical cancer always identifies malignant cells. Stage 0 is the least invasive, and stage IVB indicates spread to distant organs.
25. c. Rationale: Conization (an excision of a cone-shaped section of the cervix) and laser treatment both are effective in locally removing or destroying malignant cells of the cervix and preserve fertility. Radiation treatments frequently impair ovarian and uterine function and lead to sterility. A subtotal hysterectomy would be contraindicated in treatment of cervical cancer because the cervix would be left intact in this procedure.
26. b. Rationale: Postmenopausal vaginal bleeding is the first sign of endometrial cancer, and when it occurs, a sample of endometrial tissue must be taken to exclude cancer. An endometrial biopsy can be done as an office procedure and is indicated in this case. Abdominal x-rays and Pap smears are not reliable tests for endometrial cancer, and laser treatment of the cervix is indicated only for cervical dysplasia.
27. b. Rationale: Treatment of ovarian cancer is determined by staging from the results of laparoscopy with multiple biopsies of the ovaries and other tissue throughout the pelvis and lower abdomen. Although diagnosis of ovarian tumors may be made by ultrasound or CT scan, the treatment of ovarian cancer depends on the staging of the tumor. The patient's desire for fertility is not a consideration, because of the high mortality rate associated with ovarian cancer.
28. a. E; b. O; c. C; d. C; e. V; f. E; g. C; h. O; i. C; j. O
29. a. Rationale: Early signs of cancer of the vulva include pruritus, soreness of vulva, unusual odor, and discharge or bleeding of the vulva, with edema of the vulva and lymphadenopathy occurring as the disease progresses. Labial lesions and excoriation more commonly occur with infections, and nodules are more often cysts or lipomas.
30. c. Rationale: A total hysterectomy involves the removal of the uterus and the cervix, but the fallopian tubes and ovaries are left intact. Although menstruation is terminated, normal ovarian production of estrogen continues. A panhysterectomy is the procedure in which the uterus and cervix as well as the tubes and ovaries are removed.
31. b. Rationale: Lower leg pain, especially on extension or with dorsiflexion, is a sign of thrombophlebitis, which is a common complication of hysterectomy or other pelvic surgery and requires immediate medical attention. Abdominal distention with gas pains and depression are expected complications that are treated symptomatically, and interventions may be necessary if patients do not void for 8 hours following removal of an indwelling catheter.
32. c. Rationale: A pelvic exenteration is the most radical gynecologic surgery and results in removal of the uterus, ovaries, fallopian tubes, vagina, bladder, urethra, and pelvic lymph nodes and, in some situations, also the descending colon, rectum, and anal canal. There are urinary and fecal diversions on the abdominal wall, the absence of a vagina, and the onset of menopausal symptoms, all of which result in severe altered body structure.
33. d. Rationale: To prevent displacement of the intrauterine implant, the patient is maintained on absolute bed rest with turning from side to side. Bowel elimination is discouraged during the treatment by cleaning the colon before implantation, and urinary elimination is maintained by an indwelling catheter. Because the patient is radioactive, any one nurse should not spend more than 30 minutes daily with the patient, and visitors are restricted to less than 3 hours a day at a minimum of 6 feet from the patient.
34. a. Rationale: Kegel exercises help strengthen muscular support of the perineum, pelvic floor, and bladder and are beneficial for problems with pelvic support and stress incontinence. The muscles that should be exercised are those affected by trying to stop a flow of urine.
35. a. 5; b. 3; c. 2; d. 1; e. 4
36. a. Rationale: An anterior colporrhaphy involves repair of a cystocele, and an indwelling urinary catheter is left in place for several days postoperatively while healing occurs. Bowel function should not be altered and is maintained with a low-residue diet and a stool softener if necessary.

Case Study

1. The gonococcus spreads directly along the endometrium to the tubes and into the peritoneum, resulting in salpingitis, pelvic peritonitis, or tuboovarian abscesses.
2. Clinical manifestations include crampy or continuous bilateral lower abdominal pain that is increased with movement or ambulation; irregular menstrual bleeding and vaginal discharge that is yellow, green, or brownish with a foul odor;

dyspareunia; fever; and chills, with possible nausea and vomiting.
3. Outpatient management would include oral antibiotics, increased fluid intake, good nutrition, restriction of activities, and rest with the head elevated. She should also be instructed to avoid intercourse and douching.
4. Chronic PID is less acute, with increased cramps with menses, irregular bleeding, and moderate pain with intercourse.
5. Elevating the head of the bed promotes drainage of the pelvic cavity by gravity and may prevent the development of abscesses high in the abdomen. Application of heat with heating pads or sitz baths may help localize the infection.
6. Clarify the possible course and outcomes of the disease with the patient. Although early treatment may help prevent complications, it is realistic that sterility often results from PID because of adhesions and strictures of the fallopian tubes, and she is at increased risk for ectopic pregnancies. Discuss and listen to her concerns about her future childbearing ability.
7. *Nursing diagnoses:*
   - Ineffective health maintenance related to lack of protective measures against STDs
   - Anxiety related to outcome of disease on reproductive status
   - Risk for impaired skin integrity related to vaginal drainage

   Collaborative problems:

   Potential complications: peritonitis; septic shock; thromboembolism

CHAPTER 53

1. d. Rationale: Hyperplasia is an increase in the number of cells, and in BPH it is thought that the enlargement caused by the increase in new cells results from endocrine changes associated with aging. Hypertrophy refers to an increase in the size of existing cells. The hyperplasia is not considered a tumor, nor does BPH predispose to cancer of the prostate.
2. c. Rationale: Classic symptoms of uncomplicated BPH are those associated with urinary obstruction and include diminished caliber and force of the urinary stream, hesitancy, dribbling at the end of urination, and a feeling of incomplete bladder emptying because of urinary retention. Irritative symptoms, including nocturia, dysuria, urgency, or hematuria, occur if infection results from urinary retention.
3. c. Rationale: Urinary flow meters are used to measure the urinary flow rate, which is decreased in vesicle neck obstruction. Cystourethroscopy may also evaluate the degree of obstruction, but a cystometrogram measures bladder tone, postvoiding catheterization measures residual urine, and a rectal ultrasound may determine the size and configuration of the prostate gland.
4. a. Rationale: Finasteride results in suppression of androgen formation by inhibiting the formation of the testosterone metabolite dihydroxytestosterone, the principle prostatic androgen, and results in a decrease in the size of the prostate gland. Alpha-adrenergic blockers are used to cause smooth muscle relaxation in the treatment of BPH, but drugs affecting bladder tone are not indicated.
5. c. Rationale: Placement of stainless steel stents in the prostatic urethra hold back the walls of the prostate to allow for the unobstructed flow of urine in patients with BPH and is done under local anesthetic on an outpatient basis. Temporary incontinence may result from the procedure.
6. a. 3; b. 5; c. 1; d. 6; e. 1; f. 2; g. 1; h. 4; i. 5; j. 3; k. 2; l. 4
7. d. Rationale: The prostate gland can be easily palpated by rectal examination, and enlargement of the gland is detected early if yearly examinations are performed. If symptoms of prostatic hyperplasia are present, further diagnostic testing, including a UA, PSA, and cystoscopy, may be indicated.
8. b. Rationale: Because of injury to the internal urinary sphincter, there is usually some degree of retrograde ejaculation following any prostate surgery. The semen is ejaculated into the bladder and is eliminated with the next voiding. It is not harmful but may affect fertility because of a smaller amount or absence of normal ejaculate. Urinary incontinence may occur with a prostatectomy but not in all cases, and a vasectomy performed at the time of a prostatectomy does not affect erectile function. Long-term use of a urinary catheter depends on the patient and is not a routine procedure.
9. d. Rationale: Bleeding and blood clots from the bladder are expected after prostatectomy, and continuous irrigation is used to keep clots from obstructing the urinary tract. The rate of the irrigation may be increased to keep the clots from forming if ordered, but the nurse should also check the vital signs because hemorrhage is the most common complication of prostatectomy. The traction on the catheter applies pressure to the operative site to control bleeding and should only be relieved with specific orders. The catheter does not need to be manually irrigated unless there are signs the catheter is obstructed, and clamping the drainage tube is contraindicated because it would cause distention of the bladder.

10. b. Rationale: Bladder spasms often occur after a TURP or suprapubic prostatectomy and are caused by bladder irritation, presence of the catheter, or clots leading to obstruction of the catheter. The nurse should first check for the presence of clots obstructing the catheter or tubing and then may administer a B&O suppository if ordered. The patient should not try to void around the catheter because this will increase the spasms. The flow rate on the irrigation fluid may be decreased if orders permit because fast-flowing, cold fluid may also contribute to spasms.
11. c. Rationale: Activities that increase intraabdominal pressure should be avoided until the surgeon approves these activities at a follow-up visit. Stool softeners and high-fiber diets may be used to promote bowel elimination, but enemas should not be used, because they increase intraabdominal pressure and may initiate bleeding. Because a TURP does not remove the entire prostate gland, the patient needs annual prostatic examinations to screen for cancer of the prostate. Fluid intake should be high, but caffeine and alcohol should not be used, because they have a diuretic effect and increase bladder distention.
12. a. Hard, with asymmetric enlargement with areas of induration or nodules
    b. Prostate-specific antigen (PSA) higher than that usually seen in BPH; increased prostatic acid phosphatase (PAP), especially with metastasis; elevated alkaline phosphatase in advanced disease
    c. Pelvic or perineal pain, pain of metastasis, fatigue, malaise
13. c. Rationale: A prostatectomy performed with a perineal approach has the highest incidence of residual damage to the nerves needed for erection, and patients should be aware of this complication. Urinary incontinence also frequently occurs after radical prostatectomy. Wound infection is a possibility with a perineal approach because of the proximity of the wound to the anus but can be prevented with frequent perineal care. Loss of libido and gynecomastia are effects of antiandrogen drugs.
14. a. T; b. F, luteinizing hormone-releasing hormone (LHRH) agonists (such as leuprolide [Lupron] or goserelin [Zoladex]) and androgen receptor blockers; c. F, serum PSA measurements; d. T; e. F, African American; f. F, acute bacterial prostatitis; g. T
15. a. 4; b. 8; c. 6; d. 10; e. 12; f. 11; g. 9; h. 1; i. 3; j. 2; k. 7; l. 5
16. b. Rationale: Alpha-fetoprotein (AFP) and human chorionic gonadotropin (HCG) are glycoproteins that may be elevated in testicular cancer. If they are elevated before surgical treatment, the levels are noted, and if response to therapy is positive, the levels will decrease. PSA and PAP are used for screening of prostatic cancer; tumor necrosis factor (TNF) is a normal cytokine responsible for tumor surveillance and destruction; C-reactive protein (CRP) is found in inflammatory conditions and widespread malignancies; carcinoembryonic antigen (CEA) is a tumor marker for cancers of the gastrointestinal system; and antinuclear antibody (ANA) is found most frequently in autoimmune disorders.
17. d. Rationale: Testicular tumors most often present on the testis as a lump or nodule that is very firm, is nontender, and cannot be transilluminated. There may also be scrotal swelling and a feeling of heaviness. All of the other options are normal findings.
18. c. Rationale: Until sperm distal to the anastomotic site are ejaculated or absorbed by the body, the semen will contain sperm, and alternative contraceptive methods must be used. When a postoperative semen examination reveals no sperm, the patient is considered sterile. Following vasectomy there is rarely noticeable difference in the amount of ejaculate because ejaculate is primarily seminal fluid. Vasectomy does not affect testicular production of sperm or hormones, nor does it cause erectile dysfunction.
19. a. Rationale: Only a small percentage of erectile dysfunction is caused by psychologic factors, and before treatment for erectile dysfunction is initiated, the cause must be determined so that appropriate treatment can be planned. In the case of the 80% to 90% of erectile dysfunction that is of physiologic causes, interventions are directed at correcting or eliminating the cause or restoring function by medical means. New invasive or experimental treatments are not widely used and should be limited to research centers, and patients with systemic diseases can be treated with medical means if the cause cannot be eliminated.
20. There are many appropriate answers for this question, including these examples:
    a. Depression, stress, fear of failure, fatigue, antiandrogens decrease libido
    b. Atherosclerosis, antihypertensive drugs, diabetes
    c. Peripheral neuropathies, sympathectomy, spinal cord injuries/tumors, multiple sclerosis
    d. Antiandrogens, estrogen, thyroid, testosterone deficiency, pituitary tumors
21. a. 3; b. 1; c. 5; d. 2; e. 4; f. 5; g. 1; h. 3

Case Study

1. Testicular tumors develop either from the cellular components of the testis (very rare and usually benign) or from the embryonal precursors (germinal tumors that are almost always malignant). Risk factors include age between 15 and 35, a history of cryptorchidism, family history of testicular cancer, orchitis, HIV infection, maternal exposure to DES, and testicular cancer in the contralateral testis.
2. The primary difference on testicular examination between a spermatocele and a testicular cancer is that spermatocele will transilluminate, whereas cancer cannot be transilluminated.
3. About 95% of patients with testicular cancer that is found in early stages obtain a complete remission. He has no back pain or gynecomastia, which would indicate metastatic disease. His prognosis is positive, but he will need careful monitoring to detect any relapse early.
4. Alpha-fetoprotein (AFP) and human chorionic gonadotropin (hCG) are frequently elevated in testicular cancer and should be noted before treatment. If these markers are elevated before treatment and then decrease after treatment, it indicates a positive response to treatment. The levels of AFP and hCG are monitored during long-term follow-up to detect any relapse of the tumor.
5. Initiate conversation with him about his concerns, and allow him to talk about them. It is important to discuss the option of sperm banking before his surgery in case he later wants to have children.
6. The orchiectomy and lymph node resection will most likely be followed with radiation of the remaining lymph nodes and/or a single or multiple chemotherapy regimen. Germ-cell tumors are very sensitive to systemic chemotherapy, and its use is recommended. All of these processes will cause sterility, but the surgery and additional treatment should not alter his sexual function.
7. *Nursing diagnoses:*
    - Anxiety related to effects of surgery
    - Fear related to outcome of disease process and prognosis

    No preoperative collaborative problems

CHAPTER 54

1. a. Golgi apparatus; b. mitochondrion; c. nucleolus; d. nucleus; e. Nissl bodies; f. gemmule; g. axon hillock; h. axon; i. Schwann cell; j. myelin sheath; k. collateral axon; l. node of Ranvier; m. telodendria; n. synaptic knobs; o. neuron cell body; p. dendrites
2. a. posterior horn; b. central canal; c. anterior horn; d. anterior corticospinal tract; e. anterior spinothalamic tract; f. lateral spinothalamic tract; g. anterior spinocerebellar tract; h. lateral corticospinal tract; i. posterior spinocerebellar tract; j. posterolateral tract of Lissauer; k. fasciculus cuneatus; l. fasciculus gracilis
3. *Across:* 3. clefts; 6. synapse; 9. oligodendroglia; 11. myelin; 12. nucleus; 14. potential; 15. pia; 16. pons; 17. LOC; 18. neuron
    Down: 1. node of Ranvier; 2. astrocyte; 3. CSF; 4. LE; 5. Schwann cell; 7. axon; 8. regeneration; 10. dendrite; 13. limbic; 14. pain; 15. PO; 16. PO
4. a. F, ependymal cells; b. T; c. F, out of the cell; into the cell; d. F, inhibitory; e. T
5. b. Rationale: The fasciculus gracilis and fasciculus cuneatus tracts carry information and transmit impulses concerned with touch, deep pressure, vibration, position sense, and kinesthesia. Spinothalamic tracts carry pain and temperature sensations; the spinocerebellar tracts carry subconscious information about muscle tension and body position; and descending corticobulbar tracts carry impulses responsible for voluntary impulses from the cortex to the cranial nerves.
6. a. Rationale: The cell bodies of lower motor neurons that send impulses to skeletal muscles in the arms, legs, and trunk are located in the anterior horn of the spinal cord, and lesions generally cause weakness or paralysis and decreased muscle tone. Upper motor neurons include the brainstem and cerebral cortex motor neurons that influence skeletal muscle movement, and lesions at this point cause weakness and paralysis with hyperreflexia and spasticity.
7. a. 8; b. 10; c. 7; d. 1; e. 11; f. 2; g. 12; h. 4; i. 3; j. 5; k. 9; l. 6
8. d. Rationale: Some cranial nerves are only efferent motor nerves (e.g., III, IV, VI, VII, XI, XII), some are only afferent sensory nerves (e.g., I, II, VIII), and some have both motor and sensory functions (e.g., V, IX, X), but spinal nerves always have both sensory and motor fibers. Both cranial and spinal nerves occur in pairs, and while most cell bodies of cranial nerves are located in the brain, the primary cell bodies of CN I, II, and XI are located outside of the brain.

9. a. S; b. S; c. P; d. P; e. S; f. P; g. S; h. P; i. P; j. P; k. P
10. b. Rationale: The circle of Willis is a vascular circle formed by the basilar artery and the internal carotid arteries and may act as an anastomotic pathway when occlusion of a major artery on one side of the brain occurs. The middle cerebral arteries supply the outer portions of the frontal, parietal, and superior temporal lobes, but the circle of Willis may accommodate for plaquing in this artery.
11. a. 6; b. 4; c. 9; d. 7; e. 1; f. 8; g. 2; h. 5; i. 3
12. c. Rationale: A decrease in sensory receptors caused by degenerative changes leads to diminished sense of touch, temperature, and peripheral vibrations in the older adult. Reflexes are decreased but not normally absent, and intelligence does not decrease, although there may be some loss of memory. Hypothalamic modifications lead to increased frequency of spontaneous awakening with interrupted sleep and insomnia.
13. a. Avoid suggesting symptoms.
    b. The onset and cause of illness are especially important aspects of the nursing history.
    c. The mental status must be accurately assessed to ensure that the reported history is factual.
14. c. Rationale: Headaches are a common symptom of neurologic problems, and the use of aspirin may impair coagulation and lead to gastric bleeding. Fainting or a brief loss of consciousness that can be attributed to vasomotor events is not indicative of neurologic impairment, and there is no relationship between kidney stones or gallbladder disease and neurologic problems.
15. a. Uncontrolled hypertension, lack of appropriate helmet use, family history of neurologic problems
    b. Difficulty chewing and swallowing, B-vitamin deficiency
    c. Bowel or bladder incontinence, constipation
    d. Problems in mobility, strength, and coordination; history of falling
    e. Sleep disturbances from pain or immobility; insomnia, frequently awakening
    f. Sensory changes, dizziness; cognitive changes; language difficulties
    g. Decreased self-worth and body image; unkempt physical appearance and hygiene
    h. Changes in roles at work or in family from neurologic problems
    i. Decreased sexual desire, stimulation, function, or response
    j. Sense of being overwhelmed, inadequate coping patterns
    k. Religious or cultural beliefs that interfere or assist with planned treatment
16. a. Rationale: During the nursing history the nurse should be assessing mental functioning to determine whether the history is factual and whether the patient can remember historical events, assessments that are included in the determination of mental status. Because much of the area covered in the mental status examination is assessed during the history, it does not need to be evaluated further.
17. a. 7; b. 4; c. 8; d. 9; e. 3, 6; f. 12; g. 2, 6, 10; h. 13; i. 11; j. 11; k. 1; l. 5
18. a. Rationale: The primary purposes of the nursing neurologic examination are to determine the effects of neurologic dysfunction on daily living and the patient's and the family's ability to cope with neurologic deficits. The examination should be viewed in terms of functional disabilities, rather than dysfunction, of component parts of the nervous system, and findings of the examination should be used to plan appropriate care for deficits in self-care and in activities of daily living.
19. a. 6; b. 8; c. 5; d. 9; e. 10; f. 1; g. 4; h. 7; i. 2; j. 3
20. b. Rationale: The normal response of the triceps reflex is extension of the arm or visible contraction of the triceps. The normal response of the biceps reflex is flexion of the arm at the elbow, while the presence of the brachioradialis reflex is seen with flexion and supination at the elbow.
21. b. Rationale: Deep tendon grading is as follows: 0/5 = absent; 1/5 = weak response; 2/5 = normal response; 3/5 = exaggerated response; 4/5 = hyperreflexia with clonus.
22. d. Rationale: To facilitate insertion of the spinal needle between the third and fourth lumbar vertebrae, the patient should round the spine by flexing the knees, hips, and neck while in a lateral position. Sitting on the edge of the bed and bending only the spine does not separate the vertebrae as efficiently. Stimulants are withheld for 8 hours before an EEG, and sedation is used for more invasive tests, such as myelograms and angiography.
23. a. Rationale: A spinal headache, which may be caused by loss of CSF at the puncture site, is common following a lumbar puncture or a myelogram, and nuchal rigidity may also occur as a result of meningeal irritation. The patient is not in danger of paralysis with a lumbar puncture, nor does hemorrhage from the site occur. Contrast media are not used with a lumbar puncture.
24. c. Rationale: Following a myelogram (and a lumbar puncture) the patient is positioned flat in bed for several hours to avoid a spinal headache, and fluids are encouraged to help in the excretion of the contrast medium. Pain at the insertion site is rare, and the most common complaint after a myelogram is a headache.

25. b. Rationale: Cerebral angiography involves the injection of contrast media through a catheter inserted into the femoral or brachial artery and passed into the base of a carotid or vertebral artery and is performed when vascular lesions or tumors are suspected. Allergic reactions to the contrast medium may occur, and vascular spasms or dislodgement of plaques is possible. Neurologic and vital signs must be monitored every 15 to 30 minutes for 2 hours, every hour for the next 6 hours, and then every 2 hours for 24 hours following the test. Electroencephalograms and transcranial Doppler sonography are not invasive studies.
26. d. Rationale: Normal glucose levels in cerebrospinal fluid are 45-75 mg/dl. All types of organisms consume glucose, and decreased glucose reflects bacterial activity. Increased levels are associated with diabetes. The other values are all normal.

CHAPTER 55

1. a. Increased absorption, decreased production, displacement into spinal canal; b. Collapse of veins and dural sinuses, increased venous outflow and decreased blood flow; c. Distention of dura, slight compression of tissue
2. a. 0 to 15
   b. 50, ischemic; 150, constricted
   c. 70–100 mm Hg
      56 mm Hg: MAP = DBP + 1/3 (SBP-DBP) = 52 + 18 = 70
      CPP = MAP – ICP = 70 – 14 = 56
   d. 45 mm Hg: MAP = DBP + 1/3 (SBP-DBP) = 64 + 15 = 79
      CPP = MAP – ICP = 79 – 34 = 45
   e. 50; 30
3. b. Rationale: Compliance is the expansability of the brain, and as volume and pressure increase, compliance is lowered, and elastance increases. Elastance is the inverse of compliance and represents the brain's stiffness and ability to accommodate changes in volume. Elastance increases as volume in the brain increases. With high elastance, or stiffness, large increases in pressure occur with only small increases in volume, and with high compliance, small increases in volume are accommodated.
4. a. D; b. I; c. D; d. D; e. I
5. a. 2; b. 1; c. 2; d. 1; e. 3
6. a. CO; b. CO; c. CB; d. CO; e. CB
7. c. Rationale: One of the most sensitive signs of increased intracranial pressure is a decreasing LOC. A decrease in LOC will occur before changes in vital signs, ocular signs, or projectile vomiting occur.
8. c. Rationale: Cushing triad consists of three vital sign measures that reflect ICP and its effect on the medulla, the hypothalamus, the pons, and the thalamus. Because these structures are very deep, Cushing triad is usually a late sign of ICP. The signs include an increasing systolic blood pressure with a widening pulse pressure, a bradycardia with a full and bounding pulse, and irregular respirations.
9. c. Rationale: The dural structures that separate the two hemispheres and the cerebral hemispheres from the cerebellum influence the patterns of cerebral herniation. A cingulated herniation occurs where there is lateral displacement of brain tissue beneath the falx cerebri.
10. a. Rationale: An intraventricular catheter is a fluid-coupled system that can provide direct access for microorganisms to enter the ventricles of the brain, and aseptic technique is a very high nursing priority to decrease the risk for infection. Constant monitoring of ICP wave forms is not usually necessary, and removal of CSF for sampling or to maintain normal ICP is done only when specifically ordered.
11. a. T; b. F, cardiac; c. T; d. T
12. a. 3; b. 5; c. 4; d. 1; e. 6; f. 2
13. d. Rationale: A patient with increased intracranial pressure is in a hypermetabolic and hypercatabolic state and needs adequate glucose to maintain fuel for the brain and other nutrients to meet metabolic needs. Malnutrition promotes cerebral edema, and if a patient cannot take oral nutrition, other means of providing nutrition should be used, such as tube feedings or total parenteral nutrition. Glucose alone is not adequate to meet nutritional requirements, and 5% dextrose solutions may increase cerebral edema by lowering serum osmolarity. A fluid restriction to reduce cerebral edema must be balanced against a hypovolemia that could decrease cerebral perfusion, and it is a controversial therapy.
14. a. to speak; b. obey commands; c. open eyes to verbal or painful stimuli
15. b. Rationale: No opening of eyes = 1; incomprehensible words = 3; flexion withdrawal = 4; total = 8
16. d. Rationale: Of the body functions that should be assessed in an unconscious patient, cardiopulmonary status is the most vital function and gives priorities to the ABCs.
17. c. Rationale: One of the functions of CN III, the oculomotor nerve, is pupillary constriction, and testing for pupillary constriction is important to identify patients at risk for brainstem herniation caused by increased intracranial pressure. The corneal reflex is used to assess the functions of

CN V and VII, and the oculocephalic reflex tests all cranial nerves involved with eye movement. Nystagmus is commonly associated with specific lesions or chemical toxicities and is not a definitive sign of ICP.

18. a. Rationale: Nursing care activities that increase intracranial pressure include hip and neck flexion, suctioning, clustering care activities, and noxious stimuli and should be avoided or performed as little as possible in the patient with increased ICP. Lowering the $PaCO_2$ below 20 mm Hg can cause ischemia and worsening of ICP, and if hyperventilation is used, the $PaCO_2$ should be maintained at 30 to 35 mm Hg.
19. d. Rationale: Elevation of the head of the bed is indicated in the patient with increased intracranial pressure to promote venous drainage from the head and decrease vascular congestion unless the elevation contributes to decreased cerebral perfusion. Decreased cerebral perfusion is indicated by a decreasing level of consciousness, and the patient should be positioned so that ICP is lowered while still maintaining the CPP. Ptosis of the eyelid, unexpected vomiting, and decreased motor functions are signs of ICP.
20. c. Rationale: A PaO_2 of 50 mm Hg reflects a hypoxemia that may lead to further decreased cerebral perfusion and hypoxia and must be corrected. The pH and SaO_2 are within normal range, and a $PaCO_2$ of 30 mm Hg reflects an acceptable value for the patient with moderate hyperventilation.
21. b. Rationale: Pituitary gland secretion may be affected by increased ICP, and observation for pituitary disturbances is important. A decreased urinary output with an increased specific gravity reflects water retention that is characteristic of SIADH. SIADH results in a dilutional hyponatremia, which may contribute to increased cerebral edema, changes in LOC, seizures, and coma. Diabetes insipidus is reflected by increased urinary output and a dilute urine indicated by a decreased urine specific gravity and may result in severe dehydration and decreased cerebral circulation.
22. c. Rationale: If reflex posturing occurs during ROM or positioning of the patient, these activities should be done less frequently until the patient's condition stabilizes, because posturing can causes increases in ICP. Neither restraints nor CNS depressants would be indicated.
23. a. 4; b. 9; c. 1; d. 7; e. 6; f. 10; g. 3; h. 8; i. 12; j. 11; k. 2; l. 5
24. c. Rationale: Testing clear drainage for CSF in nasal or ear drainage may be done with a Dextrostik or Tes-Tape strip, but if blood is present, the glucose in the blood will produce an unreliable result. To test bloody drainage, the nurse should test the fluid for a "halo" or "ring" that occurs when a yellowish ring encircles blood dripped onto a white pad or towel.
25. d. Rationale: An arterial epidural hematoma is the most acute neurologic emergency, and typical symptoms include unconsciousness at the scene, with a brief lucid interval followed by a decrease in LOC. An acute subdural hematoma manifests signs within 48 hours of an injury, while a chronic subdural hematoma develops over weeks or months.
26. d. Rationale: A craniotomy is indicated when there is a depressed fracture and fractures with loose fragments in order to elevate the depressed bone and remove free fragments. A craniotomy is also indicated in cases of acute subdural and epidural hematomas in order to remove the blood and control the bleeding. Burr holes may be used in an extreme emergency for rapid decompression, but with a depressed fracture, surgery would be the treatment of choice.
27. a. Rationale: In addition to monitoring for a patent airway during emergency care of the patient with a head injury, the nurse must always assume that a patient with a head injury may have a cervical spine injury. Maintaining cervical spine precautions in all assessment and treatment activities with the patient is essential to prevent additional neurologic damage.
28. c. Rationale: Residual mental and emotional changes of brain trauma with personality changes are often the most incapacitating problems following head injury and are common in those patients who have been comatose for more than 6 hours. Families must be prepared for changes in the patient's behavior in order to avoid family-patient friction and maintain family functioning, and professional assistance may be required. There is no indication he will be dependent on others for care, but it is likely he will not return to pretrauma status.
29. a. F, all; b. F, occipital; c. F, glioblastoma multiforme; d. T; e. T
30. b. Rationale: Frontal lobe tumors often lead to loss of emotional control, confusion, memory loss, disorientation, and personality changes that are very disturbing and frightening to the family. Physical symptoms, such as blindness, disturbances in sensation and perception, and even seizures, that occur with other tumors are more likely to be understood and accepted by the family.
31. a. 4; b. 6; c. 1; d. 5; e. 2; f. 3
32. a. Rationale: To prevent undue concern and anxiety about hair loss and postoperative self-esteem

disturbances, a patient undergoing cranial surgery should be informed preoperatively that the head is usually shaved in surgery while the patient is anesthetized and that methods can be used after the dressings are removed postoperatively to disguise the hair loss. In the immediate postoperative period the patient is very ill, and the focus is on maintaining neurologic function, but preoperatively the nurse should anticipate the patient's postoperative need for self-esteem and maintenance of appearance.

33. d. Rationale: A craniectomy involves the removal of a bone flap, and postoperatively the patient should not be positioned on the operative side, but the patient with an anterior or middle fossae incision will have a midline incision and have the head of the bed elevated 30 to 45 degrees. If the incision is in the posterior fossa, the patient is usually kept flat or at a slight elevation with avoidance of neck flexion.
34. d. Rationale: The primary goal after cranial surgery is prevention of increased ICP, and interventions to prevent ICP and infection postoperatively are nursing priorities. The residual deficits, rehabilitation potential, and ultimate function of the patient depend on the reason for surgery, the postoperative course, and the patient's general state of health.
35. a. M; b. E; c. E; d. M; e. E; f. M; g. M; h. E; i. M
36. d. Rationale: Meningitis is often secondary to an upper respiratory infection or middle ear infection, where organisms gain entry to the CNS. Epidemic encephalitis is transmitted by ticks and mosquitoes, and nonepidemic encephalitis may occur as a complication of measles, chickenpox, or mumps. Encephalitis caused by the herpes simplex virus carries a high fatality rate.
37. b. Rationale: High fever, severe headache, nuchal rigidity, and positive Brudzinski's and Kernig's signs are such classic symptoms of meningitis that they are usually considered diagnostic for meningitis. Other symptoms, such as papilledema, generalized seizures, hemiparesis, and decreased LOC, may occur as complications of increased intracranial pressure and cranial nerve dysfunction.
38. a. Rationale: Because rapid diagnosis and treatment are crucial in meningitis, diagnosis is made based on history and physical examination, and antibiotic therapy with penicillins or cephalosporins is started after the collection of CSF and blood cultures, even before the diagnosis is confirmed with positive cultures. Few drugs are available to treat encephalitis, but the antiviral agent vidarabine (Vira-A) is used in the treatment of herpes simplex encephalitis.
39. a. Increased seizures; b. Increased ICP; c. Dehydration; d. Direct neurologic damage
40. c. Rationale: The symptoms of brain abscess closely resemble those of meningitis and encephalitis, including fever, headache, and increased ICP, except that the patient also usually has some focal symptoms that reflect the local area of the abscess.

Case Study

1. The temperature elevation and nuchal rigidity in the presence of increased intracranial pressure and decreasing level of consciousness indicate that Steven has developed a meningeal infection.
2. The risks for meningitis after head injury and surgery include penetrations into the intracranial cavity with the compound fracture that involves a depressed skull fracture with scalp lacerations with a communicating pathway to the intracranial cavity and the incisions necessary for craniotomy for hematoma evacuation. Postoperative drains, invasive monitoring, environmental pathogens, as well as impaired immune response, also contribute to the development of meningitis.
3. Acute inflammation and infection of the pia mater and the arachnoid membrane cause nuchal rigidity, a sign of meningeal irritation, and fever. The inflammatory response increases CSF production with an increase in pressure, and as the purulent secretion produced by microbial infection spreads to other areas of the brain, cerebral edema and increased ICP occur. Increased ICP is thought to be a result of swelling around the dura, increased CSF volume, and endotoxins produced by the bacteria.
4. Priority interventions include reduction of fever, reduction of ICP, maintaining antibiotic schedule to keep therapeutic levels, maintaining fluid balance, protection from injury if seizures occur, and minimizing environmental stimuli.
5. Access to the meninges could have occurred from facial and cranial fractures and the surgical incisions.
6. *Nursing diagnoses:*
   - Ineffective cerebral tissue perfusion related to cerebral tissue swelling
   - Hyperthermia related to infection and abnormal temperature regulation
   - Risk for ineffective breathing pattern related to decreased LOC and immobility
   - Risk for injury related to potential for seizures
   - Imbalanced nutrition: less than body requirements related to hypermetabolism and inability to ingest food and fluids

- Risk for impaired skin integrity related to immobility

Collaborative problems:
Potential complications: increased intracranial pressure; seizures; hydrocephalus; disseminated intravascular coagulation; brain herniation

CHAPTER 56

1. c. Rationale: The highest risk factors for thrombotic stroke are hypertension and diabetes. African Americans have a higher risk for stroke than do Caucasians but probably because they have a greater incidence of hypertension. Factors such as obesity, diet high in saturated fats and cholesterol, cigarette smoking, and excessive alcohol use are also risk factors but carry less risk than hypertension.
2. c. Rationale: The communication between cerebral arteries in the circle of Willis provides a collateral circulation, which may maintain circulation to an area of the brain if its original blood supply is obstructed. All areas of the brain require constant blood supply, and atherosclerotic plaques are not readily reversed. Neurologic deficits can result from ischemia caused by many factors.
3. d. Rationale: A TIA is a temporary focal loss of neurologic function caused by ischemia of an area of the brain, usually lasting only 3 hours. TIAs may be due to microemboli from heart disease or carotid or cerebral thrombi and are a warning of progressive disease. Evaluation is necessary to determine the cause of the neurologic deficit and provide prophylactic treatment if possible.
4. a. 2; b. 3; c. 3; d. 1; e. 4; f. 3; g. 4; h. 1; i. 2; j. 4; k. 1; l. 4; m. 2
5. c. Rationale: When cerebral infarction occurs, the ischemic cascade causes an inflammatory response that leads to edema and extension of tissue damage. In ischemic strokes, symptoms may progress in the first 72 hours as infarction and cerebral edema increase. Repositioning and passive range of motion should be started the first day to prevent complications, but aggressive rehabilitation is not started until the patient's condition is stable.
6. c. Rationale: Clinical manifestations of altered neurologic function differ, depending primarily on the specific cerebral artery involved and the area of the brain that is perfused by the artery. The degree of impairment depends on rapidity of onset, the size of the lesion, and the presence of collateral circulation.
7. a. L; b. R; c. R; d. R; e. L; f. R
8. a. T; b. F, expressive aphasia; c. T; d. F, fluent dysphagia; e. F, spasticity
9. a. Rationale: A CT scan is the most commonly used diagnostic test to determine the size and location of the lesion and to differentiate a thrombotic stroke from a hemorrhagic stroke. A PET will show the metabolic activity of the brain and provides a depiction of the extent of tissue damage after a stroke. Lumbar punctures are not performed routinely, because of the chance of increased intracranial pressure causing herniation. Cerebral arteriograms are invasive and may dislodge an embolism or cause further hemorrhage and are performed only when no other test can provide the needed information.
10. c. Rationale: An endarterectomy is a removal of an atherosclerotic plaque, and a plaque in the carotid artery may impair circulation enough to cause a stroke. A carotid endarterectomy is performed to prevent a CVA, as are most other surgical procedures. An extracranial-intracranial bypass involves cranial surgery to bypass a sclerotic intracranial artery. Percutaneous transluminal angioplasty uses a balloon to compress stenotic areas in the carotid and vertebrobasilar arteries and often includes inserting a stent to hold the artery open.
11. c. Rationale: The administration of antiplatelet agents, such as aspirin, dipyridamole (Persantine), and ticlopidine (Ticlid), reduces the incidence of stroke in those at risk. Anticoagulants are also used for prevention of embolic strokes but increase the risk for hemorrhage. Diuretics are not indicated for stroke prevention, other than for their role in controlling blood pressure, and antilipemic agents have not been found to have a significant effect on stroke prevention. The calcium channel blocker nimodipine is used in patients with subarachnoid hemorrhage to decrease the effects of vasospasm and minimize tissue damage.
12. d. Rationale: The first priority in acute management of the patient with a stroke is preservation of life. Because the patient with a stroke may be unconscious or have a reduced gag reflex, it is most important to maintain a patent airway for the patient and provide oxygen if respiratory effort is impaired. IV fluid replacement, treatment with osmotic diuretics, and perhaps hypothermia may be used for further treatment.
13. b. Rationale: Surgical management with clipping of an aneurysm or wrapping or reinforcing the aneurysm to decrease rebleeding and vasospasm is an option for a stroke caused by rupture of a cerebral aneurysm. Hyperventilation therapy would increase vasodilation and the potential for hemorrhage. Thrombolytic therapy would be absolutely

contraindicated, and if a vessel is patent, osmotic diuretics may leak into tissue, pulling fluid out of the vessel and increasing edema.

14. a. Rationale: The body responds to the vasospasm and decreased circulation to the brain that occurs with a stroke by increasing the blood pressure, frequently resulting in hypertension. The other options are important cardiovascular factors to assess, but they do not result from impaired cerebral blood flow.
15. a. Self-care deficit; b. Unilateral neglect; c. Impaired swallowing; d. Risk for aspiration *Also:* Impaired urinary elimination; risk for impaired skin integrity; ineffective airway clearance; impaired physical mobility
16. d. Rationale: Active ROM should be initiated on the unaffected side as soon as possible, and passive ROM of the affected side should be started on the first day. Having the patient actively exercise the unaffected side provides the patient with active and passive ROM as needed. Use of footboards is controversial because they stimulate plantar flexion. The unaffected arm should be supported, but immobilization may precipitate a painful shoulder-hand syndrome. The patient should be positioned with each joint higher than the joint proximal to it to prevent dependent edema.
17. a. Rationale: The presence of homonymous hemianopia in a patient with right-hemisphere brain damage causes a loss of vision in the left field. Early in the care of the patient, objects should be placed on the right side of the patient in the field of vision, and the nurse should approach the patient from the right side. Later in treatment, patients should be taught to turn the head and scan the environment and should be approached from the affected side to encourage head turning. Eye patches are used if patients have diplopia (double vision).
18. a. Rationale: The first step in providing oral feedings for a patient with a stroke is ensuring that the patient has an intact gag reflex, because feedings will not be provided if the gag reflex is impaired. Then the nurse should evaluate the patient's ability to swallow ice chips or ice water after placing the patient in an upright position.
19. c. Rationale: Soft foods that provide enough texture, flavor, and bulk to stimulate swallowing should be used for the patient with dysphasia. Thin liquids are difficult to swallow, and patients may not be able to control them in the mouth. Pureed foods are often too bland and too smooth, and milk products should be avoided because they tend to increase the viscosity of mucus and increase salivation.
20. c. Rationale: In most patients with a stroke confined to one hemisphere, the urinary reflex arc remains intact, a partial sensation of bladder filling remains, and the patient maintains partial voluntary control over urination. Initially the patient may experience frequency, urgency, and incontinence, but the use of indwelling catheters impairs bladder training. The nurse should first assess the patient's urinary patterns to determine whether there is reflex emptying, retention, or mobility problems that interfere with elimination. Fluids should be maintained at 2000 ml/day, and urinals or bedpans should be offered q2hr. Incontinence pads may lead to the patient's acceptance of urinary incontinence.
21. b. Rationale: During rehabilitation the patient with aphasia needs frequent, meaningful verbal stimulation that has relevance for him. Conversation by the nurse and family should address activities of daily living that are familiar to the patient. Gestures, pictures, and simple statements are more appropriate in the acute phase, when patients may be overwhelmed by verbal stimuli. Flash cards are often perceived by the patient as childish and meaningless.
22. c. Rationale: Unilateral neglect, or neglect syndrome, occurs when the patient with a stroke is unaware of the affected side of the body and puts the patient at risk for injury. During the acute phase the affected side is cared for by the nurse with positioning and support, but during rehabilitation the patient is taught to consciously care for and attend to the affected side of the body to protect it from injury. Patients may be positioned on the affected side for up to 30 minutes.
23. c. Rationale: Patients with left-brain damage from stroke often experience emotional lability, inappropriate emotional responses, mood swings, and uncontrolled tears or laughter that are out of context with the situation. The behavior is upsetting and embarrassing to both the patient and the family, and the patient should be distracted to minimize its presence. Patients with right-brain damage often have impulsive, rapid behavior that requires supervision and direction.
24. d. Rationale: The patient and family need accurate and complete information about the effects of the stroke in order to problem solve and make plans for chronic care of the patient. It is uncommon for patients with major strokes to return completely to prestroke function, behaviors, and role, and both the patient and family will grieve these losses. The patient's specific needs for care must be identified, and rehabilitation efforts should be continued at home. Family therapy and support groups may be helpful for some patients and families.

Case Study

1. A CT scan or MRI would be able to determine the size and location of a lesion and differentiate between an infarction and a hemorrhage. A lumbar puncture would not be indicated, because of the chance that hemorrhage had increased intracranial pressure. Other tests that might be used when hemorrhage is evident include intraarterial angiography, digital subtraction angiography, and transcranial Doppler sonography.
2. Unconsciousness, GCS score of 5, and wide pulse pressure with a decrease in pulse and respiration all indicate increased intracranial pressure.
3. The loss of consciousness is associated with a poor prognosis for recovery, and the family should be told that her condition is very guarded.
4. The highest priorities for interventions are those that support her life processes: airway and respiratory function with oxygen administration, fluid management without overloading the vascular system, and measures that decrease intracranial pressure.
5. Anything that impairs clotting is contraindicated in a hemorrhagic stroke: anticoagulants, antiplatelet agents, thrombolytic therapy. Hyperosmolar diuretics are also contraindicated because they may escape from an injured vessel, causing increased edema in brain tissue.
6. Hypothermia and barbiturate therapy may be used, but these treatments have not proved effective. Surgery is the only other option, and clipping of an aneurysm may be performed, or the aneurysm may be wrapped or reinforced with muscle.
7. *Nursing diagnoses:*
   - Ineffective cerebral tissue perfusion related to hemorrhage
   - Ineffective airway clearance related to unconsciousness
   - Self-care deficit related to altered mental state
   - Risk for injury related to inability to monitor personal safety
   - Risk for infection related to immobility

   Collaborative problems:
   Potential complications: increased intracranial pressure; brain herniation; seizures

CHAPTER 57

1. a. 3; b. 1; c. 2; d. 1; e. 3; f. 1; g. 3; h. 3; i. 2; j. 3; k. 2; l. 2
2. d. Rationale: The primary way to diagnose and differentiate between functional headaches is with a careful history of the headaches, requiring assessment of specific details related to the headache. EMGs may reveal contraction of the neck, scalp, or facial muscles in tension-type headaches, but this is not seen in all patients. CT scans and cerebral angiography are used to rule out organic causes of the headaches.
3. d. Rationale: Both migraine headaches and cluster headaches appear to be related to vasodilation of cranial vessels, and drugs that have a vasopressor action, especially ergotamine and sumatriptan, are useful in treatment of migraine and cluster headaches. Methysergide is an ergot alkaloid that blocks serotonin receptors in the central and peripheral nervous systems and is used for treatment of migraine headaches and prevention of cluster headaches. Beta blockers and tricyclic antidepressants are used prophylactically for migraine headaches but are not effective for cluster headaches.
4. a. Rationale: When the anxiety is related to a lack of knowledge about the etiology and treatment of a headache, helping the patient to identify stressful lifestyles and other precipitating factors and ways of avoiding them is an appropriate nursing intervention for the anxiety. Interventions that teach alternative therapies to supplement drug therapy also give the patient some control over pain and are appropriate teaching regarding treatment of the headache. The other interventions may help reduce anxiety generally, but they do not address the etiologic factor of the anxiety.
5. a. Rationale: Projectile vomiting is characteristic of brain tumors and other causes of increased intracranial pressure and is not associated with functional headaches. Nausea with vomiting may be present with migraine headaches, however, in addition to visual disturbances, weakness and paralysis, and paresthesias and confusion.
6. d. Rationale: Generalized seizures have bilateral synchronous epileptic discharge affecting the entire brain at the onset of the seizure, preventing any warning or aura. Loss of consciousness is also characteristic, but many partial seizures also include a loss of consciousness. Partial seizures begin in one side of the brain but may spread to involve the entire brain. Partial seizures that start with a local focus and spread to the entire brain, causing a secondary generalized seizure, are associated with a transient residual neurologic deficit postictally known as Todd's paralysis.
7. a. 2; b. 4; c. 7; d. 1; e. 3; f. 6; g. 1; h. 5; i. 2; j. 7; k. 7; l. 1; m. 7; n. 4
8. a. F, kindling; b. T; c. T; d. F, patient history and description of seizure; e. F, first time or status; f. T
9. c. Rationale: A seizure is a paroxysmal, uncontrolled discharge of neurons in the brain, which interrupts normal function, but the factor that

causes the abnormal firing is not clear. Seizures may be precipitated by many factors, and although scar tissue may stimulate seizures, it is not the usual cause of seizures. Epilepsy is established only by a pattern of spontaneous, recurring seizures.

10. b. Rationale: Most patients with seizure disorders maintain seizure control with medications, but if surgery is considered, three requirements must be met: the diagnosis of epilepsy must be confirmed, there must have been an adequate trial with drug therapy without satisfactory results, and the electroclinical syndrome must be defined. The focal point must be localized, but the presence of scar tissue is not required.
11. d. Rationale: Serum levels of antiseizure drugs are monitored regularly to maintain therapeutic levels of the drug, above which patients are likely to experience toxic effects and below which seizures are likely to occur. EEGs have limited value in diagnosis of seizures and even less in monitoring seizure control.
12. c. Rationale: If antiseizure drugs are discontinued abruptly, seizures can be precipitated, and patients should never just stop their medication. Missed doses should be made up if the omission is remembered within 24 hours, and patients should not adjust medications without professional guidance because this, too, can increase seizure frequency and may cause status epilepticus. If side effects occur, the physician should be notified and drug regimens evaluated. Antiseizure drugs have numerous interactions with other drugs, and the use of other medications should be evaluated by health professionals.
13. a. Rationale: Maintaining an airway during a seizure is important and may involve turning the patient to the side, supporting and protecting the head, or loosening constrictive clothing. Oral airways should not be inserted during the seizure, and restraining a patient during a seizure may cause injury. Suctioning and oxygen administration may be required after the seizure has ended.
14. b. Rationale: In the postictal phase of generalized tonic-clonic seizures, patients are usually very tired and may sleep for several hours, and the nurse should allow the patient to sleep as long as necessary. Suctioning is performed only if it is needed, and decreased level of consciousness is not a problem postictally unless a head injury has occurred during the seizure.
15. b. Rationale: One of the most common complications of a seizure disorder is the effect it has on the patient's lifestyle. This is because of the social stigma attached to seizures, causing patients to hide their diagnosis and to prefer not to be identified as having epilepsy. Job discrimination against the handicapped is prevented by federal and state laws, and patients need to identify their disease in case of medical emergencies. Medication regimens usually require only once- or twice-daily dosing, and the major restrictions of lifestyle usually involve driving and high-risk environments.
16. a. 3; b. 5; c. 4; d. 2; e. 1
17. b. Rationale: Most patients with MS have remissions and exacerbations of neurologic dysfunction that eventually cause progressive loss of motor, sensory, and cerebellar functions. Intellectual function generally remains intact, but patients may experience anger, depression, or euphoria. A few people have chronic progressive deterioration, and some may experience only occasional and mild symptoms for several years after onset.
18. c. Rationale: Motor and sensory dysfunctions, including paresthesias as well as patchy blindness, blurred vision, and hearing loss, are the most common manifestations of MS. Bowel and bladder dysfunctions and ataxia also occur, but excessive involuntary movements, tremors, and memory loss are not seen in MS.
19. d. Rationale: There is no specific diagnostic test for MS, and a diagnosis is made primarily by history and clinical manifestations. In later MS, CT and MRI may detect sclerotic plaques. Some patients have elevations of oligoclonal immunoglobulin G, lymphocytes, and monocytes in cerebrospinal fluid, but these findings do not establish a diagnosis of MS.
20. b. Rationale: Mitoxantrone (Novantrone) is an immunosuppressant drug that reduces both B and T lymphocytes and impairs antigen presentation. It is similar to other immunosuppressants in that it increases the risk for infection, but it cannot be used for more than 2 to 3 years because it causes cardiac toxicity. It is administered IV monthly.
21. c. Rationale: The main goal in care of the patient with MS is to keep the patient active and maximally functional, promoting self-care as much as possible to maintain independence. Assistive devices encourage independence while preserving the patient's energy. No care that patients can do for themselves should be performed by others. Involvement of the family in the patient's care and maintenance of social interactions are also important but are not the priority in care.
22. b. Rationale: Corticosteroids used in treating acute exacerbations should not be abruptly stopped by the patient, because adrenal insufficiency may result, and prescribed tapering doses should be followed. Infections may cause exacer-

bations of symptoms and should be avoided, and high-protein diets with vitamin supplements are advocated. Long-term planning for increasing disability is also important.

23. a. Tremor: impaired handwriting and hand activities
    b. Rigidity: muscle soreness and pain; slowness of movement
    c. Bradykinesia: lack of blinking, arm swinging while walking, and facial expression; shuffling gait; difficulty initiating movement
24. b. Rationale: Although clinical manifestations are characteristic in Parkinson's disease, there are no laboratory or diagnostic tests specific for the condition. A diagnosis is made when there are at least two of the three signs of the classic triad, and it is confirmed with a positive response to antiparkinsonian medication. Essential tremors increase during voluntary movement, while the tremors of Parkinson's disease are more prominent at rest.
25. c. Rationale: The bradykinesia of Parkinson's disease prevents automatic movements, and such activities as beginning to walk, rising from a chair, or even swallowing saliva cannot be executed unless they are consciously willed. Handwriting is affected by the tremor and results in the writing trailing off at the end of words. Specific limb weakness and muscle spasms are not characteristic of Parkinson's disease.
26. c. Rationale: Peripheral dopamine does not cross the blood-brain barrier, but its precursor, levodopa, is able to enter the brain, where it is converted to dopamine, increasing the supply that is deficient in Parkinson's disease. Other drugs used to treat Parkinson's disease include bromocriptine, which stimulates dopamine receptors in the basal ganglia, and amantadine, which is believed to promote the release of dopamine from brain neurons. Carbidopa is an agent that is usually administered with levodopa to prevent the levodopa from being metabolized in peripheral tissues before it can reach the brain.
27. a. Rationale: Speech and swallowing in the patient with Parkinson's disease can be facilitated by massaging the patient's facial and neck muscles to reduce the rigidity that makes chewing, swallowing, and talking difficult for the patient. An upright position and suctioning if secretions are present are necessary to prevent aspiration during eating.
28. c. Rationale: The shuffling gait of Parkinson's disease causes the patient to be off balance and at risk for falling. Teaching the patient to use a wide stance with the feet apart, to lift the toes when walking, and to look ahead helps promote a more balanced gait. Use of an elevated toilet seat and rocking from side to side will enable a patient to initiate movement. Canes and walkers are difficult for patients with Parkinson's disease to maneuver and may make the patient more prone to injury.
29. b. Rationale: The reduction of acetylcholine (ACh) effect in myasthenia gravis (MG) is treated with acetylcholinesterase inhibitors, which prolong the action of ACh at the neuromuscular synapse, but too much of these drugs causes a cholinergic crisis with symptoms very similar to those of MG. To determine whether the patient's manifestations are due to a deficiency of ACh or too much anticholinesterase drug, the anticholinesterase drug edrophonium chloride (Tensilon) is administered. If the patient is in cholinergic crisis, the patient's symptoms will become worse, but if the patient is in a myasthenic crisis, the patient will improve.
30. c. Rationale: The patient in myasthenic crisis has severe weakness and fatigability of all skeletal muscles, affecting the patient's ability to swallow, talk, move, and breathe, but the priority of nursing care is monitoring and maintaining adequate ventilation.
31. c. Rationale: Restless legs syndrome that is not related to other pathologic processes, such as diabetes mellitus or rheumatic disorders, may be caused by an alteration in dopaminergic transmission in the basal ganglia because dopaminergic agents, such as those used for parkinsonism, are effective in managing sensory and motor symptoms. Polysomnography studies during sleep are the only tests that have diagnostic value, and although exercise should be encouraged, excessive leg exercise does not have an effect on the symptoms.
32. b. Rationale: In ALS there is gradual degeneration of motor neurons with extreme muscle wasting from lack of stimulation and use. However, cognitive function is not impaired, and patients feel trapped in a dying body. Chorea manifested by writhing, involuntary movements is characteristic of Huntington's disease. As an autosomal dominant genetic disease, Huntington's disease also has a 50% chance of being passed to each offspring.
33. c. Rationale: Many chronic neurologic diseases involve progressive deterioration in physical or mental capabilities and have no cure, with devastating results for patients and families. Health care providers can only attempt to alleviate physical symptoms, prevent complications, and assist patients in maximizing function and self-care abilities as long as possible.

Case Study

1. The cause of MS is unknown, although research findings suggest MS is related to infectious (viral), immunologic, and genetic factors. T cells are activated by some unknown factor, and these T cells migrate to the CNS and cause a disruption in the blood-brain barrier. Subsequent antigen-antibody reaction within the CNS results in activation of the inflammatory response, and through multiple mechanisms, destruction of the myelin of axons occurs. There is loss of myelin, disappearance of oligodendrocytes, and proliferation of astrocytes. These changes result in characteristic plaque formation, or sclerosis, scattered through the CNS and loss of nerve impulse transmission.
2. The role of precipitating factors, such as exposure to pathogenic agents, in the etiology of MS is controversial. It is possible that their association with MS is random and that there is no cause-and-effect relationship. Possible precipitating factors include emotional stress, excessive fatigue, pregnancy, and a poorer state of health. In Ms. S.'s case, it is possible that the viral neuritis was a precipitating factor.
3. Because there is no definitive diagnostic test for MS, diagnosis is based primarily on history and clinical manifestations. Although MRI can detect sclerotic plaques, Ms. S.'s initial symptoms were so non-specific and transient that often a "wait-and-see" approach is taken.
4. Patient education should focus on preventing exacerbations or worsening of the disease. Building general resistance to illness, including avoiding fatigue, stress, extremes of heat and cold, and exposure to infection, are important measures in maintaining general health. Vigorous and early treatment of infection is critical if it does occur. It is important to teach the patient to (1) achieve a good balance of exercise and rest, (2) eat nutritious and well-balanced meals, and (3) avoid the hazards of immobility (contractures and pressure sores). Patients should know their treatment regimens, the side effects of medications and how to watch for them, and drug interactions with over-the-counter medications. The patient should consult a health care provider before taking nonprescription medications.
5. Because there is no cure for MS, treatment is aimed at slowing the disease process and providing symptomatic relief. The disease process is treated with drugs, and the symptoms are controlled with a variety of medications and other forms of therapy. Corticosteroids are helpful in treating acute exacerbations of the disease, probably by reducing edema and acute inflammation at the site of demyelination. Immunosuppressive drugs, such as azathioprine (Imuran), cyclosporine (Sandimmune), and cyclophosphamide (Cytoxan), have been shown to produce some beneficial effects in patients with severe and relapsing MS. A new immunosuppressant drug, mitoxantrone (Novantrone), reduces both B and T lymphocytes. However, the potential benefits of these drugs in patients with MS need to be counterbalanced against the potentially serious side effects. Immunomodulator drugs, such as interferon β-1b (Betaseron), interferon β-1a (Avonex), and glatiramer acetate (Copaxone), have been effective in reducing frequency and severity of exacerbations, but all of these agents must be administered parenterally. Physical therapy and speech therapy may also help improve neurologic function.
6. *Nursing diagnoses:*
   - Ineffective role performance
   - Anxiety
   - Disturbed sensory perception: visual
   - Risk for impaired parenting

   Collaborative problems:
   Potential complication: blindness

CHAPTER 58

1. a. Rationale: Conditions that decrease the CNS production of acetylcholine are believed to be a critical factor in the development of delirium. Patients with Parkinson's disease are treated with anticholinergics to help balance the deficiency of dopamine characteristic of Parkinson's disease, and these anticholinergics decrease the acetylcholine in the brain. It is true that delirium and Parkinson's disease are seen in older people, but the relationship is more specific than just age.
2. d. Rationale: Cytokines, such as interferons and interleukins, that are increased during infection, inflammation, and cancer, and even treatment of various disorders with cytokines, are believed to be related to the development of delirium.
3. a. age; b. infection (cytokines); c. hypoxemia (lung disease); d. ICU hospitalization (change in environment, sensory overload); e. preexisting dementia; f. dehydration; g. hyperthermia
4. d. Rationale: Delirium is an acute problem that usually has a rapid onset in response to a precipitating event, especially when the patient has underlying health problems, such as heart disease and sensory limitations. In the absence of prior cognitive impairment, a sudden onset of confusion, disorientation, and agitation is usually delirium. Delirium may manifest with both hypo- and hyperactive symptoms.

5. c. Rationale: Care of the patient with delirium is focused on identifying and eliminating precipitating factors if possible. Treatment of underlying medical conditions, changing environmental conditions, and discontinuing medications that induce delirium are important. Drug therapy is reserved for those patients with severe agitation, because the drugs themselves may worsen delirium.
6. a. DL; b. DM; c. DL; d. DL; e. DM; f. DL; g. DM; h. DM; i. DL; j. DM
7. a. T; b. F, vascular; c. T; d. T; e. F, amyloid-beta protein
8. a. Rationale: Depression is often associated with Alzheimer's disease, especially early in the disease when the patient has awareness of the diagnosis and the progression of the disease. When dementia and depression occur together, intellectual deterioration may be more extreme. Depression is treatable, and use of antidepressants often improves cognitive function.
9. c. Rationale: The only definitive diagnosis of Alzheimer's disease can be made on examination of brain tissue on autopsy, but a clinical diagnosis is made when all other possible causes of dementia have been eliminated. Patient's with Alzheimer's disease may have amyloid-beta proteins in the blood, brain atrophy, or isoprostanes in the urine, but these findings are not exclusive to those with Alzheimer's disease.
10. c. Rationale: The Mini-Mental State Examination is a tool to document the degree of cognitive impairment and can be used to determine a baseline from which changes over time can be evaluated. It does not evaluate mood or thought processes but can detect dementia and delirium and differentiate these from psychiatric mental illness. A score of 30 indicates full cognitive function.
11. b. Rationale: Because there is no cure for AD, collaborative management is aimed at improving or controlling decline in cognition and controlling the undesirable manifestations that the patient may exhibit. Anticholinesterase agents help increase acetylcholine in the brain, but a variety of other drugs are also used to control behavior. Memory enhancement techniques have little or no effect in patients with Alzheimer's disease, especially as the disease progresses. Patients with Alzheimer's disease have limited ability to communicate health symptoms and problems, leading to lack of professional attention for acute and other chronic illnesses.
12. a. 3, 10; b. 4, 9; c. 1, 8; d. 6, 8; e. 5, 9; f. 7, 11; g. 3, 8; h. 2, 10; i. 5, 9; j. 1, 8; k. 2, 10
13. c. Rationale: Adhering to a regular, consistent daily schedule helps the patient avoid confusion and anxiety and is important both during hospitalization and at home. Clocks and calendars may be useful in early Alzheimer's disease, but they have little meaning to a patient as the disease progresses. Questioning the patient about activities and events they cannot remember is threatening and may cause severe anxiety. Maintaining a safe environment for the patient is important but does not change the disturbed thought processes.
14. b. Rationale: Caregiver role strain is characterized by such symptoms of stress as inability to sleep, make decisions, or concentrate and is frequently seen in family members who are responsible for the care of the patient with Alzheimer's disease. Assessment of the caregiver may reveal a need for assistance to increase coping skills, effectively use community resources, or maintain social relationships. Eventually the demands on a caregiver exceed the resources, and the person with Alzheimer's disease may be placed in an institutional setting.
15. a. Rationale: Adult day care is an option to provide respite for caregivers and a protective environment for the patient during the early and middle stages of AD. The respite from the demands of care allows the caregiver to maintain social contacts and perform normal tasks of living and be more responsive to the patient's needs. Visits by home care nurses involve the caregiver and cannot provide adequate respite. Institutional placement is not always an acceptable option at earlier stages of AD, nor is hospitalization an acceptable form of respite care.

Case Study

1. The pathophysiology of Alzheimer's disease includes cellular changes with neurofibrillary tangles with altered tau proteins and neuritic plaques containing amyloid-beta protein in the cerebral cortex and hippocampus. Excessive loss of cholinergic neurons is also present, and other neurotransmitters, such as serotonin and norepinephrine, are also lost over time.
2. Alzheimer's disease is diagnosed by exclusion. When all other possible causes of mental impairment and persistence of dementia are ruled out, the diagnosis of Alzheimer's remains. Brain atrophy and enlarged ventricles seen in some patients with Alzheimer's disease are also seen in normal people and in other conditions. Only on autopsy can Alzheimer's disease be confirmed by the presence of neurofibrillary tangles in brain tissue.

3. All functions of mental capacity and ability to care for oneself are lost as the disease progresses. There will be deterioration of personal hygiene and all activities of daily living, progression of psychotic symptoms now evidenced by his hallucinations, loss of long-term memory and recognition of his family, and loss of communication.
4. Assess what she is doing now to manage his care. Teach her about the expected progression of the disease, and assist her in planning respite care or arranging for home health assistants. Help her identify problem areas. Encourage her to keep Mr. D. awake and busy during the day so that he will sleep better at night, and so will she.
5. Community resources may include Alzheimer's support groups, adult day care, home health assistants and home nursing, and various forms of assisted living and long-term care facilities.
6. *Nursing diagnoses:*
   - Risk for injury related to impaired judgment, nighttime wandering
   - Risk for other-directed violence related to misinterpretation of environmental stimuli
   - Disturbed thought processes related to effects of dementia
   - Wandering related to cognitive impairment
   - Disturbed sleep pattern related to circadian asynchrony

   Collaborative problems:
   Potential complication: psychosis
7. Nursing diagnoses:
   - Anxiety related to erratic behavioral patterns and cognitive decline of husband
   - Altered health maintenance related to fatigue and chronic stress
   - Caregiver role strain related to grieving the family member's illness
   - Risk for other-directed violence (patient abuse) related to ineffective coping

   Collaborative problems:
   Potential complication: depression

CHAPTER 59

1. a. T; b. F, Bell's palsy; c. F, corticosteroids; d. F, Bell's palsy; e. T; f. T
2. a. Rationale: The pain of trigeminal neuralgia is excruciating, and it may occur in clusters that continue for hours. The condition is considered benign with no major effects except the pain. Corneal exposure is a problem in Bell's palsy, or it may occur following surgery for treatment of trigeminal neuralgia. Maintenance of nutrition is important but not urgent, because chewing may trigger trigeminal neuralgia and patients avoid eating. Except during an attack, there is no change in facial appearance in a patient with trigeminal neuralgia, and body image is more disturbed in response to the paralysis typical of Bell's palsy.
3. a. Rationale: Although percutaneous radiofrequency rhizotomy and microvascular decompression provide the greatest relief of pain, glycerol rhizotomy causes less sensory loss and fewer sensory aberrations with comparable or better pain relief. The suboccipital craniotomy and microvascular decompression require a cranial incision and carry the highest risk for complications.
4. c. Rationale: Because attacks of trigeminal neuralgia may be precipitated by hot or cold air movement on the face, jarring movements, or talking, the environment should be of moderate temperature and free of drafts, and patients should not be expected to converse during the acute period. Patients often prefer to carry out their own care because they are afraid someone else may inadvertently injure them or precipitate an attack. The nurse should stress that oral hygiene be performed because patients often avoid it, but residual food in the mouth after eating occurs more frequently with Bell's palsy.
5. a. Rationale: The most serious complication of Guillain-Barré syndrome is respiratory failure, and it is essential that vital capacity and ABGs are monitored to detect involvement of the nerves that affect respiration. Corticosteroids may be used in treatment but do not appear to have an effect on the prognosis or duration of the disease. Rather, plasmapheresis or administration of high-dose immunoglobulin does result in shortening recovery time. The peripheral nerves of both the sympathetic and parasympathetic nervous systems are involved in the disease and may lead to orthostatic hypotension, hypertension, and abnormal vagal responses affecting the heart. Guillain-Barré syndrome may affect the lower brainstem and CNs VII, VI, III, XII, V, and X, affecting facial, eye, and swallowing functions.
6. c. Rationale: As nerve involvement ascends, it is very frightening for the patient, but more than 85% of patients with Guillain-Barré syndrome recover completely with care. Patients also recover if ventilatory support is provided during respiratory failure, although 5% to 10% of patients die from respiratory failure or cardiac arrhythmias. Guillain-Barré syndrome affects only peripheral nerves and does not affect the brain.
7. a. 3; b. 1; c. 2; d. 1; e. 2; f. 3; g. 2; h. 1; i. 2; j. 3; k. 1
8. d. Rationale: Spinal cord injuries are highest in young adult men between the ages of 15 and 30

and those who are impulsive or risk takers in daily living. Other risk factors include alcohol and drug abuse as well as participation in sports and occupational exposure to trauma or violence.

9. b. Rationale: Tetraplegia with motor and sensory loss is characteristic of a complete cord injury at the level of C8, with paraplegia with motor and sensory loss at the level of T1. A hemiplegia occurs with central (brain) lesions affecting motor and sensory function, and any partial loss of function is associated with incomplete spinal cord lesions.
10. a. 5; b. 4; c. 1; d. 3; e. 2
11. c. Rationale: The primary injury of the spinal cord rarely affects the entire cord, but the pathophysiology of secondary injury may result in damage that is the same as mechanical severance of the cord. Complete cord dissolution occurs through autodestruction of the cord by hemorrhage, edema, and the presence of metabolites and norepinephrine, resulting in anoxia and infarction of the cord. Edema secondary to the inflammatory response may increase the damage as it extends above and below the injury site.
12. c. Rationale: Spinal shock occurs in about half of all people with acute spinal cord injury. In spinal shock, the entire cord below the level of the lesion fails to function, resulting in a flaccid paralysis and hypomotility of most processes without any reflex activity. Return of reflex activity signals the end of spinal shock. Sympathetic function is impaired below the level of the injury because sympathetic nerves leave the spinal cord at the thoracic and lumbar areas, and cranial parasympathetic nerves predominate in control over respirations, heart, and all vessels and organs below the injury. Neurogenic shock results from loss of vascular tone caused by the injury and is manifested by hypotension, peripheral vasodilation, and decreased cardiac output. Rehabilitation activities are not contraindicated during spinal shock and should be instituted if the patient's cardiopulmonary status is stable.
13. b. Rationale: Until the edema and necrosis at the site of the injury are resolved in 72 hours to 1 week after the injury, it is not possible to determine how much cord damage is present from the initial injury, how much secondary injury occurred, or how much the cord was damaged by edema that extended above the level of the original injury. The return of reflexes signals only the end of spinal shock, and the reflexes may be inappropriate and excessive, causing spasms that complicate rehabilitation.
14. a. Above T5; b. Above C4; c. Below C4; d. Above L3
15. b. Rationale: Care of the patient during the acute phase, when the influence of the sympathetic nervous system is decreased, includes monitoring for bradycardia that can compromise cardiac output and lead to hypoxemia because of the effect of the vagus nerve on the heart and vessels. Anything that causes vagal stimulation may cause cardiac arrest, and cardiovascular instability is a major complication of unopposed vagal stimulation. Return of reflexes, effects of sensory deprivation, and fluctuations in body temperature should also be monitored, but they do not have the priority that cardiovascular status does.
16. a. 7; b. 3; c. 9; d. 7; e. 1; f. 6
17. d. Rationale: Although surgical treatment of spinal cord injuries often depends on the preference of the physician, surgery is usually indicated when there is continued compression of the cord by extrinsic forces or when there is evidence of cord compression. Other indications may include progressive neurologic deficit, compound fracture of the vertebra, bony fragments, and penetrating wounds of the cord.
18. a. Rationale: The need for a patent airway is the first priority for any injured patient, and a high cervical injury may decrease gag reflex and ability to maintain an airway, as well as the ability to breathe. Maintaining cervical stability is then a consideration, along with assessing for other injuries and the patient's neurologic status.
19. c. Rationale: Cervical injuries usually require skeletal traction with the use of Crutchfield, Vinke, or other types of skull tongs to immobilize the cervical vertebrae, even if fracture has not occurred. Hard cervical collars are used for minor injuries or for stabilization during emergency transport of the patient. Sandbags are also used temporarily to stabilize the neck during insertion of tongs or during diagnostic testing immediately following the injury. Special turning or kinetic beds may be used to turn and mobilize patients who are in cervical traction.
20. d. Rationale: Early, large-dose methylprednisolone is standard treatment for spinal cord injuries because it has been found to improve blood flow and reduce edema in the spinal cord following injury. Tirilazad (Freedox) has the same use as methylprednisolone with perhaps fewer adverse effects. Other vasoactive drugs for spinal cord damage are currently being studied. Dopamine and IV fluids are used to maintain blood pressure during the initial stage of injury.
21. b. Rationale: Because pneumonia and atelectasis are potential problems related to ineffective coughing and the loss of intercostal and abdominal muscle function, the nurse should frequently

monitor the patient for breath sounds and respiratory function to determine whether secretions are being retained or whether there is progression of respiratory impairment. Suctioning is not indicated unless lung sounds indicate retained secretions, and the prone position, although used for positioning patients with spinal cord injuries, can compromise respiratory function. Intubation and mechanical ventilation are used if the patient becomes exhausted from labored breathing or if ABGs deteriorate.

22. c. Rationale: During the first 2-3 days after a spinal cord injury, paralytic ileus may occur, and nasogastric suction must be used to remove secretions and gas from the gastrointestinal tract until peristalsis resumes. IV fluids are used to maintain fluid balance but do not specifically relate to paralytic ileus. Tube feedings would be used only for patients who had difficulty swallowing and not until peristalsis returned, and TPN would be used only if the paralytic ileus was unusually prolonged.
23. a. Rationale: During the acute phase of spinal cord injury, the bladder is hypotonic, causing urinary retention with the risk for reflux into the kidney or rupture of the bladder. An indwelling catheter is used to keep the bladder empty and closely monitor urinary output. Intermittent catheterization and/or other urinary drainage methods may be used in long-term bladder management. Use of incontinent pads is inappropriate because the bladder fails to empty.
24. b. Rationale: In 1 week following a spinal cord injury, there may be a resolution of the edema of the injury and an end to spinal shock. When spinal shock ends, reflex movement and spasms will occur, which may be mistaken for return of function, but with the resolution of edema, some normal function may also occur. It is important when movement occurs to determine whether the movement is voluntary and can be consciously controlled, which would indicate some return of function.
25. b. Rationale: Manifestations of autonomic dysreflexia include severe hypertension, bradycardia, headache, blurred vision, and flushing and diaphoresis above the level of the lesion, and it is a life-threatening situation. At the first indication, the nurse should check the patient's blood pressure, raise the head of the bed to 45 degrees, check for the stimulus that is causing the reaction (usually a distended bladder or rectum), and notify the physician if it is apparent that the problem is autonomic dysreflexia.
26. d. Rationale: A neurogenic bladder is any type of bladder dysfunction related to abnormal or absent bladder innervation and occurs not only with spinal cord injury but also with many other conditions as well. To determine what function the bladder has, diagnostic evaluation must be performed with cystometrograms and perhaps an IV pyelogram and urine culture before appropriate interventions can be instituted. The bladder may have various degrees of flaccidity or spasticity.
27. d. Rationale: Intermittent catheterization five to six times a day is the recommended method of bladder management for the patient with a spinal cord injury because it more closely mimics normal emptying and has less potential for infection. The patient and family should be taught the procedure using clean technique, and if the patient has use of the arms, self-catheterization should be performed. Indwelling catheterization is used during the acute phase to prevent overdistention of the bladder, and suprapubic indwelling catheters and surgical urinary diversions are used if urinary complications occur.
28. d. Rationale: Most patients with a complete lower motor neuron lesion are unable to have either psychogenic or reflexogenic erections, and alternative methods of obtaining sexual satisfaction may be suggested. Patients with incomplete lower motor neuron lesions have the highest possibility of successful psychogenic erections with ejaculation, while patients with incomplete upper motor neuron lesions are more likely to experience reflexogenic erections with ejaculation. Patients with complete upper motor neuron lesions usually only have reflex sexual function with rare ejaculation.
29. a. Rationale: Working through the grief process is a lifelong process that is triggered by new experiences, such as marriage, child rearing, employment, or illness, which the patient must adjust to throughout life within the context of his or her disability. The goal of recovery is related to adjustment, rather than acceptance, and many patients do not experience all components of the grief process. During the anger phase, patients should be allowed outbursts, and the nurse should use humor to displace some of the patient's anger.
30. b. Rationale: Most metastatic tumors are extradural lesions that may be successfully removed surgically. Most tumors of the spinal cord are slow-growing, do not cause autodestruction and, with the exception of intradural-intramedullary tumors, can be removed with complete functional restoration. Radiation is used

to treat metastatic tumors that are sensitive to radiation and that have caused only minor neurologic deficits in the patient; radiation also is used as adjuvant therapy to surgery for intramedullary tumors.

Case Study

1. Susan is experiencing central cord syndrome of the cervical cord, in which there is compression on anterior horn cells. It usually occurs as a result of hyperextension.
2. The cell bodies of lower motor neurons, which send axons to innervate the skeletal muscles of arms, trunk, and legs, are located in the anterior horn of the spinal cord. The cervical segments of the spinal cord contain the lower motor neurons for the arms, and a cervical injury that affects the anterior horn will affect the arms to a greater extent than the legs.
3. Injury to the cord may occur without fracture of the vertebrae, with traumatic twisting or stretching of the cord. The response to the trauma includes secondary injury leading to edema, hemorrhage, and ischemia of the cord, impairing function.
4. Methylprednisolone has been found to improve blood flow and reduce edema in the spinal cord, with the effects of reduction of posttraumatic spinal cord ischemia, improvement of energy balance, restoration of extracellular calcium, improvement of nerve impulse condition, and repression of the release of free fatty acids from spinal cord tissues.
5. Shock and denial are common first reactions to the loss of function with spinal cord injuries, followed by anger and depression. During the acute phase, Susan will probably have unrealistic expectations concerning her recovery, sleep a lot, and withdraw. As she progresses she will become angry and refuse to discuss her limitations. Altered body image will be a big problem because she will see herself as different from her peers, an important developmental issue during adolescence.
6. Intensive rehabilitation that focuses on refined retraining of physiologic function of her limbs should be planned and will involve much physical therapy over time. She should be mobilized as quickly as appropriate to prevent hazards of immobility and to encourage her in her progress.
7. *Nursing diagnoses:*
   - Impaired physical mobility related to spinal cord injury and prescribed bed rest
   - Risk for disuse syndrome related to immobilization
   - Self-care deficit: feeding, bathing/hygiene, and grooming related to upper extremity weakness
   - Risk for injury related to sensory deficit and lack of self-protective abilities

   Collaborative problems:
   Potential complications: progression of lesion; hypoventilation; spinal shock

CHAPTER 60

1. a. epiphysis; b. metaphysis; c. diaphysis; d. periosteum; e. compact bone; f. bone marrow; g. medullary cavity; h. epiphyseal growth plate; i. cancellous bone; j. articular cartilage
2. a. periosteum; b. canaliculi; c. haversian canal; d. blood vessels; e. haversian system (osteon)
3. a. joint cavity; b. bursa; c. articular cartilage; d. periosteum; e. joint capsule; f. nerve; g. blood vessel; h. synovial membrane; i. bone

4. a. haversian; b. sarcomere; c. epiphysis; d. osteocyte; e. tendon; f. periosteum; g. synovium; h. isometric; i. calcium; j. canaliculi; k. osteoclast; l. atrophy; m. actin; n. bursae; o. osteoblast; p. cartilage; q. ligament; r. fascia; s. hyaline; t. striated

```
M I T I S O M E T R I C E T
P N A I S R E V A H T P E O
R A D E T A I R T S I E R L
S T B U R S A E A P U M E I
O R A R S N I L H V D U M G
S O S T E O C Y T E L G O A
S P E R I O S T E U M A C M
C H E L E I A E N M A H R E
A Y R T S F F W D A L Y A N
L U S B O S T E O B L A S T
C O W A A C T I N E O L U X
I M C A N A L I C U L I S T
U L Y T A M M U I V O N Y S
M S E G A L I T R A C E N S
```

5. a. 1; b. 1, 2, 3; c. 1, 2, 3; d. 4; e. 1, 2, 3; f. 1; g. 1, 2, 3
6. d. Rationale: Loss of water from disks between vertebrae, vertebral disk compression, and narrowing of intervertebral spaces all contribute to a loss of height in the older adult. Although bone density decreases and cartilage is lost from joints, these do not affect the long bones or the height of the person.
7. c. Rationale: Cartilage disruption and overgrowth of bone around joint margins that occur with aging result in joint stiffness and pain that most often affect physical mobility. Changes in the bones lead to decreased bone mass and the possibility of fractures. Fatigue and a high risk for impaired skin integrity are not directly related to changes in the musculoskeletal system that are associated with aging.
8. a. Rationale: Corticosteroids cause protein catabolism with skeletal muscle wasting and increased osteoclast activity with loss of bone mass, which can have a marked detrimental effect on mobility and activity. Potassium-depleting diuretics may cause hypokalemia, which is associated with muscle weakness and cramps. Oral hypoglycemic drugs and NSAIDs are not known to have an effect on the musculoskeletal system.
9. a. History of musculoskeletal injuries, poor use of body mechanics or excessive muscular stress, family history of joint and bone disease
   b. Presence of obesity, inadequate calcium, vitamin D or C, or protein intake
   c. Inability to physically access toilet; constipation
   d. Limitation of movement; pain, weakness, crepitus; extremes of occupational activity—sedentary or heavy use of body
   e. Pain interfering with sleep; frequent position changes
   f. Musculoskeletal pain; pain management measures
   g. Loss of body image or self-worth, caused by musculoskeletal deformity
   h. Change in work and family roles and responsibilities, caused by immobility or pain
   i. Decreased sexual activity and satisfaction because of pain, deformity
   j. Decreased coping ability related to effect of musculoskeletal problems

10. c. Rationale: Muscle strength is graded on a scale of 0 to 5, with 0 = no detection of muscle strength and 5 = active movement against full resistance (normal). Active movement against gravity and some resistance = 4.
11. b. Rationale: There is no indication to measure the length of limbs during assessment unless a gait disturbance or limb-length discrepancy is noted, and then the limb should be measured between two bony prominences and compared with the measurement of the opposite extremity. Muscle mass measurement and joint movement may affect gait, but differences in limb length will always affect gait. Palpating for crepitus will identify friction between bones, usually at joints.
12. c. Rationale: A goniometer is a protractor device that measures the angle of joints and can be used to determine specific degrees of joint range of motion. It is used when a specific musculoskeletal problem has been identified that affects ROM.
13. a. 10; b. 7; c. 9; d. 1; e. 6; f. 8; g. 5; h. 4; i. 2; j. 3
14. a. Standard x-ray; b. Arthrocentesis; c. Diskogram; d. Dual-energy x-ray absorptiometry (DEXA); e. Electromyogram; f. Creatine kinase
15. a. Rheumatoid factor (RF); b. Erythrocyte sedimentation rate (ESR); c. Antinuclear antibody (ANA)

CHAPTER 61

1. d. Rationale: Musculoskeletal problems in the older adult can be prevented with appropriate strategies, especially exercise. Almost all older adults have some degree of decreased muscle strength, joint stiffness, and pain with motion. The use of mild antiinflammatory agents decreases inflammation and pain and can help the patient maintain activity and prevent further deconditioning. Stair walking can create enough stress on fragile bones to cause a hip fracture, and use of ramps may help prevent falls. Walkers and canes should be used as necessary to decrease stress on joints so that activity can be maintained.
2. c. Rationale: Warm-up exercises "prelengthen" potentially strained tissues by avoiding the quick stretch often encountered in sports and also increase the temperature of muscle, resulting in increased speed of cell metabolism, increased speed of nerve impulses, and improved oxygenation of muscle fibers. Stretching is also thought to improve kinesthetic awareness, lessening the chance of uncoordinated movement. Taping or wrapping joints may actually predispose a person to injury, and muscle strength is not a key factor in soft tissue injuries.
3. a. 8; b. 10; c. 6; d. 2; e. 9; f. 1; g. 3; h. 7; i. 4; j. 5
4. b. Rationale: Application of cold, compression, and elevation is indicated to prevent edema resulting from sprain and strain injury. Muscle spasms are usually treated with heat applications and massage, and repetitive strain injuries require cessation of the precipitating activity and physical therapy. Dislocations or subluxations require immediate reduction and immobilization to prevent vascular impairment and bone cell death.
5. a. Rationale: Immobilization of a joint after the acute damage leads to muscle shortening, atrophy, and possible contractures. Gentle, progressive exercise is indicated to promote circulation and healing and increase muscle strength and function. Immobilization and rest, alternating use of heat and cold, and administration of antiinflammatory drugs are indicated for management of acute soft tissue injury.
6. a. 4; b. 8; c. 5; d. 6; e. 1; f. 9; g. 2; h. 7; i. 10; j. 3
7. a. 3; b. 5; c. 1; d. 6; e. 2; f. 6; g. 2; h. 4; i. 6; j. 2; k. 5
8. b. Rationale: Deformity is the cardinal sign of fracture but may not be apparent in all fractures. Other supporting signs include edema and swelling, pain and tenderness, muscle spasm, ecchymosis, loss of function, and crepitation.
9. a. Rationale: A malunion occurs when the bone heals in the expected time but in an unsatisfactory position, possibly resulting in deformity or dysfunction. Nonunion occurs when the fracture fails to heal properly despite treatment, and delayed union is healing of the fracture at a slower rate than expected. The loss of bone substances as a result of immobilization occurs in posttraumatic osteoporosis.
10. a. F, reduction; b. T; c. F, infection; d. F, skin; e. F, foot of the bed; f. T
11. d. Rationale: The suspension of the extremity provided by the use of a Thomas splint and Pearson attachment in balanced suspension traction allows the patient to raise the body off the bed with the support of a trapeze and the unaffected leg. The patient is not allowed to turn from side to side, but care is enhanced by upward elevation of the body. Because the other skeletal and skin traction do not suspend the affected limbs, this movement is not possible.
12. a. Rationale: Basic maintenance of traction requires that weights hang free and consist of the prescribed amount of weight, ropes are intact and ride in the pulleys, knots are secure, and pulley clamps are firmly fastened to the bedframe. The patient should be in direct alignment with the

traction and should exercise the unaffected limb as much as possible to prevent complications of immobility.

13. d. Rationale: Complaints of abdominal pain or pressure, nausea, and vomiting are signs of cast syndrome that occur when body casts are applied too tightly, causing compression of the superior mesenteric artery against the duodenum. The cast may need to be split or removed, and the physician should be notified. Elevation is not indicated for a spica cast, and the patient with a spica cast should not be placed in the prone position during the initial drying stage, because the cast is so large and heavy it may break. A cast should never be covered with a blanket, because heat builds up in the cast and may increase edema.
14. b. Rationale: Infection is the greatest risk with an open fracture, and all open fractures are considered contaminated. Tetanus prevention is always indicated if the patient has not been immunized or does not have current boosters. Prophylactic antibiotics are often used in management of open fractures, but recent antibiotic therapy is not relevant, nor are previous injuries to the site.
15. d. Rationale: Pulses distal to the injury should be checked before and after splinting to assess for nerve or vascular damage and documented to avoid doubts about whether a problem discovered later was missed during the original examination or was caused by the treatment. Elevation of the limb and application of ice should be instituted after the extremity is splinted.
16. b. Rationale: Neurologic assessment includes evaluation of motor and sensory function and, in the upper extremity, includes abduction and adduction of the fingers, opposition of the fingers, and suppination and pronation of the hands. It would also include sensory perception in the fingers. Evaluation of the feet would occur in lower extremity injuries. Assessment of color, temperature, capillary refill, peripheral pulses, and edema evaluates vascular status.
17. b. Rationale: A patient with any type of cast should exercise the joints above and below the cast frequently, and moving the fingers frequently will improve circulation and help prevent edema. Unlike plaster casts, thermoplastic resin or fiberglass casts are relatively waterproof and, if they become wet, can be dried with a hair dryer on low setting. Tape petals are used on plaster casts to protect the edges from breaking and crumbling but are not necessary for synthetic casts. After the cast is applied, the extremity should be elevated at about the level of the heart to promote venous return, and ice may be used to prevent edema.
18. a. Rationale: A swing-to gait is a three-point gait in which the patient places the crutches ahead of the unaffected leg and swings up to the level of the crutches, keeping weight off the affected leg. It is safer than a swing-through gait because it provides better balance and stability. Two-point and four-point gaits are used when at least partial weight bearing is allowed on the limb.
19. c. Rationale: Progressive pain that is distal to the injury and is unrelieved by usual analgesics is the earliest sign of compartment syndrome. Paralysis and absence of peripheral pulses will eventually occur if it is not treated, but these are late signs that often appear after permanent damage has occurred. The overlying skin may appear normal because the surface vessels are not occluded.
20. a. Paresthesia; b. Pain; c. Pressure; d. Pallor; e. Paralysis; f. Pulselessness
21. a. Rationale: Soft tissue edema in the area of the injury may cause an increase of pressure within the closed spaces of the tissue compartments formed by the nonelastic fascia, creating a compartment syndrome. If symptoms occur, it may be necessary to surgically incise the fascia, a procedure known as a fasciotomy. Amputation is usually necessary only if the limb becomes septic because of untreated compartment syndrome.
22. a. Rationale: Initial manifestations of fat embolism usually occur 12 to 72 hours after injury and are associated with fractures of long bones and multiple fractures related to pelvic injuries, including fractures of the femur, tibia, ribs, and pelvis.
23. d. Rationale: Patients with fractures are at risk for both fat embolism and pulmonary embolism from peripheral thromboses, but there is a difference in the time of occurrence, with fat embolism occurring shortly after the injury and thrombotic embolism occurring several days after immobilization. They both may cause pulmonary symptoms of chest pain, tachypnea, dyspnea, apprehension, tachycardia, and cyanosis, but fat embolism may cause petechiae located around the neck, anterior chest wall, axilla, buccal membrane of the mouth, and conjunctiva of the eye, which differentiate it from thrombotic embolism.
24. a. 2; b. 3; c. 1; d. 7; e. 4; f. 2; g. 6; h. 5; i. 7; j. 1; k. 6; l. 3; m. 5; n. 4; o. 6
25. a. F, intracapsular; b. T; c. F, intracapsular; d. T; e. T
26. d. Rationale: The classic signs of a hip fracture are shortening of the leg and external rotation accompanied by severe pain at the fracture site. The patient may not be able to move the hip or the knee, but movement in the ankle and toes is not affected.

27. c. Rationale: Although surgical repair is the preferred method of managing intracapsular and extracapsular hip fractures, initially patients are frequently treated with skin traction, such as Buck's extension or Russell's traction, to temporarily immobilize the limb and relieve the painful muscle spasms before surgery is performed. Prolonged traction would be required to reduce the fracture or immobilize it for healing, creating a very high risk for complications of immobility.
28. a. Rationale: Because the fracture site is internally fixed with pins or plates, the fracture site is stable, and the patient is moved from the bed to the chair on the first postoperative day, with ambulation beginning on the first or second postoperative day, without weight bearing on the affected leg. Weight bearing on the affected extremity is usually restricted for 3 to 5 months until adequate healing is evident on x-ray. The patient may be positioned on the operative side following internal fixation, and abductor pillows are used for patients who have total hip replacements.
29. d. Rationale: Patients with hip prostheses must avoid extreme flexion, adduction, or internal rotation for at least 6 weeks to prevent dislocation of the prosthesis. Gradual weight bearing on the limb is allowed, and ambulation should be encouraged.
30. c. Rationale: The low-bulk, high-carbohydrate liquid diet and intake of air through a straw required during mandibular fixation often lead to constipation and flatus, which may be relieved with bulk-forming laxatives, prune juice, or ambulation. Wires or rubber bands should be cut only in the case of cardiac or respiratory arrest, and patients should be taught to clear their mouth of vomitus or secretions. The mouth should be thoroughly cleaned with water, saline, or alkaline mouthwashes or with the use of a Water Pik as necessary to remove food debris. Hard candy should not be held in the mouth.
31. b. Rationale: Patients with peripheral vascular disease often have extensive arterial impairment that necessitates removal of a limb much higher than is indicated by external signs of ischemia, in order for healing to occur. Preoperative arteriography and transcutaneous Doppler studies help determine the point at which blood supply is adequate for healing. As much limb as possible is preserved to enhance rehabilitation. Amputation does not alter the underlying vascular disease.
32. b. Rationale: The disruption in body image caused by an amputation often causes a patient to go through psychologic stages of grieving, and the patient should be allowed to go through a period of depression as a normal consequence of the amputation. The grieving process is not ineffective coping or impaired adjustment but a normal process of adjusting to loss.
33. b. Rationale: Phantom sensation or phantom pain may occur following amputation, especially if pain was present in the affected limb preoperatively. The pain is a real sensation to the patient and should be treated with analgesics and other pain interventions. As recovery and ambulation progress, phantom limb sensation usually subsides.
34. b. Rationale: An immediate prosthetic fitting involves the application of a rigid plastic bandage with a prosthetic pylon and ankle-foot assembly. Because the device covers the residual limb, the surgical site cannot be directly seen, and postoperative hemorrhage is not apparent on dressings, requiring vigilant assessment of vital signs for signs of bleeding. Elevation of the residual limb with an immediate prosthetic fitting is not necessary because the device itself prevents edema formation. Exercises to the leg are not performed in the immediate postoperative period, in order to prevent disruption of ligatures and the suture line.
35. a. Rationale: Flexion contractures, especially of the hip, may be debilitating and delay rehabilitation of the patient with a leg amputation. To prevent hip flexion, the patient should avoid sitting in a chair with the hips flexed or having pillows under the surgical extremity for prolonged periods, and the patient should lie on the abdomen for 30 minutes three to four times a day to extend the hip.
36. a. Rationale: Skin breakdown on the residual limb can prevent the use of a prosthesis, and the limb should be inspected every day for signs of irritation or pressure areas. No substances except water and mild soap should be used on the residual limb, and ROM exercises are not necessary when the patient is using a prosthesis. A residual limb shrinker is an elastic stocking that is used to mold the limb in preparation for prosthesis use, but a cotton residual limb sock is worn with the prosthesis.
37. a. 3; b. 4; c. 5; d. 1; e. 2
38. d. Rationale: Physical therapy is initiated one day postoperatively with ambulation and weight bearing with a walker for a patient with a cemented prosthesis and non-weight bearing on the operative side for an uncemented prosthesis. In addition, the patient is turned to both sides and back with support of the operative leg and sits in the chair at least twice a day.

39. b. Rationale: Following a total hip arthroplasty, extremes of internal rotation, adduction, and 90-degree flexion of the hip must be avoided for 4 to 6 weeks postoperatively to prevent dislocation of the prosthesis. During hospitalization an abduction pillow is placed between the legs to maintain abduction, and the leg is extended.
40. b. Rationale: Continuous passive motion machines are frequently used following knee surgery to promote earlier joint mobility, and because joint dislocation is not a problem with knee replacements, early exercise with straight leg raises and gentle ROM is also encouraged postoperatively.
41. b. Rationale: Neurovascular checks of the fingers following surgery of the hands are essential to detect compromised vascular and neurologic function due to trauma or edema. Postoperatively the hands are elevated with a bulky dressing in place, and when the dressing is removed, a guided splinting program is started. Exercises are performed three to four times a day when the splints are removed and the patient is discharged. Before surgery, it must be made clear to the patient that the goal of the surgery is to restore function related to grasp, pinch, stability, and strength, and the hands will not necessarily have good cosmetic appearance.

Case Study

1. The knee and ankle should be immobilized with the splint. Unless the joints above and below the site are immobilized, the affected area is unstable.
2. The five Ps should be assessed: pulses, paresthesias, pallor, paralysis, and pain, especially unrelieved pain, which may indicate compartment syndrome.
3. The wound should be cleaned with extensive irrigation with normal saline, and if the wound is highly contaminated, surgical debridement may be necessary. Tetanus immunization is required if a dose of tetanus toxoid has not been given in the past 5 years, or if the patient has had fewer than three doses of toxoid, tetanus immunoglobulin should be administered. Bleeding should be controlled with sterile dressings.
4. Measures to relieve pain include elevating the limb and applying ice to decrease swelling, administering analgesics, and keeping the limb immobilized.
5. It will take about 20 weeks for complete healing of the fracture, but ossification should take place in 2 to 3 weeks. At that time the limb can be casted, and he can be mobile with crutches with no weight bearing on the affected limb. Weight bearing will be restricted for 6 to 12 weeks, depending on the rate of healing. His return to work will depend on how he is able to perform his responsibilities on crutches.
6. Mrs. A. should be called and informed of her husband's accident, and she should be told that Mr. A. is alert and oriented but that he has a fractured leg and will require hospitalization. Care should be taken not to panic her and to reassure her that he is stable.
7. *Nursing diagnoses:*
   - Acute pain related to edema and muscle spasms
   - Risk for peripheral neurovascular dysfunction related to edema
   - Risk for infection related to disruption of skin integrity and presence of environmental pathogens
   - Anxiety related to unknown outcome and restrictions

   Collaborative problems:
   Potential complications: fat embolism; compartment syndrome; infection; malunion or nonunion

CHAPTER 62

1. c. Rationale: Chronic infection of the bone leads to formation of scar tissue from the granulation tissue. This avascular scar tissue provides an ideal site for continued microorganism growth and is impenetrable to antibiotics. Surgical debridement is often necessary to remove the poorly vascularized tissue and dead bone and instill antibiotics directly to the area. Involucrum is new bone laid down at the infection site, which seals off areas of sequestra. Antibiotics can be effective during acute osteomyelitis, and prevention of chronic osteomyelitis requires early antibiotic treatment. Bone and skin grafting may be necessary following surgical removal of infection if destruction is extensive.
2. b. Rationale: The patient with osteomyelitis is at risk for pathologic fractures at the site of the infection because of weakened, devitalized bone, and careful handling of the extremity is necessary. Range-of-motion exercises should be limited because of the possibility of spread of infection, and edema is not a common finding in osteomyelitis. Careful handling of dressings is necessary to prevent the spread of infection to others.
3. c. Rationale: Because large doses of appropriate antibiotics are necessary in treatment of acute osteomyelitis, it is important to identify the causative microorganism. The definitive way to

determine the causative agent is by bone biopsy or biopsy of the soft tissue surrounding the site. The other tests may help establish the diagnosis but do not identify the causative agent.

4. d. Rationale: Activities such as exercise or heat application, which increase circulation and serve as stimuli for the spread of infection, should be avoided by patients with acute osteomyelitis. Oral or IV antibiotic therapy is continued at home for 4 to 8 weeks, and weight bearing is contra-indicated to prevent pathologic fractures.
5. b. Rationale: One of the most common adverse effects of prolonged and high-dose antibiotic therapy is overgrowth of *Candida albicans* in the oral cavity and genitourinary tract. These infections are manifested by whitish-yellow, curdlike lesions of the mucosa. A dry, cracked, furrowed tongue is characteristic of severe dehydration, vesicles are characteristic of herpes simplex infections, and mouth and lip ulcers are characteristic of aphthous somatitis, or canker sores.
6. a. 4; b. 1; c. 3; d. 2; e. 1; f. 2; g. 3
7. b. Rationale: Promotion of muscle activity is important in any patient with muscular dystrophy, but when the disease has progressed to cardiomyopathy and/or respiratory failure, activity must be balanced with oxygen supply. At this stage of the disease, care should be taken to prevent skin or respiratory complications. The patient should be encouraged to perform as much self-care and exercise as energy allows, but this will be limited.
8. a. T; b. F, mechanical strain of paravertebral muscles; c. T; d. F, herniated lumbar intervertebral disk; e. T; f. T
9. a. Rationale: Proper daily exercise is an important part of the prevention of back injury, with the goal of maintaining mobility and strength in the back. Patients should sit with the knees higher than the hips and should sleep in a side-lying position, with knees and hips bent, or on the back, with a device to flex the hips and knees. Although some occupations, such as those requiring prolonged driving and heavy, repetitive lifting, pose a high risk for acute back pain, most jobs require body use. Good body mechanics with proper transfer and turning techniques are necessary in all activities.
10. b. Rationale: Patients with chronic back pain may develop sick role behavior because of poor self-esteem and inability to adjust to the chronic pain condition, and the nurse should encourage activity within the patient's limitation to maintain physical mobility and independence in order to prevent assumption of this behavior. Coping is improved if the patient understands the nature of the pain and can make lifestyle adjustments for the pain. Pain control may require use of NSAIDs and other methods.
11. d. Rationale: During acute back pain, the head of the bed should be kept elevated 20 degrees and the knees slightly flexed to prevent strain on the back muscles. Exercise of the legs increases pain and should be avoided, and neurovascular, not neurologic, assessment of the legs is indicated. This is not an appropriate time to assess body mechanics, because frequently the patient cannot even stand upright.
12. b. Rationale: Urinary incontinence following spinal surgery may indicate nerve damage and should be reported to the physician. Paralytic ileus is common following surgery and is expected. Pain at the graft site, usually the iliac crest or the fibula, often is more severe than pain from the fused area, and although movement and sensation of the arms and legs should not be more impaired than before surgery, they often are not relieved immediately after surgery.
13. c. Rationale: After spinal surgery, patients are logrolled to maintain straight alignment of the spine at all times, requiring the patient to be turned with a pillow between the legs and moving the body as a unit. The head of the bed is usually kept flat, and the legs are extended.
14. a. 4; b. 7; c. 5; d. 2; e. 3; f. 1; g. 2; h. 5; i. 1; j. 6
15. c. Rationale: Poorly fitted shoes selected for fashion rather than comfort are the primary factor in the development of foot problems. A few congenital problems predispose to foot problems, and poor hygiene in patients with peripheral vascular disease may lead to foot infections, but these factors are in the minority in comparison with the effect of ill-fitting shoes.
16. a. 3; b. 1; c. 2; d. 1; e. 3; f. 2; g. 2
17. d. Rationale: Risk factors for osteoporosis include female gender, Caucasian and Asian race, prolonged immobility, insufficient calcium intake, smoking and alcoholism, and estrogen deficiency. Decreased risk is associated with physical activity, especially stress on bones, and fluoride and vitamin D intake.
18. a. Increased calcium intake and vitamin D; b. Weight-bearing exercise; c. Postmenopausal estrogen replacement therapy; d. Biphosphonates (e.g., etidronate [Didronel], alendronate [Fosamax])

Case Study

1. Risk factors for back pain in Mr. Brown include excess body weight, cigarette smoking, and a job that requires heavy lifting and prolonged periods of sitting.
2. Preoperative preparation includes teaching about the restrictions on positioning and movement required following surgery, measures for pain control, and assessments that will be carried out postoperatively. The nurse should ensure that Mr. Brown has received information about the procedure from the surgeon and understands the benefits and risks of the surgery.
3. Mr. Brown will probably be restricted to flat bed rest for at least the first 24 hours to avoid straining the surgical area. Pillows may be used under the thigh of each leg to prevent strain on the back muscles. When turning is allowed, he must be turned with the help of several personnel to avoid changing the alignment of the spine, or log-rolled. Depending on the surgeon's preference, ambulation will usually begin by the second postoperative day, again keeping the spine in alignment.
4. These postoperative assessments should be carried out by the nurse q2-4hr during the first 24-48 hours:
   - Sensation: in all extremities in all appropriate dermatomes
   - Movement: of all extremities
   - Muscle strength: note any weakness of the extremities
   - Wound: assess dressing for drainage and note amount, color, characteristics; clear or light yellow drainage should be tested for the presence of glucose, which would indicate spinal fluid leakage
   - Pain: document location and intensity of pain; evaluate pain after administration of analgesia
   - Bowel activity: assess bowel sounds, passage of flatus, and abdomen; paralytic ileus is common for several days
   - Urinary function: incontinence or retention may indicate nerve damage and should be reported. Intermittent catheterization may be required for bladder emptying, especially until Mr. Brown is allowed to stand to void.
5. Discharge instructions include teaching Mr. Brown to report any persistent limb weakness, abnormal sensations, or pain to the health care provider. He should be instructed to avoid standing or sitting for prolonged periods of time. Walking, lying down, and shifting weight from one foot to another should be encouraged. Twisting of the spine is harmful, and he should be taught to think through any activity before bending, lifting, or stooping. A firm mattress or bed board should be used at home. To prevent further back problems, weight loss and smoking cessation should be encouraged. He should be taught correct body mechanics and to do strengthening back exercises after recovery from the surgery (Tables 62-5 and 62-6).
6. *Nursing diagnoses:*
   - Acute pain related to nerve root compression, muscle spasms, and surgical incision
   - Impaired physical mobility related to pain
   - Ineffective therapeutic regimen management related to lack of knowledge regarding posture, exercises, body mechanics, and weight reduction

   Collaborative problems:
   Potential complication: paralysis

CHAPTER 63

1. d. Rationale: Cartilage destruction in the joints affects 90% of people by the age of 40, and when the destruction becomes symptomatic, osteoarthritis is said to be present. Because degenerative changes cause symptoms in only about 60% of those over the age of 65, joint pain and functional disability should not be considered a normal finding in aging persons. Osteoarthritis is not a systemic disease, and although degenerative changes can be accelerated by excessive use of or stress on a joint, many people with joint pain have no history of previous joint stress or injury.
2. a. 3; b. 5; c. 6; d. 1; e. 4; f. 2
3. a. F, Heberden's; b. F, bone surfaces rubbing together; c. T; d. F, acetaminophen; e. T
4. b. Rationale: Principles of joint protection and energy conservation are critical in being able to maintain functional mobility in the patient with osteoarthritis, and patients should be helped to find ways to perform activities and tasks with less stress. Range-of-motion, isotonic, and isometric exercises of the affected joints should be balanced with joint rest and protection, but during an acute flare of joint inflammation, the joints should be rested. If a joint is painful, it should be used only to the point of pain, and masking the pain with analgesics may lead to greater joint injury.
5. c. Rationale: Common side effects of NSAIDs include GI irritation and bleeding, dizziness, rash, headache, and tinnitus. Oral lesions and blood dyscrasias are common in patients receiving immunosuppressive agents and disease-modifying agents. Fluid retention, hypertension, and bruising from capillary fragility are frequently seen in patients using systemic corticosteroids.

6. b. Rationale: There are promising results from the use of glucosamine and chondroitin sulfate in the treatment of arthritis, and overall, these substances have few side effects. The one identified contraindication to the use of glucosamine is diabetes mellitus because glucosamine may enhance the effects of hypoglycemic drugs.
7. a. Rationale: Alternatives to traditional NSAIDs that are not tolerated because of their GI effects are newer, selective COX-2 inhibitors, which include celecoxib, valdecoxib, and rofecoxib. These drugs inhibit COX-2 without affecting COX-1, an enzyme that primarily protects the stomach lining. Indomethocin, naproxen, and diclofenac are all traditional NSAIDs that inhibit both COX-1 and COX-2.
8. d. Rationale: In rheumatoid arthritis (RA), autoantibodies known as rheumatoid factors are formed against abnormal IgG, which is stimulated by an unknown factor. When the autoantibodies and the abnormal IgG combine, they form immune complexes that are deposited in the joints, blood vessels, and pleura and cause activation of complement with a resulting inflammatory response. The joint and systemic manifestations of RA are a result of the action of inflammatory mediators and cells. Some patients with RA have a prevalence of the HLA-DR4 antigen, but it does not directly cause damage.
9. a. RA; b. OA; c. OA; d. B; e. RA; f. B; g. RA; h. OA; i. B; j. O; k. RA
10. a. 3; b. 6; c. 2; d. 1; e. 4; f. 5; g. 7
11. c. Rationale: A patient with moderate RA has no joint deformities but may have limited joint mobility, adjacent muscle atrophy, and inflammation of the joints. Synovial hypertrophy and thickening of the joint capsule may cause spindle-shaped fingers. Splenomegaly may be found with RA, and crepitus on movement and Heberden's nodes are associated with osteoarthritis.
12. c. Rationale: The inflammatory reactions of RA cause an elevation in C-reactive protein (CRP), a finding that is useful in monitoring the response to therapy. The WBC count may be increased in response to inflammation and is also elevated in synovial fluid. Anemia, rather than polycythemia, is common, and normal IgG levels are not affected.
13. a. Rheumatoid nodules: firm, nontender, subcutaneous masses occurring over the extensor surfaces of joints, such as fingers and elbows
    b. Sjögren's syndrome: diminished lacrimal and salivary gland secretions
    c. Felty's syndrome: inflammatory eye disorders, splenomegaly, lymphadenopathy, pulmonary disease, and blood dyscrasias
14. a. 7; b. 6; c. 5; d. 1; e. 9; f. 2; g. 3; h. 1; i. 7; j. 2; k. 5; l. 4; m. 8; n. 2
15. c. Rationale: Because older adults are more likely to take many drugs, the use of multidrug therapy in RA is particularly problematic because of the increased likelihood of untoward drug interactions and toxicity. Rheumatic disorders do occur in older adults but usually in milder form. Interpretation of laboratory values in older adults is more difficult in diagnosing RA because of age-related serologic changes, but the disease can be diagnosed. Older adults are not less compliant with drug regimens but may need help with complex regimens.
16. b. Rationale: Most patients with RA experience morning stiffness, and morning activities should be scheduled later in the day after the stiffness subsides. A warm shower in the morning and time to become more mobile before activity are advised. Management of RA includes daily exercises for the affected joints and protection of joints with devices and movements that prevent joint stress. Splinting should be done during an acute flare to rest the joint and prevent further damage.
17. b. Rationale: Pacing activities and alternating rest with activity are important in maintaining self-care and independence of the patient with RA, in addition to preventing deconditioning and a negative attitude. The nurse should not carry out activities for patients that they can do for themselves but should support and assist patients as necessary.
18. d. Rationale: Cold therapy is indicated to relieve pain during an acute inflammation, can be applied with frozen packages of vegetables, and should only last 10-15 minutes at a time. Heat in the form of heating pads, moist warm packs, paraffin baths, or warm baths or showers is indicated to relieve stiffness and muscle spasm. Heat should not be applied for more than 20 minutes at a time.
19. c. Rationale: Aquatic exercises in warm water allow easier joint movement because of the buoyancy of the water, yet water produces more resistance and can strengthen the muscles. Tai Chi is also a good form of gentle, stretching exercise that would be appropriate. Dancing and even walking impact the joints of the feet, and even low-impact aerobics could be damaging. Exercises for those with RA should be gentle.
20. d. Rationale: An unusually high frequency of HLA-B27 is found in patients with ankylosing spondylitis, psoriatic arthritis, and Reiter's syndrome, and these diseases have a predilection for involvement of the spine, peripheral joints, and

periarticular structures, as well as an absence of rheumatoid factor and autoantibodies.

21. d. Rationale: Kyphosis and involvement of costovertebral joints in ankylosing spondylitis lead to a bent-over posture and a decrease in chest expansion, manifestations that are managed with chest expansion and deep-breathing exercises. Postural training emphasizes avoiding forward flexion during any activities, and the patient should sleep on the back without the use of pillows.
22. a. 6; b. 4; c. 1; d. 2; e. 3; f. 5; g. 6; h. 1; i. 3; j. 5; k. 4; l. 2
23. d. Rationale: The diagnosis of gout is established by finding monosodium urate monohydrate crystals in the synovial fluid of an inflamed joint or tophus. Hyperuricemia and elevated urine uric acid are not diagnostic for gout, because they may be related to a variety of drugs or may exist as a totally asymptomatic abnormality in the general population. Although there is a familial predisposition to hyperuricemia, both environmental and genetic factors contribute to gout.
24. b. Rationale: Colchicine has an antiinflammatory action specific for gout and is the treatment of choice during an acute attack, often producing dramatic pain relief in 24 to 48 hours. It may also be used prophylactically to reduce the frequency of attacks. Probenecid is a uricosuric drug that is used to control hyperuricemia by increasing the excretion of uric acid through the kidney, and allopurinol is also used to control hyperuricemia by blocking production of uric acid. Aspirin inactivates the effect of uricosuric drugs and should not be used when patients are taking probenecid and other uricosuric drugs.
25. b. Rationale: During therapy with probenecid or allopurinol, the patient must have periodic determination of blood uric acid levels to evaluate the effectiveness of the therapy and to ensure that levels are kept low enough to prevent future attacks of gout. Patients should not alter their doses of medications without medical direction, and the drugs used for control of gout are not useful in the treatment of an acute attack. With the use of medications, strict dietary restrictions of alcohol and high-purine foods are usually not necessary. When the patient is taking probenecid, urine output should be maintained at 2-3 L to prevent urate from precipitating in the urinary tract and causing kidney stones.
26. a. Rationale: In systemic lupus erythematosus (SLE), autoantibodies are produced against nuclear antigens, cytoplasmic antigens, and blood cell surface antigens, and the clinical manifestations of SLE depend on which cell types or organs are involved. Overproduction of collagen is characteristic of systemic sclerosis, and abnormal IgG reactions with autoantibodies is characteristic of rheumatoid arthritis.
27. a. Cutaneous vascular lesions on sun-exposed skin with classic butterfly rash on face; b. Polyarthralgia and polyarthritis; c. Arrythmias; d. Restrictive lung disease with cough, tachypnea and pleurisy; e. Proteinuria resulting from nephritis; f. Seizures, peripheral neuropathy; g. Anemia, leukopenia, and thrombocytopenia
28. b. Rationale: Patients with SLE often find that one of the most difficult facets of the disease is its extreme variability in severity and progression. There is no characteristic pattern of progressive organ involvement, nor is it predictable as to which systems may become affected. SLE is now associated with a normal lifespan, but patients must be helped to adjust to the unknown course of the disease.
29. c. Rationale: Efficacy of treatment with corticosteroids or immunosuppressive drugs is best monitored by serial serum complement levels and anti-DNA titers, both of which will decrease as the drugs have an effect. A reduction in ESR is not as specific, and the patient with SLE often has a chronic anemia that is not affected by drug therapy.
30. a. Rationale: Acute exacerbations of SLE may be precipitated by overexposure to ultraviolet light, physical and emotional stress, fatigue, and infection or surgery. The major concern in planning a pregnancy is that exacerbations are also common following delivery, and there are increased risks for the mother and fetus during pregnancy. Although SLE has an identified genetic association with HLA-DR2 and HLA-DR3, genetic counseling is not usually recommended. Dietary recommendations include small, frequent meals and adequate iron intake. Although nonpharmacologic methods of pain control are encouraged, the use of NSAIDs is often necessary to help control inflammation and pain.
31. a. Rationale: Skin lesions of SLE include discoid lesions and diffuse maculopapular rashes, and it is important to keep the skin clean and dry to prevent infection. Unprescribed ointments, lotions, or cosmetics often exacerbate existing conditions and should not be used.
32. d. Rationale: Systemic sclerosis is a disorder of connective tissue that causes skin thickening and tightening, resulting in expressionless facial features, puckering of the mouth, and a small oral orifice. It also causes symmetric, painless swelling or thickening of the skin of the fingers and hands. It does not cause the swan-neck or

ulnar drift deformities seen in RA or SLE, and low back pain and spinal stiffness are associated with ankylosing spondylitis.

33. d. Rationale: One of the most common and early manifestations of CREST syndrome is Raynaud's phenomenon, which causes paroxysmal vasospasms of the digits with diminished blood flow to the fingers and toes on exposure to cold, followed by cyanosis and then erythema on rewarming. The hands and feet must be protected from cold exposure and possible burns or cuts that might heal slowly, and smoking is contraindicated. Ultraviolet light sensitivity is not a factor in systemic sclerosis, nor is fluid intake. Cardiovascular involvement may occur, but it does not require patient monitoring.
34. c. Rationale: Dermatomyositis produces symmetric weakness of striated muscle, and weak neck and pharyngeal muscles may produce dysphasia. Deglutition impairment contributes to death from dermatomyositis and requires special attention during mealtime to prevent aspiration. Muscle tenderness or pain is uncommon, as is joint involvement. During an acute attack the patient is so weak that bed rest is needed, and passive ROM is usually required.
35. b. Rationale: The diagnosis of dermatomyositis in older men is frequently associated with concurrent malignant disease, and a careful search for possible malignant lesions should be made. The disease is more common in the fifth and sixth decades of life and can be diagnosed with serum muscle enzymes.
36. b. Rationale: People with FMS typically experience nonrestorative sleep, morning stiffness, irritable bowel syndrome, and anxiety in addition to the widespread, nonarticular musculoskeletal pain and fatigue. FMS is nondegenerative, nonprogressive, and noninflammatory. Neither muscle weakness nor muscle spasms are associated with the disease, although there may be tics in the muscle at the tender points.
37. d. Rationale: Two criteria for the diagnosis of FMS are that (1) pain is experienced in 11 of the 18 tender points on palpation and (2) the patient has a history of widespread pain for at least 3 months. The other findings may also be present but are not diagnostic for FMS.
38. c. Rationale: The pain and related symptoms of FMS cause significant stress, and anxiety is a common finding. Stress management is an important part of the treatment and may include any of the commonly used relaxation strategies as well as psychologic counseling.
39. a. Unexplained, persistent, or relapsing chronic fatigue that is of new and definite onset
    b. Fatigue is not due to ongoing exertion.
    c. Fatigue is not substantially alleviated by rest.
    d. Fatigue results in substantial reduction in occupational, educational, social, or personal activities.

Case Study

1. Mrs. M. should be told that rheumatoid arthritis is a disease that affects all of her body, even though her joints are primarily affected at this time. She needs to know that it is not known what causes RA but that antibodies are formed which react with substances causing inflammation and damage to a variety of organs. Joint changes include inflammation of the lining of the joints and eventual filling of the joint with bone, completely immobilizing the joint and causing deformities similar to those she is developing in her hands. She should be told that the fatigue and low-grade fever she has are part of the disease and that with disease control these symptoms will improve.
2. The painful, stiff hands and feet, the fatigue, the low-grade fever, and the ulnar drift deviation are all manifestations of RA.
3. Methotrexate is a chemotherapeutic agent that has an antiinflammatory effect but causes bone marrow suppression and hepatotoxicity. Its dosage in RA is much smaller than that used for cancer therapy, and side effects are not as common. When used in RA, it frequently reduces clinical symptoms in days to weeks with few, if any, adverse effects. Teaching Mrs. M. about methotrexate is an important nursing responsibility. Periodic blood chemistry and hematology tests must be done, the patient should take a daily supplement of folic acid, and the patient should report signs of anemia or any infection. Methotrexate is teratogenic, and Mrs. M. should be informed that contraception must be used during and 3 months after treatment.
4. Protection of her joints will be enhanced if she can maintain a normal weight, avoid tasks that cause pain, use assistive devices to prevent joint stress, and avoid forceful, repetitive movements. She should plan regularly scheduled rest periods alternated with activity throughout the day and should develop organizing and pacing techniques that spread tasks through the day or the week. Suggesting that she take a warm shower or bath in the morning to relieve her morning stiffness may be helpful. Exercise regimens will be prescribed for Mrs. M., and she should be encouraged to follow the regimens daily.

5. Because of the chronicity and disability associated with arthritis, patients are often vulnerable to claims of unproven remedies. The nurse should recognize that the copper bracelet will do no harm but may be a waste of money for Mrs. M. It is important to encourage her to recognize that regular, proven methods of treatment used on a consistent basis are the best way to control her condition. The more she is taught about the disease and its management, the more compliant she will be with treatment regimens.
6. Additional sources of information and sharing are available from the Arthritis Foundation and should be suggested to Mrs. M.
7. *Nursing diagnoses:*
   - Acute and chronic pain related to joint inflammation
   - Impaired physical mobility related to joint pain, stiffness, and deformity
   - Fatigue related to disease activity
   - Ineffective therapeutic regimen management related to use of unproven remedies
   - Risk for infection related to altered immune function

   Collaborative problems:
   Potential complication: bone marrow suppression

CHAPTER 64

1. d. Rationale: One of the primary characteristics of critical care nurses that is different from those of generalist medical-surgical nurses is the use of advanced technology to accurately measure physiologic parameters and manage life-threatening complications. All nursing addresses human responses to health problems and requires knowledge of physiology, pathophysiology, pharmacology, and psychologic support to the patient and family. Diagnosis and treatment of life-threatening diseases are roles of medicine.
2. a. Physiologically unstable; b. Risk for serious complications; c. Risk for serious complications; d. Intensive nursing support
3. a. Rationale: When anxiety in the ICU patient is related to the environment that has unfamiliar equipment, high noise and light levels, and an intense pace of activity, which leads to sensory overload, the nurse should eliminate as much of this source of stress as possible by muting phones, limiting overhead paging, setting alarms appropriate to the patient's condition, and eliminating unnecessary alarms. Flexible visiting schedules for family members and providing as much autonomy in decisions about care as possible are indicated when impaired communication and loss of control contribute to the anxiety. Use of sedation to reduce anxiety should be carefully evaluated and implemented when nursing measures are not effective.
4. c. Rationale: The family of the critically ill patient is very important in the recovery and well-being of the patient, and the extent to which the family is involved and supported affects the patient's clinical course. Although the cost of planning and providing critical care is a concern to families, it is not the major reason that family members are included in the patient's care. Family members may be responsible for making decisions about the patient's care only when the patient is unable to make personal decisions. Most families have questions regarding the patient's quality of care, because of anxiety and lack of information about the patient's condition.
5. a. Decreased; b. Increased; c. Decrease; d. Increase; e. Increased; f. Increases
6. d. Rationale: Cardiac output is dependent on heart rate and stroke volume, and stroke volume is determined by preload, afterload, and contractility. If cardiac output is decreased and heart rate is unchanged, stroke volume is the variable factor. If the preload determined by PAWP and the afterload determined by SVR are unchanged, the factor that is changed is contractility of the myocardium.
7. b. Rationale: Referencing hemodynamic monitoring equipment means positioning the monitoring equipment so that the zero reference point is at the vertical level of the left atrium of the heart. The port of the stopcock nearest the transducer is placed at the phlebostatic axis, the external landmark of the left atrium. The phlebostatic axis is the intersection of two planes: a horizontal line midchest, halfway between the outermost anterior and posterior surfaces, transecting a vertical line through the fourth intercostal space at the sternum.
8. a. T; b. F, pulmonary artery; c. F, left ventricle; d. T; e. T
9. c. Rationale: During insertion of a pulmonary artery catheter, it is necessary to monitor the ECG continuously because of the risk for arrhythmias, particularly when the catheter reaches the right ventricle. It is the physician's responsibility to obtain informed consent regarding the catheter insertion. During the catheter insertion the patient is placed supine with the head of the bed flat. An Allen test to confirm adequate ulnar artery perfusion is performed before insertion of an arterial catheter in the radial artery for arterial pressure monitoring.
10. a. Slowly inflate the pulmonary artery catheter balloon with 1.0 to 1.5 ml of air while observ-

ing the pressure tracing, and measure the PAWP at the end of expiration, limiting the balloon inflation to less than four respiratory cycles.

b. Rapidly inject the prescribed amount and temperature of solution into the right atrial lumen of the pulmonary artery catheter, and read the computer display of the cardiac output.

11. a. MAP—75 mm Hg (90 + 136/3)
PAP—26 mm Hg (20 + 1/3 of 18)
SV—25.8 ml/beat (3.2 x 1000/124)
SVR—1625 dyne sec/cm^5 (75 – 10 x 80/3.2)

b. All of the changes in the hemodynamic parameters are characteristic findings in the patient with heart failure: increased pulmonary congestion and pressures; increased pressure in the left atrium and ventricle; increased systemic vascular resistance; and decreased stroke volume, cardiac output, and systemic blood pressure.

12. b. Rationale: The normal mixed venous oxygen saturation of 60%-80% becomes decreased with decreased arterial oxygenation, low cardiac output, low hemoglobin, or increased oxygen consumption. With normal cardiac output, arterial oxygenation, and hemoglobin, the factor that is responsible for decreased SvO_2 is increased oxygen consumption, which can result from increased metabolic rate, pain, movement, or fever.

13. d. Rationale: When a pulmonary artery pressure tracing indicates a wedged wave form when the balloon is deflated, this indicates that the catheter has advanced and has become spontaneously wedged. If the catheter is not repositioned immediately, a pulmonary infarction or a rupture of a pulmonary artery may occur. If the catheter is becoming occluded, the pressure tracing becomes blunted, and pulmonary edema and increased pulmonary congestion increase the pulmonary artery wave form. Balloon leaks that are found when injected air does not flow back into the syringe do not alter wave forms.

14. c. Rationale: The counterpulsation of the intra-aortic balloon pump increases diastolic arterial pressure, forcing blood back into the coronary arteries and main branches of the aortic arch, increasing coronary artery perfusion pressure and blood flow to the myocardium. The balloon pump also causes a drop in aortic pressure just before systole, decreasing afterload and myocardial oxygen consumption. These effects make the IABP valuable in treating unstable angina, acute myocardial infarction, and a variety of surgical heart situations. Its use is contraindicated in incompetent aortic valves, dissecting aortic aneurysms, and generalized peripheral vascular disease.

15. a. F, afterload; b. T; c. F, diastolic

16. c. Rationale: Because the IABP is inserted into the femoral artery and advanced to the descending thoracic aorta, compromised distal extremity circulation is common and requires that the cannulated extremity be extended at all times. Repositioning the patient is limited to side-lying or supine positions with the head of the bed elevated no more than 30 to 45 degrees. Assessment for bleeding is important because the IABP may cause platelet destruction, and occlusive dressings are used to prevent site infection.

17. d. Rationale: Weaning from the IABP involves reducing the pumping to every second or third heart beat or gradually decreasing the augmentation pressure until the IABP catheter is removed. The pumping and infusion flow are continued to reduce the risk for thrombus formation around the catheter until it is removed.

18. b. Rationale: Ventricular assist devices are temporary devices that can partially or totally support circulation until the heart recovers and can be weaned from cardiopulmonary bypass or a donor heart can be obtained. The devices currently available do not permanently support circulation, and many patients die while awaiting a donor heart.

19. c. Rationale: A nasal endotracheal tube is longer and smaller in diameter than an oral endotracheal tube, creating more airway resistance and increasing the work of breathing. Suctioning and secretion removal are also more difficult with a nasal endotracheal tube, and they are more subject to kinking than are oral tubes. Oral tubes require a bite block to stop the patient from biting the tube and may cause more laryngeal damage because of their larger size.

20. b. Rationale: An alert patient should be informed of the sensations likely to be experienced during endotracheal intubation, in order to help prevent anxiety and panic when feelings of suffocation are experienced. The patient may be asked to extrude the tongue during nasal intubation. The patient is positioned with the mouth, pharynx, and trachea in direct alignment, with the head extended in the "sniffing position," but the head must not hang over the edge of the bed. Talking is not possible during intubation or while the tube is in place, because the tube splits the vocal cords.

21. d. Rationale: The first action by the nurse following endotracheal intubation is to auscultate the chest to confirm bilateral breath sounds and observe to confirm bilateral chest expansion. If this evidence is present, the tube is secured and connected to an O_2 source. Then the placement is confirmed immediately with x-ray, and the tube is

marked where it exits the mouth. Then the patient should be suctioned as needed.

22. c. Rationale: The minimal occluding volume (MOV) involves adding air to the endotracheal tube cuff until no leak is heard at peak inspiratory pressure but ensures that minimal pressure is applied to the tracheal wall to prevent pressure necrosis of the trachea. The minimal occluding volume should apply between 20 to 25 mm Hg pressure on the trachea to prevent injury. The cuff does not secure the tube in place but rather prevents escape of ventilating gases through the upper airway.
23. a. 8, between 20 and 25 mm Hg; b. suctioning; bag-valve mask (BVM); c. half; d. 100 to 120 mm Hg; e. 10 seconds or less; f. hyperoxygenates, hyperventilates
24. c. Rationale: Suctioning an endotracheal tube is performed when adventitious sounds over the trachea and/or bronchi confirm the presence of secretions that can be removed by suctioning. Visible secretions in the ET tube, respiratory distress, suspected aspiration, increase in peak airway pressures, and changes in oxygen status are other indications. Peripheral crackles are not an indication for suctioning, and suctioning as a means of inducing a cough is not recommended, because of the complications associated with suctioning.
25. d. Rationale: If serious arrhythmias occur during suctioning, the suctioning should be stopped, and the patient should be slowly ventilated via MRB with 100% oxygen until the arrhythmia subsides. Patients with bradycardia should not be suctioned excessively. Ventilation of the patient with slow, small-volume breaths using the MRB is performed when severe coughing results from suctioning.
26. a. Use two nurses—one to hold the tube while it is untaped or the holder is loosened and another to perform care.
    b. After completion of care, confirm the presence of bilateral breath sounds to ensure that the position of the tube was not changed.
27. c. Rationale: Because the patient with an ET tube cannot protect the airway from aspiration and cannot swallow, the cuff should always be inflated and the head of the bed elevated while the patient is receiving tube feedings or mouth care is being performed. Patients with ET tubes cannot phonate, and clearing the ventilatory tubing of condensed water is important to prevent respiratory infection. The mouth and oropharynx should be suctioned with a Yankauer or tonsil suction to remove accumulated secretions that cannot be swallowed.
28. a. Rationale: The nurse should carefully observe the patient for respiratory distress and laryngospasm following extubation that may indicate a need for immediate reintubation. The tube and the oropharynx are suctioned before removal of the tube, and the patient is encouraged to cough after the tube is removed. ABGs are not routinely assessed after tube removal, but SpO_2 may be monitored.
29. d. Rationale: A maximal inspiratory pressure of –15 cm H_2O indicates that the patient does not have enough negative inspiratory force, or muscular strength, to promote effective ventilation and is an indication for mechanical ventilation. Other indications for mechanical ventilation include $PaCO_2$ greater than 55 mm Hg, tidal volume less than 5 ml/kg, and resting minute ventilation greater than 10 L/min.
30. a. N; b. P; c. B; d. N; e. N; f. B; g. P; h. N
31. a. 2; b. 1; c. 2; d. 2; e. 1
32. a. CPAP—continuous positive airway pressure; b. SIMV—synchronized intermittent mandatory ventilation; c. CMV—controlled mechanical ventilation; d. PSV—pressure support ventilation; e. ACV—assist-control ventilation; f. PEEP—positive end-expiratory pressure; g. HFV—high-frequency ventilation; h. PC/IRV—pressure-controlled/inverse-ratio ventilation
33. c. Rationale: Positive pressure ventilation, especially with end-expiratory pressure, increases intrathoracic pressure with compression of thoracic vessels, resulting in decreased venous return to the heart, decreased left ventricular end-diastolic volume (preload), decreased cardiac output, and lowered blood pressure. None of the other factors are related to increased intrathoracic pressure.
34. d. Rationale: Decreased cardiac output associated with positive pressure ventilation and PEEP results in decreased renal perfusion, release of renin, and increased aldosterone secretion, which causes sodium and water retention. ADH may be released because of stress, but ADH is responsible only for water retention, and increased intrathoracic pressure decreases, not increases, the release of atrial natriuretic factor, causing sodium retention. There is decreased, not increased, insensible water loss via the airway during mechanical ventilation.
35. b. Rationale: The ABGs reflect a trend toward respiratory alkalosis, and although the $PaCO_2$ is within normal limits, if a patient with COPD is ventilated with a return to a normal $PaCO_2$, the patient will develop an alkalosis because of chronically retained bicarbonate. The patient is being overventilated, and the rate or volume of

respirations should be decreased to maintain the $PaCO_2$ at the patient's normal value. PEEP is generally contraindicated or used with extreme caution in patients with COPD, and these patients usually do better with a short inspiratory and longer expiratory time.

36. c. Rationale: Neuromuscular blocking agents produce a paralysis that facilitates ventilation, but they do not sedate the patient. It is important for the nurse to remember that the patient can hear, see, think, and feel and should be addressed and given explanations accordingly. Communication with the patient is possible, especially from the nurse, but visitors for an anxious and agitated patient should provide a calming, restful effect on the patient.
37. a. Anemia resulting in poor O_2 transport; b. Decreased respiratory strength; c. Delayed weaning; d. Decreased resistance to infection; e. Decreased recovery
38. b. Rationale: A leaking cuff can lower the tidal volume delivered by the ventilator, resulting in hypoventilation. Other causes are low Tv or respiratory rates, an SIMV rate tht is too low, presence of lung secretions, or obstruction. A decreased $PaCO_2$ and increased pH indicate a respiratory alkalosis from hyperventilation, and cardiac arrhythmias can occur with either hyper- or hypoventilation.
39. b. Rationale: A variety of ventilator weaning methods is used, but all should provide for weaning trials with adequate rest between weaning trials to prevent respiratory muscle fatigue. Weaning is usually carried out during the day, with the patient ventilated at night until there is sufficient spontaneous ventilation without excess fatigue. In all methods, patients usually require a 10% increase in FIO_2 to maintain arterial oxygen tension. If the patient becomes hypoxemic, ventilator support is indicated.
40. c. Rationale: Care of a ventilator-dependent patient in the home usually requires extensive nursing care and financial and time commitments. The nurse should ensure that family members understand the potential sacrifices they may have to make and the impact that home mechanical ventilation will have over time, before final decisions and arrangements are made.

Case Study

1. The best indicators to use to monitor Mr. V.'s hemodynamic status are the values determined from the pulmonary artery catheter, the urinary output, and the blood pressure, because infectious processes are altering his level of consciousness, skin temperature, and other vital signs that may commonly be used to monitor hemodynamic status. Of the hemodynamic parameters, it is most important to monitor CO, SVR, and SVO_2 because these parameters are the most out of range and suggest septic shock.
2. PEEP is used for Mr. V. to increase his oxygenation because his PaO_2 is decreased, but it can increase intrathoracic pressure, suppressing venous return and increasing intracranial pressure.
3. Mr. V.'s MAP is 64 mm Hg (46 + 1/3 of 54). The MAP necessary to promote tissue and cerebral perfusion and yet not increase ICP would be a MAP that maintains a CPP of 70 mm Hg. With an intracranial pressure of 22 mm Hg, MAP needs to be 92 mm Hg to maintain cerebral perfusion, yet not increase ICP. (CPP = MAP – ICP, or 70 = 92 – 22.) His current MAP results in a cerebral perfusion pressure of 42, which is inadequate to maintain cerebral perfusion.
4. Fluid therapy would include rapid administration of 0.9% sodium chloride, colloids, or both to expand vascular volume and maintain tissue perfusion, with monitoring of PAP, PAWP, and CO to evaluate fluid replacement. Lactated Ringer's is contraindicated because of the patient's elevated lactate levels. Antibiotics specific for cryptococcal infections, such as fluconazole (Diflucan), should be initiated immediately, and a broad-spectrum antibiotic, such as an aminoglycoside, is indicated for bacterial prophylaxis. Vasopressor agents, such as norepinephrine (Levophed), dopamine (Intropin), or phenylephrine (Neo-Synephrine), are indicated to promote vasoconstriction and increase systemic vascular resistance. After fluid therapy has been initiated, an osmotic diuretic, such as mannitol, may be used to pull water out of the brain tissue and decrease intracranial pressure. Aspirin or other antipyretics should be given to control his temperature, because increased temperature increases metabolic rate and oxygen need. Sodium bicarbonate is not indicated to correct the patient's acidosis unless the pH is below 7.20.
5. Gastrointestinal ischemia may cause translocation of bowel bacteria into the systemic circulation, creating a source of further infection and sepsis. Early institution of enteral tube feedings may help promote perfusion of the gastrointestinal tract and prevent bacterial translocation.
6. *Subjective assessment findings:*
Seizures reflect the cerebral irritation caused by the inflammation of the meninges and the increased intracranial pressure.

Objective assessment findings:
- Increased intracranial pressure is responsible for the GCS score of 6 and is reflected by the ICP of 22 mm Hg.
- The infectious process of the meningitis is reflected by the increased body temperature and the WBC count of 18,500/μl.
- The response of the sympathetic nervous system to the inflammation and sepsis is seen in the elevated blood glucose level.
- Most of the other findings reflect the development of septic shock, systemic inflammatory response syndrome (SIRS), and possible development of multiple organ dysfunction syndrome (MODS).
- Shock is evident from the lowered blood pressure, metabolic acidosis, markedly reduced systemic vascular resistance (SVR), and decreased urinary output resulting from poor renal perfusion.
- Septic shock is characterized by activation of mediators that cause widespread vasodilation and increased capillary permeability, resulting in decreased systemic vascular resistance (SVR) and high cardiac output (CO) because of the decreased peripheral resistance. The vasodilation causes the skin to be warm and dry. Septic shock also results in poor oxygen utilization, resulting in elevated mixed venous oxygen saturation (SVO_2). All of these processes are reflected in the assessment findings in this patient.
- The ABGs and increased lactate indicate the metabolic acidosis resulting from anaerobic metabolism of cells. The $PaCO_2$ and HCO_3^- are low, and the respiratory rate is increased, indicating the body's attempt to compensate for the metabolic acidosis by using bicarbonate to buffer lactic acid and by hyperventilation to blow off extra carbon dioxide.
- The decreased urinary output and decreased arterial oxygenation may reflect not only poor perfusion to the kidneys and lungs but also initial organ damage and development of MODS.

7. *Nursing diagnoses:*
   - Ineffective cerebral tissue perfusion related to cerebral tissue swelling
   - Ineffective peripheral tissue perfusion related to deficit in capillary blood supply
   - Ineffective protection related to neurosensory alterations
   - Hyperthermia related to inflammatory process
   - Ineffective airway clearance related to unconsciousness and presence of artificial airway
   - Risk for injury related to endotracheal intubation, mechanical ventilation, seizure activity, and environmental hazards
   - Risk for aspiration related to presence of artificial airway
   - Imbalanced nutrition: less than body requirements related to increased caloric demands and inability to take nourishment orally
   - Risk for decreased cardiac output related to impeded venous return by PEEP

   Collaborative problems:
   Potential complications: ARDS; DIC; organ ischemia—neurologic, renal, GI, respiratory; pneumothorax or pneumomediastinum; MODS

CHAPTER 65

1. d. Rationale: Although all of the factors may be present, regardless of the cause, the end result is inadequate supply of oxygen and nutrients to body cells from inadequate tissue perfusion.
2. a. 1; b. 2; c. 1; d. 2; e. 2
3. a. 2; b. 3; c. 5; d. 1; e. 2; f. 1; g. 5; h. 4; i. 3; j. 5; k. 1; l. 5; m. 5; n. 2
4. a. F, hypovolemic; b. T; c. T; d. T; e. F, absolute
5. a. Decreased capillary hydrostatic pressure; b. Alpha-adrenergic stimulation; c. Beta-adrenergic stimulation, increased heart strength and rate; d. Renin release; e. Aldosterone secretion; f. Increased venous return to heart, increased blood pressure; g. Increased serum osmolality, release of ADH; h. Renal water reabsorption
6. a. Increased heart rate (beta-adrenergic stimulation); b. Cool, pale skin (alpha-adrenergic stimulation); c. Thirst (with fluid shift to intravascular space); d. Decreased urinary output (ADH and aldosterone); e. Fluctuating blood pressure; f. Decreased bowel sounds (alpha-adrenergic stimulation); Others: abdominal distention, edema (sodium retention)
7. a. Rationale: When sepsis is the cause of shock, the endotoxins stimulate a cascade of inflammatory responses that start with release of TNF and IL-1, which stimulate other inflammatory mediators that increase neutrophil and platelet aggregation and adhesion to the endothelium. There is an increase in coagulation and inflammation and fibrinolysis, and platelet-activating factor causes formation of microthrombi and vessel obstruction. The process does not occur in other types of shock until late stages.
8. a. Renin-angiotensin activation causes arteriolar constriction, decreasing perfusion.
   b. Vasoconstriction of the pulmonary arterioles decreases the blood flow to pulmonary capillaries, and a ventilation-perfusion mismatch

occurs. Areas of the lung that are oxygenated are not perfused by blood, because of the decreased blood flow, resulting in additional hypoxemia and decreased oxygen for cells.

c. Capillary permeability and profound vasoconstriction cause increased hydrostatic pressure with shift of fluid to interstitial spaces and decreased circulating blood volume.

d. Decreased myocardial perfusion occurs as the heart fails, leading to arrhythmias and myocardial ischemia, further decreasing cardiac output and oxygen delivery to cells.

9. d. Rationale: During both the compensated and progressive stages of shock, the sympathetic nervous system is activated in an attempt to maintain cardiac output and systemic vascular resistance, and clinical manifestations reflect the effects of this stimulation. In the refractory or irreversible stage of shock, the sympathetic nervous system can no longer compensate to maintain homeostasis, and a loss of vasomotor tone affects perfusion to all vital organs, causing increasing cellular hypoxia, metabolic acidosis, and cellular death.

10. c. Rationale: In every type of shock there is a deficiency of oxygen to the cells, and high-flow oxygen therapy is indicated. Vasopressor therapy may be indicated in some cases but only after fluid replacement has been established. Fluid therapy is not indicated for cardiogenic shock, and not all patients require intubation and ventilation.

11. b. Rationale: In early compensated shock, activation of the renin-angiotensin system stimulates the release of aldosterone, which causes sodium reabsorption and potassium excretion by the kidney, elevating serum sodium levels and decreasing serum potassium levels. Blood glucose levels are elevated during the compensated stage of shock in response to catecholamine stimulation of the liver, which releases its glycogen stores in the form of glucose. Metabolic acidosis does not occur until the progressive stage of shock, when compensatory mechanisms become ineffective and anaerobic cellular metabolism causes lactic acid production.

12. b. Rationale: In late irreversible shock, progressive cellular destruction causes an elevation of liver enzymes and other laboratory findings that indicate organ damage. Metabolic acidosis is usually severe as cells continue anaerobic metabolism, and the respiratory alkalosis that may occur in the progressive stage has failed to compensate for the acidosis. Urine specific gravity becomes fixed or increased as the kidneys fail, and hemoglobin and hematocrit are usually increased in a patient with burns as fluid leaves the vascular space.

13. a. Rationale: Lactated Ringer's solution may increase lactate levels, which a damaged liver cannot convert to bicarbonate, and may intensify the metabolic lactic acidosis that occurs in progressive shock, necessitating careful attention to the patient's acid-base balance. Sodium and potassium levels as well as hemoglobin and hematocrit levels should be monitored in all patients receiving fluid replacement therapy.

14. 90 ml/hr. Adequate fluid replacement is indicated by a urinary output of 1 ml/kg/hr.

15. b. Rationale: When large amounts of crystalloid fluids are given to critically ill patients to maintain vascular volume, about two-thirds of the volume will diffuse out of the vascular space into the interstitial space, causing systemic edema. Increased vascular volume from the fluids will increase CO, PAWP, and urinary output.

16. a. Rationale: A decreased mixed venous oxygen saturation (SvO_2) indicates that the patient has used the venous oxygen reserve and is at greater risk for anaerobic metabolism. The SvO_2 decreases when more oxygen is used by the cells, as in activity or hypermetabolism. All of the other values indicate an improvement in the patient's condition.

17. d. Rationale: As a vasopressor, norepinephrine may cause severe vasoconstriction, which would further decrease tissue perfusion, especially if fluid replacement is inadequate. Vasopressors generally cause hypertension, reflex bradycardia, and decreased urine output, because of decreased renal blood flow; they do not directly affect acid-base balance.

18. b. Rationale: Vasoactive drugs are those that can either dilate or constrict blood vessels, and both are used in various stages of shock treatment. When using either vasodilators or vasoconstrictors, it is important to maintain a MAP of at least 60 mm Hg so that adequate perfusion is maintained.

19. a. Restore coronary artery blood flow with thrombolytic therapy, angioplasty, emergency revascularization; increase cardiac output with inotropic agents; reduce workload by dilating coronary arteries, decreasing preload and afterload; use circulatory assist devices, such as an intraaortic balloon pump

b. Fluid and blood replacement, control of bleeding with pressure, surgery

c. Fluid resuscitation, antimicrobial agents, inotropic agents with vasopressors

d. Epinephrine, inhaled bronchodilators, colloidal fluid replacement, diphenhydramine, corticosteroids

20. a. Dobutamine (Dobutrex) increases myocardial contractility and causes mild vasodilation by α1-adrenergic stimulation.
    b. Milrinone (Primacor) increases cardiac contractility and output and decreases preload and afterload by directly relaxing vascular smooth muscles.
    c. Nitroglycerine (Nitrol, Tridil) primarily dilates veins, reducing preload.
    d. Nitroprusside (Nipride) acts as a potent vasodilator of veins and arteries and may increase or decrease CO, depending on the extent of preload and afterload reduction.
    Others: diuretics, ACE inhibitors, β-adrenergic blockers
21. c. Rationale: Prevention of shock necessitates identification of persons who are at risk and a thorough baseline nursing assessment with frequent ongoing assessments to monitor and detect changes in patients at risk. Frequent monitoring of all patients' vital signs is not necessary. Aseptic technique for all invasive procedures should always be implemented but will not prevent all types of shock. Health promotion activities that reduce the risk for precipitating conditions, such as coronary artery disease or anaphylaxis, may help prevent shock in some selected cases.
22. Vital signs, level of consciousness, skin, urine output, peripheral pulses with capillary refill
23. a. 3; b. 2; c. 3; d. 5; e. 2; f. 1; g. 3; h. 1; i. 2; j. 5
24. c. Rationale: If the metabolic acidosis is compensated, the pH will be within the normal range, and if the patient is hyperventilating to blow off carbon dioxide to reduce the acid load of the blood, $PaCO_2$ will be decreased.
25. d. Rationale: Although some patients in shock may be treated with antianxiety and sedative drugs to control anxiety and apprehension, the nurse should always acknowledge the patient's feelings and explain procedures before they are carried out and inform the patient of the plan of care and its rationale. Members of the clergy should be called only if the patient requests or agrees to a visit, and while visits by family may have a therapeutic effect on some patients, family visits may increase stress in others.
26. a. T; b. F, results; c. F, SIRS; d. T; e. T; f. F, lungs
27. a. 4; b. 2; c. 4; d. 2; e. 1; f. 3; g. 1; h. 3; i. 5; j. 5; k. 6
28. d. Rationale: A respiratory rate above 20/min and a WBC count of less than 4000/μl or more than 12,000/μl meet the clinical manifestation and laboratory finding criteria for determining the presence of SIRS. Other criteria include $PaCO_2$ less than 32 mm Hg, heart rate greater than 90/min, and temperature greater than 101.4° F (38° C) or less than 97° F (36° C).
29. a. Rationale: It is believed that early enteral feedings in the patient in shock increase the blood supply to the GI tract and help prevent translocation of GI bacteria and endotoxins into the blood, preventing initial or additional infection in patients in shock. Surgical removal of necrotic tissue, especially from burns, eliminates a source of infection in critically ill patients, as does the use of strict aseptic technique in all patient procedures. Known infections are treated with specific agents, and broad-spectrum agents are used only until organisms are identified.
30. d. Rationale: The presence of MODS is confirmed when there is defined clinical evidence of failure of more than one organ. Elevated serum lipase and amylase levels indicate pancreatic failure, a serum creatinine of 3.8 mg/dl indicates kidney failure, and a platelet count of 15,000/μl indicates hematologic failure. Other criteria include urine output less than 0.5 ml/kg/hr, BUN 100 mg/dl or greater, WBC count 1000/μl, upper or lower GI bleeding, Glasgow Coma Scale score 6 or less, and hematocrit 20% or less. A respiratory rate of 45/min, $PaCO_2$ of 60, and a chest x-ray with bilateral diffuse, patchy infiltrates indicate respiratory failure but not other organ damage.

Case Study

1. Indwelling catheter leading to urinary tract infection; compromised patient—elderly, chronic illnesses of diabetes and heart failure
2. Aseptic technique in catheter placement; increased fluid intake to flush catheter; consult with physician regarding prophylactic antimicrobials; early detection of changes in urine, temperature
3. Release of endotoxins by gram-negative bacteria that cause inflammatory responses is the initial insult. The endotoxins bind to monocytes and lymphocytes, stimulating the release of tumor necrosis factor and interleuken 1 (IL-1), which in turn cause release or activation of platelet-activating factor, prostaglandins, leukotrienes, thromboxane A-2, kinins, and complement. The result is widespread vasodilation and increased capillary permeability. Histamine also is released, which causes increased capillary permeability. The end result is decreased systemic vascular resistance (SVR) and normal or increased cardiac output (CO) as a result of the decreased SVR. Myocardial function is also suppressed by myocardial depressant factor. Death is associated with persistent increase in heart rate and CO,

with low SVR and refractory hypotension with progression to MODS.

4. The widespread vasodilation caused by the inflammatory processes and increased capillary permeability causing fluid loss to the interstitium cause hypotension.
5. Decreased LOC—decreased tissue perfusion to the brain and hypoxia of brain cells
Warm, dry, and flushed skin—massive vasodilation
Tachycardia—activation of sympathetic nervous system with beta-adrenergic stimulation increasing heart rate
Tachypnea—compensation for tissue hypoxia and metabolic acidosis
Fever—bacterial infection
Decreased SVR—profound vasodilation
Increased cardiac output—occurs as a result of decreased vascular resistance
Oliguria—inadequate renal perfusion and possible renal failure
Hyperglycemia—sympathetic nervous system stimulation causes glycogenolysis by the liver
6. To monitor fluid replacement and cardiac function because of multiple system involvement
7. Blood gases:
   - pH—indicates an acidosis, typical of the metabolic acidosis of anaerobic metabolism of shock
   - PaO_2—very low, indicating a marked hypoxemia
   - $PaCO_2$—also low as a result of hyperventilation to compensate for the metabolic acidosis
   - HCO_3^-—the bicarbonate is low because it is used to neutralize the acids of anaerobic metabolism.
   - SaO_2—a very low oxygen saturation. Normal should be 96%-100%, and the patient's level indicates severe hypoxemia.
8. Hemodynamic pressures:
   - Right atrial pressure (RAP)—normal is 2 to 8 mm Hg. Marked vasodilation would decrease venous return to the heart, and it would be expected to be decreased.
   - Pulmonary artery pressure (PAP)—normal is 10 to 20 mm Hg and is an indicator of afterload or systemic vascular resistance. The patient's PAP would be expected to be decreased in septic shock, where there is profound vasodilation.
   - Pulmonary artery wedge pressure (PAWP)—normal is 6 to 12 mm Hg and is an indicator of afterload or systemic vascular resistance. The patient's PAWP would be expected to be low.
   - Cardiac output (CO)—normal is 4 to 8 L/min. The patient's CO would be expected to be elevated, illustrating the high cardiac output typical of septic shock.
   - Systemic vascular resistance (SVR)—normal is 900 to 1400 dynes/sec/cm^{-5}. Vasodilation would produce a decreased SVR.
9. Fluid therapy is used to increase vascular volume and blood pressure to increase tissue perfusion. Dopamine is used to increase vasoconstriction and strengthen myocardial contractions to elevate systemic vascular resistance.
10. *Nursing diagnoses:*
    - Altered tissue perfusion related to deficit in capillary blood supply
    - Altered protection related to neurosensory alterations
    - Hyperthermia related to inflammatory process
    - Risk for disuse syndrome related to perceptual-cognitive impairment

    Collaborative problems:
    Potential complications: heart failure; ARDS; DIC; organ ischemia—neurologic, renal, GI; MODS

CHAPTER 66

1. c. Rationale: Respiratory failure results when the transfer of oxygen or carbon dioxide functions of the respiratory system are impaired, and although the definition is determined by PaO_2 and $PaCO_2$ levels, the major factor in respiratory failure is inadequate gas exchange to meet tissue O_2 needs. Absence of ventilation is respiratory arrest, and partial airway obstruction may not necessarily cause respiratory failure. Acute hypoxemia may be caused by factors other than pulmonary dysfunction.
2. a. HO; b. HO; c. HC; d. HO; e. HO; f. HC; g. HC; h. HO; i. HC
3. a. T; b. F, 1 or less; c. T; d. F, air in the lung from passing into the blood; e. F, V/Q mismatch; f. F, diffusion limitation
4. a. 3; b. 4; c. 2; d. 5; e. 1
5. a. 3; b. 1; c. 2; d. 4
6. b. Rationale: Hypercapnic respiratory failure is associated with alveolar hypoventilation with increases in alveolar and arterial CO_2 and often is caused by problems outside the lungs. A patient with slow, shallow respirations is not exchanging enough gas volume to eliminate CO_2. Deep, rapid respirations reflect hyperventilation and often accompany lung problems that cause hypoxemic respiratory failure. Pulmonary edema and large airway resistance cause obstruction of oxygenation and result in a V/Q mismatch or shunt typical of hypoxemic respiratory failure.

7. d. Rationale: In a patient with normal lung function, respiratory failure is commonly defined as a PaO_2 ≤60 mm Hg or a $PaCO_2$ >45 mm Hg or both, but because the patient with chronic pulmonary disease normally maintains low PaO_2 and high $PaCO_2$, acute respiratory failure in these patients can be defined as an acute decrease in PaO_2 or increase in $PaCO_2$ from the patient's baseline parameters, accompanied by an acid pH. The pH of 7.28 reflects an acidemia and a loss of compensation in the patient with chronic lung disease.
8. a. HO; b. HC; c. HC; d. HO; e. HO; f. HC; g. HC
9. a. Rationale: Because the brain is very sensitive to a decrease in oxygen delivery, restlessness, agitation, disorientation, and confusion are early signs of hypoxemia, for which the nurse should be alert. Mild hypertension is also an early sign, accompanied by tachycardia. Central cyanosis is an unreliable, late sign of hypoxemia, and cardiac arrhythmias also occur later.
10. d. Rationale: The increase in respiratory rate required to blow off accumulated CO_2 predisposes to respiratory muscle fatigue, and the slowing of a rapid rate in a patient in acute distress indicates tiring and the possibility of respiratory arrest unless ventilatory assistance is provided. A decreased I/E ratio, orthopnea, and accessory muscle use are common findings in respiratory distress but do not necessarily signal respiratory fatigue or arrest.
11. a. Rationale: Patients with a shunt are usually more hypoxemic than are patients with a V/Q mismatch, because the alveoli are filled with fluid, which prevents gas exchange. Hypoxemia secondary to an intrapulmonary shunt is usually not responsive to high O_2 concentrations, and the patient will usually require positive pressure ventilation. Hypoxemia associated with a V/Q mismatch usually responds favorably to oxygen administration at 1 to 3 L/min by nasal cannula. Removal of secretions with coughing and suctioning is not generally effective in reversing an acute hypoxemia secondary to a shunt.
12. a. Rationale: When there is impaired function of the one lung, the patient should be positioned with the unaffected lung in the dependent position to promote perfusion to the functioning tissue. If the diseased lung is positioned dependently, more V/Q mismatch would occur. The head of the bed may be elevated, or a reclining chair may be used, with the patient positioned on the unaffected side, to maximize thoracic expansion if the patient has increased work of breathing.
13. b. Rationale: Augmented coughing by applying pressure on the thorax or abdominal muscles at the beginning of expiration helps produce muscle movement, increases pleural pressure and expiratory flows, and assists the cough to remove secretions in the patient who is exhausted. An oral airway is used only if there is a possibility that the tongue will obstruct the airway. Huff coughing is indicated for patients with problems with endotracheal tubes in place, which prevent glottal closure, and slow, pursed-lip breathing is used to prevent air trapping and give the patient a sense of control over breathing.
14. c. Rationale: Hemodynamic monitoring with a pulmonary artery catheter is instituted in severe respiratory failure to determine the amount of blood flow to tissues and the response of the lung and heart to hypoxemia. Continuous blood pressure monitoring may be performed, but blood pressure is a reflection of cardiac activity, which can be determined by the pulmonary artery catheter findings. Arterial blood gas values are important to evaluate oxygenation and ventilation status and V/Q mismatches.
15. d. Rationale: Drug therapy indicated for acute respiratory failure depends on the symptoms that are present and the underlying cause of the respiratory failure. Brochodilators and IV corticosteroids are used if bronchospasm and inflammation are present; antibiotics are used if infection is present; diuretics are used if pulmonary congestion is caused by heart failure; and sedatives may be used if anxiety and agitation increase the degree of hypoxemia.
16. d. Rationale: NIPPV involves the application of a face mask and delivery of a volume of air under inspiratory pressure. Because the device is worn externally, the patient must be able to cooperate in its use, and frequent access to the airway for suctioning or inhaled medications must not be necessary. It is not indicated when high levels of oxygen are needed or respirations are absent.
17. a. Rationale: Although ARDS may occur in the patient who has virtually any severe illness or trauma and may be both a cause and result of SIRS, the most common precipitating insults of ARDS are septic shock and gastric aspiration.
18. a. Interstitial and alveolar edema from damage to vascular endothelium and increased capillary permeability
    b. Atelectasis from destruction of type II cells, resulting in inactivation of surfactant
    c. Hyaline membrane formation from exudation of high molecular weight substances in the edema fluid

19. c. Rationale: In the fibrotic phase of ARDS, diffuse scarring and fibrosis of the lungs occur, resulting in decreased surface area for gas exchange and continued hypoxemia due to diffusion limitation. Although edema is resolved, lung compliance is decreased because of interstitial fibrosis, and long-term mechanical ventilation is required with a poor prognosis for survival.
20. a. Rationale: Hypoxemia that does not respond to oxygenation by any route is a hallmark of ARDS and is always present. $PaCO_2$ levels may be normal until the patient is no longer able to compensate in response to the hypoxemia. Bronchial breath sounds may be associated with the progression of ARDS. Pulmonary capillary wedge pressures that are normally elevated in cardiogenic pulmonary edema are normal in the pulmonary edema of ARDS.
21. c. Rationale: Early signs of ARDS are insidious and difficult to detect, but the nurse should be alert for any early signs of hypoxemia, such as restlessness, dyspnea, and decreased mentation, in patients at risk for ARDS. Abnormal findings on physical examination or diagnostic studies, such as adventitious lung sounds, signs of respiratory distress, respiratory alkalosis, or decreasing PaO_2, are usually indications that ARDS has progressed beyond the initial stages.
22. b. Rationale: Nosocomial pneumonia is one of the most common complications of ARDS, and early detection requires frequent monitoring of sputum smears and cultures and assessment of the quality, quantity, and consistency of sputum. Blood in gastric aspirate may indicate a stress ulcer, and subcutaneous emphysema of the face, neck, and chest occurs with barotrauma during mechanical ventilation. Oral infections may result from prophylactic antibiotics and impaired host defenses but are not common.
23. a. Rationale: Because ARDS is precipitated by a physiologic insult, a critical factor in its prevention and early management is treatment of the underlying condition. Prophylactic antibiotics, treatment with diuretics and fluid restriction, and mechanical ventilation are also used as ARDS progresses.
24. a. Rationale: PEEP used with mechanical ventilation applies positive pressure to the airway and lungs at the end of exhalation, keeping the lung partially expanded and preventing collapse of the alveoli and helping to open up collapsed alveoli. Permissive hypercapnia is allowed when the patient with ARDS is ventilated with smaller tidal volumes to prevent barotrauma. Extracorporeal membrane oxygenation and extracorporeal CO_2 removal involve passing blood across a gas-exchanging membrane outside the body and then returning oxygenated blood back to the body.
25. c. Rationale: PEEP increases intrathoracic and intrapulmonic pressures, compresses the pulmonary capillary bed, and reduces blood return to both the right and left side of the heart. Preload (CVP) and cardiac output are decreased, often with a dramatic decrease in blood pressure.
26. d. Rationale: When a patient with ARDS is supine, alveoli in the posterior areas of the lung are dependent and fluid-filled, and the heart and mediastinal contents place more pressure on the lungs, predisposing to atelectasis. If the patient is turned prone, air-filled, nonatelectic alveoli in the anterior portion of the lung receive more blood, and perfusion may be better matched to ventilation, causing less V/Q mismatch. Lateral rotation therapy is used to stimulate postural drainage and help mobilize pulmonary secretions.

Case Study

1. The patient is experiencing hypercapnic respiratory failure, reflected by the elevated $PaCO_2$ and pH of 7.3. In this case severe COPD, with destruction of alveoli and terminal respiratory units, has led to hypoventilation, with less removal of CO_2 and less space for O_2 in the alveoli. The patient with severe COPD always has some degree of decompensation resulting in chronic respiratory failure, but an acute exacerbation or infection may cause an acute decompensation, thus producing an acute or chronic respiratory failure.
2. The primary contributing factor to the onset of the acute failure is the pneumonia, but other factors include the presence of chronic lung disease, her age, and immunosuppression with steroids.
3. The primary pathophysiologic effects of hypercapnia are a respiratory acidosis resulting from retained CO_2 and a hypoxemia resulting from alveolar retention of CO_2. Clinical manifestations of hypercapnic respiratory failure that Mrs. C. is experiencing include the dyspnea, shortness of breath, sitting in a tripod position, and using pursed-lip breathing, in addition to her ABG values. Other manifestations of hypercapnia that the nurse should assess Mrs. C. for include morning headache, somnolence, confusion, arrhythmias, and muscle weakness. Because she is also hypoxemic, she should be assessed for mild hypertension, tachycardia, prolonged expiration, and accessory respiratory muscle use.
4. The tripod position helps decrease the work of breathing, because propping the arms up increases the anterior-posterior diameter of the

chest and changes pressures in the thorax. Pursed-lip breathing causes an increase in SaO_2 because it slows respiration, allows more time for expiration, and prevents the small bronchioles from collapsing.

5. Noninvasive positive pressure ventilation (NIPPV) is delivered by placing a mask over the patient's nose or nose and mouth, and the patient breathes spontaneously while positive pressure is delivered. It may be used as a treatment for patients with acute or chronic respiratory failure and helps decrease the work of breathing, without the need for endotracheal intubation. It is not appropriate for the patient who has absent respirations, excessive secretions, a decreased level of consciousness, high O_2 requirements, facial trauma, or hemodynamic instability.
6. Treatment of acute respiratory failure is directed toward reversing the disease process that resulted in the failure. Mrs. C.'s COPD is chronic and irreversible, but the IV antibiotics are critical in treating the pneumonia that precipitated the acute or chronic respiratory failure. The bronchodilators and corticosteroids will help with airway inflammation and spasm, but it cannot be expected that she will recover without treatment of the infection.
7. *Nursing diagnoses:*
   - Ineffective breathing pattern related to expiratory obstruction to airflow
   - Ineffective airway clearance related to increased airway resistance
   - Impaired gas exchange related to alveolar hypoventilation
   - Risk for impaired skin integrity related to NIPPV mask

   Collaborative problems:
   Potential complications: hypoxia; hypercapnia; respiratory and metabolic acidosis; arrhythmias

CHAPTER 67

1. a. U; b. E; c. U; d. N; e. E; f. E; g. U
2. b. Rationale: During the primary survey of emergency care, assessment and immediate interventions for life-threatening problems affecting airway, breathing, circulation, and disability are performed. The triage system is used initially to determine the priority of care for patients, and history of the illness or accident is part of the secondary survey. Any emergency department should be able to stabilize and initially treat a patient if the patient requires specialized care unavailable at the admitting facility.
3. a. Inhalation injury, airway obstruction, upper airway wounds or trauma
   Interventions: Jaw-thrust, artificial airway, suctioning
   b. Anaphylaxis, flail chest, hemothorax, open or tension pneumothorax
   Interventions: Ventilate with bag-valve mask at 100% oxygen, chest tube insertion or needle thoracostomy, endotracheal intubation
   c. Cardiac injury, pericardial tamponade, shock, uncontrolled external hemorrhage
   Interventions: CPR and ALS if no pulse, two large-bore IVs with infusions of fluids or blood, pneumatic antishock garment for pelvic fracture, direct pressure to bleeding
   d. Head injury, stroke
   Interventions: Monitor LOC, hyperventilation if increased ICP, elevate head of bed 30 degrees
4. a. Rationale: Specific injuries are associated with specific types of accidents and events surrounding an incident, and details of the incident and the trajectory of penetrating injuries are important in identifying and treating injury. Alcohol use is assessed with blood testing, and although information may be used for regulatory agencies, the primary use of the information is for treatment of the patient.
5. a. Cardiac monitoring; b. Pulse oximetry monitoring; c. Indwelling urinary catheter; d. Oro- or nasogastric tube; e. Laboratory studies
6. b. Rationale: A nasally placed tube is contraindicated if the patient has facial fractures or a possible basilar skull fracture, because the tube could enter the brain. It would not be contraindicated in the other conditions.
7. a. Allergies; b. Medications; c. Past health history, pregnancy status; d. Last meal; e. Events of the illness or injury
8. b. Rationale: Tetanus immunoglobulin provides passive immunity for tetanus and is used in treatment of a tetanus-prone wound if the patient has not had at least three doses of active tetanus toxoid. The patient would also receive tetanus toxoid to initiate active immunity in the case of tetanus-prone wounds. If the patient has fewer than three doses of tetanus toxoid and a non–tetanus-prone wound, only tetanus toxoid would be administered to initiate active immunity. In the actively immunized patient, tetanus toxoid is administered for tetanus-prone wounds if it has been more than 5 years since the last dose, and it is also administered for non–tetanus-prone wounds if it has been more than 10 years since the last dose.

9. a. Rationale: Before organ procurement agencies are notified, the family members should be made aware of the possibility of organ donation and have a chance to discuss the issue. The best way is just to question them about the possibility without influencing them to make a decision they would later question. If there is interest, the organ procurement agent can be notified to assist in screening, counseling, and obtaining consent.
10. a. 4; b. 5; c. 2; d. 5; e. 4; f. 5; g. 3; h. 5; i. 4; j. 1
11. c. Rationale: Rewarming of frostbitten tissue is extremely painful, and analgesia should be administered during the process. The affected part is submerged in a warm water bath at approximately 104° to 108° F (40° to 42° C), and massage or scrubbing of the tissue should be avoided because of the potential for tissue damage. Blisters form in hours to days following the injury and are not an immediate concern.
12. a. Rationale: Unconsciousness, bradycardia, and slowed respiratory rate are signs of moderate hypothermia, and movement of the patient should be avoided to prevent ventricular fibrillation, a common complication of hypothermia and rewarming. Active core rewarming is indicated for moderate to severe hypothermia. Axillary temperatures are inadequate to monitor core temperature, so esophageal, rectal, or indwelling urinary catheter thermometers are used. The patient should be assessed for other injuries but should not be exposed, in order to prevent further loss of heat.
13. b. Rationale: Patients with profound hypothermia appear dead on presentation and exhibit fixed, dilated pupils, no obtainable vital signs, unconsciousness, and apnea. Shivering is seen in mild hypothermia, and moderate hypothermia is characterized by slowed respirations, blood pressure obtainable only by Doppler, and rigidity.
14. a. F; b. B; c. S; d. B; e. S; f. B
15. a. Rationale: The most important life-threatening consequence of near-drowning of any type is hypoxia from fluid-filled and poorly ventilated alveoli, and airway and oxygenation are first priorities. Correction of metabolic (anaerobic) acidosis occurs with effective ventilation and oxygenation; lactated Ringer's or normal saline solution is started to manage fluid balance; and mannitol or furosemide may be used to treat free-water and cerebral edema.
16. d. Rationale: As edema increases with the response to snake or insect bites, watches, rings, or constrictive clothing on an affected part may cause circulatory obstruction and should be removed before the onset of edema. Ice and tourniquets are not recommended, because both may cause tissue necrosis, and elevation of the extremity causes increased absorption and circulation of venom.
17. a. Rationale: Wood ticks or dog ticks release a neurotoxin as long as the tick head is attached to the body, and tick removal is essential for effective treatment. Tick removal leads to return of muscle movement, usually within 48 to 72 hours. There is no antidote, and hemodialysis is not known to remove the neurotoxin. Antibiotics are used to treat Lyme disease and Rocky Mountain spotted fever, infections spread by tick bites.
18. a. F, human; b. T; c. F, washing with large amounts of water; d. F, water or milk; e. T
19. a, c, d
20. a. 3; b. 1; c. 4; d. 3
21. c. Rationale: Gastric lavage with a large-gauge oral-gastric tube is indicated to remove any drug that is not already absorbed from the stomach. Vomiting should never be induced in a patient who is unconscious, and activated charcoal does not absorb lithium. Cathartics are usually given with activated charcoal to increase elimination of the toxins absorbed by the charcoal.

22.

Agent	Bacterial	Viral	Person-to-Person Spread	Antibiotic Treatment	Active Vaccine	Passive Vaccine/ Antitoxin
Botulism	X					X
Anthrax	X			X	X	
Plague	X		X	X (if early)		
Hemorrhagic Fever		X	X			
Tularemia	X			X		
Smallpox		X	X		X	X

23. a. 6; b. 4; c. 2; d. 1; e. 4; f. 6; g. 3; h. 2; i. 6; j. 5; k. 3; l. 1
24. b. Rationale: Ionizing radiation exposure in a sublethal dose will cause nausea and vomiting within 2-4 hours of exposure, hair loss in 2 days to 2 weeks, and coagulopathies in 2 days to 2 weeks.

Case Study

1. Advanced age and prolonged exposure to heat over several days are risk factors for Mr. M.'s development of heatstroke.
2. ABGs—decreased PaO_2; electrolytes—decreased serum sodium, chloride, potassium; CBC—hemoconcentration with elevated hemoglobin and hematocrit; BUN and creatinine—elevated; serum glucose—decreased; coagulation studies—decreased prothrombin time, decreased bleeding times; liver function tests—elevated enzymes; UA—elevated specific gravity, protein, possible microscopic hematuria
3. Clothing would be removed, and fans and tepid water mist may be used, as well as ice water baths. If the temperature is not reduced by these methods, ice water lavage or cold water peritoneal dialysis may be used.
4. 100% oxygen to compensate for the hypermetabolic state, with intubation and mechanical ventilation if necessary; IV crystalloid salt solution with CVC or PA catheter to monitor fluid status; cooling methods with monitoring of core temperature; indwelling catheter and I&O; administration of chlorpromazine (Thorazine) to control shivering during cooling process
5. Mrs. M. should be told that Mr. M. is very seriously ill and that there is a chance he might not recover, because heatstroke has a very high morbidity and mortality rate. She should be kept informed of the treatment he is receiving and his response to treatment, and she should be provided with emotional support.
6. *Nursing diagnoses:*
   - Hyperthermia related to environmental exposure
   - Decreased cardiac output related to hypermetabolic process
   - Deficient fluid volume related to fluid loss excessive of intake
   - Altered protection related to altered mental state
   - Risk for injury related to seizure activity
   - Risk for impaired skin integrity related to immobility

   Collaborative problems:
   Potential complications: hypovolemic shock; cerebral edema; seizures; hypoxia; electrolyte imbalance; renal failure